MANAGING CLINICALLY IMPORTANT DRUG INTERACTIONS

AUTHORS

Philip D. Hansten, PharmD
University of Washington, Seattle

John R. Horn, PharmD
University of Washington, Seattle

FACTS AND COMPARISONS® PUBLISHING GROUP

Executive Vice President	Kenneth H. Killion
Publisher	Cathy H. Reilly
Senior Managing Editor	Renée M. Wickersham
Managing Editor	Jill A. O'Dell
Associate Editors	Sarah Lenzini Sharon M. McCarron
Assistant Editor	John G. Hall
Quality Control Editor	Susan H. Sunderman
Senior Composition Specialist	Beverly A. Donnell
Senior SGML Specialist	Linda M. Jones
Purchasing Specialist	Heather L. Guyott
General Manager, Disease and Drug Information	Renée Rivard, PharmD
Drug Information Specialists	Lori A. Buss, PharmD Kim S. Dufner, PharmD Cathy A. Meives, PharmD Larry Schreiber, Jr., RPh Nicole E. Williams, PharmD
Acquisitions Editor	Teri Hines Burnham
Cover Design	Mark L. Wickersham
Director of Marketing	Mark A. Sohasky

Facts and Comparisons®
part of Wolters Kluwer Health
111 West Port Plaza Dr., Suite 300
St. Louis, Missouri 63146-3098
(314) 216-2100
(800) 223-0554 Customer Service
(314) 878-5563 Fax
www.drugfacts.com

MANAGING CLINICALLY IMPORTANT DRUG INTERACTIONS

FACTS AND COMPARISONS® EDITORIAL ADVISORY PANEL

MANAGING
CLINICALLY IMPORTANT
DRUG INTERACTIONS

TABLE OF CONTENTS

MANAGING CLINICALLY IMPORTANT DRUG INTERACTIONS

PREFACE

Hansten and Horn Managing Clinically Important Drug Interactions is derived from our more comprehensive book, *Drug Interactions Analysis and Management.* Given that the latter book has more than 1000 pages, users have requested a smaller book with a focus on those drug interactions that have the most potential for causing harm. Accordingly, this book does not contain Class 4 or Class 5 interactions. To save additional space, we have also removed the "Mechanism" and "Clinical Evaluation" sections from the monographs.

The management of drug interactions is emphasized in this book. Unlike adverse drug reactions to individual drugs, adverse drug *interactions* are almost completely preventable. Hence, we have devoted considerable effort to providing management options for each interaction. These options allow the health care provider to select one or more courses of action that are designed to reduce the likelihood that the patient will suffer an adverse consequence from the interaction.

We also designed this book to be used by health care providers who prescribe, dispense, or administer medications. We have included prescription and non-prescription medications, as well as herbal remedies. Nonetheless, there are a few types of drug interactions that one is *not* likely to find in this book: drugs used primarily in the practice of anesthesiology, drugs of abuse, and some well-known and predictable pharmacodynamic interactions such as combinations of CNS depressants.

We would like to thank our students and colleagues for their many helpful suggestions on previous editions of this book. Special thanks go to Edward Hartshorn, PhD, who has shown an unflagging commitment to providing timely updates of the drug interaction literature for over a third of a century. We would also like to thank the Drug Interaction Foundation for the five-step classification system used in this book. The foundation has made this classification available to anyone who would like to use it, and many health care providers have found it to be a particularly useful system.

Philip D. Hansten, PharmD
John R. Horn, PharmD
Authors

MANAGING CLINICALLY IMPORTANT DRUG INTERACTIONS

INTRODUCTION

Instructions to Users

Originally, the abridged monograph format of *Hansten and Horn Managing Clinically Important Drug Interactions* was based on the authors' evaluation of the interaction's clinical significance. The clinical significance was established by considering the potential harm to the patient and the degree of documentation available. Each interaction was assigned to one of three classes: Major, Moderate, or Minor. While this classification system has been adapted by many other providers of drug interaction information, the authors became increasingly dissatisfied with the utility of this system. By emphasizing the "clinical significance" of an interaction, the format did not focus on the most important aspect of drug interaction assessment: **prevention of patient harm**.

Knowing the clinical significance of an interaction provides only minimal information for selection of appropriate management strategies for a particular patient. Thus, we have revised the format of the monographs to emphasize the management options available for a patient receiving an interacting pair of drugs. This change enables the reader to quickly select one or more appropriate standardized management options. These options still are based, in part, on the severity of the potential interaction outcomes, but other factors such as the availability of alternative, noninteracting drugs also contribute. The goal of each monograph is to provide the reader with information necessary to assess the degree of risk to the patient, and to prevent an adverse outcome as a result of exposure to the interacting drugs.

Interacting drugs are assigned to one of three classes based on the intervention needed to minimize the risk of the interaction. This classification system originally was developed by the Drug Interaction Foundation. The interactions are assigned the following Significance numbers:

1 = **Avoid Combination.** Risk always outweighs benefit.
AVOID

2 = **Usually Avoid Combination.** Use combination only under special circumstances.

3 = **Minimize Risk.** Take action as necessary to reduce risk.

The goal of *Hansten and Horn Managing Clinically Important Drug Interactions* is to provide the reader with an abstract of each significant interaction based on the authors' analysis of the interaction and its potential to harm the patient. The purpose of each of the monograph sections is detailed below.

Summary provides a concise description of the potential outcome of the interaction and its clinical significance.

Risk Factors outlines patient or drug specific factors that have been identified as contributing to the magnitude or severity of the interaction. Obvious factors that apply universally are not listed. For example, virtually all drug interactions are dose dependent, or more precisely, dependent on the concentration of the precipitant drug at the site of the interaction. The larger dose or the higher the concentration of the precipitant drug, the greater the magnitude of the interaction and the larger the risk that an adverse outcome may result. If the literature provides specific data on dose- or concentration-effect relationships, they are included here.

Related Drugs cites examples of closely related agents that would be expected to interact in a similar manner as the monograph agents. Related drugs usually are confined to the chemical class as those in the monograph that have similar pharmacokinetic or pharmacodynamic interaction potential. This listing aids in selecting alternative therapy by noting those drugs that should be eliminated from consideration as alternatives. Prediction of potential interactions that are as yet undocumented are simplified by consulting this section. When specific data are available, related drugs also appear in individual monographs.

Management Options includes different options for patient management based on the actions necessary to avoid patient harm. These management options are placed into three classifications that assist the reader in eliminating or minimizing the risk to the patient. Each drug interaction in the Index identifies the management class to which it has been assigned.

Class 1 Interactions. Avoid administration of the drug combination. The risk of adverse patient outcome precludes the concomitant administration of the drugs.

Class 2 Interactions. Should avoid administration unless it is determined that the benefit of coadministration of the drugs outweighs the risk to the patient. The use of an alternative to one of the interacting drugs is recommended when appropriate. Patients should be monitored carefully if the drugs are coadministered.

Class 3 Interactions. Several potential management options are available for class 3 interactions. When an alternative agent should be considered, examples of documented noninteracting drugs are provided. Changes in drug dosage or route of administration that can circumvent or minimize the potential interaction are suggested. Again, patient monitoring is suggested in case the interacting drugs are administered.

References will contain pertinent citations that provide meaningful insight for the interaction.

Monographs are organized alphabetically and both interacting drugs are placed in the Index. All drugs are listed by generic name and not pharmacological class except combination products like antacids that are listed under "Antacids" as well as brand name. The few exceptions are, from the standpoint of drug interactions, homogenous (eg, thyroid, oral contraceptives, and thiazides) where interactions apply equally to all members of the class.

The monograph profiling the drug interaction between Erythromycin and Simvastatin that follows illustrates the organization and format used throughout *Hansten and Horn Managing Clinically Important Drug Interactions.*

Erythromycin (eg, *E-Mycin*)

Simvastatin (*Zocor*)

SUMMARY: Erythromycin administration may markedly increase simvastatin concentrations; avoid using the drugs together to avoid the risk of increased side effects.

RISK FACTORS: No specific risk factors are known.

RELATED DRUGS: Erythromycin will likely affect lovastatin (*Mevacor*) plasma concentrations in a similar manner. Atorvastatin (*Lipitor*) plasma concentrations are increased to a lesser degree by erythromycin administration. While no data are available, erythromycin may also increase the plasma concentrations of cerivastatin (*Baycol*). Clarithromycin (*Biaxin*) and troleandomycin (*TAO*) would probably reduce the metabolism of simvastatin. Azithromycin (*Zithromax*) and dirithromycin (*Dynabac*) would not likely inhibit the metabolism of simvastatin. The metabolism of pravastatin (*Pravachol*) and fluvastatin (*Lescol*) would not be expected to be affected by erythromycin.

MANAGEMENT OPTIONS:

➥ *Use Alternative.* Consider the use of a HMG-CoA reductase inhibitor other than simvastatin or lovastatin for patients receiving erythromycin. Atorvastatin and cerivastatin plasma concentrations are likely to be increased by a smaller amount during erythromycin coadministration. Pravastatin and fluvastatin metabolism should not be altered by erythromycin. Azithromycin or dirithromycin are macrolides that will not affect simvastatin metabolism.

REFERENCES:

Kantola T, et al. Erythromycin and verapamil considerably increase serum simvastatin and simvastatin acid concentrations. *Clin Pharmacol Ther.* 1988;64:177.

MONOGRAPHS

Acetaminophen (eg, *Tylenol*)

Cholestyramine (eg, *Questran*)

SUMMARY: Cholestyramine markedly reduces plasma acetaminophen concentrations and probably reduces acetaminophen therapeutic response.

RISK FACTORS: No specific risk factors are known.

RELATED DRUGS: Colestipol (*Colestid*) probably would reduce plasma acetaminophen concentrations also, but clinical studies are lacking.

MANAGEMENT OPTIONS:

➥ *Circumvent/Minimize.* Give acetaminophen 2 hours before or 6 hours after cholestyramine.

➥ *Monitor.* Monitor patients for reduced acetaminophen effects if this combination is given.

REFERENCES:
Dordoni B, et al. Reduction of absorption of paracetamol by activated charcoal and cholestyramine: a possible therapeutic measure. *BMJ.* 1973;3:86.

Acetaminophen (eg, *Tylenol*)

Ethanol (Ethyl Alcohol)

SUMMARY: Substantial evidence indicates that chronic, excessive alcohol ingestion increases the toxicity of high therapeutic doses or overdoses of acetaminophen, while preliminary evidence indicates that acute alcohol intoxication protects against acetaminophen overdose toxicity.

RISK FACTORS:

➥ *Dosage Regimen.* The increased risk of acetaminophen hepatotoxicity occurs primarily with excessive doses of acetaminophen in the presence of chronic, excessive alcohol ingestion.

RELATED DRUGS: No information is available.

MANAGEMENT OPTIONS:

➥ *Circumvent/Minimize.* Warn patients who chronically ingest large amounts of alcohol (eg, several drinks a day or more) to avoid taking large or prolonged doses of acetaminophen.

➥ *Monitor.* When monitoring serum acetaminophen following acute acetaminophen overdose in alcohol abusers, be aware that acetylcysteine may be indicated even if the serum acetaminophen concentration is below the "action line" on the standard nomogram. This is probably because of the ability of alcohol to enhance acetaminophen metabolism. (Some have recommended that the serum acetaminophen threshold for acetylcysteine therapy should be reduced by as much as 70% in patients who chronically ingest large amounts of alcohol.)

REFERENCES:
Emby DJ, et al. Hepatotoxicity of paracetamol enhanced by ingestion of alcohol: report of two cases. *S Afr Med J.* 1977;51:208.

Barker JD Jr, et al. Chronic excessive acetaminophen use and liver damage. *Ann Intern Med.* 1977;87:299.

McClain CJ, et al. Potentiation of acetaminophen hepatotoxicity by alcohol. *JAMA*. 1980;244:251.

Johnson MW, et al. Alcoholism, nonprescription drugs and hepatotoxicity. The risk from unknown acetaminophen ingestion. *Am J Gastroenterol*. 1981;76:530.

McJunkin B, et al. Fatal massive hepatic necrosis following acetaminophen overdose. *JAMA*. 1976;236:1874.

Dietz AJ Jr, et al. Acetaminophen kinetics in the alcoholic. *Clin Pharmacol Ther*. 1982;31:218.

Licht J, et al. Apparent potentiation of acetaminophen hepatotoxicity by alcohol. *Ann Intern Med*. 1980;92:511.

Sato C, et al. Prevention of acetaminophen-induced hepatotoxicity by acute ethanol administration in the rat: comparison with carbon tetrachloride-induced hepatotoxicity. *J Pharmacol Exp Ther*. 1981;218:805.

Sato C, et al. Mechanism of the preventive effect of ethanol on acetaminophen-induced hepatotoxicity. *J Pharmacol Exp Ther*. 1981;218:811.

Lyons L, et al. Treatment of acetaminophen overdosage with N-acetylcysteine. *N Engl J Med*. 1977;296:174.

McClements BM, et al. Management of paracetamol poisoning complicated by enzyme induction due to alcohol or drugs. *Lancet*. 1990;1:1526.

Skinner MH, et al. Acetaminophen metabolism in recovering alcoholics. *Clin Pharmacol Ther*. 1990;47:160.

Wootton FT, et al. Acetaminophen hepatotoxicity in the alcoholic. *South Med J*. 1990;83:1047.

Seifert CF, et al. Patterns of acetaminophen use in alcoholic patients. *Pharmacotherapy*. 1993;13:391.

Kumar S, et al. Failure of physicians to recognize acetaminophen hepatotoxicity in chronic alcoholics. *Arch Intern Med*. 1991;151:1189.

Cheung L, et al. Acetaminophen treatment nomogram. *New Engl J Med*. 1994;330:1907.

Acetaminophen (eg, *Tylenol*)

Isoniazid (eg, *Nydrazid*)

SUMMARY: Acetaminophen concentrations were increased by isoniazid; cases of hepatotoxicity have been reported following administration of isoniazid and acetaminophen.

RISK FACTORS: No specific risk factors are known.

RELATED DRUGS: No information is available.

MANAGEMENT OPTIONS:

➡ *Circumvent/Minimize.* Until further data are available, it would be prudent for patients taking isoniazid to limit their consumption of acetaminophen. Aspirin or an NSAID could be used instead of acetaminophen.

➡ *Monitor.* Until further data are available, monitor patients taking isoniazid and acetaminophen for hepatotoxicity.

REFERENCES:

Murphy R, et al. Severe acetaminophen toxicity in a patient receiving isoniazid. *Ann Intern Med*. 1990;113:799.

Moulding TS, et al. Acetaminophen, isoniazid, and hepatic toxicity. *Ann Intern Med*. 1991;114:431.

Epstein MM, et al. Inhibition of the metabolism of paracetamol by isoniazid. *Br J Clin Pharmacol*. 1991;31:139.

Zand R, et al. Inhibition and induction of cytochrome p450e1-catalyzed oxidation by isoniazid in humans. *Clin Pharmacol Ther*. 1993;54:142.

Acetaminophen (eg, *Tylenol*)

Phenobarbital (eg, *Solfoton*)

SUMMARY: Barbiturates may enhance the hepatotoxic potential of overdoses (and possibly large therapeutic doses) of acetaminophen; it is also possible that barbiturates reduce the therapeutic response to acetaminophen.

RISK FACTORS:

➡ **Dosage Regimen.** The danger of hepatotoxicity is primarily with overdoses or large or prolonged use of acetaminophen.

RELATED DRUGS: Enzyme inducers other than phenobarbital (eg, other barbiturates, carbamazepine [eg, *Tegretol*], phenytoin [eg, *Dilantin*], primidone [eg, *Mysoline*], rifabutin [eg, *Mycobutin*], and rifampin [eg, *Rifadin*]) may interact similarly.

MANAGEMENT OPTIONS:

➡ **Circumvent/Minimize.** Patients on barbiturate therapy should probably avoid taking large or prolonged doses of acetaminophen. With acute acetaminophen overdoses, acetylcysteine may be indicated even if the serum acetaminophen concentration is below the "action line" on the standard nomogram. (Some have recommended that the serum acetaminophen threshold for acetylcysteine therapy should be reduced by as much as 70% in patients who are taking enzyme inducers such as barbiturates.)

➡ **Monitor.** Monitor patients for reduced acetaminophen effect. In patients taking large or prolonged doses of acetaminophen, watch for evidence of hepatotoxicity.

REFERENCES:

Perucca E, et al. Paracetamol disposition in normal subjects treated with antiepileptic drugs. *Br J Clin Pharmacol.* 1979;7:201.

Pessayre E, et al. Additive effects of inducers and fasting on acetaminophen hepatotoxicity. *Biochem Pharmacol.* 1980;29:2219.

McLean AEM, et al. Dietary factors in renal & hepatic toxicity of paracetamol. *J Int Med Res.* 1976;4(Suppl.4):79.

Wilson JT, et al. Death in an adolescent following an overdose of acetaminophen and phenobarbital. *Am J Dis Child.* 1978;132:466.

Boyer TD, et al. Acetaminophen-induced hepatic necrosis and renal failure. *JAMA.* 1971;218:440.

Neuvonen PJ, et al. Antipyretic analgesics in patients on antiepileptic drug therapy. *Eur J Clin Pharmacol.* 1979;15:263.

Minton NA, et al. Fatal paracetamol poisoning in an epileptic. *Hum Toxicol.* 1988;7:33.

McClements BM, et al. Management of paracetamol poisoning complicated by enzyme induction due to alcohol or drugs. *Lancet.* 1990;1:1526.

Acetaminophen (eg, *Tylenol*)

Phenytoin (eg, *Dilantin*)

SUMMARY: Phenytoin may enhance the hepatotoxic potential of overdoses (and possibly large therapeutic doses) of acetaminophen; it is also possible that phenytoin reduces the therapeutic response to acetaminophen.

RISK FACTORS: No specific risk factors are known.

RELATED DRUGS: Other enzyme-inducing anticonvulsants such as carbamazepine (eg, *Tegretol*), phenobarbital (eg, *Solfoton*), and primidone (eg, *Mysoline*) probably also increase acetaminophen hepatotoxicity.

MANAGEMENT OPTIONS:

➦ *Circumvent/Minimize.* Patients on phenytoin therapy should probably avoid taking large or prolonged doses of acetaminophen. In cases of acute acetaminophen overdoses, acetylcysteine may be indicated even if the serum acetaminophen concentration is below the "action line" on the standard nomogram. (Some have recommended that the serum acetaminophen threshold for acetylcysteine therapy should be reduced by as much as 70% in patients who are taking enzyme inducers such as phenytoin.)

➦ *Monitor.* Monitor patients taking this combination for evidence of hepatotoxicity.

REFERENCES:

Perucca E, et al. Paracetamol disposition in normal subjects and in patients treated with antiepileptic drugs. *Br J Clin Pharmacol.* 1971;7:201.

Neuvonen PJ, et al. Antipyretic analgesics in patients on antiepileptic drug therapy. *Eur J Clin Pharmacol.* 1979;15:263.

McClements BM, et al. Management of paracetamol poisoning complicated by enzyme induction due to alcohol or drugs. *Lancet.* 1990;1:1526.

Minton NA, et al. Fatal paracetamol poisoning in an epileptic. *Hum Toxicol.* 1988;7:33.

Acetaminophen (eg, *Tylenol*)

Warfarin (eg, *Coumadin*)

SUMMARY: Repeated doses of acetaminophen may increase the hypoprothrombinemic response to oral anticoagulants like warfarin in some patients.

RISK FACTORS:

➦ *Dosage Regimen.* Although the dose relationship is not clearly established, an interaction appears more likely with daily acetaminophen doses of more than 2 g/day for at least 1 week. Maximal effects on the hypoprothrombinemic response have occurred 1 to 3 weeks after starting acetaminophen. Occasional doses of acetaminophen do not appear likely to interact.

RELATED DRUGS: Although most data on this interaction involve warfarin, limited clinical information suggests that other oral anticoagulants such as acenocoumarol and phenprocoumon may interact with acetaminophen as well. Most alternative analgesics (eg, aspirin, NSAIDs) would not be suitable alternatives to acetaminophen in patients receiving oral anticoagulants.

MANAGEMENT OPTIONS:

➦ *Circumvent/Minimize.* Warn patients receiving warfarin or other oral anticoagulants to limit their intake of acetaminophen-containing products. Although a "safe" amount cannot be determined with certainty, it would be prudent to limit acetaminophen intake to 2 g/day or less for no more than a few days. Aspirin-containing products should not be used as alternatives; acetaminophen lacks the adverse effects of aspirin on the gastric mucosa and platelets, and it is considered safer than aspirin in anticoagulated patients.

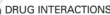

➡ ***Monitor.*** Monitor patients taking amounts of acetaminophen larger than recommended above for enhanced hypoprothrombinemic response and the anticoagulant dose adjusted as needed.

REFERENCES:
Antlitz AM, et al. Potentiation of oral anticoagulant therapy by acetaminophen. *Curr Ther Res.* 1968;10:501.

Rubin RN, et al. Potentiation of anticoagulant effect of warfarin by acetaminophen (*Tylenol*). *Clin Res.* 1984;32:698a.

Boeijinga JJ, et al. Interaction between paracetamol and coumarin anticoagulants. *Lancet.* 1982;1:506.

Bartle WR, et al. Potentiation of warfarin anticoagulant by acetaminophen. *JAMA.* 1991;265:1260.

Udall JA. Drug interference with warfarin therapy. *Clin Med.* 1970;77:20.

Antlitz AM, et al. A double-blind study of acetaminophen used in conjunction with oral anticoagulant therapy. *Curr Ther Res.* 1969;11:360.

Orme M, et al. Warfarin and distalgesic interaction. *BMJ.* 1976;1:200.

Jones RV. Warfarin and distalgesic interaction. *BMJ.* 1976;1:460.

Kaye L. Warfarin and paracetamol. *Pharmaceutical J.* 1991;246:692.

Weibert RT. Warfarin-acetaminophen interaction. ASHP Midyear Clinical Meeting, Dec. 1994.

Kwan D, et al. The effects of acute and chronic acetaminophen dosing on the pharmacodynamics and pharmacokinetics of (R)- and (S) warfarin. *Clin Pharmacol Ther.* 1995;57:212.

Acetazolamide (*Diamox*)

Aspirin

SUMMARY: Aspirin increases the plasma concentrations of acetazolamide, leading to CNS toxicity.

RISK FACTORS: No specific risk factors are known.

RELATED DRUGS: Theoretically, salicylates other than aspirin would also interact with acetazolamide. The effect of salicylates on carbonic anhydrase inhibitors other than acetazolamide is not established.

MANAGEMENT OPTIONS:

➡ ***Avoid Unless Benefit Outweighs Risk.*** Avoid concurrent use of salicylates and acetazolamide if possible, particularly in patients with renal dysfunction.

➡ ***Monitor.*** If the combination is used, monitor the patient carefully for symptoms of CNS toxicity, such as lethargy, confusion, somnolence, tinnitus, and anorexia.

REFERENCES:
Hill JB. Experimental salicylate poisoning: observations on effects of altering blood pH on tissue and plasma salicylate concentrations. *Pediatrics.* 1971;47:658.

Anderson CJ, et al. Toxicity of combined therapy with carbonic anhydrase inhibitors and aspirin. *Am J Ophthalmol.* 1978;86:516.

Acetazolamide (eg, *Diamox*)

Methenamine (eg, *Urised*)

SUMMARY: Acetazolamide interferes with the urinary antibacterial activity of methenamine compounds.

RISK FACTORS: No specific risk factors are known.

RELATED DRUGS: Other drugs that alkalinize the urine, such as sodium bicarbonate or large doses of antacids, would be expected to have a similar effect on methenamine compounds.

MANAGEMENT OPTIONS:

➡ *Monitor.* Monitor patients to keep the urine pH at approximately 5.5 or lower during methenamine use.

REFERENCES:

Product Information. Methenamine Mandelate (*Mandelamine*). Warner Chilcott. 1997.

Kevorkian CG, et al. Methenamine mandelate with acidification: an effective urinary antiseptic in patients with neurogenic bladder. *Mayo Clin Proc.* 1984;59:523.

Pearman JW, et al. The antimicrobial activity of urine of paraplegic patients receiving methenamine mandelate. *Invest Urol.* 1978;16:91.

Acetazolamide (*Diamox*)

Phenytoin (*Dilantin*)

SUMMARY: Acetazolamide may increase the risk of osteomalacia in patients receiving anticonvulsants.

RISK FACTORS: No specific risk factors are known.

RELATED DRUGS: Other carbonic anhydrase inhibitors when prescribed with an anticonvulsant could increase the risk of osteomalacia.

MANAGEMENT OPTIONS:

➡ *Monitor.* Give special attention to early detection of osteomalacia to patients receiving acetazolamide (or other carbonic anhydrase inhibitors) in addition to an anticonvulsant such as phenytoin, phenobarbital, or primidone. If osteomalacia does occur under these conditions, stopping the acetazolamide and instituting replacement therapy with phosphate or vitamin D may be beneficial.

REFERENCES:

Matsuda I, et al. Renal tubular acidosis and skeletal demineralization in patients on long-term anticonvulsant therapy. *J Pediatr.* 1975;87:202.

Mallette LE. Anticonvulsants, acetazolamide, and osteomalacia. *N Engl J Med.* 1975;293:668.

Mallette LE. Acetazolamide-accelerated anticonvulsant osteomalacia. *Arch Intern Med.* 1977;137:1013.

Acetazolamide (eg, *Diamox*)

Primidone (eg, *Mysoline*)

SUMMARY: A few case reports suggest that acetazolamide may reduce primidone serum concentrations and its anticonvulsant effect.

RISK FACTORS: No specific risk factors are known.

RELATED DRUGS: The effect of other carbonic anhydrase inhibitors on primidone is unknown.

MANAGEMENT OPTIONS:

➡ *Monitor.* It appears unnecessary to avoid the concomitant use of acetazolamide and primidone. However, until this interaction is better described, monitor patients receiving primidone and acetazolamide for a decreased primidone effect.

REFERENCES:

Syversen BG, et al. Acetazolamide-induced interference with primidone absorption. *Arch Neurol.* 1977;34:80.

Acetazolamide (eg, *Diamox*)

Quinidine (eg, *Quinora*)

SUMMARY: Alkalinization of the urine by acetazolamide tends to increase plasma quinidine concentrations.

RISK FACTORS: No specific risk factors are known.

RELATED DRUGS: Other drugs that alkalinize the urine (eg, sodium bicarbonate) would produce similar effects on quinidine serum concentrations. Acetazolamide may increase quinine concentrations.

MANAGEMENT OPTIONS:

➡ *Monitor.* Initiation, discontinuation, or a change in dose of acetazolamide in a patient receiving quinidine may necessitate a change in the quinidine dose. Monitor for altered quinidine response of urine pH changes.

REFERENCES:

Knouss RF, et al. Variation in quinidine excretion with changing urine pH. *Ann Intern Med.* 1968;68:1157.

Gerhardt RE, et al. Quinidine excretion in aciduria and alkaluria. *Ann Intern Med.* 1969;71:927.

Acetohexamide (eg, *Dymelor*)

Potassium

SUMMARY: Treatment of hypokalemia with potassium may result in a tendency toward hypoglycemia.

RISK FACTORS: No specific risk factors are known.

RELATED DRUGS: A similar reaction may occur with all hypoglycemic agents.

MANAGEMENT OPTIONS:

➡ *Monitor.* The effect of potassium on the response to antidiabetic agents is unlikely to be large enough to warrant any precautionary measures. However, monitor hypokalemic diabetic patients treated with potassium supplementation for reduced blood glucose.

REFERENCES:

Gershberg H, et al. Antidiabetic effect of acetohexamide. Effect of potassium supplements. *NY J Med.* 1969;69:1287.

Spergel G, et al. The effect of potassium on the impaired glucose tolerance in chronic uremia. *Metabolism.* 1967;16:581.

Levine R. Mechanisms of insulin secretion. *N Engl J Med.* 1970;283:522.

Grunfeld C, et al. Hypokalemia and diabetes mellitus. *Am J Med.* 1983;75:553.

Helderman JN, et al. Prevention of the glucose intolerance of thiazide diuretics by maintenance of body potassium. *Diabetes.* 1983;32:106.

Acitretin (*Soriatane*)

AVOID Ethanol (Ethyl Alcohol)

SUMMARY: Ethanol can result in the conversion of acitretin to etretinate, and the latter substance may remain in the body for years, thus increasing the risk of teratogenic effects. Women on acitretin should totally abstain from alcohol.

RISK FACTORS:

➡ **Gender.** The teratogenic risk applies only to women.

RELATED DRUGS: It is not known if other drugs or substances can also promote the conversion of acitretin to etretinate.

MANAGEMENT OPTIONS:

➡ **AVOID COMBINATION.** Warn women on acitretin to totally abstain from alcohol during and for at least 2 months after stopping the drug.

REFERENCES:

Product information. Acitretin (*Soriatane*). Roche Pharmaceuticals. 1997.

 ### Acitretin (*Soriatane*)

Methotrexate (*Mexate*)

SUMMARY: Combined use of acitretin and methotrexate reportedly increases the risk of hepatotoxicity.

RISK FACTORS: No specific risk factors are known.

RELATED DRUGS: No information is available.

MANAGEMENT OPTIONS:

➡ **Avoid Unless Benefit Outweighs Risk.** Although the risk of hepatotoxicity with concurrent use of acitretin and methotrexate is unknown, the manufacturer states that the combination should be avoided.

➡ **Monitor.** If the combination is used, monitor for clinical and laboratory evidence of hepatotoxicity.

REFERENCES:

Product information. Acitretin (*Soriatane*). Roche Pharmaceuticals. 1997.

 ### Acitretin (*Soriatane*)

AVOID Norethindrone (*Micronor*)

SUMMARY: Acitretin appears to inhibit the contraceptive efficacy of progestin "minipill" preparations and the latter should not be used in patients receiving acitretin.

RISK FACTORS: No specific risk factors are known.

RELATED DRUGS: The effect of acitretin on other progestin contraceptives (eg, implants, injectables) or standard combined oral contraceptives is unknown.

MANAGEMENT OPTIONS:

→ *AVOID COMBINATION.* Progestin "minipill" contraceptives should not be relied upon to prevent pregnancy in patients taking acitretin. Instead, suggest the use of at least 2 reliable forms of contraception at the same time to prevent pregnancy during acitretin therapy.

REFERENCES:

Product information. Acitretin (*Soriatane*). Roche Pharmaceuticals. 1997.

Acitretin (*Soriatane*)

Vitamin A

SUMMARY: Since acitretin is a retinoid (a vitamin A derivative), it is recommended that large doses of vitamin A be avoided.

RISK FACTORS: No specific risk factors are known.

RELATED DRUGS: Large doses of vitamin A should probably also be avoided with other retinoids such as etretinate (*Tegison*).

MANAGEMENT OPTIONS:

→ *Circumvent/Minimize.* The manufacturer recommends against taking vitamin A in doses greater than the minimum recommended daily allowances while taking acitretin.

REFERENCES:

Product information. Acitretin (*Soriatane*). Roche Pharmaceuticals. 1997.

Adenosine (eg, *Adenocard*)

Dipyridamole (eg, *Persantine*)

SUMMARY: Dipyridamole increases the serum concentrations of endogenous and exogenous adenosine, thereby potentiating its pharmacologic effects.

RISK FACTORS: No specific risk factors are known.

RELATED DRUGS: No information is available.

MANAGEMENT OPTIONS:

→ *Circumvent/Minimize.* Patients taking dipyridamole should receive reduced doses of adenosine for the treatment of arrhythmias or diagnostic tests.

→ *Monitor.* Be alert for bradycardia and prolonged AV conduction when dipyridamole and adenosine are coadministered. The enhancement of adenosine effects on AV conduction (eg, bradycardia) by dipyridamole may be reversed by aminophylline.

REFERENCES:

Lerman BB, et al. Electrophysiologic effects of dipyridamole on atrioventricular nodal conduction and supraventricular tachycardia. *Circulation.* 1989;80:1536-1543.

German DC, et al. Oral dipyridamole increases plasma adenosine levels in human beings. *Clin Pharmacol Ther.* 1989;45:80-84.

Watt AH, et al. Intravenous adenosine in the treatment of supraventricular tachycardia; a dose-ranging study and interaction with dipyridamole. *Br J Clin Pharmacol.* 1986;21:227-230.

Biaggioni I, et al. Cardiovascular effects of adenosine infusion in man and their modulation by dipyridamole. *Life Sci.* 1986;39:2229-2236.

Conradson TB, et al. Cardiovascular effects of infused adenosine in man: potentiation by dipyridamole. *Acta Physiol Scand.* 1987;129:387-391.

McCollam PL, et al. Adenosine-related ventricular asystole. *Ann Intern Med.* 1993;118:315-316.

Littmann L, et al. Adenosine and *Aggrenox*: a hazardous combination. *Ann Intern Med.* 2002;137:W1.

▼ 3   Adenosine (eg, *Adenocard*)

Nicotine (eg, *Nicorette*)

SUMMARY: Nicotine increases the hemodynamic and atrioventricular (AV) blocking effects of adenosine, resulting in low blood pressure and change in heart rate.

RISK FACTORS: No specific risk factors are known.

RELATED DRUGS: It is likely that other nicotine products would produce similar effects on adenosine.

MANAGEMENT OPTIONS:

➡ *Monitor.* Monitor cigarette smokers and those using nicotine gum or transdermal patches for a greater hemodynamic response to adenosine than nonsmokers. Enhanced hypotension or chest pain may result.

REFERENCES:

Smits P, et al. Nicotine enhances the circulatory effects of adenosine in human beings. *Clin Pharmacol Ther.* 1989;46:272-278.

Sylven C, et al. Nicotine enhances angina pectoris-like chest pain and atrioventricular blockade provoked by intravenous bolus of adenosine in healthy volunteers. *J Cardiovasc Pharmacol.* 1990;16:962–965.

▼ 3   Adenosine (*Adenocard*)

Theophylline (eg, *Slo-Phyllin*)

SUMMARY: Theophylline inhibits the hemodynamic effects of adenosine and may increase adenosine dosage requirements.

RISK FACTORS: No specific risk factors are known.

RELATED DRUGS: Caffeine produces similar effects on adenosine hemodynamics.

MANAGEMENT OPTIONS:

➡ *Circumvent/Minimize.* Patients maintained on theophylline may require greater than normal doses of adenosine to control arrhythmias.

➡ *Monitor.* Watch for decreased therapeutic response to adenosine when theophylline is initiated and for adenosine toxicity (eg, bradycardia) when theophylline is discontinued.

REFERENCES:

Fredholm BB. On the mechanism of action of theophylline and caffeine. *Acta Med Scand.* 1985;217:149-153.

Taddei S, et al. Theophylline antagonizes the vasorelaxant action of adenosine in human forearm arterioles of hypertensive patients. *Clin Pharmacol Ther.* 1990;47:144.

Smits P, et al. Caffeine and theophylline attenuate adenosine-induced vasodilation in humans. *Clin Pharmacol Ther.* 1990;48:410-418.

Lerman BB, et al. Electrophysiologic effects of dipyridamole on atrioventricular nodal conduction and supraventricular tachycardia. *Circulation*. 1989;80:1536-1543.

Heller GV, et al. Pretreatment with theophylline does not affect adenosine-induced thallium-201 myocardial imaging. *Am Heart J*. 1993;126:1077-1083.

Product information. Adenosine (*Adenocard*). Lyphomed, Inc. 1989.

Minton NA, et al. Pharmacodynamic interactions between infused adenosine and oral theophylline. *Hum Exp Toxicol*. 1991;10:411-418.

Alendronate (*Fosamax*)

Naproxen (*Naprosyn*)

SUMMARY: Preliminary clinical evidence suggests that the risk of gastric ulcers with combined use of alendronate and naproxen is substantially greater than with use of either drug alone.

RISK FACTORS: No specific risk factors are known.

RELATED DRUGS: Theoretically, one would expect other NSAIDs to have a similar effect if combined with alendronate. COX-2 inhibitors such as celecoxib (*Celebrex*) and rofecoxib (*Vioxx*) might be less likely to interact, but clinical data are lacking.

MANAGEMENT OPTIONS:

➡ *Consider Alternative.* Consider using an alternative to one of the drugs (see Related Drugs).

➡ *Monitor.* Monitor patients on alendronate and NSAIDs for clinical evidence of gastric ulcers.

REFERENCES:
Graham DY, et al. Alendronate and naproxen are synergistic for development of gastric ulcers. *Arch Intern Med*. 2001;161:107.

Alfentanil (*Alfenta*)

Cimetidine (eg, *Tagamet*)

SUMMARY: Cimetidine appears to substantially increase serum concentrations of alfentanil, but it is not known how often this leads to adverse effects.

RISK FACTORS: No specific risk factors are known.

RELATED DRUGS: Preliminary evidence suggests that ranitidine (eg, *Zantac*) does not seem to affect the pharmacokinetics of alfentanil. The effect of famotidine (eg, *Pepcid*) and nizatidine (*Axid*) on alfentanil is not established, but theoretically they would not be expected to interact.

MANAGEMENT OPTIONS:

➡ *Consider Alternative.* Consider using H_2-receptor antagonists other than cimetidine.

➡ *Monitor.* If alfentanil is used in a patient receiving cimetidine, monitor for excessive or prolonged alfentanil effect. Adjust alfentanil dose as needed.

REFERENCES:
Keinlen J, et al. Pharmacokinetics of alfentanil in patients treated with either cimetidine or ranitidine. *Drug Invest*. 1993;6:257.

Alfentanil (*Alfenta*)

Diltiazem (eg, *Cardizem*)

SUMMARY: Diltiazem increases alfentanil plasma concentrations and may prolong sedation and respiratory depression.

RISK FACTORS: No specific risk factors are known.

RELATED DRUGS: Diltiazem is likely to affect other analgesics that are metabolized by CYP3A4 including fentanyl (*Sublimaze*) and sufentanil (*Sufenta*). Verapamil (*Calan*) and mibefradil (*Posicor*) may inhibit the metabolism of alfentanil.

MANAGEMENT OPTIONS:

➡ *Consider Alternative.* The use of a dihydropyridine calcium channel blocker (eg, amlodipine [*Norvasc*] or felodipine [*Plendil*]) would probably avoid the interaction.

➡ *Monitor.* Monitor patients receiving diltiazem and alfentanil for prolonged sedation and respiratory depression.

REFERENCES:
Ahonen J, et al. Effect of diltiazem on midazolam and alfentanil disposition in patients undergoing coronary artery bypass grafting. *Anesthesiology.* 1996;85:1246.

Alfentanil (*Alfenta*)

Erythromycin (eg, *E-Mycin*)

SUMMARY: Patients taking erythromycin may experience prolonged anesthesia or increased respiratory depression when given alfentanil.

RISK FACTORS: No specific risk factors are known.

RELATED DRUGS: Other macrolides such as troleandomycin (*TAO*) or clarithromycin (*Biaxin*) also may inhibit alfentanil. Azithromycin (*Zithromax*) and dirithromycin (*Dynabac*) would be unlikely to inhibit alfentanil metabolism.

MANAGEMENT OPTIONS:

➡ *Circumvent/Minimize.* Erythromycin has no effect on sufentanil serum concentrations. Consider using azithromycin or dirithromycin with alfentanil.

➡ *Monitor.* Until further information is available, monitor patients taking erythromycin for enhanced effects following usual doses of alfentanil.

REFERENCES:
Bartkowski RR, et al. Inhibition of alfentanil metabolism by erythromycin. *Clin Pharmacol Ther.* 1989;46:99.

Mansuy D. Formation of reactive intermediates and metabolites: effects of macrolide antibiotics on cytochrome P-450. *Pharmacol Ther.* 1987;33:41.

Barkowski RR, et al. Prolonged alfentanil effect following erythromycin administration. *Anesthesiology.* 1990;73:566.

Barkowski RR, et al. Sufentanil disposition. Is it affected by erythromycin? *Anesthesiology.* 1993;78:260.

Alfentanil (*Alfenta*)
Fluconazole (*Diflucan*)

SUMMARY: Fluconazole increases alfentanil plasma concentrations; increased or prolonged respiratory depression may result.

RISK FACTORS: No specific risk factors are known.

RELATED DRUGS: Other antifungal agents such as ketoconazole (*Nizoral*) and itraconazole (*Sporanox*) that are known to inhibit CYP3A4 may decrease alfentanil metabolism. Other analgesics such as fentanyl (*Sublimaze*) and sufentanil (*Sufenta*) may be affected by fluconazole or other antifungal agents that inhibit CYP3A4.

MANAGEMENT OPTIONS:

➡ *Monitor.* Be alert for altered opioid effects including increased or prolonged respiratory depression when alfentanil is administered to patients taking drugs known to inhibit CYP3A4 activity.

REFERENCES:
Palkama VJ, et al. The effect of intravenous and oral fluconazole on the pharmacokinetics and pharmacodynamics of intravenous alfentanil. *Anesth Analg.* 1998;87:190.

Allopurinol (eg, *Zyloprim*)
Antacids

SUMMARY: Aluminum hydroxide appeared to inhibit the response to allopurinol considerably in several patients.

RISK FACTORS: No specific risk factors are known.

RELATED DRUGS: Pending additional information, consider all *aluminum*-containing antacids capable of inhibiting allopurinol absorption. Although little is known regarding *magnesium*- or *calcium*-containing antacids, assume that they also inhibit allopurinol absorption until proven otherwise.

MANAGEMENT OPTIONS:

➡ *Circumvent/Minimize.* Until more information is available, administer allopurinol at least 3 hours before or 6 hours after aluminum hydroxide.

➡ *Monitor.* Also, monitor patients for reduced allopurinol response. The same precautions would apply to other antacids until information on their effect on allopurinol is available.

REFERENCES:
Weissman I, et al. Interaction of aluminum hydroxide and allopurinol in patients on chronic hemodialysis. *Ann Intern Med.* 1987;107:787.

Allopurinol (eg, *Zyloprim*)
Azathioprine (eg, *Imuran*)

SUMMARY: Allopurinol may increase the toxicity of azathioprine; careful dosage adjustment is necessary.

RISK FACTORS: No specific risk factors are known.

RELATED DRUGS: Mercaptopurine (*Purinethol*) interacts similarly with allopurinol.

MANAGEMENT OPTIONS:

➡ ***Avoid Unless Benefit Outweighs Risk.*** Several authors have recommended that the azathioprine dose be reduced to one-fourth of the recommended dose when it is used concurrently with allopurinol.

➡ ***Monitor.*** Allopurinol and azathioprine should never be given together without meticulous attention to adjusting the dosage of the azathioprine.

REFERENCES:

Anon. Clinicopathologic conference: hypertension and the lupus syndrome. *Am J Med*. 1970;49:519.

Nies AS, Oates JA. Clinicopathologic conference: hypertension and the lupus syndrome revisited. *Am J Med*. 1971;51:812.

 Allopurinol (eg, *Zyloprim*)

Captopril (eg, *Capoten*)

SUMMARY: Isolated case reports indicate that patients on allopurinol and angiotensin-converting enzyme (ACE) inhibitors such as captopril or enalapril may be predisposed to hypersensitivity reactions including Stevens-Johnson syndrome, anaphylaxis, skin eruptions, fever, and arthralgias, but a causal relationship has not been established.

RISK FACTORS:

➡ ***Concurrent Diseases.*** Impaired renal function has been proposed as a risk factor, but more study is needed.

RELATED DRUGS: It is not known whether ACE inhibitors other than captopril and enalapril would produce similar reactions if combined with allopurinol.

MANAGEMENT OPTIONS:

➡ ***Avoid Unless Benefit Outweighs Risk.*** Although it is not firmly established that these reactions resulted from the combined effects of ACE inhibitors and allopurinol, the severity of the potential reactions suggests that the combinations generally should be avoided until more information is available.

➡ ***Monitor.*** Monitor patients receiving the combination carefully for hypersensitivity reactions. Prompt discontinuation of the offending drugs is important.

REFERENCES:

Pennell DJ, et al. Fatal Stevens-Johnson syndrome in a patient on captopril and allopurinol. *Lancet*. 1984;1:463.

Sanamta A, et al. Fever, myalgia, and arthralgia in a patient on captopril and allopurinol. *Lancet*. 1984;1:679.

Lupton GP, et al. The allopurinol hypersensitivity syndrome. *J Am Acad Dermatol*. 1979;1:365.

Burkle WS. Allopurinol hypersensitivity. *Drug Intell Clin Pharm*. 1979;13:218.

Al-Kawas FH, et al. Allopurinol hepatotoxicity. Report of two cases and review of the literature. *Ann Intern Med*. 1981;95:588.

Ahmad S. Allopurinol and enalapril: drug induced anaphylactic coronary spasm and acute myocardial infarction. *Chest*. 1995;108:586.

Allopurinol (eg, *Zyloprim*)

Cyclophosphamide (eg, *Cytoxan*)

SUMMARY: Some evidence indicates that allopurinol increases cyclophosphamide toxicity, but this has not been a consistent finding.

RISK FACTORS: No specific risk factors are known.

RELATED DRUGS: No information is available.

MANAGEMENT OPTIONS:

➥ *Monitor.* It has been proposed that the appropriateness of routine prophylactic use of allopurinol in patients receiving cytotoxic drugs be re-evaluated. When it is necessary to give allopurinol and cyclophosphamide concomitantly, be alert for evidence of excessive cyclophosphamide effect.

REFERENCES:

Boston Collaborative Drug Surveillance Program. Allopurinol and cytotoxic drugs. Interaction in relation to bone marrow depression. *JAMA.* 1974;227:1036.

Stolbach L, et al. Evaluation of bone marrow toxic reaction in patients treated with allopurinol. *JAMA.* 1982;247:334.

Bagley CM Jr, et al. Clinical pharmacology of cyclophosphamide. *Cancer Res.* 1973;33:226.

Witten J, et al. The pharmacokinetics of cyclophosphamide in man after treatment with allopurinol. *Acta Pharmacol et Toxicol.* 1980;46:392–94.

Allopurinol (eg, *Zyloprim*)

Cyclosporine (eg, *Sandimmune*)

SUMMARY: Case reports suggest that allopurinol may increase cyclosporine blood concentrations and increase the risk of cyclosporine toxicity.

RISK FACTORS: No specific risk factors are known.

RELATED DRUGS: The effect of allopurinol on tacrolimus (*Prograf*) is not established. Given the similarity in the metabolism of cyclosporine and tacrolimus, it is possible that allopurinol affects them similarly.

MANAGEMENT OPTIONS:

➥ *Circumvent/Minimize.* Adjustments of cyclosporine dosage may be needed.

➥ *Monitor.* Monitor for altered cyclosporine concentrations and renal function if allopurinol is initiated, discontinued, or changed in dosage.

REFERENCES:

Stevens SL, et al. Cyclosporine toxicity associated with allopurinol. *South Med J.* 1992;85:1265.

Gorrie M, et al. Allopurinol interaction with cyclosporin. *BMJ.* 1994;308:113.

Allopurinol (eg, *Zyloprim*)

Mercaptopurine (*Purinethol*)

SUMMARY: Allopurinol increases the effect of mercaptopurine; reduce mercaptopurine dose and monitor the patient for toxicity.

RISK FACTORS: No specific risk factors are known.

RELATED DRUGS: Azathioprine (eg, *Imuran*) interacts in a similar manner with allopurinol.

MANAGEMENT OPTIONS:

➡ ***Circumvent/Minimize.*** When allopurinol and mercaptopurine are given concomitantly, the mercaptopurine dose may need to be reduced to as little as 25% of the usual dose.

➡ ***Monitor.*** Monitor for both excessive bone marrow suppression and adequate therapeutic response during cotherapy with these drugs.

REFERENCES:

Calabro JJ, et al. Case records of the Massachusetts General Hospital (Case 4–1972). *N Engl J Med.* 1972;286:205.

Coffey JJ, et al. Effect of allopurinol on the pharmacokinetics of 6-mercaptopurine (NSC 755) in cancer patients. *Cancer Res.* 1972;32:1283.

Allopurinol (eg, *Zyloprim*)

Theophylline (eg, *Slo-Phyllin*)

SUMMARY: Allopurinol, especially in large doses, may increase serum theophylline concentrations, but the incidence of theophylline toxicity in patients receiving the combination is not known.

RISK FACTORS:

➡ ***Dosage Regimen.*** Allopurinol doses at least 600 mg/day may inhibit the hepatic metabolism of theophylline.

RELATED DRUGS: No information is available.

MANAGEMENT OPTIONS:

➡ ***Monitor.*** Monitor for evidence of altered theophylline effect if allopurinol therapy is initiated or discontinued, especially if large doses of allopurinol are used. Alteration of theophylline dose may be needed.

REFERENCES:

Barry M, et al. Allopurinol influences aminophenazone elimination. *Clin Pharmacokinet.* 1990;19:167.

Jacobs MH, et al. Theophylline toxicity due to impaired theophylline degradation. *Am Rev Resp Dis.* 1974;110:342.

Marlin GE, et al. Assessment of combined oral theophylline and inhaled beta-adrenoceptor agonist bronchodilator therapy. *Br J Clin Pharmacol.* 1978;5:45.

Vozeh S, et al. Influence of allopurinol on theophylline disposition in adults. *Clin Pharmacol Ther.* 1980;27:194.

Grygiel JJ, et al. Effects of allopurinol on theophylline metabolism and clearance. *Clin Pharmacol Ther.* 1979;26:660.

Manfredi RL, et al. Inhibition of theophylline metabolism by longterm allopurinol administration. *Clin Pharmacol Ther*. 1981;29:224.

Matheson LE, et al. Drug interference with the Schack and Waxler plasma theophylline assay. *Am J Hosp Pharm*. 1977;34:496.

Allopurinol (eg, *Zyloprim*)

Vidarabine (*Vira-A*)

SUMMARY: Allopurinol may increase vidarabine toxicity.

RISK FACTORS: No specific risk factors are known.

RELATED DRUGS: No information is available.

MANAGEMENT OPTIONS:

➡ ***Monitor.*** Until additional information regarding this interaction is available, carefully monitor patients receiving allopurinol and vidarabine for signs of vidarabine toxicity.

REFERENCES:

Friedman HM, et al. Adenine arabinoside and allopurinol-possible adverse drug interaction. *N Engl J Med*. 1981;304:423.

Allopurinol (eg, *Zyloprim*)

Warfarin (eg, *Coumadin*)

SUMMARY: Although the evidence is conflicting, allopurinol appears to enhance the hypoprothrombinemic response to oral anticoagulants in some patients; bleeding episodes have been reported in some cases.

RISK FACTORS: No specific risk factors are known.

RELATED DRUGS: Although data are limited, assume that all oral anticoagulants interact with allopurinol until proven otherwise.

MANAGEMENT OPTIONS:

➡ ***Monitor.*** Watch for an alteration in the hypoprothrombinemic response to oral anticoagulants when allopurinol is started, stopped, or changed in dosage; adjust oral anticoagulant dosage as needed.

REFERENCES:

Vesell ES, et al. Impairment of drug metabolism in man by allopurinol and nortriptyline. *N Engl J Med*. 1970;283:1484.

Pond SM, et al. The effects of allopurinol and clofibrate on the elimination of coumarin anticoagulants in man. *Aust NZ J Med*. 1975;5:324.

Rawlins MD, et al. Influence of allopurinol on drug metabolism in man. *Br J Pharmacol*. 1973;48:693.

Jahnchen E, et al. Interaction of allopurinol with phenprocoumon in man. *Klin Wochenschr*. 1977;55:759.

Self TH, et al. Drug-enhancement of warfarin activity. *Lancet*. 1975;2:557.

Weart CW. Coumarin and allopurinol: a drug interaction case report. Contributed paper, 32nd annual meeting ASHP, 1975.

McInnes GT, et al. Acute adverse reactions attributed to allopurinol in hospitalized patients. *Ann Rheum Dis*. 1981;40:245.

Barry M, et al. Allopurinol influences aminophenazone elimination. *Clin Pharmacokinet*. 1990;19:167.

Almotriptan (*Axert*)

Ketoconazole (eg, *Nizoral*)

SUMMARY: Ketoconazole administration increases the plasma concentration of almotriptan; increased side effects caused by vasoconstriction may occur in some patients.

RISK FACTORS:

➥ **Pharmacogenetics.** Since almotriptan is metabolized by CYP3A4, CYP2D6 and mono-amine oxidase, the effect of a CYP3A4 inhibitor like ketoconazole may be greater in patients who are deficient in CYP2D6 and do not have this metabolic pathway for almotriptan elimination.

RELATED DRUGS: Itraconazole (*Sporanox*), voriconazole (*Vfend*), and fluconazole (*Diflucan*) are known to inhibit CYP3A4 and could increase almotriptan plasma concentrations.

MANAGEMENT OPTIONS:

➥ **Consider Alternative.** Terbinafine (*Lamisil*) does not inhibit CYP3A4 but it does inhibit CYP2D6. It is unknown how much CYP2D6 contributes to the metabolism of almotriptan. Although data are lacking, other selective serotonin 1B/1D receptor antagonists (naratriptan [*Amerge*], sumatriptan [*Imitrex*], rizatriptan [*Maxalt*], zolmitriptan [*Zomig*]) that do not rely on CYP3A4 for their metabolism may not be affected in a similar manner by ketoconazole.

➥ **Monitor.** Carefully monitor patients taking chronic antifungal therapy if almotriptan is administered. Almotriptan doses should probably start with 6.25 mg and repeated only with caution.

REFERENCES:

Fleishaker JC, et al. Effect of ketoconazole on the clearance of the antimigraine compound, almotriptan, in humans. *Clin Pharmacol Ther.* 2001;69:P25.

Alprazolam (eg, *Xanax*)

Digoxin (eg, *Lanoxin*)

SUMMARY: A case report indicates that alprazolam may increase digoxin serum concentrations, but this has not been a consistent finding.

RISK FACTORS:

➥ **Dosage Regimen.** Alprazolam doses more than 0.5 mg/day may increase digoxin serum concentrations.

RELATED DRUGS: No information is available.

MANAGEMENT OPTIONS:

➥ **Monitor.** Pending further information, monitor patients stabilized on digoxin for increased digoxin concentrations and effect when alprazolam is added to their therapy.

REFERENCES:

Ochs HR, et al. Effect of alprazolam on digoxin kinetics and creatinine clearance. *Clin Pharmacol Ther.* 1985;38:595.

Tollefson G, et al. Alprazolam-related digoxin toxicity. *Am J Psych.* 1984;141:1612.

Guven H, et al. Age-related digoxin-alprazolam interaction. *Clin Pharmacol Ther.* 1993;54:42.

Alprazolam (*Xanax*)

Erythromycin (eg, *E-Mycin*)

SUMMARY: Erythromycin increases the plasma concentration and half-life of alprazolam. An increase in alprazolam effects may occur in some patients.

RISK FACTORS: No specific risk factors are known.

RELATED DRUGS: Erythromycin is known to increase the plasma concentrations of other benzodiazepines including triazolam (*Halcion*) and midazolam (*Versed*). Clarithromycin (*Biaxin*) or troleandomycin (*TAO*) may produce similar reductions in the clearance of alprazolam.

MANAGEMENT OPTIONS:

➡ *Consider Alternative.* Selection of a noninhibiting macrolide (eg, azithromycin [*Zithromax*] or dirithromycin [*Dynabac*]) is likely to limit changes in alprazolam pharmacokinetics. Anxiolytics not metabolized by CYP3A4 such as lorazepam (*Ativan*) or temazepam (*Restoril*) could be substituted for alprazolam.

➡ *Monitor.* Monitor patients taking alprazolam chronically for increased sedation during erythromycin administration.

REFERENCES:

Yasui N, et al. A kinetic and dynamic study of oral alprazolam with and without erythromycin in humans: in vivo evidence for the involvement of CYP3A4 in alprazolam metabolism. *Clin Pharmacol Ther.* 1996;59:514.

Alprazolam (eg, *Xanax*)

Fluoxetine (eg, *Prozac*)

SUMMARY: In healthy subjects, fluoxetine appears to increase alprazolam plasma concentrations, resulting in an increase in alprazolam-induced psychomotor impairment.

RISK FACTORS: No specific risk factors are known.

RELATED DRUGS: The effect of selective serotonin reuptake inhibitors other than fluoxetine on alprazolam is not established, but fluvoxamine (eg, *Luvox*) is known to inhibit CYP3A4, an isozyme important in the metabolism of alprazolam.

MANAGEMENT OPTIONS:

➡ *Circumvent/Minimize.* It would be prudent to use conservative doses of alprazolam in the presence of fluoxetine until patient response is assessed. Advise patients receiving combined therapy to watch for excessive sedation.

➡ *Monitor.* Monitor for altered alprazolam effect if fluoxetine is initiated, discontinued, or changed in dosage. Adjust alprazolam dose as needed.

REFERENCES:

Greenblatt DJ, et al. Fluoxetine impairs clearance of alprazolam but not of clonazepam. *Clin Pharmacol Ther.* 1992;52:479-486.

Lasher TA, et al. Pharmacokinetic pharmacodynamic evaluation of the combined administration of alprazolam and fluoxetine. *Psychopharmacology.* 1991;104:323-327.

Alprazolam (eg, _Xanax_)

Fluvoxamine (eg, _Luvox_)

SUMMARY: Fluvoxamine increases alprazolam plasma concentrations and may increase alprazolam sedation.

RISK FACTORS:

➡ **_Pharmacogenetics._** The increases in alprazolam concentrations were greater in patients with higher CYP2C19 activity (0 or 1 mutated allele) than in patients with low CYP2C19 activity (2 mutated alleles).

RELATED DRUGS: Fluoxetine (eg, _Prozac_) can also increase alprazolam plasma concentrations, but other selective serotonin reuptake inhibitors (SSRIs) would theoretically be less likely to interact.

MANAGEMENT OPTIONS:

➡ **_Consider Alternative._** Theoretically, fluvoxamine would be less likely to interact with benzodiazepines that are largely glucuronidated, such as temazepam (eg, _Restoril_), oxazepam (eg, _Serax_), estazolam (eg, _ProSom_), and lorazepam (eg, _Ativan_). SSRIs that would theoretically be unlikely to interact with alprazolam include citalopram (_Celexa_), escitalopram (_Lexapro_), paroxetine (_Paxil_), and sertraline (_Zoloft_).

➡ **_Monitor._** Be alert for evidence of excessive sedation in patients who receive alprazolam and fluvoxamine (or fluoxetine) concurrently.

REFERENCES:

Suzuki Y, et al. Effects of concomitant fluvoxamine on the metabolism of alprazolam in Japanese psychiatric patients: interaction with CYP2C19 mutated alleles. _Eur J Clin Pharmacol._ 2003;58:829-833.

 Alprenolol

Pentobarbital (eg, _Nembutal_)

SUMMARY: Barbiturates may reduce the plasma concentrations of some beta-blockers.

RISK FACTORS: No specific risk factors are known.

RELATED DRUGS: Pentobarbital also reduced the area under the concentration-time curve for metoprolol (eg, _Lopressor_) 32%. In 68 patients receiving propranolol (eg, _Inderal_) or sotalol (eg, _Betapace_), the 3 patients on enzyme inducers (phenobarbital or phenytoin) had a higher plasma clearance of propanolol than the other patients. Sotalol, which undergoes minimal metabolism, was not influenced by the inducers. Atenolol (eg, _Tenormin_) and nadolol (eg, _Corgard_), which are excreted primarily unchanged by the kidneys, are unlikely to interact with barbiturates. Phenobarbital (eg, _Solfoton_) and other barbiturates probably will increase the metabolism of beta-blockers that are extensively metabolized.

MANAGEMENT OPTIONS:

➡ **_Consider Alternative._** Beta-blockers excreted primarily unchanged by the kidneys (eg, atenolol, nadolol) are unlikely to interact with barbiturates and could be used to avoid the interaction.

➥ *Monitor.* Watch for evidence of altered response to beta-blockers metabolized by the liver (eg, propranolol, metoprolol, alprenolol) when barbiturate therapy is initiated or discontinued.

REFERENCES:

Alvan G, et al. Effect of pentobarbital on the disposition of alprenolol. *Clin Pharmacol Ther.* 1977;22:316-321.

Seideman P, et al. Decreased plasma concentrations and clinical effects of alprenolol during combined treatment with pentobarbitone in hypertension. *Br J Clin Pharmacol.* 1987;23:267-271.

Collste P, et al. Influence of pentobarbital on effect and plasma levels of alprenolol and 4-hydroxy-alprenolol. *Clin Pharmacol Ther.* 1979;25:423-427.

Haglund K, et al. Influence of pentobarbital on metoprolol plasma levels. *Clin Pharmacol Ther.* 1979;26:326-329.

Sotaniemi EA, et al. Plasma clearance of propranolol and sotalol and hepatic drug-metabolizing enyzme activity. *Clin Pharmacol Ther.* 1979;26:153-161.

Altretamine (*Hexalen*)

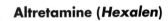

Imipramine (eg, *Tofranil*)

SUMMARY: Altretamine appears to increase the incidence of orthostatic hypotension caused by tricyclic antidepressants or MAO inhibitors.

RISK FACTORS: No specific risk factors are known.

RELATED DRUGS: Theoretically, other tricyclic antidepressants or MAO inhibitors might interact with altretamine.

MANAGEMENT OPTIONS:

➥ *Consider Alternative.* Antidepressants which are normally associated with a low incidence of orthostatic hypotension, such as nortriptyline or selective serotonin reuptake inhibitors, could be considered.

➥ *Circumvent/Minimize.* Warn patients requiring an antidepressant and receiving altretamine about orthostatic hypotension.

➥ *Monitor.* Monitor for orthostatic hypotension in patients receiving altretamine with either tricyclic antidepressants or MAO inhibitors.

REFERENCES:

Bruckner HW, et al. Orthostatic hypotension as a complication of hexamethylmelamine antidepressant interaction. *Cancer Treat Rep.* 1983;67:516.

Aluminum

Cyclosporine (eg, *Sandimmune*)

SUMMARY: Clinical observations in pediatric patients suggest that aluminum hydroxide reduces cyclosporine blood concentrations, but additional study is needed.

RISK FACTORS: No specific risk factors are known.

RELATED DRUGS: The effect of other antacids on cyclosporine is not established, but assume that they may interact until it is proven otherwise.

MANAGEMENT OPTIONS:

➤ *Circumvent/Minimize.* Until more information is available, it would be prudent to give cyclosporine at least 2 hours before or 6 hours after aluminum hydroxide or other antacids.

➤ *Monitor.* Monitor for reduced cyclosporine blood concentrations if aluminum hydroxide or other antacids are given concurrently.

REFERENCES:

Ichisawa M, et al. The effect of dried aluminum hydroxide gel on the blood concentration of cyclosporine-A. *Jpn J Hosp Pharm.* 1997;23:407.

Amantadine (eg, *Symmetrel*)

Bupropion (eg, *Wellbutrin*)

SUMMARY: Bupropion may increase the risk of amantadine neurotoxicity, but more study is needed to establish a causal relationship.

RISK FACTORS: No specific risk factors are known.

RELATED DRUGS: No information is available.

MANAGEMENT OPTIONS:

➤ *Circumvent/Minimize.* If amantadine use is short-term for influenza, consider stopping the bupropion temporarily during the amantadine therapy.

➤ *Monitor.* If the combination is used, monitor for evidence of neurotoxicity. If neurotoxicity occurs, temporary discontinuation of both drugs may be required.

REFERENCES:

Trappler B, et al. Bupropion-amantadine-associated neurotoxicity. *J Clin Psychiatry.* 2000;61:61-62.

Amantadine (eg, *Symmetrel*)

Triamterene (*Dyrenium*)

SUMMARY: Triamterene-hydrochlorothiazide (eg, *Dyazide*) has been reported to increase serum concentrations and toxicity of amantadine.

RISK FACTORS: No specific risk factors are known.

RELATED DRUGS: It is possible that rimantadine (*Flumadine*) is similarly affected by triamterene.

MANAGEMENT OPTIONS:

➤ *Circumvent/Minimize.* Amantadine dosage may need to be reduced when triamterene is coadministered.

➤ *Monitor.* In patients receiving amantadine, use triamterene or thiazides with caution and watch for signs of amantadine toxicity including nausea, dizziness, and dry mouth.

REFERENCES:

Wilson TW, et al. Amantadine-dyazide interaction. *Can Med Assoc J.* 1983;129:974-975.

Amantadine (eg, *Symmetrel*)

Trihexyphenidyl (eg, *Trihexy*)

SUMMARY: Trihexyphenidyl and other anticholinergic drugs may potentiate CNS side effects of amantadine.

RISK FACTORS: No specific risk factors are known.

RELATED DRUGS: It is possible that rimantadine (*Flumadine*) would be similarly affected by trihexyphenidyl. Amantadine also can potentiate the anticholinergic effects of other anticholinergic drugs such as benztropine (eg, *Cogentin*).

MANAGEMENT OPTIONS:

➡ *Circumvent/Minimize.* Although more information is needed, consider reducing high-dose anticholinergic therapy before administering amantadine.

➡ *Monitor.* Be alert for confusion and hallucinations when amantadine is combined with other anticholinergics.

REFERENCES:

Schwab RS, et al. Amantadine in the treatment of Parkinson's disease. *JAMA*. 1969;208:1168-1170.

Parkes JD, et al. Treatment of Parkinson's disease with amantadine and levodopa. A one-year study. *Lancet*. 1971;1:1083-1086.

Postma JU, et al. Visual hallucinations and delirium during treatment with amantadine (*Symmetrel*). *J Am Geriatr Soc*. 1975;23:212-215.

Amiloride (*Midamor*)

Candesartan (*Atacand*)

SUMMARY: Combining amiloride with candesartan or other angiotensin II receptor blockers (ARBs) may increase the risk of hyperkalemia, especially in patients with 1 or more risk factors.

RISK FACTORS:

➡ *Other Drugs.* The addition of other hyperkalemic drugs may increase the risk of hyperkalemia in patients on amiloride and ARBs. Hyperkalemic drugs include ACE inhibitors, potassium supplements, cyclosporine, tacrolimus, NSAIDs, COX-2 inhibitors, nonselective beta-adrenergic blockers, trimethoprim, and pentamidine.

➡ *Concurrent Diseases.* Diseases that increase the risk of hyperkalemia for this interaction include diabetes and significant renal impairment.

➡ *Diet/Food.* A diet high in potassium may increase the risk of hyperkalemia from this interaction. Salt substitutes may contain potassium.

RELATED DRUGS: Amiloride would be expected to increase the risk of hyperkalemia when combined with other ARBs, including eprosartan (*Teveten*), irbesartan (*Avapro*), losartan (*Cozaar*), telmisartan (*Micardis*), and valsartan (*Diovan*).

MANAGEMENT OPTIONS:

➡ *Monitor.* In patients receiving amiloride and an ARB, monitor serum potassium and renal function, particularly if the patient has 1 or more of the risk factors listed above.

REFERENCES:

Wrenger E, et al. Interaction of spironolactone with ACE inhibitors or angiotensin receptor blockers: analysis of 44 cases. *BMJ.* 2003;327:147-149.

Amiloride (*Midamor*)

Enalapril (eg, *Vasotec*)

SUMMARY: Combining amiloride with enalapril or other ACE inhibitors increases the risk of hyperkalemia, especially in patients with 1 or more risk factors.

RISK FACTORS:

➡ *Other Drugs.* In patients on amiloride and ACE inhibitors, the addition of other hyperkalemic drugs can increase the risk. Such drugs include potassium supplements, nonselective beta-adrenergic blockers, cyclosporine, tacrolimus, NSAIDs, COX-2 inhibitors, trimethoprim, and pentamidine.

➡ *Concurrent Diseases.* Diseases that increase the risk of hyperkalemia for this interaction include diabetes and significant renal impairment.

➡ *Diet/Food.* A diet high in potassium may increase the risk of hyperkalemia from this interaction. Some salt substitutes contain potassium.

RELATED DRUGS: Amiloride would also be expected to interact with other ACE inhibitors, including benazepril (*Lotensin*), captopril (eg, *Capoten*), fosinopril (*Monopril*), lisinopril (eg, *Prinivil*), moexipril (eg, *Univasc*), quinapril (*Accupril*), ramipril (*Altace*), and trandolapril (*Mavik*).

MANAGEMENT OPTIONS:

➡ *Monitor.* In patients receiving amiloride and an ACE inhibitor, monitor serum potassium and renal function, particularly if the patient has 1 or more of the risk factors listed above.

REFERENCES:

Chiu TF, et al. Rapid life-threatening hyperkalemia after addition of amiloride HCl/hydrochlorothiazide to angiotensin-converting enzyme inhibitor therapy. *Ann Emerg Med.* 1997;30:612-615.

Schepkens H, et al. Life-threatening hyperkalemia during combined therapy with angiotensin-converting enzyme inhibitors and spironolactone. *Am J Med.* 2001;110:438-441.

Berry C, McMurray J. Life-threatening hyperkalemia during combined therapy with angiotensin-converting enzyme inhibitors and spironolactone. *Am J Med.* 2001;111:587.

Blaustein DA, et al. Estimation of glomerular filtration rate to prevent life-threatening hyperkalemia due to combined therapy with spironolactone and angiotensin-converting enzyme inhibition or angiotensin receptor blockade. *Am J Cardiol.* 2002;90:662-663.

Wrenger E, et al. Interaction of spironolactone with ACE inhibitors or angiotensin receptor blockers: analysis of 44 cases. *BMJ.* 2003;327:147-149.

Weber EW, et al. Incidence of hyperkalemia in chronic heart failure patients taking spironolactone in a VA medical center. *Pharmacotherapy.* 2003;23:391.

Amiloride (*Midamor*)

Quinidine

SUMMARY: Coadministration of amiloride with quinidine appears to increase the risk of arrhythmias in patients with ventricular tachycardia.

RISK FACTORS: No specific risk factors are known.

RELATED DRUGS: No information is available.

MANAGEMENT OPTIONS:

➥ *Consider Alternative.* Until more information is available, patients taking quinidine should avoid the use of amiloride. Thiazides have not been reported to produce proarrhythmic effects with quinidine.

➥ *Monitor.* If amiloride and quinidine are coadministered, carefully monitor patients for evidence of prolonged ventricular conduction (QRS prolongation) in excess of QRS changes produced by quinidine monotherapy.

REFERENCES:

Wang L, et al. Amiloride-quinidine interaction: adverse outcomes. *Clin Pharmacol Ther.* 1994;56:659-667.

Aminoglutethimide (*Cytadren*)

Dexamethasone (eg, *Decadron*)

SUMMARY: Aminoglutethimide enhances the elimination of dexamethasone (and probably other corticosteroids), resulting in a marked reduction in corticosteroid response.

RISK FACTORS: No specific risk factors are known.

RELATED DRUGS: Theoretically, the metabolism of corticosteroids other than dexamethasone (eg, hydrocortisone [eg, *Cortef*], cortisone, prednisone [eg, *Deltasone*], prednisolone [eg, *Prelone*], methylprednisolone [eg, *Medrol*]) also would be enhanced by aminoglutethimide, but it is not known whether they would be affected to the same degree as dexamethasone.

MANAGEMENT OPTIONS:

➥ *Monitor.* Dexamethasone dosage requirements are likely to increase considerably (eg, up to at least 2-fold) in the presence of aminoglutethimide. Give careful attention to dexamethasone response when aminoglutethimide is initiated, discontinued, or changed in dosage.

REFERENCES:

Kvinnsland S, et al. Aminoglutethimide as an inducer of microsomal enzymes. Part 1: Pharmacological aspects. *Breast Cancer Res Treat.* 1986;7(suppl):573-576.

Santen RJ, et al. Successful medical adrenalectomy with amino-glutethimide. Role of altered drug metabolism. *JAMA.* 1974;230:1661-1665.

Halpern J, et al. A call for caution in the use of aminoglutethimide: negative interaction with dexamethasone and beta blocker treatment. *J Med.* 1984;15:59-63.

Aminoglutethimide (*Cytadren*)

Digitoxin†

SUMMARY: Aminoglutethimide administration reduced the serum concentration of digitoxin in several patients.

RISK FACTORS: No specific risk factors are known.

RELATED DRUGS: Because the primary route of elimination is renal, digoxin (eg, *Lanoxin*), is not likely to interact with aminoglutethimide to the same degree as digitoxin.

MANAGEMENT OPTIONS:

➥ *Consider Alternative.* Theoretically, the substitution of digoxin for digitoxin would reduce the likelihood of an interaction.

➥ *Monitor.* Monitor digitoxin concentrations for several weeks when patients are maintained on digitoxin following the addition of aminoglutethimide. Increased digitoxin doses may be required to maintain the serum concentrations in the therapeutic range following aminoglutethimide administration.

REFERENCES:

Lonning PE, et al. Mechanisms of action of aminoglutethimide as endocrine therapy of breast cancer. *Drugs.* 1988;35:685-710.

Lonning E, et al. Effect of aminoglutethimide on antipyrine, theophylline, and digitoxin disposition in breast cancer. *Clin Pharmacol Ther.* 1984;36:796-802.

† Not available in the United States.

 Aminoglutethimide (*Cytadren*)

Medroxyprogesterone (*Provera*)

SUMMARY: Aminoglutethimide substantially lowers plasma medroxyprogesterone concentrations, but more study is needed to determine the degree to which this reduces the therapeutic response.

RISK FACTORS: No specific risk factors are known.

RELATED DRUGS: It is not known to what extent aminoglutethimide enhances the metabolism of progestins other than medroxyprogesterone, but consider the possibility.

MANAGEMENT OPTIONS:

➥ *Monitor.* Monitor for altered medroxyprogesterone effect if aminoglutethimide is initiated, discontinued, or changed in dosage.

REFERENCES:

Kvinssland S, et al. Aminoglutethimide as an inducer of microsomal enzymes. Part 1. Pharmacological aspects. *Breast Cancer Res Treat.* 1986;7(Suppl.):73.

Van Deijk WA, et al. Influence of aminoglutethimide on plasma levels of medroxyprogesterone acetate: its correlation with serum cortisol. *Cancer Treat Rep.* 1985;69:85.

2 Aminoglutethimide (*Cytadren*)

Tamoxifen (*Nolvadex*)

SUMMARY: Aminoglutethimide reduces tamoxifen concentrations and may reduce its clinical effect.

RISK FACTORS: No specific risk factors are known.

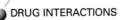

RELATED DRUGS: No information is available.

MANAGEMENT OPTIONS:

➡ *Avoid Unless Benefit Outweighs Risk.* Generally, do no administer aminoglutethimide with tamoxifen since it lowers tamoxifen concentrations and does not enhance the response of breast cancer patients to tamoxifen therapy.

➡ *Monitor.* If the combination is used, monitor tamoxifen response carefully.

REFERENCES:

Lien EA, et al. Decreased serum concentrations of tamoxifen and its metabolites induced by amino-glutethimide. *Cancer Res.* 1990;50:5851.

Aminoglutethimide (*Cytadren*)

Theophylline (eg, *Slo-Phyllin*)

SUMMARY: Preliminary evidence from a limited number of patients indicates that aminoglutethimide reduces the serum concentration of theophylline.

RISK FACTORS: No specific risk factors are known.

RELATED DRUGS: No information is available.

MANAGEMENT OPTIONS:

➡ *Monitor.* Patients maintained on theophylline should have their theophylline concentrations monitored for several weeks following the initiation or discontinuation of aminoglutethimide. Adjustment of theophylline doses may be required for some patients to maintain their serum concentrations in the therapeutic range following the initiation or discontinuation of aminoglutethimide.

REFERENCES:

Lonning PE, et al. Mechanisms of action of aminoglutethimide as endocrine therapy of breast cancer. *Drugs.* 1988;35:685.

Lonning PE, et al. Effect of aminoglutethimide on antipyrine, theophylline, and digitoxin disposition in breast cancer. *Clin Pharmacol Ther.* 1984;6:796.

Aminoglutethimide (*Cytadren*)

Warfarin (eg, *Coumadin*)

SUMMARY: Aminoglutethimide enhances the elimination of warfarin and other oral anticoagulants and can considerably reduce the hypoprothrombinemic response.

RISK FACTORS:

➡ *Dosage Regimen.* The interaction appears to be dose related. In one study, plasma warfarin clearance was increased 41% by 250 mg/day of aminoglutethimide and 91% by 1000 mg/day of aminoglutethimide.

RELATED DRUGS: Although the reports involved warfarin and acenocoumarol, it is likely that other oral anticoagulants interact similarly with aminoglutethimide.

MANAGEMENT OPTIONS:

➡ *Monitor.* In patients receiving warfarin or other oral anticoagulants, monitor the hypoprothrombinemic response carefully if aminoglutethimide is initiated, discontinued, or changed in dosage; oral anticoagulant dosage requirements are likely to change substantially. Warn patients accordingly.

REFERENCES:

Kvinssland S, et al. Aminoglutethimide as an inducer of microsomal enzymes. Part 1. Pharmacological aspects. *Breast Cancer Res Treat.* 1986;7(Suppl):73.

Murray RML, et al. Medical adrenalectomy with aminoglutethimide in the management of advanced breast cancer. *Med J Aust.* 1981;1:179.

Bruning PF. Aminoglutethimide and oral anticoagulant therapy. *Lancet.* 1983;2:582.

Lonning PE, et al. Aminoglutethimide and warfarin. A new important drug interaction. *Cancer Chemother Pharmacol.* 1984;12:10.

Lonning PE, et al. The influence of a graded dose schedule of aminoglutethimide on the disposition of the optical enantiomers of warfarin in patients with breast cancer. *Cancer Chemother Pharmacol.* 1986;17:177.

Aminosalicylic Acid (PAS)

Rifampin (eg, *Rifadin*)

SUMMARY: Aminosalicylic acid reduces serum concentrations of rifampin.

RISK FACTORS: No specific risk factors are known.

RELATED DRUGS: Other drugs containing bentonite probably inhibit rifampin absorption.

MANAGEMENT OPTIONS:

➡ *Circumvent/Minimize.* Separate doses of PAS and rifampin by 8 to 12 hours if possible.

➡ *Monitor.* Monitor rifampin concentrations if it is administered with bentonite.

REFERENCES:

Boman G, et al. Drug interaction: decreased serum concentrations of rifampicin when given with P.A.S. *Lancet.* 1971;1:800.

Boman G, et al. Mechanism of the inhibitory effect of PAS granules on the absorption of rifampicin: absorption of rifampicin by an excipient, bentonite. *Eur J Clin Pharmacol.* 1975;8:293.

Amiodarone (*Cordarone*)

Aprindine (*Fibocil*)

SUMMARY: Amiodarone may increase the plasma concentrations of aprindine.

RISK FACTORS: No specific risk factors are known.

RELATED DRUGS: No information is available.

MANAGEMENT OPTIONS:

➡ *Circumvent/Minimize.* Patients receiving both drugs may require less aprindine than those receiving aprindine alone.

➡ *Monitor.* Watch for evidence of altered aprindine response when amiodarone therapy is initiated or discontinued.

REFERENCES:

Southworth W, et al. Possible amiodarone-aprindine interaction. *Am Heart J.* 1982;104:323.

Amiodarone (*Cordarone*)

Cholestyramine (*Questran*)

SUMMARY: Cholestyramine can decrease amiodarone plasma concentrations and antiarrhythmic efficacy.

RISK FACTORS: No specific risk factors are known.

RELATED DRUGS: Colestipol (*Colestid*) also probably decreases amiodarone plasma concentrations.

MANAGEMENT OPTIONS:

➡ *Monitor.* Observe patients receiving cholestyramine and amiodarone for increased amiodarone dosage requirements. Discontinuation of cholestyramine may result in excessive accumulation of amiodarone and toxicity (eg, arrhythmia, pneumonitis, thyroid abnormalities).

REFERENCES:

Nitsch J, et al. Enhanced elimination of amidoarone by cholestyramine. *Dtsch Med Wochenschr.* 1986;111:1241.

Amiodarone (eg, *Cordarone*)

Cimetidine (eg, *Tagamet*)

SUMMARY: Cimetidine administration to patients stabilized on amiodarone can increase amiodarone serum concentrations and possibly enhance amiodarone toxicity.

RISK FACTORS: No specific risk factors are known.

RELATED DRUGS: The effects of other H_2-receptor antagonists, such as ranitidine (eg, *Zantac*), famotidine (eg, *Pepcid*), and nizatidine (*Axid*), on amiodarone are unknown, but they probably would not affect amiodarone metabolism.

MANAGEMENT OPTIONS:

➡ *Monitor.* Monitor amiodarone serum concentrations in amiodarone-treated patients following the institution of cimetidine. Many weeks may be required for the maximum effects of this interaction to become evident. It also may take several weeks for amiodarone concentrations to return to normal after cimetidine is discontinued.

REFERENCES:

Landau S, et al. Cimetidine-amiodarone interaction. *J Clin Pharmacol.* 1988;38:909.

Amiodarone (eg, *Cordarone*)

Cyclosporine (eg, *Sandimmune*)

SUMMARY: An increase in cyclosporine concentrations following the addition of amiodarone therapy has been reported.

RISK FACTORS: No specific risk factors are known.

RELATED DRUGS: It is possible that tacrolimus (*Prograf*) also may be affected by amiodarone.

MANAGEMENT OPTIONS:

➡ **Monitor.** Watch for increased cyclosporine concentrations and evidence of toxicity (renal dysfunction) in patients started on amiodarone therapy.

REFERENCES:

Nicolau DP, et al. Amiodarone-cyclosporine interaction in heart transplant patient. *J Heart Lung Transplant.* 1992;11:564.

Chitwood KK, et al. Cyclosporine-amiodarone interaction. *Ann Pharmacother.* 1993;27:569.

Mamprin F, et al. Amiodarone-cyclosporine interaction in cardiac transplantation. *Am Heart J.* 1992;123:1725.

Amiodarone (eg, *Cordarone*)

Digoxin (eg, *Lanoxin*)

SUMMARY: Amiodarone can cause digoxin to accumulate in the serum to concentrations that often are associated with toxicity.

RISK FACTORS: No specific risk factors are known.

RELATED DRUGS: The effect of amiodarone on digitoxin (*Crystodigin*) is not established but probably would be similar.

MANAGEMENT OPTIONS:

➡ **Circumvent/Minimize.** Digoxin doses probably will need to be reduced when amiodarone is added to therapy.

➡ **Monitor.** Monitor patients for changes in digoxin serum concentrations when amiodarone is initiated or discontinued during concurrent therapy. Several weeks may be required before new steady-state digoxin concentrations are achieved.

REFERENCES:

Moysey JO, et al. Amiodarone increases plasma digoxin concentrations. *BMJ.* 1981;282:272.

Klein HO, et al. Asystole produced by the combination of amiodarone and digoxin. *Am Heart J.* 1987;113(Part 1):399.

McGovern B, et al. Sinus arrest during treatment with amiodarone. *BMJ.* 1982;284:160.

Santostasi G, et al. Effects of amiodarone on oral and intravenous digoxin kinetics in healthy subjects. *J Cardiovasc Pharmacol.* 1987;9:385.

Fenster PE, et al. Pharmacokinetic evaluation of the digoxin-amiodarone interaction. *J Am Coll Cardiol.* 1985;5:108.

Nademanee K, et al. Amiodarone-digoxin interaction: clinical significance, time course of development, potential pharmacokinetic mechanisms and therapeutic implications. *J Am Coll Cardiol.* 1984;4:111.

Johnston A, et al. The digoxin-amiodarone interaction. *Br J Clin Pharmacol.* 1987;24:253P.

Koren G, et al. Digoxin toxicity associated with amiodarone therapy in children. *J Pediatr.* 1984;104:467.

Ben-chetrit E, et al. Case report: amiodarone-associated hypothyroidism—a possible cause of digoxin intoxication. *Am J Med Sci.* 1985;289:114.

Robinson K, et al. The digoxin-amiodarone interaction. *Cardiovasc Drugs Ther.* 1989;3:25.

Amiodarone (eg, *Cordarone*)

Diltiazem (eg, *Cardizem*)

SUMMARY: Amiodarone and diltiazem may result in cardiotoxicity with bradycardia and decreased cardiac output.

RISK FACTORS: No specific risk factors are known.

RELATED DRUGS: Verapamil (eg, *Calan*) may produce similar effects when used with amiodarone. Dihydropyridine calcium channel blockers (eg, nifedipine [eg, *Procardia*], amlodipine [*Norvasc*], felodipine [*Plendil*]) would be unlikely to interact with amiodarone.

MANAGEMENT OPTIONS:

➡ *Monitor.* Until more information is available, monitor patients receiving amiodarone for signs of cardiac toxicity when diltiazem is coadministered.

REFERENCES:

Lee TH, et al. Sinus arrest and hypotension with combined amiodarone-diltiazem therapy. *Am Heart J.* 1985;109:163.

Amiodarone (eg, *Cordarone*)

Flecainide (*Tambocor*)

SUMMARY: When amiodarone is administered in conjunction with flecainide, the dose of flecainide required to maintain therapeutic plasma concentrations may be one-third less than that required when flecainide is administered alone.

RISK FACTORS: No specific risk factors are known.

RELATED DRUGS: Amiodarone may affect encainide (*Enkaid*) in a similar manner.

MANAGEMENT OPTIONS:

➡ *Circumvent/Minimize.* Until more information is available, consider reducing the dose of flecainide by 33% to 50% when it is used in patients who already are being treated with amiodarone.

➡ *Monitor.* Observe patients for signs and symptoms consistent with altered flecainide serum concentrations when amiodarone is added to or discontinued from the regimens of patients taking flecainide. Because amiodarone has a long half-life, monitor patients for several weeks.

REFERENCES:

Shea P, et al. Flecainide and amiodarone interaction. *J Am Coll Cardiol.* 1986;7:1127.

Funck-Brentano C, et al. Variable disposition kinetics and electrocardiographic effects of flecainide during repeated dosing in humans: contribution of genetic factors, dose-dependent clearance, and interaction with amiodarone. *Clin Pharmacol Ther.* 1994;55:256.

Amiodarone (eg, *Cordarone*)

Indinavir (*Crixivan*)

SUMMARY: Indinavir appears to increase amiodarone concentrations; increased effects on cardiac conduction may occur in some patients.

RISK FACTORS: No specific risk factors are known.

RELATED DRUGS: Nelfinavir (*Viracept*), saquinavir (*Fortovase*), and ritonavir (*Norvir*) also inhibit CYP3A4 and may reduce amiodarone metabolism.

MANAGEMENT OPTIONS:

➡ *Monitor.* Carefully monitor patients receiving amiodarone for increased antiarrhythmic effects during indinavir administration.

REFERENCES:

Lohman JJ, et al. Antiretroviral therapy increases serum concentrations of amiodarone. *Ann Pharmacother.* 1999;33:645-646.

Amiodarone (eg, *Cordarone*)

Metoprolol (eg, *Lopressor*)

SUMMARY: The administration of metoprolol or propranolol (eg, *Inderal*) to patients maintained on amiodarone may lead to bradycardia, cardiac arrest, or ventricular arrhythmia shortly after initiation of the beta blocker.

RISK FACTORS: No specific risk factors are known.

RELATED DRUGS: Two patients receiving amiodarone (1 for atrial flutter, 1 for ischemia) developed cardiac arrest or ventricular fibrillation within 2 hours following 1 or 2 oral doses of propranolol. If additive pharmacodynamic effects are partially responsible, all beta blockers (eg, propranolol [*Inderal*]) would be expected to interact in a similar manner. If reduction in beta blocker metabolism is responsible for this interaction, renally eliminated beta blockers (eg, atenolol [*Tenormin*]) would be expected to be less likely to interact.

MANAGEMENT OPTIONS:

➡ *Monitor.* Until additional information is available, carefully observe patients maintained on amiodarone when beta blockers that undergo extensive hepatic metabolism are initiated. Although atenolol did not appear to interact with amiodarone in one case, there is insufficient evidence to recommend atenolol as an alternative.

REFERENCES:

Leor J, et al. Amiodarone and beta-adrenergic blockers: an interaction with metoprolol but not with atenolol. *Am Heart J.* 1988;116:206.

Derrida JP, et al. Amiodarone and propranolol, a dangerous association. *Nouv Presse Med.* 1979;8:1429.

Amiodarone (eg, *Cordarone*)

Phenytoin (eg, *Dilantin*)

SUMMARY: The serum concentration of phenytoin can be increased considerably during concomitant amiodarone therapy and the serum concentration of amiodarone can be reduced by phenytoin coadministration.

RISK FACTORS: No specific risk factors are known.

RELATED DRUGS: Mephenytoin (*Mesantoin*) has been reported not to interact with amiodarone.

MANAGEMENT OPTIONS:

➡ *Monitor.* Patients being treated with phenytoin should have their phenytoin serum concentrations monitored carefully when amiodarone is added to or removed from their drug regimen. This drug interaction may take several weeks to become fully apparent. In addition, monitor patients taking amiodarone for reduced anti-arrhythmic efficacy, and monitor amiodarone serum concentrations if phenytoin is added to their drug regimen.

REFERENCES:

Gore JM, et al. Interaction of amiodarone and diphenylhydantoin. *Am J Cardiol.* 1984;54:1145.

MacGovern B, et al. Possible interaction between amiodarone and phenytoin. *Ann Intern Med.* 1984;101:650.

Shackleford EJ, et al. Amiodarone-phenytoin interaction. *Drug Intell Clin Pharm.* 1987;21:921.

Nolan PE Jr., et al. Pharmacokinetic interaction between intravenous phenytoin and amiodarone in healthy volunteers. *Clin Pharmacol Ther.* 1989;46:43.

Nolan PE, et al. Evidence for an effect of phenytoin on the pharmacokinetics of amiodarone. *J Clin Pharmacol.* 1990;30:1112.

Nolan PE, et al. Steady-state interaction between amiodarone and phenytoin in normal subjects. *Am J Cardiol.* 1990;65:1252.

Amiodarone (eg, *Cordarone*)

Procainamide (eg, *Procan SR*)

SUMMARY: Amiodarone increases procainamide concentrations and may enhance toxicity.

RISK FACTORS: No specific risk factors known.

RELATED DRUGS: No information is available.

MANAGEMENT OPTIONS:

➡ *Circumvent/Minimize.* Procainamide dosages may need to be reduced by 25% to avoid toxicity.

➡ *Monitor.* Monitor procainamide concentrations and the patient observed for hypotension or arrhythmias when amiodarone is added to therapy.

REFERENCES:

Windle J, et al. Pharmacokinetic and electrophysiologic interaction of amiodarone and procainamide. *Clin Pharmacol Ther.* 1987;41:603.

Saal AK, et al. Effect of amiodarone on serum quinidine and procainamide levels. *Am J Cardiol.* 1984;53:1264.

Amiodarone (eg, *Cordarone*)

Quinidine (eg, *Quinora*)

SUMMARY: Amiodarone increases quinidine plasma concentrations, and the combination can excessively prolong cardiac conduction.

RISK FACTORS: No specific risk factors are known.

RELATED DRUGS: No information is available.

MANAGEMENT OPTIONS:

➡ *Monitor.* When amiodarone is added to quinidine therapy, monitor the cardiac status (eg, QT interval prolongation) and plasma quinidine concentrations.

REFERENCES:

Tartini R, et al. Dangerous interaction between amiodarone and quinidine. *Lancet.* 1982;1:1327.

Saal AK, et al. Effect of amiodarone on serum quinidine and procainamide levels. *Am J Cardiol.* 1984;53:1264.

Kerin NZ, et al. The effectiveness and safety of the simultaneous administration of quinidine and amiodarone in the conversion of chronic atrial fibrillation. *Am Heart J.* 1993;125:1017.

Amiodarone (eg, *Cordarone*)

Rifampin (eg, *Rifadin*)

SUMMARY: Rifampin reduces amiodarone plasma concentrations; a reduction or loss of therapeutic efficacy may result.

RISK FACTORS: No specific risk factors are known.

RELATED DRUGS: Rifabutin (*Mycobutin*) may affect amiodarone in a similar manner.

MANAGEMENT OPTIONS:

➡ *Consider Alternative.* An alternative antiarrhythmic agent could be considered for patients receiving rifampin. However, rifampin is known to induce the metabolism of quinidine (eg, *Quinora*), disopyramide (eg, *Norpace*), propafenone (*Rythmol*), and verapamil (eg, *Isoptin*).

➡ *Monitor.* Monitor amiodarone and DEA concentrations in patients receiving concurrent rifampin or rifabutin.

REFERENCES:

Zarembski DG, et al. Impact of rifampin on serum amiodarone concentrations in a patient with congenital heart disease. *Pharmacotherapy.* 1999;19:249-51.

Amiodarone (eg, *Cordarone*)

Sotalol (*Betapace*)

SUMMARY: A patient given amiodarone following chronic sotalol therapy developed hypotension and bradycardia, but a causal relationship for an interaction between the drugs was not established.

RISK FACTORS: No specific risk factors are known.

RELATED DRUGS: Beta blockers, including metoprolol (eg, *Lopressor*) and propranolol (eg, *Inderal*), have been noted to produce bradycardia when administered with amiodarone.

MANAGEMENT OPTIONS:

➡ *Circumvent/Minimize.* It may be prudent to avoid the administration of amiodarone for several days to patients previously receiving drugs that depress myocardial conduction and contractility.

➡ *Monitor.* Until further information is available, carefully monitor patients receiving sotalol (and perhaps other beta blockers) and amiodarone for hemodynamic depression.

REFERENCES:

Warren R, et al. Serious interaction of sotalol with amiodarone and flecainide. *Med J Aust.* 1990;152:227.

Amiodarone (eg, *Cordarone*)
Theophylline (eg, *Slo-Phyllin*)

SUMMARY: Amiodarone may increase the concentration of theophylline, resulting in toxicity.

RISK FACTORS: No specific risk factors are known.

RELATED DRUGS: No information is available.

MANAGEMENT OPTIONS:

➡ *Monitor.* Carefully observe patients maintained on theophylline for the development of theophylline toxicity (eg, nausea, tachycardia, nervousness, tremor, seizures) following the addition of amiodarone. One or more weeks may be required for the onset and offset of this interaction because of the long half-life of amiodarone.

REFERENCES:

Soto J, et al. Possible theophylline-amiodarone interaction. *DICP.* 1990;24:1115.

Amiodarone (eg, *Cordarone*)
Thioridazine (eg, *Mellaril*) AVOID

SUMMARY: Amiodarone may increase thioridazine serum concentrations and produce additive prolongation of the QT interval, thus increasing the risk of ventricular arrhythmias; avoid concurrent use.

RISK FACTORS:

➡ *Pharmacogenetics.* Only patients with the extensive metabolizer CYP2D6 phenotype (EMs) would be expected to experience increased thioridazine serum concentrations. Poor metabolizers (PMs) do not have the gene for production of CYP2D6, and would likely already have high serum concentrations of thioridazine. Approximately 8% of whites are deficient in CYP2D6, but the deficiency is rare in Asians—usually 1% or less.

➡ *Hypokalemia.* The corrected QT interval (QTc) may be prolonged in patients with hypokalemia, thus increasing the risk of this interaction. Any other factor that may prolong the QTc interval would also increase the risk of this interaction.

RELATED DRUGS: Other antiarrhythmics such as disopyramide (eg, *Norpace*), procain-amide (eg, *Procan SR*), and quinidine can also increase the QT interval, and may increase the risk of arrhythmias. Also, propafenone (*Rythmol*) and quinidine are known inhibitors of CYP2D6, and may increase thioridazine serum concentrations. Although a number of antipsychotic drugs have, like thioridazine, been shown to prolong the QT interval, clinical evidence suggests that thioridazine may produce the greatest risk.

MANAGEMENT OPTIONS:

➡ *AVOID COMBINATION.* Although the risk of this combination is not well established, it would be prudent to avoid concurrent use.

REFERENCES:

Hartigan-Go K, et al. Concentration-related pharmacodynamic effects of thioridazine and its metabolites in humans. *Clin Pharmacol Ther.* 1996;60:543-53.

'Dear Doctor or Pharmacist' Letter, Novartis Pharmaceuticals, July 7, 2000.

Amiodarone (eg, *Cordarone*)

Warfarin (eg, *Coumadin*)

SUMMARY: Amiodarone enhances the hypoprothrombinemic response to warfarin.

RISK FACTORS: No specific risk factors are known.

RELATED DRUGS: Acenocoumarol interacts in a similar manner with amiodarone.

MANAGEMENT OPTIONS:

➡ *Circumvent/Minimize.* A decrease in the warfarin dose by 33% to 50% may be necessary to maintain the INR within the therapeutic range.

➡ *Monitor.* When amiodarone is administered to patients requiring oral anticoagulant therapy, carefully monitor the hypoprothrombinemic response. Because the onset and offset of this interaction is delayed, continue to closely monitor for a month or two following the initiation or discontinuation of amiodarone.

REFERENCES:

Hamer A, et al. The potentiation of warfarin anticoagulation by amiodarone. *Circulation.* 1982;65:1025-1029.

Fondevila C, et al. Amiodarone potentiates acenocoumarin. *Thromb Res Suppl.* 1989;53:203-208.

Sanoski CA, et al. Clinical observations with the amiodarone/warfarin interaction: dosing relationships with long-term therapy. *Chest.* 2002;121:19-23.

O'Reilly RA, et al. Interaction of amiodarone with racemic warfarin and its separated enantiomorphs in humans. *Clin Pharmacol Ther.* 1987;42:290-294.

Kerin NZ, et al. The incidence, magnitude, and time course of the amiodarone-warfarin interaction. *Arch Intern Med.* 1988;148:1779-1781.

Amitriptyline (eg, *Elavil*)

Bethanidine

SUMMARY: Amitriptyline and other tricyclic antidepressants (TCAs) inhibit the antihypertensive effect of bethanidine.

RISK FACTORS: No specific risk factors are known.

RELATED DRUGS: Desipramine and imipramine have been shown to reduce bethanidine's antihypertensive effect. Assume that all TCAs inhibit bethanidine effect until proven otherwise. TCAs also may inhibit the antihypertensive effect of clonidine (*Catapres*), guanabenz (*Wytensin*), guanethidine (*Ismelin*), guanfacine (*Tenex*), guanadrel (*Hylorel*), and debrisoquin. The effect of selective serotonin reuptake inhibitors on bethanidine is not established.

MANAGEMENT OPTIONS:

➡ *Use Alternative.* Avoid combined therapy with TCAs and bethanidine. Doxepin might be less likely to interact than other TCAs. If tricyclics are to be used, consider selecting an alternative antihypertensive agent. But, keep in mind that TCAs also may inhibit the effect of clonidine, guanabenz, guanfacine, guanethidine, and debrisoquin.

REFERENCES:

Oates JA, et al. Effect of doxepin on the norepinephrine pump. A preliminary report. *Psychosomatics.* 1969;10:12.

Mitchell JR, et al. Antagonism of the antihypertensive action of guanethidine sulfate by desipramine hydrochloride. *JAMA.* 1967;202:973.

Feagin OT, et al. Uptake and release of guanethidine and bethanidine by the adrenergic neuron. *J Clin Invest.* 1969;48:23a.

Mitchell JR, et al. Guanethidine and related agents. III. Antagonism by drugs which inhibit the norepinephrine pump in man. *J Clin Invest.* 1970;49:1596.

Skinner C, et al. Antagonism of the hypotensive action of bethanidine and debrisoquine by tricyclic antidepressants. *Lancet.* 1969;2:564.

Amitriptyline (eg, *Elavil*)

Ethanol (Ethyl Alcohol)

SUMMARY: Combined use of ethanol and tricyclic antidepressants (TCAs), such as amitriptyline, may result in additive impairment of motor skills; abstinent alcoholics may eliminate TCAs more rapidly than nonalcoholics.

RISK FACTORS: No specific risk factors are known.

RELATED DRUGS: Doxepin (eg, *Sinequan*) adds to the deleterious effect of ethanol on motor skills. However, the evidence for doxepin is conflicting; some evidence suggests that it is less likely to interact. Trazodone also produced additive impairment of manual dexterity in the presence of alcohol. Nortriptyline (eg, *Pamelor*) and clomipramine (eg, *Anafranil*) are less sedating than amitriptyline, which may account for reports that they are less likely to enhance the adverse effects of ethanol on psychomotor skills. Imipramine and desipramine elimination is increased in detoxified alcoholics.

MANAGEMENT OPTIONS:

➡ *Circumvent/Minimize.* Inform patients receiving tricyclic or related antidepressants that ethanol may produce a greater-than-expected impairment in psychomotor skills, especially during the first week of treatment. This warning probably is more important for the more sedative tricyclics, such as amitriptyline and, possibly, doxepin.

➥ **Monitor.** In abstinent alcoholics, monitor for an inadequate antidepressant effect and adjust the antidepressant dosage as needed. Measurement of antidepressant serum concentrations may be useful in selected cases.

REFERENCES:

Lockett MF, et al. Combining the antidepressant drugs. *BMJ.* 1965;1:921.

Laurie W. Alcohol as a cause of sudden unexpected death. *Med J Aust.* 1971;1:1224-1227.

Dorian P, et al. Amitriptyline and ethanol: pharmacokinetic and pharmacodynamic interaction. *Eur J Clin Pharmacol.* 1983;25:325-331.

Ciraulo DA, et al. Clinical pharmacokinetics of imipramine and desipramine in alcoholics and normal volunteers. *Clin Pharmacol Ther.* 1988;43:509-518.

Sandoz M, et al. Biotransformation of amitriptyline in alcoholic depressive patients. *Eur J Clin Pharmacol.* 1983;24:615-621.

Hall RC, et al. The effect of desmethylimipramine on the absorption of alcohol and paracetamol. *Postgrad Med J.* 1976;52:139-142.

Landauer AA, et al. Alcohol and amitriptyline effects on skills related to driving behavior. *Science.* 1969;163:1467-1468.

Seppala T, et al. Effect of tricyclic antidepressants and alcohol on psychomotor skills related to driving. *Clin Pharmacol Ther.* 1975;17:515-522.

Seppala T. Psychomotor skills during acute and two-week treatment with mianserin (ORG GB 94) and amitriptyline, and their combined effects with alcohol. *Ann Clin Res.* 1977;9:66-72.

Warrington SJ, et al. Evaluation of possible interactions between ethanol and trazodone or amitriptyline. *Neuropsychobiology.* 1986;15(Suppl 1):31-37.

Milner G. Gastrointestinal side effects and psychotropic drugs. *Med J Aust.* 1969;2:153-155. Review.

Milner G, et al. The effects of doxepin, alone and together with alcohol, in relation to driving safety. *Med J Aust.* 1973;1:837-841.

Amitriptyline (eg, *Elavil*)

Fluconazole (*Diflucan*)

SUMMARY: Fluconazole repeatedly resulted in syncope in a boy receiving amitriptyline, but it is not known how often this combination would result in adverse effects.

RISK FACTORS: No specific risk factors are known.

RELATED DRUGS: Other tricyclic antidepressants are metabolized by CYP2C19 or CYP3A4; theoretically, these may interact with fluconazole, but little clinical information is available.

MANAGEMENT OPTIONS:

➥ **Monitor.** Monitor for altered amitriptyline effect if fluconazole is initiated, discontinued, or changed in dosage.

REFERENCES:

Robinson RF, et al. Syncope associated with concurrent amitriptyline and fluconazole therapy. *Ann Pharmacother.* 2000;34:1406-1409.

Amitriptyline (eg, *Elavil*)

Fluoxetine (eg, *Prozac*)

SUMMARY: Fluoxetine increases amitriptyline serum concentrations and markedly increases the serum concentrations of its active metabolite, nortriptyline. The death of a man was attributed to fluoxetine-induced amitriptyline toxicity, but a causal relationship was not established.

RISK FACTORS: No specific risk factors are known.

RELATED DRUGS: Because fluoxetine-induced inhibition of CYP2D6 is the likely mechanism, one would expect paroxetine (*Paxil*), which is also a potent CYP2D6 inhibitor, to interact with amitriptyline in a similar manner. Sertraline (*Zoloft*) is only a weak CYP2D6 inhibitor and would theoretically be less likely to interact. Fluvoxamine (eg, *Luvox*) has little or no effect on CYP2D6, but its ability to inhibit other cytochrome P450 isozymes might affect the metabolism of tricyclic antidepressants.

MANAGEMENT OPTIONS:

➡ *Monitor.* Although combinations of tricyclic antidepressants and selective serotonin reuptake inhibitors are frequently used with positive results, the patient's response to the tricyclic antidepressant must be carefully monitored if a selective serotonin reuptake inhibitor is initiated, discontinued, or changed in dosage.

REFERENCES:

el-Yazigi A, et al. Steady-state kinetics of fluoxetine and amitriptyline in patients treated with a combination of these drugs as compared with those treated with amitriptyline alone. *J Clin Pharmacol.* 1995;35:17-21.

Preskorn SH, et al. Fatality associated with combined fluoxetine-amitriptyline therapy. *JAMA.* 1997;277:1682.

Amitriptyline (eg, *Elavil*)

Guanfacine (eg, *Tenex*)

SUMMARY: Limited clinical information and theoretical considerations suggest that tricyclic antidepressants (TCAs) can inhibit the antihypertensive response to guanfacine.

RISK FACTORS: No specific risk factors are known.

RELATED DRUGS: Theoretically, any combination of a TCA and a centrally acting alpha agonist (eg, clonidine [eg, *Catapres*], guanabenz [eg, *Wytensin*]) would interact.

MANAGEMENT OPTIONS:

➡ *Consider Alternative.* If tricyclics are to be used, consider selecting an alternative antihypertensive agent. But, keep in mind that TCAs also may inhibit the effect of clonidine, guanabenz, guanethidine, bethanidine, and debrisoquin.

➥ **Monitor.** Until more clinical evidence is available, monitor for reduced antihypertensive response when TCAs are added to guanfacine therapy. If guanfacine is withdrawn in the presence of TCAs, monitor for exaggerated rebound hypertension.

REFERENCES:

Buckley M, et al. Antagonism of antihypertensive effect of guanfacine by tricyclic antidepressants. *Lancet.* 1991;337:1173-1174.

 Amitriptyline (*Elavil*)

Isoproterenol (*Isuprel*)

SUMMARY: Isolated case reports indicate that the combined use of isoproterenol and tricyclic antidepressants (TCAs) may predispose patients to cardiac arrhythmias, but the clinical importance of this interaction is not established.

RISK FACTORS:

➥ **Dosage Regimen.** It is possible that the risk is primarily in patients who take large doses of isoproterenol.

RELATED DRUGS: Little is known regarding the effect of beta agonists other than isoproterenol (eg, albuterol [eg, *Proventil*], metaproterenol [*Alupent*], terbutaline [eg, *Brethaire*]) in patients receiving TCAs. To the extent that these agents have less cardiac effects than isoproterenol, one would expect a reduced likelihood of cardiac interactions with TCAs.

MANAGEMENT OPTIONS:

➥ **Circumvent/Minimize.** Avoid excessive use of isoproterenol or other beta-agonists in any case, but it may be particularly important in patients receiving TCAs.

➥ **Monitor.** Although this interaction is not well documented, it would be prudent to monitor for cardiac arrhythmias if isoproterenol or other beta-agonists (especially in large doses) are used with TCAs.

REFERENCES:

Kadar D. Amitriptyline and isoproterenol: fatal drug combinations. *Can Med Assoc J.* 1975;112:556.

Boakes AJ, et al. Interactions between sympathomimetic amines and antidepressant agents in man. *BMJ.* 1973;1:311.

Amitriptyline (*Elavil*)

Lithium (eg, *Eskalith*)

SUMMARY: Although lithium and tricyclic antidepressants (TCAs) are frequently used together with good results, there is some evidence that their concurrent use may increase the risk for neurotoxicity (eg, tremors, ataxia, seizures), particularly in the elderly.

RISK FACTORS:

➥ **Effects of Age.** Elderly patients may be at higher risk.

RELATED DRUGS: TCAs other than amitriptyline probably have a similar effect when combined with lithium.

MANAGEMENT OPTIONS:

➥ *Circumvent/Minimize.* Limited information suggests that using low doses of lithium may reduce the risk of neurotoxicity in geriatric patients without compromising its therapeutic effect.

➥ *Monitor.* Until further information is available, cautiously use lithium and TCAs in elderly patients. Monitor for evidence of neurotoxicity such as tremors, disorders of mentation, ataxia, and seizures.

REFERENCES:

Price LH, et al. Variability of response to lithium augmentation in refractory depression. *Am J Psychiatry.* 1986;143:1387.

Feder R. Lithium augmentation of clomipramine. *J Clin Psychiatry.* 1988;49:11.

Camara EG. Lithium potentiation of antidepressant treatment in panic disorder. *J Clin Psychopharmacol.* 1990;10:225.

Austin LS, et al. Toxicity resulting from lithium augmentation of antidepressant treatment in elderly patients. *J Clin Psychiatry.* 1990;51:344.

Lafferman J, et al. Lithium augmentation for treatment-resistant depression in the elderly. *J Geriatric Psychiatry Neurol.* 1988;1:49.

Solomon JG. Seizures during lithium-amitriptyline therapy. *Postgrad Med.* 1979;66:145.

Kushnir SL. Lithium: antidepressant combinations in the treatment of depressed, physically ill geriatric patients. *Am J Psychiatry.* 1986;143:378.

Amitriptyline (eg, *Elavil*)

Propantheline (eg, *Pro-Banthine*)

SUMMARY: Combined use of anticholinergic tricyclic antidepressants (TCAs) such as amitriptyline and anticholinergics such as propantheline may result in excessive anticholinergic effects.

RISK FACTORS:

➥ *Effects of Age.* The elderly possibly are at greater risk.

RELATED DRUGS: Additive anticholinergic effects are more likely to be associated with TCAs possessing significant anticholinergic activity (eg, amitriptyline, nortriptyline [*Pamelor*], imipramine [*Tofranil*], trimipramine [*Surmontil*], doxepin [*Sinequan*], and maprotiline [*Ludiomil*]). Antidepressants with modest anticholinergic effects (eg, trazodone [*Desyrel*], protriptyline [*Vivactil*], desipramine [*Norpramin*], and amoxapine [*Asendin*]) are less likely to interact. Nevertheless, 1 patient receiving an anticholinergic (isopropamide iodide) developed acute urinary retention on 2 occasions when trazodone was taken. A number of other drugs (eg, antihistamines, neuroleptics, disopyramide [*Norpace*], antiparkinsonian drugs, glutethimide, and meperidine [*Demerol*]) possess anticholinergic activity.

MANAGEMENT OPTIONS:

➥ *Consider Alternative.* If additive anticholinergic effects become troublesome, consider use of an antidepressant with low anticholinergic activity. Also, an alternative drug often can be found for the agent that is adding to the anticholinergic effect of the TCA.

➥ *Circumvent/Minimize.* A method has been described by which drug-induced dry mouth may be treated with a pilocarpine syrup. Pyridoxine may prevent some of the anticholinergic side effects of TCAs.

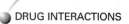
➡ *Monitor.* Serious complications are unlikely to occur if alert to the possibility of excessive anticholinergic activity.

REFERENCES:

Kessell A, et al. Side effects with a new hypnotic: drug potentiation. *Med J Aust.* 1967;2:1194.

Milner G. Gastro-intestinal side effects and psychotropic drugs. *Med J Aust.* 1969;2:153-155.

Blazer DG, et al. The risk of anticholinergic toxicity in the elderly: a study of prescribing practices in two populations. *J Gerontol.* 1983;38:31-35.

Chan CH, et al. Anticholinergic side effects of trazodone combined with another pharmacologic agent. *Am J Psychiatry.* 1990;147:533.

Ayd FJ. Rx tip: relieving drug-induced oral and pharyngeal dryness. *Int Drug Ther Newsl.* 1967;2:24.

Arnold SE, et al. Tricyclic antidepressant and peripheral anticholinergic activity. *Psychopharmacology.* 1981;74:325-328.

 Amlodipine (*Norvasc*)

Diltiazem (eg, *Cardizem*)

SUMMARY: Diltiazem administration resulted in an increase in amlodipine plasma concentrations and hypotensive effect.

RISK FACTORS: No specific risk factors are known.

RELATED DRUGS: Diltiazem has been noted to increase the plasma concentration of immediate-release nifedipine (eg, *Procardia*) and enhance the hypotensive effects of other calcium channel blockers.

MANAGEMENT OPTIONS:

➡ *Monitor.* If diltiazem and amlodipine are coadministered, monitor for enhanced hypotensive effects.

REFERENCES:

Sasaki M, et al. Influence of diltiazem on the pharmacokinetics of amlodipine in elderly hypertensive patients. *Eur J Clin Pharmacol.* 2001;57:85.

 Ammonium Chloride

Spironolactone (*Aldactone*)

SUMMARY: Spironolactone may produce systemic acidosis when administered with ammonium chloride.

RISK FACTORS: No specific risk factors are known.

RELATED DRUGS: The effect of potassium-sparing diuretics other than spironolactone on ammonium chloride is not established.

MANAGEMENT OPTIONS:

➡ *Monitor.* Monitor for acidosis if spironolactone is used with acidifying doses of ammonium chloride.

REFERENCES:

Mashford ML, et al. Spironolactone and ammonium and potassium chloride. *BMJ.* 1972;4:299.

Manuel MA, et al. An effect of spironolactone on urinary acidification in normal man. *Arch Intern Med.* 1974;134:472.

Amobarbital (*Amytal*)

Tranylcypromine (*Parnate*)

SUMMARY: Limited clinical evidence suggests that tranylcypromine may prolong the effect of amobarbital, but little is known about other combinations of nonselective monoamine oxidase inhibitors (MAOIs) and barbiturates.

RISK FACTORS: No specific risk factors are known.

RELATED DRUGS: Little is known about possible effects of other nonselective MAOIs such as isocarboxazid (*Marplan*) and phenelzine (*Nardil*) on barbiturates, but consider the possibility that the barbiturate effect may be increased.

MANAGEMENT OPTIONS:

➥ *Monitor.* Until more is known about this interaction, monitor for increased barbiturate effect if nonselective MAOIs are given concurrently.

REFERENCES:

Domino EF, et al. Barbiturate intoxication in patient treated with a MAO inhibitor. *Am J Psychiatry*. 1962;118:941.

Sjoqvist F. Psychotropic drugs (2). Interaction between monoamine oxidase (MAO) inhibitors and other substances. *Proc R Soc Med*. 1965;58:967.

Amphotericin B (*Fungizone*)

Cyclosporine (eg, *Sandimmune*)

SUMMARY: The administration of amphotericin B and cyclosporine probably increases the nephrotoxicity of both drugs.

RISK FACTORS: No specific risk factors are known.

RELATED DRUGS: No information is available.

MANAGEMENT OPTIONS:

➥ *Circumvent/Minimize.* Alternative immunosuppression or antifungal therapy may be required to avoid or reverse renal toxicity.

➥ *Monitor.* Patients receiving both cyclosporine and amphotericin B should have their renal function monitored carefully.

REFERENCES:

Kennedy MS, et al. Acute renal toxicity with combined use of amphotericin B and cyclosporine after marrow transplantation. *Transplantation*. 1983;35:211.

Amphotericin B (*Fungizone*)

Digoxin (eg, *Lanoxin*)

SUMMARY: Digitalis toxicity may be enhanced by amphotericin B-induced hypokalemia.

RISK FACTORS:

➥ *Concurrent Diseases.* Diseases or drugs that cause hypokalemia may increase the risk of digitalis toxicity.

RELATED DRUGS: Digitoxin (*Crystodigin*) also will be affected by amphotericin B-induced hypokalemia.

MANAGEMENT OPTIONS:

➡ *Monitor.* Closely follow the potassium status of patients on digitalis who receive amphotericin B therapy. Promptly treat any potassium deficit that develops.

REFERENCES:

    Miller RP, et al. Amphotericin B toxicity. A follow-up report of 53 patients. *Ann Intern Med.* 1969;71:1089.

    Cushard WG, et al. Blastomycosis of bone. Treatment with intramedullary amphotericin B. *J Bone Joint Surg.* 1969;51A:704.

Amphotericin B (*Fungizone*)

Gentamicin (*Garamycin*)

SUMMARY: The combination of aminoglycosides and amphotericin B may enhance the potential for nephrotoxicity.

RISK FACTORS:

➡ *Concurrent Diseases.* Renal dysfunction may increase the risk of nephrotoxicity.

RELATED DRUGS: Other aminoglycosides may produce nephrotoxicity with amphotericin.

MANAGEMENT OPTIONS:

➡ *Consider Alternative.* The use of an alternative antibiotic or antifungal agent without nephrotoxicity would be prudent.

➡ *Monitor.* Closely monitor patients on combined therapy with an aminoglycoside and amphotericin B for deterioration of renal function.

REFERENCES:

    Churchill DN, et al. Nephrotoxicity associated with combined gentamicin-amphotericin B therapy. *Nephron.* 1977;19:176.

Amphotericin B (*Fungizone*)

Succinylcholine (eg, *Anectine*)

SUMMARY: Prolonged muscle relaxation may accompany the use of amphotericin B and neuromuscular blocking agents.

RISK FACTORS: No specific risk factors are known.

RELATED DRUGS: Other drugs causing hypokalemia may cause a similar reaction with muscle relaxants like atracurium and vecuronium.

MANAGEMENT OPTIONS:

➡ *Monitor.* Carefully check the potassium balance of patients on amphotericin B before use of neuromuscular blocking agents.

REFERENCES:

    Miller RP, et al. Amphotericin B toxicity. A follow-up report of 53 patients. *Ann Intern Med.* 1969;71:1089.

    Cushard WG, et al. Blastomycosis of bone. Treatment with intramedullary amphotericin B. *J Bone Joint Surg.* 1969;51A:704.

Ampicillin (eg, *Principen*)

Atenolol (*Tenormin*)

SUMMARY: Ampicillin may reduce atenolol serum concentrations and a reduction of beta blocker effect is possible.

RISK FACTORS:

➥ *Dosage Regimen.* Ampicillin doses more than 1 g appear to decrease the bioavailability of atenolol.

RELATED DRUGS: No information is available.

MANAGEMENT OPTIONS:

➥ *Monitor.* Until more data are available, watch for evidence of altered atenolol response when large doses of ampicillin are coadministered.

REFERENCES:

McLean AJ, et al. Dose-dependence of atenolol-ampicillin interaction. *Br J Clin Pharmacol.* 1984;18:969.

Schafer-Korting M, et al. Atenolol interaction with aspirin, allopurinol, and ampicillin. *Clin Pharmacol Ther.* 1983;33:283.

Ampicillin (eg, *Principen*)

Contraceptives, Oral

SUMMARY: Ampicillin probably impairs oral contraceptive efficacy occasionally.

RISK FACTORS: No specific risk factors are known.

RELATED DRUGS: The effect of other penicillins on oral contraceptives is not well established; however, reports of contraceptive failure have been noted with the concomitant use of a variety of antibiotics.

MANAGEMENT OPTIONS:

➥ *Circumvent/Minimize.* Since ampicillin often is given in relatively short courses, it may be best for patients to continue their oral contraceptive and use supplementary contraception during cycles in which ampicillin is used.

➥ *Monitor.* Tell patients that spotting or breakthrough bleeding may be an indication that an interaction between ampicillin and an oral contraceptive is occurring.

REFERENCES:

Boehm FH, et al. The effect of ampicillin administration on urinary estriol and serum estradiol in the normal pregnant patient. *Am J Obstet Gynecol.* 1974;119:98.

Sybulski S, et al. Effect of ampicillin administration on estradiol, estriol, and cortisol levels in maternal plasma and on estriol levels in urine. *Am J Obstet Gynecol.* 1976;124:379.

Adlercreutz H, et al. Effect of ampicillin administration on plasma conjugated and unconjugated estrogen and progesterone levels in pregnancy. *Am J Obstet Gynecol.* 1977;128:266.

Friedman CI, et al. The effect of ampicillin on oral contraceptive effectiveness. *Obstet Gynecol.* 1980;55:33.

DeSano EA, et al. Possible interactions of antihistamines and antibiotics with oral contraceptive effectiveness. *Fertil Steril.* 1982;37:853.

Back DJ, et al. The effects of ampicillin on oral contraceptive steroids in women. *Br J Clin Pharmacol.* 1982;14:43.

Amprenavir (*Agenerase*)

Delavirdine (*Rescriptor*)

SUMMARY: Chronic dosing of delavirdine increases amprenavir concentrations while chronic amprenavir administration decreases delavirdine plasma concentrations. Careful monitoring of patients on the combination of these drugs is necessary.

RISK FACTORS: No specific risk factors are known.

RELATED DRUGS: Delavirdine may reduce the clearance, and thus increase the plasma concentration, of other antiretroviral drugs metabolized by CYP3A4. The chronic administration of amprenavir may reduce the concentration of other antiretrovirals metabolized by CYP3A4.

MANAGEMENT OPTIONS:

➡ *Monitor.* Monitor plasma concentrations, antiviral response, and drug toxicity when combinations of antiretroviral drugs are administered or when one drug is discontinued from a combination regimen. The apparent mixed effect on CYP3A4 activity demonstrated by amprenavir will produce different effects on object drugs that will depend on the duration of amprenavir administration.

REFERENCES:

Tran JQ, et al. Pharmacokinetic interaction between amprenavir and delavirdine: evidence of induced clearance by amprenavir. *Clin Pharmacol Ther.* 2002;72:615-626.

Antacids

Aspirin

SUMMARY: Some antacids can decrease serum salicylate concentrations in patients receiving large doses of salicylates; in some patients, this effect may be sufficient to require salicylate dosage adjustments.

RISK FACTORS:

➡ *Dosage Regimen.* The lowering of serum salicylate concentrations by antacids is likely to occur only in patients receiving large doses of salicylate (eg, several grams per day), since it is only with such doses that the renal excretion of unchanged salicylic acid is an important elimination pathway.

RELATED DRUGS: Salicylates other than aspirin also would be affected by increases in urine pH.

MANAGEMENT OPTIONS:

➡ *Monitor.* In patients receiving large doses of salicylates (eg, for arthritis), be alert for alteration in serum salicylate concentrations if antacids are initiated, discontinued, or changed in dosage. Adjustments in salicylate dosage may be required in some cases.

REFERENCES:

Feldman S, et al. Effect of antacid on absorption of enteric-coated aspirin. *JAMA.* 1974;227:660.

Levy G, et al. Decreased serum salicylate concentrations in children with rheumatic fever treated with antacid. *N Engl J Med.* 1975;293:323.

Hansten PD, et al. Effect of antacids and ascorbic acid on serum salicylate concentration. *J Clin Pharmacol.* 1980;24:326.

Strickland-Hodge B, et al. The effects of antacids on enteric coated salicylate preparations. *Rheumatol Rehab*. 1976;15:148.

Shastri RA. Effect of antacids on salicylate kinetics. *Int J Clin Pharmacol Ther Toxicol*. 1985;23:480.

Kaniwa N, et al. The bioavailabilities of aspirin from an aspirin aluminum and aspirin tablets and the effects of food and aluminum hydroxide gel. *J Pharm Dyn*. 1981;4:860.

Nayak RK, et al. Effect of antacids on aspirin dissolution and bioavailability. *J Pharmacokinet Biopharm*. 1977;5:597.

Gibaldi M, et al. Effect of antacids on pH of urine. *Clin Pharmacol Ther*. 1974;16:520.

Gibaldi M, et al. Time course and dose dependency of antacid effect on urine pH. *J Pharmaceut Sci*. 1975;64:2003.

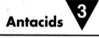

Antacids

Atenolol (*Tenormin*)

SUMMARY: The GI absorption of atenolol may be reduced by coadministration of aluminum or magnesium antacids, but the clinical importance is not established.

RISK FACTORS: No specific risk factors are known.

RELATED DRUGS: Other beta-adrenergic blockers also may be affected by antacids.

MANAGEMENT OPTIONS:

➥ *Circumvent/Minimize.* Take atenolol at least 2 hours before or 6 hours after the antacid, and try to maintain a relatively constant interval and sequence of administration of the two drugs.

➥ *Monitor.* Monitor for altered atenolol effect if antacid therapy is initiated, discontinued, or changed in dosage; adjust atenolol dose as needed.

REFERENCES:

Regardh CG, et al. The effect of antacid, metoclopramide, and propantheline on the bioavailability of metoprolol and atenolol. *Biopharm Drug Dispos*. 1981;2:79.

Kirch W, et al. Interaction of atenolol with furosemide and calcium and aluminum salts. *Clin Pharmacol Ther*. 1981;30:429.

Antacids

Atevirdine

SUMMARY: Atevirdine administration contiguous with antacid dosing reduces atevirdine concentrations; reduced antiviral efficacy could result.

RISK FACTORS: No specific risk factors are known.

RELATED DRUGS: The effect of other antacids on atevirdine is unknown, but consider all antacids to interact until more information is available.

MANAGEMENT OPTIONS:

➥ *Circumvent/Minimize.* Avoid the administration of atevirdine and antacids. Until more information is available, separate doses of atevirdine and antacids by 2 to 3 hours.

➡ **Monitor.** If patients receiving atevirdine are administered antacids, monitor for reduced antiviral effects.

REFERENCES:

Borin MT, et al. Effects of food and antacid on bioavailability of atevirdine mesylate (ATV) in HIV+ patients. *Clin Pharmacol Ther.* 1994;55:194.

Antacids

Cefpodoxime Proxetil (*Vantin*)

SUMMARY: Antacids reduce the bioavailability and serum concentrations of cefpodoxime proxetil and could reduce the efficacy of the antibiotic.

RISK FACTORS: No specific risk factors are known.

RELATED DRUGS: Theoretically, any drug that substantially increases gastric pH also would reduce cefpodoxime absorption. This would include H_2-receptor antagonists (eg, cimetidine [eg, *Tagamet*], famotidine [eg, *Pepcid*], nizatidine [*Axid*], ranitidine [*Zantac*]), proton pump inhibitors (eg, omeprazole [*Prilosec*], lansoprazole [*Prevacid*]) and other antacids.

MANAGEMENT OPTIONS:

➡ **Circumvent/Minimize.** Advise patients taking cefpodoxime to take the antibiotic between meals, preferably on an empty stomach. Do not administer antacids for at least 2 hours before or after administration of cefpodoxime.

➡ **Monitor.** Be alert for evidence of reduced cefpodoxime response if antacids are used concurrently.

REFERENCES:

Saathoff N, et al. Pharmacokinetics of cefpodoxime proxetil and interactions with an antacid and an H_2-receptor antagonist. *Antimicrob Agents Chemother.* 1992;36:796.

Hughes GS, et al. The effects of gastric pH and food on the pharmacokinetics of a new oral cephalosporin, cefpodoxime proxetil. *Clin Pharmacol Ther.* 1989;46:647.

Antacids

Ciprofloxacin (*Cipro*)

SUMMARY: Antacids reduce the serum concentration of ciprofloxacin and may inhibit its efficacy.

RISK FACTORS:

➡ **Dosage Regimen.** The effects of antacids on quinolone absorption appear to be greater when large antacid doses are administered.

➡ **Diet/Food.** Binding interactions in the GI tract tend to be greater in the fasting state than if there is food in the stomach.

RELATED DRUGS: The absorption of other quinolones is also reduced by antacids, but the absorption of lomefloxacin (*Maxaquin*) and ofloxacin (*Floxacin*) appears somewhat less affected by cations (eg, antacids) than ciprofloxacin. Since ranitidine (*Zantac*) does not appear to affect ciprofloxacin absorption,, one would assume that other H_2-receptor antagonists (eg, cimetidine [*Tagamet*], famotidine [*Pepcid*], nizatidine [*Axid*]) and proton pump inhibitors (eg, omeprazole [*Prilosec*], lansoprazole [*Pre-*

vacid]) also would have no effect. Sucralfate (*Carafate*) dramatically reduces ciprofloxacin absorption.

MANAGEMENT OPTIONS:

➥ *Consider Alternative.* Since it may be difficult to separate the doses of magnesium-aluminum-hydroxide antacids and ciprofloxacin sufficiently to prevent their interaction, consider using H_2-receptor antagonists or proton pump inhibitors.

➥ *Circumvent/Minimize.* If antacids are used with oral ciprofloxacin, give the ciprofloxacin at least 2 hours before or 6 hours after the antacid.

➥ *Monitor.* Monitor for reduced ciprofloxacin response if antacids are also taken.

REFERENCES:

Hoffken G, et al. Reduced enteral absorption of ciprofloxacin in the presence of antacids. *Eur J Clin Microbiol.* 1985;4:345.

Preheim LC, et al. Ciprofloxacin and antacids. *Lancet.* 1986;2:48.

Fleming LW, et al. Ciprofloxacin and antacids. *Lancet.* 1986:2:294.

Nix DE, et al. Effects of aluminum and magnesium antacids and ranitidine on the absorption of ciprofloxacin. *Clin Pharmacol Ther.* 1989;46:700.

Frost RW, et al. Effect of aluminum hydroxide and calcium carbonate antacids on ciprofloxacin bioavailability. *Clin Pharmacol Ther.* 1989;45:165.

Hoffken G, et al. Pharmacokinetics and bioavailability of ciprofloxacin and ofloxacin: effect of food and antacid intake. *Rev Infect Dis.* 1988;10:S138.

Frost RW, et al. Ciprofloxacin pharmacokinetics after a standard or high-fat/high-calcium breakfast. *J Clin Pharmacol.* 1989;29:953.

Yek JHJ, et al. Relative bioavailability in healthy volunteers of ciprofloxacin administration through a nasogastric tube with and without enteral feeding. *Antimicrob Agents Chemother.* 1989;22:1118.

Watson WA, et al. Effects of timing of Maalox administration and ranitidine on ciprofloxacin (*Cipro*) absorption. *Pharm Res.* 1988:5(Suppl):S164.

Brouwers JRBJ, et al. Important reduction of ciprofloxacin absorption by sucralfate and magnesium citrate solution. *Drug Invest.* 1990;2:197.

Navarro AS, et al. Comparative study of the influence of CA^{2+} on absorption parameters of ciprofloxacin and ofloxacin. *J Antimicrob Chemother.* 1994;34:119.

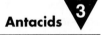

Antacids

Dextroamphetamine (eg, *Dextrostat*)

SUMMARY: Large sodium bicarbonate doses can inhibit the elimination and increase the effect of dextroamphetamine.

RISK FACTORS: No specific risk factors are known.

RELATED DRUGS: Any drug that substantially alkalinizes the urine (eg, carbonic anhydrase inhibitors) would be expected to inhibit amphetamine elimination. Some antacids other than sodium bicarbonate (eg, aluminum-, magnesium-, and calcium-containing antacids) may slightly alkalinize the urine, but their effect on dextroamphetamine excretion is probably not large. Sympathomimetic amines other than dextroamphetamine have been shown to demonstrate pH dependent urinary excretion.

MANAGEMENT OPTIONS:

➡ *Monitor.* Monitor for altered dextroamphetamine effect if sodium bicarbonate is initiated, discontinued or changed in dosage. Alteration in dextroamphetamine dose may be necessary.

REFERENCES:

Anggard E, et al. Amphetamine metabolism in amphetamine psychosis. *Clin Pharmacol Ther.* 1973;14:870.

Rowland M. Amphetamine blood and urine levels in man. *J Pharm Sci.* 1969;58:508.

Milne MD. Influence of acid-base balance on efficacy and toxicity of drugs. *Proc R Soc Med.* 1965;58:961.

 Antacids

Enoxacin (*Penetrex*)

SUMMARY: Antacids reduce the serum concentration of enoxacin and may inhibit its efficacy.

RISK FACTORS:

➡ *Dosage Regimen.* The effects of antacids on quinolone absorption appear to be greater when large antacid doses are administered.

➡ *Diet/Food.* Binding interactions in the GI tract tend to be greater in the fasting state than if there is food in the stomach.

RELATED DRUGS: The absorption of other quinolones also is reduced by antacids. Given the effect of ranitidine on enoxacin absorption, other H_2-receptor antagonists (eg, cimetidine [*Tagamet*], famotidine [*Pepcid*), nizatidine [*Axid*]) and proton pump inhibitors (eg, omeprazole [*Prilosec*], lansoprazole [*Prevacid*]) should be expected to reduce enoxacin absorption as well.

MANAGEMENT OPTIONS:

➡ *Circumvent/Minimize.* If antacids are used with oral enoxacin, give the enoxacin at least 2 hours before or 6 hours after the antacid.

➡ *Monitor.* Monitor for reduced enoxacin response if antacids are also taken.

REFERENCES:

Grasela TH, et al. Inhibition of enoxacin absorption by antacids or ranitidine. *Antimicrob Agents Chemother.* 1989;33:615.

Lebsack M, et al. Impact of gastric pH on ranitidine-enoxacin drugdrug interaction. *J Clin Pharmacol.* 1988;28:939.

 Antacids

Ephedrine

SUMMARY: Large doses of sodium bicarbonate may increase serum concentrations of ephedrine.

RISK FACTORS: No specific risk factors are known.

RELATED DRUGS: Any drug that substantially alkalinizes the urine (eg, carbonic anhydrase inhibitors) would be expected to inhibit ephedrine elimination. Some antacids other than sodium bicarbonate (eg, aluminum-, magnesium-, and calcium-containing antacids) may slightly alkalinize the urine, but their effect on ephedrine excretion is probably not large. Sympathomimetic amines other than ephedrine have been shown to demonstrate pH dependent urinary excretion.

MANAGEMENT OPTIONS:

➡ *Monitor.* Monitor for evidence of ephedrine toxicity (eg, nervousness, insomnia, excitability) if the urine remains alkaline for more than a day or two. Monitor for altered ephedrine effect if sodium bicarbonate therapy is initiated, discontinued, or changed in dosage; adjust ephedrine dose as needed.

REFERENCES:

Wilkinson GR, et al. Absorption, metabolism and excretion of the ephedrines in man I. The influence of urinary pH and urine volume output. *J Pharmacol Exp Ther.* 1968;162:139.

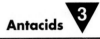

Antacids

Fleroxacin

SUMMARY: Limited data demonstrate a small effect of aluminum hydroxide on fleroxacin concentrations.

RISK FACTORS:

➡ *Dosage Regimen.* The effects of antacids on quinolone absorption appear to be greater when large antacid doses are administered.

➡ *Diet/Food.* Binding interactions in the GI tract tend to be greater in the fasting state than if there is food in the stomach.

RELATED DRUGS: The absorption of other quinolones also is reduced by antacids. H_2-receptor antagonists (eg, cimetidine [eg, *Tagamet*], famotidine [eg, *Pepcid*], nizatidine [eg, *Axid*], ranitidine [eg, *Zantac*]) and proton pump inhibitors (eg, omeprazole [eg, *Prilosec*], lansoprazole [*Prevacid*]) are not known to affect fleroxacin absorption.

MANAGEMENT OPTIONS:

➡ *Consider Alternative.* Because it may be difficult to separate the doses of antacid and fleroxacin sufficiently to prevent an interaction, the use of H_2-receptor antagonists or proton pump inhibitors may be necessary for severe infections when patients require gastric acid reduction.

➡ *Circumvent/Minimize.* If antacids are used with oral fleroxacin, give the fleroxacin at least 2 hours before or 6 hours after the antacid.

➡ *Monitor.* Monitor for reduced fleroxacin response if antacids are also taken.

REFERENCES:

Shiba K, et al. Interactions of fleroxacin with dried aluminum hydroxide gel and probenecid. *Rev Infect Dis.* 1989;11(suppl 5):S1097.

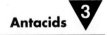

Antacids

Gatifloxacin (*Tequin*)

SUMMARY: Antacids can lower the absorption of gatifloxacin, resulting in reduced serum concentrations and possibly loss of antibiotic efficacy.

RISK FACTORS: No specific risk factors are known.

RELATED DRUGS: Aluminum and magnesium containing antacids inhibit the absorption of other quinolone antibiotics including ciprofloxacin (eg, *Cipro*), ofloxacin (*Floxin*), and trovafloxacin (*Trovan*).

MANAGEMENT OPTIONS:

➡ *Consider Alternative.* Patients taking quinolone antibiotics should utilize other acid-suppressant drugs, such as H_2-antagonists or proton pump inhibitors.

➡ *Circumvent/Minimize.* Administration of the gatifloxacin more than 2 hours before the antacid will minimize the magnitude of the interaction.

➡ *Monitor.* Monitor patients taking gatifloxacin and antacid products containing di- or trivalent cations for adequate antibiotic response.

REFERENCES:

Lober S, et al. Pharmacokinetics of gatifloxacin and interaction with an antacid containing aluminum and magnesium. *Antimicrob Agents Chemother.* 1999;43:1067-1071.

 Antacids

Glipizide (eg, *Glucotrol*)

SUMMARY: Magnesium hydroxide or sodium bicarbonate may enhance the rate of absorption of glipizide, but the clinical importance is not established.

RISK FACTORS: No specific risk factors are known.

RELATED DRUGS: H_2-receptor antagonists (eg, cimetidine [eg, *Tagamet*], famotidine [eg, *Pepcid*], nizatidine [eg, *Axid*], ranitidine [eg, *Zantac*]) also have been reported to increase the hypoglycemic effect of glipizide. Glyburide (eg, *DiaBeta*) absorption also appears to be increased by elevating gastric pH.

MANAGEMENT OPTIONS:

➡ *Circumvent/Minimize.* Until more information is available, it would be prudent to give glipizide 2 hours before or after antacids.

➡ *Monitor.* Monitor for altered hypoglycemic effect of glipizide if antacids are initiated, discontinued, changed in dosage, or if the dosage interval between the antacid and glipizide is changed.

REFERENCES:

Kivisto KT, et al. Enhancement of absorption and effect of glipizide by magnesium hydroxide. *Clin Pharmacol Ther.* 1991;49:39–43.

Kivisto KT, et al. Differential effects of sodium bicarbonate and aluminum hydroxide on the absorption and activity of glipizide. *Eur J Clin Pharmacol.* 1991;40:383-386.

 Antacids

Glyburide (eg, *DiaBeta*)

SUMMARY: Antacid (aluminum-magnesium hydroxides) increased glyburide serum concentrations, but the clinical importance of this effect is not established.

RISK FACTORS: No specific risk factors are known.

RELATED DRUGS: If the increased glyburide levels are caused by increased gastric pH, all antacids would be expected to interact, as would H_2-receptor antagonists (eg, cimetidine [eg, *Tagamet*], famotidine [eg, *Pepcid*], nizatidine [eg, *Axid*]) and proton pump inhibitors (eg, lansoprazole [*Prevacid*], omeprazole [eg, *Prilosec*]). Ranitidine does not alter glyburide pharmacokinetics.

MANAGEMENT OPTIONS:

➥ *Circumvent/Minimize.* Because the interaction is most likely caused by the increased gastric pH, one would expect that giving the glyburide at least 2 hours before or after the antacid should minimize the effect. If antacids are taken regularly, maintain a relatively constant interval between the antacid and glyburide so that any interaction will remain relatively constant.

➥ *Monitor.* Monitor for altered hypoglycemic effect of glyburide if antacids are initiated, discontinued, changed in dosage, or if the dosing interval between the antacid and glyburide is changed.

REFERENCES:

Zuccaro P, et al. Influence of antacids on the bioavailability of glibenclamide. *Drugs Exp Clin Res.* 1989;15:165-169.

Antacids (eg, magnesium carbonate [eg, *Marblen*]

Halofantrine (*Halfan*)

SUMMARY: Magnesium carbonate, and possibly other antacids, may reduce the bioavailability of halofantrine.

RISK FACTORS: No specific risk factors are known.

RELATED DRUGS: Although the effect of other antacids on halofantrine bioavailability is not established, assume that they interact until proven otherwise.

MANAGEMENT OPTIONS:

➥ *Consider Alternative.* Theoretically, H_2-receptor antagonists other than cimetidine (eg, *Tagamet*) would be unlikely to interact with halofantrine.

➥ *Circumvent/Minimize.* Although the effect of spacing doses of halofantrine and antacids is not known, it would be prudent to give the halofantrine at least 2 hours before or 6 hours after the antacid.

REFERENCES:

Aideloje SO, et al. Altered halofantrine by an antacid, magnesium carbonate. *Eur J Pharm Biopharm.* 1998;46:299-303.

Antacids

Iron

SUMMARY: Some antacids reduce the GI absorption of iron; inhibition of the hematological response to iron has been reported.

RISK FACTORS: No specific risk factors are known.

RELATED DRUGS: Until more information is available, assume that all antacids can reduce iron absorption.

MANAGEMENT OPTIONS:

➡ *Circumvent/Minimize.* Space antacids containing magnesium trisilicate, calcium carbonate, or sodium bicarbonate as far apart as possible from oral iron preparations. Until further information is available, observe the same precaution with other antacids.

➡ *Monitor.* Monitor for reduced iron response if antacids are also taken.

REFERENCES:

Azarnoff DL, et al. Drug interactions. *Pharmacol Physicians.* 1970;4 (Feb):1.

Hall GJL, et al. Inhibition of iron absorption by magnesium trisilicate. *Med J Aust.* 1969;2:95.

Coste JF, et al. *In vitro* interactions of oral hematinics and antacid suspensions. *Curr Ther Res.* 1977;22:205.

O'Neil-Cutting MA, et al. The effect of antacids on the absorption of simultaneously ingested iron. *JAMA.* 1986;255:1468.

 Antacids

Isoniazid (INH; eg, *Nydrazid*)

SUMMARY: Some antacids may reduce the plasma concentration of INH.

RISK FACTORS: No specific risk factors are known.

RELATED DRUGS: Until more information is available, assume that all antacids can reduce INH absorption.

MANAGEMENT OPTIONS:

➡ *Circumvent/Minimize.* Give isoniazid 2 hours before or 6 hours after antacids.

➡ *Monitor.* Monitor for reduced isoniazid response if antacids are also used.

REFERENCES:

Hurwitz A, et al. Effects of antacids on gastrointestinal absorption of isoniazid in rat and man. *Am Rev Respir Dis.* 1974;109:41.

Gallicano K, et al. Effect of antacids in didanosine tablet on bioavailability of isoniazid. *Antimicrob Agents Chemother.* 1994;38:894.

Antacids

Ketoconazole (*Nizoral*)

SUMMARY: Antacids may reduce ketoconazole concentrations.

RISK FACTORS: No specific risk factors are known.

RELATED DRUGS: Any agents that substantially increase gastric pH (eg, H_2-receptor antagonists, proton pump inhibitors, and antacids containing aluminum, magnesium, or calcium) are likely to reduce the absorption of ketoconazole. Itraconazole absorption is similarly reduced by increased gastric pH, but fluconazole (*Diflucan*) is not.

MANAGEMENT OPTIONS:

➡ *Circumvent/Minimize.* Avoid antacids 2 hours before or after administration of ketoconazole.

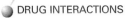

➡ **Monitor.** Monitor for reduced ketoconazole effect if antacids are also given.

REFERENCES:

Van Der Meer JWM, et al. The influence of gastric acidity on the bioavailability of ketoconazole. *J Antimicrob Chemother.* 1980;6:552.

Lelawongs P, et al. Effect of food and gastric acidity on absorption of orally administered ketoconazole. *Clin Pharm.* 1988;7:228.

Carlson JA, et al. Effect of pH on disintegration and dissolution of ketoconazole tablets. *Am J Hosp Pharm.* 1983;40:1334.

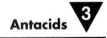

Antacids

Levofloxacin (*Levaquin*)

SUMMARY: Antacids containing aluminum, calcium, or magnesium may reduce the plasma concentrations of levofloxacin. A reduction in antibiotic effect may occur.

RISK FACTORS: No specific risk factors are known.

RELATED DRUGS: Antacids are known to reduce the absorption of other quinolone antibiotics including ciprofloxacin (*Cipro*) and lomefloxacin (*Maxaquin*). Other drugs that contain divalent cations (eg, sucralfate [*Carafate*], iron) would be expected to interact with levofloxacin in a similar manner.

MANAGEMENT OPTIONS:

➡ **Circumvent/Minimize.** Administration of levofloxacin 2 hours prior to the cation-containing drug will ensure optimal absorption of the quinolone.

➡ **Monitor.** Monitor patients taking levofloxacin for a reduced therapeutic response if antacids are coadministered.

REFERENCES:

Product information. Levofloxacin (*Levaquin*). McNeil Pharmaceutical. 1997.

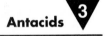

Antacids

Lomefloxacin (*Maxaquin*)

SUMMARY: Antacids reduce the serum concentration of lomefloxacin and may inhibit its efficacy.

RISK FACTORS:

➡ **Dosage Regimen.** The effects of antacids on quinolone absorption appear to be greater when large antacid doses are administered.

➡ **Diet/Food.** Binding interactions in the GI tract tend to be greater in the fasting state than if there is food in the stomach.

RELATED DRUGS: The absorption of other quinolones also is reduced by antacids. Lomefloxacin absorption appears somewhat less affected by cations (eg, antacids) than ciprofloxacin (*Cipro*) or norfloxacin (*Noroxin*). H_2-receptor antagonists (eg, cimetidine [eg, *Tagamet*], famotidine [*Pepcid*], nizatidine [*Axid*], ranitidine [*Zantac*]) and proton pump inhibitors (eg, omeprazole [*Prilosec*], lansoprazole [*Prevacid*]) are not known to affect lomefloxacin absorption.

MANAGEMENT OPTIONS:

➡ *Consider Alternative.* Because it may be difficult to separate the doses of antacid and lomefloxacin sufficiently to prevent their interaction, the use of H_2-receptor antagonists or proton pump inhibitors may be necessary for severe infections when patients require gastric acid reduction.

➡ *Circumvent/Minimize.* If antacids are used with oral lomefloxacin, give the lomefloxacin at least 2 hours before or 6 hours after the antacid.

➡ *Monitor.* Monitor for reduced lomefloxacin response if antacids are also taken.

REFERENCES:

Kunka RL, et al. Effect of antacid on the pharmacokinetics of lomefloxacin. *Pharm Res.* 1988;10(suppl):S165.

 ## Antacids (eg, *Maalox*)

Moxifloxacin (*Avelox*)

SUMMARY: The administration of antacid (eg, *Maalox*) reduced the plasma concentrations of moxifloxacin; some loss of efficacy may result.

RISK FACTORS: No specific risk factors are known.

RELATED DRUGS: Other quinolone antibiotics such as ciprofloxacin (*Cipro*) and lomefloxacin (*Maxaquin*) are affected in a similar manner by antacids. Other antacids containing di- or trivalent cations would be expected to affect moxifloxacin in a similar manner.

MANAGEMENT OPTIONS:

➡ *Consider Alternative.* Because it may be difficult to separate the doses of antacid and moxifloxacin sufficiently to prevent the interaction, consider using H_2-receptor antagonists or proton pump inhibitors to reduce gastric acidity.

➡ *Circumvent/Minimize.* If antacids are used with moxifloxacin, administer the moxifloxacin at least 2 hours before or 6 hours after the antacid.

➡ *Monitor.* Watch for reduced antibiotic efficacy if moxifloxacin and antacids are coadministered.

REFERENCES:

Stass H, et al. Evaluation of the influence of antacids and H_2 antagonists on the absorption of moxifloxacin after oral administration of a 400 mg dose to health volunteers. *Clin Pharmacokinet.* 2001;40(suppl 1):39.

 ## Antacids

Norfloxacin (*Noroxin*)

SUMMARY: Antacids reduce the serum concentration of norfloxacin and probably inhibit its efficacy.

RISK FACTORS:

➡ *Dosage Regimen.* The effects of antacids on quinolone absorption appear to be greater when large antacid doses are coadministered.

➡ *Diet/Food.* Binding interactions in the GI tract tend to be greater in the fasting state than if there is food in the stomach.

RELATED DRUGS: The absorption of other quinolones also is reduced by antacids, but the absorption of lomefloxacin (*Maxaquin*) and ofloxacin (*Floxin*) appears somewhat less affected by cations (eg, antacids) than norfloxacin. H_2-receptor antagonists (eg, cimetidine [eg, *Tagamet*], famotidine [*Pepcid*], nizatidine [*Axid*], ranitidine [*Zantac*]) and proton pump inhibitors (eg, omeprazole [*Prilosec*]), lansoprazole [*Prevacid*]) are not known to affect norfloxacin absorption.

MANAGEMENT OPTIONS:

➡ **Consider Alternative.** Since it may be difficult to separate the doses of antacid and norfloxacin sufficiently to prevent their interaction, the use of H_2-receptor antagonists or proton pump inhibitors may be necessary for severe infections when patients require gastric acid reduction.

➡ **Circumvent/Minimize.** If antacids are used with oral norfloxacin, give the norfloxacin at least 3 hours before or 6 hours after the antacid.

➡ **Monitor.** Monitor for reduced norfloxacin response if antacids are also given.

REFERENCES:

Nix DE, et al. Inhibition of norfloxacin absorption by antacids. *Antimicrob Agents Chemother*. 1990;34:432.

Noyes M, et al. Norfloxacin and absorption of magnesium-aluminum. *Ann Intern Med*. 1988;109:168.

Campbell NRC, et al. Norfloxacin interaction with antacids and minerals. *Br J Clin Pharmacol*. 1992;33:115.

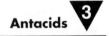

Antacids 3

Ofloxacin (*Floxin*)

SUMMARY: Antacids reduce the serum concentration of ofloxacin and may inhibit its efficacy.

RISK FACTORS:

➡ **Dosage Regimen.** Larger doses of antacids produce a greater reduction in ofloxacin absorption.

➡ **Diet/Food.** Binding interactions in the GI tract tend to be greater in the fasting state than if there is food in the stomach.

RELATED DRUGS: The absorption of other quinolones also is reduced by antacids. Ofloxacin absorption appears somewhat less affected by cations (eg, antacids) than ciprofloxacin (*Cipro*) or norfloxacin (*Noroxin*). H_2-receptor antagonists (eg, cimetidine [eg, *Tagamet*], famotidine [*Pepcid*], nizatidine [*Axid*], ranitidine [*Zantac*]) and proton pump inhibitors (eg, omeprazole [*Prilosec*], lansoprazole [*Prevacid*]) are not known to affect ofloxacin absorption.

MANAGEMENT OPTIONS:

➡ **Consider Alternative.** Calcium antacids, at least in small doses, appear to have little effect on the absorption of ofloxacin. Also consider the use of H_2-receptor antagonists or proton pump inhibitors in place of antacids.

➡ **Circumvent/Minimize.** If antacids are used with oral ofloxacin, give the ofloxacin at least 2 hours before or 6 hours after the antacid.

➡ **Monitor.** Monitor for reduced ofloxacin response if antacids are also given.

REFERENCES:

Maesen FPV, et al. Ofloxacin and antacids. *J Antimicrob Chemother*. 1987;19:848.

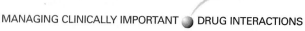

Hoffken G, et al. Pharmacokinetics and bioavailability of ciprofloxacin and ofloxacin: effect of food and antacid intake. *Rev Infect Dis.* 1988;10:S138.

Flor D, et al. Effects of magnesium-aluminum hydroxide and calcium carbonate antacids on bioavailability of ofloxacin. *Antimicrob Agents Chemother.* 1990;34:2436.

Cabarga MM, et al. Effects of two cations on gastrointestinal absorption of ofloxacin. *Antimicrob Agents Chemother.* 1991;35:2102.

Akerele JO, et al. Influence of oral coadministered metallic drugs on ofloxacin pharmacokinetics. *J Antimicrob Chemother.* 1991;28:87.

Navarro AS, et al. Comparative study of the influence of Ca^{2+} on absorption parameters of ciprofloxacin and ofloxacin. *J Antimicrob Chemother.* 1994;34:119.

 Antacids

Pefloxacin

SUMMARY: Antacids reduce the serum concentration of pefloxacin and may inhibit its efficacy.

RISK FACTORS:

➥ *Dosage Regimen.* The effects of antacids on quinolone absorption appear to be greater when large antacid doses are coadministered.

➥ *Diet/Food.* Binding interactions in the GI tract tend to be greater in the fasting state than if there is food in the stomach.

RELATED DRUGS: The absorption of other quinolones also is reduced by antacids. H$_2$-receptor antagonists (eg, cimetidine [eg, *Tagamet*], famotidine [*Pepcid*], nizatidine [*Axid*], ranitidine [*Zantac*]) and proton pump inhibitors (eg, omeprazole [*Prilosec*], lansoprazole [*Prevacid*]) are not known to affect pefloxacin absorption.

MANAGEMENT OPTIONS:

➥ *Consider Alternative.* Since it may be difficult to separate the doses of antacid and pefloxacin sufficiently to prevent their interaction, the use of H$_2$-receptor antagonists or proton pump inhibitors may be considered in place of the antacid.

➥ *Circumvent/Minimize.* If antacids are used with oral pefloxacin, give the pefloxacin at least 2 hours before or 6 hours after the antacid.

➥ *Monitor.* Monitor for reduced pefloxacin effect if antacids are also given.

REFERENCES:

Jaehde U, et al. Effect of an antacid containing magnesium and aluminum on absorption, metabolism and mechanism of renal elimination of pefloxacin in humans. *Antimicrob Agents Chemother.* 1994;38:1129.

 Antacids

Penicillamine (*Cuprimine*)

SUMMARY: Magnesium-aluminum hydroxides may reduce the bioavailability of penicillamine.

RISK FACTORS: No specific risk factors are known.

RELATED DRUGS: The effect of antacids other than magnesium aluminum hydroxides on penicillamine absorption is not established.

MANAGEMENT OPTIONS:

➡ *Circumvent/Minimize.* Until more is known about this interaction, it would be prudent to give penicillamine 2 hours before or 6 hours after antacids.

➡ *Monitor.* Monitor for reduced penicillamine response if antacids are also given.

REFERENCES:

Osman MA, et al. Reduction in oral penicillamine absorption by food, antacid, and ferrous sulfate. *Clin Pharmacol Ther.* 1983;33:465.

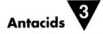

Antacids

Pseudoephedrine (eg, *Sudafed*)

SUMMARY: Sodium bicarbonate in doses sufficient to alkalinize the urine may inhibit the elimination of pseudoephedrine markedly.

RISK FACTORS: No specific risk factors are known.

RELATED DRUGS: Any drug that significantly alkalinizes the urine (eg, carbonic anhydrase inhibitors) would be expected to reduce the urinary excretion of pseudoephedrine. Nonsystemic antacids such as magnesium-aluminum hydroxides also may alkalinize the urine somewhat, but the extent to which this reduced pseudoephedrine elimination is not established. Sympathomimetic amines other than pseudoephedrine (eg, amphetamines, ephedrine) also have been shown to undergo pH dependent urinary excretion.

MANAGEMENT OPTIONS:

➡ *Consider Alternative.* If more than an occasional dose of sodium bicarbonate is used, consider using alternative antacid. (See Related Drugs.)

➡ *Monitor.* Monitor for enhanced pseudoephedrine effect (eg, anxiety, tremor, palpitations, psychiatric changes) if large doses of sodium bicarbonate are taken concurrently.

REFERENCES:

Brater DC, et al. Renal excretion of pseudoephedrine. *Clin Pharmacol Ther.* 1980;28:690.

Kuntzman RG, et al. The influence of urinary pH on the plasma halflife of pseudoephedrine in man and dog and a sensitive assay for its determination in human plasma. *Clin Pharmacol Ther.* 1971;12:62.

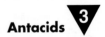

Antacids

Quinidine

SUMMARY: Antacids capable of increasing urine pH (eg, magnesium-aluminum hydroxides) may increase serum quinidine concentrations. Aluminum hydroxide probably does not impair GI quinidine absorption, but the effect of other antacids is not established.

RISK FACTORS:

➡ *Diet/Food.* Diets that increase urine pH (eg, large amounts of citrus juices) may add to the effect of antacids.

RELATED DRUGS: H$_2$-receptor antagonists (eg, famotidine [*Pepcid*], nizatidine [*Axid*], ranitidine [*Zantac*]) and proton pump inhibitors (eg, omeprazole [*Prilosec*], lansoprazole [*Prevacid*]) are not known to affect urine pH significantly, but cimetidine (eg,

Tagamet) inhibits the hepatic metabolism of quinidine and may increase its serum concentrations significantly.

MANAGEMENT OPTIONS:

➥ *Monitor.* Monitor for altered quinidine effect if antacids are initiated, discontinued or changed in dosage. Current evidence does not suggest that it is necessary to space doses of quinidine from antacids.

REFERENCES:

Gibaldi M, et al. Effect of antacids on pH of urine. *Clin Pharmacol Ther.* 1974;16:520.

Remon JP, et al. Interaction of antacids with antiarrhythmics. V. Effect of aluminum hydroxide and magnesium oxide on the bioavailability of quinidine, procainamide and propranolol in dogs. *Arzneimittelforsch.* 1983;33:117.

Romankiewicz JA, et al. The noninterference of aluminum hydroxide gel with quinidine sulfate absorption: an approach to control quinidine-induced diarrhea. *Am Heart J.* 1978;96:518.

Mauro VF, et al. Effect of aluminum hydroxide gel on quinidine gluconate absorption. *DICP.* 1990;24:252.

 Antacids

Sodium Polystyrene Sulfonate Resin (*Kayexalate*)

SUMMARY: Combined use of magnesium- or calcium-containing antacids with sodium polystyrene sulfonate resin may result in systemic alkalosis.

RISK FACTORS: No specific risk factors are known.

RELATED DRUGS: Theoretically, H_2–receptor antagonists (eg, cimetidine [eg, *Tagamet*], famotidine [*Pepcid*], nizatidine [*Axid*], ranitidine [*Zantac*]) and proton pump inhibitors (eg, lansoprazole [*Prevacid*], omeprazole [*Prilosec*]) would not be expected to interact with sodium polystyrene sulfonate resin.

MANAGEMENT OPTIONS:

➥ *Consider Alternative.* Consider use of alternative to antacids (see Related Drugs).

➥ *Circumvent/Minimize.* Separating the time of administration of doses of antacid from the oral sodium polystyrene sulfonate resin would theoretically avoid the interaction; since it is not known how much of a separation would be necessary to avoid the interaction, separate doses by as much time as possible. Administering sodium polystyrene sulfonate resin rectally also would be expected to avoid this interaction.

➥ *Monitor.* If antacids and sodium polystyrene sulfonate resin are used concurrently, be alert for clinical or laboratory evidence of alkalosis.

REFERENCES:

Schroeder ET. Alkalosis resulting from combined administration of a nonsystemic antacid and a cation-exchange resin. *Gastroenterology.* 1969;56:868.

Fernandez PC, et al. Metabolic acidosis reversed by the combination of magnesium hydroxide and a cation-exchange resin. *N Engl J Med.* 1972;286:23.

Ziessman HA. Alkalosis and seizure due to a cation-exchange resin and magnesium hydroxide. *South Med J.* 1976;69:497.

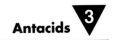

Antacids

Tetracycline

SUMMARY: Cotherapy with a tetracycline and an antacid containing divalent or trivalent cations (aluminum, calcium, magnesium) can reduce the serum concentration and efficacy of the tetracycline.

RISK FACTORS: No specific risk factors are known.

RELATED DRUGS: H$_2$-receptor antagonists (eg, cimetidine [eg, *Tagamet*], famotidine [*Pepcid*], nizatidine [*Axid*], ranitidine [*Zantac*]) and proton pump inhibitors (eg, lansoprazole [*Prevacid*], omeprazole [*Prilosec*]) are not known to affect tetracycline.

MANAGEMENT OPTIONS:

➡ *Circumvent/Minimize.* Take oral tetracyclines 2 hours before or 6 hours after antacids. This may not completely avoid the interaction, but it should minimize it.

➡ *Monitor.* Monitor for reduced tetracycline response if antacids are also used.

REFERENCES:
Scheiner J, et al. Experimental study of factors inhibiting absorption and effective therapeutic levels of declomycin. *Surg Gynecol Obstet.* 1962;114:9.

Anon. Risk of drug interaction may exist in 1 of 13 prescriptions (Medical News). *JAMA.* 1972;220:1287.

Jaffe JM, et al. Effect of altered urinary pH on tetracycline and doxycycline excretion in humans. *J Pharmacokinet Biopharm.* 1973;1:267.

Jaffe JM, et al. Influence of repetitive dosing and altered urinary pH on doxycycline excretion human. *J Pharm Sci.* 1974;63:1256.

Chin TF, et al. Drug diffusion and bioavailability: tetracycline metallic chelation. *Am J Hosp Pharm.* 1975;32:625.

Neuvonen PJ. Interactions with the absorption of tetracyclines. *Drugs.* 1976;11:45.

Rosenblatt JE, et al. Comparison of *in vitro* activity and clinical pharmacology of doxycycline with other tetracyclines. *Antimicrob Agents Chemother.* 1966:134.

Nix DE, et al. Effect of oral aluminum containing antacids on the disposition of intravenous doxycycline. *Pharm Res.* 1988;5(Suppl.):S174.

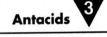

Antacids

Tocainide (*Tonocard*)

SUMMARY: In a report involving healthy subjects, antacids that increase urine pH were found to increase tocainide serum concentrations. The degree to which this effect increases the potential for adverse reactions is unknown.

RISK FACTORS: No specific risk factors are known.

RELATED DRUGS: No information is available.

MANAGEMENT OPTIONS:

➡ *Monitor.* Monitor patients taking tocainide more closely for excessive tocainide effect when antacids are coadministered.

REFERENCES:
Meneilly GP et al. The effect of antacid induced urinary alkalinization on the pharmacokinetics of tocainide. *Pharmacotherapy.* 1988;8:120.

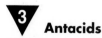
 Antacids

Trovafloxacin (*Trovan*)

SUMMARY: Antacids reduce the bioavailability of trovafloxacin; a loss of therapeutic efficacy may occur in some patients.

RISK FACTORS: No specific risk factors are known.

RELATED DRUGS: Antacids containing di- and trivalent cations similarly affect other quinolones such as ciprofloxacin (*Cipro*) and ofloxacin (*Floxin*).

MANAGEMENT OPTIONS:

➥ *Consider Alternative.* Consider the use of an OTC H_2-receptor antagonist.

➥ *Circumvent/Minimize.* Administer the antibiotic at least 2 hours before the antacid. If possible, avoid antacids during trovafloxacin administration.

➥ *Monitor.* Observe patients receiving trovafloxacin who also take antacids for a potential reduction in antibiotic effect.

REFERENCES:

Product information. Trovafloxacin (*Trovan*). Pfizer Inc. 1998.

 Antacids

Vitamin C

SUMMARY: Preliminary evidence from healthy subjects and animal studies suggests that vitamin C increases the amount of aluminum absorbed from aluminum hydroxide, but the clinical importance is not established.

RISK FACTORS: No specific risk factors are known.

RELATED DRUGS: Theoretically, any aluminum-containing antacid would interact with vitamin C in the same way.

MANAGEMENT OPTIONS:

➥ *Circumvent/Minimize.* The degree to which separating the doses of aluminum from vitamin C would circumvent the interaction is unknown, but taking the ascorbic acid at least 2 hours before or 4 hours after the aluminum antacid would be prudent.

➥ *Monitor.* There are no specific monitoring recommendations.

REFERENCES:

Domingo JL, et al. Effect of ascorbic acid on gastrointestinal aluminum absorption. *Lancet.* 1991;338:1467.

Domingo JL, et al. Influence of some dietary constituents on aluminum absorption and retention in rats. *Kidney Int.* 1991;39:598.

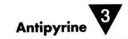

Antipyrine

Ciprofloxacin (*Cipro*)

SUMMARY: Ciprofloxacin reduces the clearance of antipyrine and probably other drugs that are metabolized in metabolic pathways similar to antipyrine.

RISK FACTORS:

➡ ***Dosage Regimen.*** Ciprofloxacin doses more than 250 mg/day are likely to reduce antipyrine clearance.

RELATED DRUGS: Ofloxacin 200 mg every 12 hours for 7 days did not alter the antipyrine clearance in 12 healthy subjects. Other quinolones reported to inhibit drug metabolism include enoxacin (*Penetrex*), norfloxacin (*Noroxin*), pipemidic acid, and pefloxacin.

MANAGEMENT OPTIONS:

➡ ***Monitor.*** While antipyrine is not used clinically, monitor patients receiving drugs that undergo similar hepatic oxidative metabolism (eg, theophylline) for reduced clearance if ciprofloxacin is prescribed.

REFERENCES:

Ludwig E, et al. The effect of ciprofloxacin on antipyrine metabolism. *J Antimicrob Chemother.* 1988;22:61.

Ludwig E, et al. Metabolic interactions of ciprofloxacin. *Diagn Microbiol Infect Dis.* 1990;13:135.

Waite NM, et al. The effect of ciprofloxacin on antipyrine pharmacokinetics in young and elderly healthy subjects. *Pharmacotherapy.* 1989;9:183.

Tan KKC, et al. Effect of ciprofloxacin on the pharmacokinetics of antipyrine. *Br J Clin Pharmacol.* 1989;27:235.

Graber H, et al. Ofloxacin does not influence antipyrine metabolism. *Rev Infect Dis.* 1989;11(Suppl. 5):S1093.

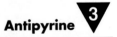

Antipyrine

Propranolol (eg, *Inderal*)

SUMMARY: Propranolol and, to a lesser extent, metoprolol and atenolol are capable of increasing antipyrine serum concentrations.

RISK FACTORS: No specific risk factors are known.

RELATED DRUGS: Other drugs metabolized by the cytochrome P450 system may be affected similarly by beta blocker administration.

MANAGEMENT OPTIONS:

➡ ***Monitor.*** Watch for increased effect of hepatically metabolized drugs when beta blockers, particularly propranolol, are coadministered.

REFERENCES:

Bax ND, et al. Inhibition of antipyrine metabolism by beta-adrenoreceptor antagonists. *Br J Clin Pharmacol.* 1981;12:779.

Bax ND, et al. Penbutolol and propranolol: a comparison of their effects on antipyrine clearance in man. *Br J Clin Pharmacol.* 1985;19:593.

Greenblatt DJ. Impairment of antipyrine clearance in humans by propranolol. *Circulation.* 1978;57:1161.

Perrild H, et al. Differential effect of continuous administration of beta-adrenoreceptor antagonists on antipyrine and phenytoin clearance. *Br J Clin Pharmacol.* 1989;28:551.

Adamska-Dyniewska H, et al. The effect of six beta-adrenolytics and labetalol on hepatic biotransformation studied by antipyrine test, in man. *Int J Clin Pharmacol Ther Toxicol.* 1986;24:303.

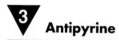
▼ Antipyrine

Verapamil (eg, *Calan*)

SUMMARY: Verapamil and diltiazem can increase antipyrine serum concentrations and inhibit the metabolism of other hepatically-eliminated drugs.

RISK FACTORS: No specific risk factors are known.

RELATED DRUGS: Other drugs that undergo oxidative metabolism by the hepatic cytochrome P450 enzyme system also may have reduced clearance in the presence of verapamil or diltiazem.

MANAGEMENT OPTIONS:

➡ *Consider Alternative.* Nifedipine or other dihydropyridine calcium channel blockers have little effect on the hepatic metabolism of other drugs.

➡ *Circumvent/Minimize.* Dose reduction may be appropriate for other drugs whose metabolism is reduced by the calcium channel blockers verapamil and diltiazem.

➡ *Monitor.* If verapamil or diltiazem are administered with other drugs that undergo hepatic metabolism, monitor for increased object drug effects and toxicity.

REFERENCES:

Bauer LA, et al. Changes in antipyrine and indocyanine green kinetics during nifedipine, verapamil and diltiazem therapy. *Clin Pharmacol Ther.* 1986;40:239.

Ohashi K, et al. The effect of diltiazem on hepatic drug oxidation assessed by antipyrine and trimethadione. *J Clin Pharmacol.* 1991;31:1132.

Dickinson TH, et al. Effects of nifedipine on hepatic drug oxidation. *Pharmacology.* 1988;36:405.

Edeki T, et al. An examination of a possible pharmacokinetic interaction between nifedipine and antipyrine. *Eur J Clin Pharmacol.* 1990;39:405.

Bach D, et al. The effect of verapamil on antipyrine pharmacokinetics and metabolism in man. *Br J Clin Pharmacol.* 1986;21:655.

Egan JM, et al. Effect of chronic oral verapamil on antipyrine metabolism. *Clin Pharmacol Ther.* 1986;39:191.

Carrum BA, et al. Diltiazem treatment impairs hepatic drug oxidation: studies of antipyrine. *Clin Pharmacol Ther.* 1986;40:140.

Rumiantsev DO, et al. The effect of oral verapamil therapy on antipyrine clearance. *Br J Clin Pharmacol.* 1986;22:606.

Rocci ML, et al. Comparative evaluation of the effects of labetalol, verapamil and diltiazem on antipyrine and indocyanine green clearances. *J Clin Pharmacol.* 1989;29:891.

Bottorff MB, et al. The effects of encainide versus diltiazem on the oxidative metabolic pathways of antipyrine. *Pharmacotherapy.* 1989;9:315.

▼ Apple Juice

Fexofenadine (*Allegra*)

SUMMARY: Ingestion of large amounts of apple juice reduces the absorption of fexofenadine and may reduce fexofenadine efficacy.

RISK FACTORS: No specific risk factors are known.

RELATED DRUGS: Orange and grapefruit juice also appear to reduce fexofenadine bioavailability.

MANAGEMENT OPTIONS:

➡ ***Circumvent/Minimize.*** Until more data are available, it would be prudent to take fexofenadine with water rather than apple juice or other fruit juices.

REFERENCES:

Dresser GK, et al. Fruit juices inhibit organic anion transporting polypeptide-mediated drug uptake to decrease the oral availability of fexofenadine. *Clin Pharmacol Ther.* 2002;71:11-20.

Aripiprazole (*Abilify*)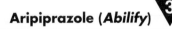

Ketoconazole (eg, *Nizoral*)

SUMMARY: Ketoconazole increases the plasma concentrations of aripiprazole and its active metabolite; aripiprazole dose reductions may be required.

RISK FACTORS:

➡ ***Pharmacogenetics.*** Patients who are poor metabolizers for CYP2D6 are likely to be most affected by this interaction.

RELATED DRUGS: Itraconazole (*Sporanox*) is a potent CYP3A4 inhibitor that is likely to produce similar increases in aripiprazole concentrations. Other antifungal agents that are known to inhibit CYP3A4 include fluconazole (*Diflucan*) and voriconazole (*Vfend*). Terbinafine (*Lamisil*) would not represent a suitable alternative antifungal agent because it inhibits CYP2D6, the other pathway for aripiprazole metabolism.

MANAGEMENT OPTIONS:

➡ ***Monitor.*** Observe patients maintained on aripiprazole for altered response if a potent inhibitor of CYP3A4 is added to or discontinued from therapy. Aripiprazole dosage adjustments may be required.

REFERENCES:

Product Information. Aripiprazole (*Abilify*). Bristol-Myers Squibb Co. 2002.

Aripiprazole (*Abilify*)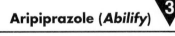

Quinidine

SUMMARY: Quinidine increases the plasma concentrations of aripiprazole and its active metabolite; aripiprazole dose reductions may be required.

RISK FACTORS:

➡ ***Pharmacogenetics.*** Patients who are rapid metabolizers for CYP2D6 are likely to be most affected by this interaction. Quinidine will have a minimal effect on aripiprazole in poor metabolizers of CYP2D6.

RELATED DRUGS: Other antiarrhythmic agents that inhibit CYP2D6 (eg, amiodarone [*Cordarone*] or propafenone [*Rythmol*]) also would be expected to inhibit the metabolism of aripiprazole.

MANAGEMENT OPTIONS:

➥ *Monitor.* Observe patients maintained on aripiprazole for altered response if a potent inhibitor of CYP2D6 is added to or discontinued from therapy. Aripiprazole dosage adjustments may be required.

REFERENCES:

Product Information. Aripiprazole (*Abilify*). Bristol-Myers Squibb Co. 2002.

 Aspirin

Captopril (*Capoten*)

SUMMARY: Aspirin appears to inhibit both the antihypertensive effects of captopril and other angiotensin-converting enzyme (ACE) inhibitors and the favorable hemodynamic effects of ACE inhibitors in patients with CHF.

RISK FACTORS:

➥ *Dosage Regimen.* The inhibitory effect of aspirin on ACE inhibitors is probably dose related.

RELATED DRUGS: The effect of aspirin is probably similar for all ACE inhibitors. Other nonsteroidal anti-inflammatory drugs probably also inhibit ACE inhibitor effect, although it is possible that sulindac (*Clinoril*) interacts to a lesser degree. The effect of salicylates other than aspirin on ACE inhibitors is not established; theoretically, nonacetylated salicylates may be less likely to interact since they tend to have less inhibitory effect on prostaglandin synthesis.

MANAGEMENT OPTIONS:

➥ *Consider Alternative.* Acetaminophen is not known to affect ACE inhibitor response and may be a suitable alternative to aspirin as an analgesic or antipyretic.

➥ *Monitor.* If more than occasional doses of aspirin are used in a patient on an ACE inhibitor, monitor for worsening of disease (hypertension or CHF). Be alert for evidence of reduced renal function.

REFERENCES:

Moore TJ, et al. Contribution of prostaglandins to the antihypertensive action of captopril in essential hypertension. *Hypertension.* 1981;3:168.

Seelig CB, et al. Nephrotoxicity associated with concomitant ACE inhibitor and NSAID therapy. *South Med J.* 1990;83:1144.

Smith SR, et al. Effect of low-dose aspirin on thromboxane production and the antihypertensive effect of captopril. *J Am Soc Nephrol.* 1993;4:1133.

Hall D, et al. Counteraction of the vasodilator effects of enalapril by aspirin in severe heart failure. *J Am Coll Cardiol.* 1992;20:1549.

van Wijngaarden J, et al. Effects of acetylsalicylic acid on peripheral hemodynamics in patients with chronic heart failure treated with angiotensin-converting enzyme inhibitors. *J Cardiovasc Pharmacol.* 1994;23:240.

Sioufi A, et al. The absence of a pharmacokinetic interaction between aspirin and the angiotensin-converting enzyme inhibitor benazepril in healthy volunteers. *Biopharm Drug Disposit.* 1994;15:451.

Chlorpropamide (*Diabinese*)

SUMMARY: Salicylate administration may enhance the hypoglycemic response to sulfonylureas, particularly chlorpropamide.

RISK FACTORS: No specific risk factors are known.

RELATED DRUGS: Similar cases of hypoglycemia have been reported with tolbutamide (*Orinase*). Aspirin also has been noted to reduce glyburide (*DiaBeta*) serum concentrations while enhancing its hypoglycemic effects. More study in diabetic patients is needed to evaluate this interaction.

MANAGEMENT OPTIONS:

➡ *Monitor.* Be alert for evidence of altered response to oral hypoglycemics and insulin when salicylate therapy is started or stopped. Monitor blood glucose concentrations and watch for symptoms of hyper- or hypoglycemia.

REFERENCES:

Peaston MJT, et al. A case of combined poisoning with chlorpropamide, acetylsalicylic acid and paracetamol. *Br J Clin Pract.* 1968;22:30.

Richardson T, et al. Enhancement by sodium salicylate of the blood glucose lowering effect of chlorpropamide—drug interaction or summation of similar effects? *Br J Clin Pharmacol.* 1986;22:43.

Wishinsky H, et al. Protein interactions of sulfonylurea compounds. *Diabetes.* 1962;2(Suppl.):18.

Cherner R, et al. Prolonged tolbutamide-induced hypoglycemia. *JAMA.* 1963;185:883.

Guigliano D, et al. Effects of salicylate, tolbutamide, and prostaglandin E2 on insulin responses to glucose in non insulin-dependent diabetes mellitus. *J Clin Endocrinol Metab.* 1985;61:160.

Kubacka RT, et al. Effects of aspirin and ibuprofen on the pharmacokinetics and pharmacodynamics of in healthy subjects. *Ann Pharmacother.* 1996;30:20.

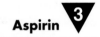

Diltiazem (*Cardizem*)

SUMMARY: Diltiazem appears to enhance the antiplatelet activity of aspirin, but the clinical importance of this effect is not established.

RISK FACTORS: No specific risk factors are known.

RELATED DRUGS: Verapamil (*Calan*) may interact similarly; patients have developed bruising or petechiae following coadministration with aspirin.

MANAGEMENT OPTIONS:

➡ *Monitor.* Until further information is available, monitor patients for prolonged bleeding times when diltiazem or verapamil is coadministered with aspirin.

REFERENCES:

Ring ME, et al. Effects of oral diltiazem on platelet function: alone and in combination with "low dose" aspirin. *Thromb Res.* 1986;44:391.

Ring ME, et al. Clinically significant antiplatelet effects of calciumchannel blockers. *J Clin Pharmacol.* 1986;26:719.

Altman R, et al. Diltiazem potentiates the inhibitory effect of aspirin on platelet aggregation. *Clin Pharmacol Ther.* 1988;44:320.

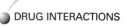

Ring ME, et al. Antiplatelet effects of oral diltiazem, propranolol, and their combination. *Br J Clin Pharmacol.* 1987;24:615.

Yamauchi K, et al. Effects of diltiazem hydrochloride on cardiovascular response, platelet aggregation and coagulating activity during exercise testing in systemic hypertension. *Am J Card.* 1986;57:609.

Cremer KF, et al. Effects of diltiazem, dipyridamole, and their combination on hemostasis. *Clin Pharmacol Ther.* 1984;34:641.

Kiyomoto A, et al. Inhibition of platelet aggregation by diltiazem: comparison with verapamil and nifedipine and inhibitory potencies of diltiazem metabolites. *Circ Res.* 1983;52(Suppl.):115.

Verzino E, et al. Verapamil-aspirin interaction. *Annals Pharmacother.* 1994;28:536.

 Aspirin

Ethanol (Ethyl Alcohol)

SUMMARY: Ethanol appears to enhance aspirin-induced gastric mucosal damage and aspirin-induced prolongation of the bleeding time.

RISK FACTORS:

➡ *Diet/Food.* Theoretically, more concentrated alcohol (eg, hard liquor) on an empty stomach would be more likely to enhance gastric mucosal damage from aspirin.

RELATED DRUGS: Theoretically, salicylate preparations which are less likely to produce gastric mucosal injury (eg, effervescent buffered salicylates [*Alka-Seltzer*], enteric-coated aspirin [eg, *Ecotrin*], and nonacetylated salicylates) would be less likely to produce additive gastric mucosal damage when administered in the presence of alcohol. Also, salicylate-induced prolongation of the bleeding time can be avoided by using nonacetylated salicylates such as choline salicylate (*Arthropan*), salsalate (*Disalcid*), choline magnesium salicylate, and sodium salicylate; ethanol induced potentiation of the salicylate-induced prolongation of the bleeding time by ethanol would not be a factor with these nonacetylated salicylates.

MANAGEMENT OPTIONS:

➡ *Consider Alternative.* Some forms of salicylate appear to be less likely to produce gastric mucosal injury than standard aspirin tablets. Such products include effervescent buffered products, enteric-coated products, and the nonacetylated salicylates. Theoretically, these preparations would be less likely to produce additive gastric mucosal damage with alcohol than standard aspirin tablets. (Also see Related Drugs for additional alternatives.)

➡ *Circumvent/Minimize.* Although concomitant use of ethanol and aspirin is not necessarily contraindicated, consider the possibility of enhanced GI bleeding. When possible, avoid aspirin use within 8 to 10 hours of heavy alcohol use.

➡ *Monitor.* Be alert for evidence of GI bleeding (eg, melena, black stools).

REFERENCES:

Goulston K, et al. Alcohol, aspirin and gastrointestinal bleeding. *BMJ.* 1968;4:664.

Bouchier IND, et al. Determination of faecal blood-loss after combined alcohol and sodium-acetylsalicylate intake. *Lancet.* 1969;1:178.

Mould G. Faecal blood-loss after sodium acetylsalicylate taken with alcohol. *Lancet.* 1969;1:1268.

Wood PHN. Faecal blood-loss after sodium acetylsalicylate taken with alcohol. *Lancet.* 1969;1:677.

Dobbing J. Faecal blood-loss after sodium acetylsalicylate taken with alcohol. *Lancet.* 1969;1:527.

DeSchepper PJ, et al. Gastrointestinal blood loss after diflunisal and after aspirin: effect of ethanol. *Clin Pharmacol Ther.* 1978;23:669.

Deykin D, et al. Ethanol potentiation of aspirin-induced prolongation of the bleeding time. *N Engl J Med.* 1982;306:852.

Needham CD, et al. Aspirin and alcohol in gastrointestinal haemorrhage. *Gut.* 1971;12:819.

Roine R, et al. Aspirin increases blood alcohol concentrations in humans after ingestion of ethanol. *JAMA.* 1990;264:2406.

Aspirin

Fluoxetine (eg, *Prozac*)

SUMMARY: The combined use of selective serotonin reuptake inhibitors (SSRIs) or clomipramine with aspirin appears to increase the risk of upper GI bleeding.

RISK FACTORS: No specific risk factors are known.

RELATED DRUGS: Assume all other drugs that inhibit serotonin reuptake (citalopram [*Effexor*], clomipramine [*Anafranil*], fluvoxamine [*Luvox*], nefazodone [*Serzone*], paroxetine [*Paxil*], sertraline [*Zoloft*], and venlafaxine [*Effexor*]) would interact with aspirin. The risk of using SSRIs with other platelet inhibitors such as clopidogrel (*Plavix*) or ticlopidine (*Ticlid*) is not known, but it is possible that the risk of GI bleeding would be increased.

MANAGEMENT OPTIONS:

➡ ***Consider Alternative.*** For analgesia, consider using a nonaspirin analgesic such as acetaminophen. If a salicylate is needed, consider a nonacetylated salicylate such as choline magnesium trisalicylate (*Trilisate*), salsalate (*Disalcid*), or magnesium salicylate (*Doan's*) since these products have minimal effects on platelets and the gastric mucosa. It is not known whether COX-2 inhibitors such as celecoxib (*Celebrex*), rofecoxib (*Vioxx*), or valdecoxib (*Bextra*) would be less likely to cause GI bleeding with SSRIs. Antidepressants with less effect on serotonin may reduce the risk of GI bleeding when combined with aspirin.

➡ ***Monitor.*** Patients receiving both a SSRI and aspirin should be alert for evidence of GI bleeding.

REFERENCES:
Dalton SO, et al. Use of selective serotonin reuptake inhibitors and risk of upper gastrointestinal tract bleeding: a population-based cohort study. *Arch Intern Med.* 2003;163:59-64.

Aspirin **2**

Ginkgo

SUMMARY: A patient on low-dose aspirin developed ocular hemorrhage after starting *Ginkgo biloba*, but the contribution of ginkgo to the bleeding was not established.

RISK FACTORS: No specific risk factors are known.

RELATED DRUGS: No information is available.

MANAGEMENT OPTIONS:

➡ ***Use Alternative.*** Although the risk of serious bleeding associated with the addition of ginkgo to aspirin therapy is not established, the combination should generally be avoided, because a) the benefit of ginkgo as a "memory aid" is questionable and b) the potential adverse outcome of the interaction is life-threatening.

REFERENCES:

Rosenblatt M, et al. Spontaneous hyphema associated with ingestion of Ginkgo biloba extract. *N Engl J Med.* 1997;336:1108.

Matthews MK Jr. Association of Ginkgo biloba with intracerebral hemorrhage. *Neurology.* 1998;50:1933-1934.

Aspirin (eg, *Bayer*)

Griseofulvin (eg, *Grisactin*)

SUMMARY: Griseofulvin administration markedly reduced the plasma concentration of salicylate in a patient taking chronic aspirin therapy.

RISK FACTORS: No specific risk factors are known.

RELATED DRUGS: No information is available.

MANAGEMENT OPTIONS:

➡ ***Circumvent/Minimize.*** Until the mechanism of this interaction is established, consider the administration of an alternative antifungal agent in patients receiving aspirin.

➡ ***Monitor.*** Based on this initial case report, monitor patients stabilized on aspirin therapy for loss of efficacy following the coadministration of griseofulvin.

REFERENCES:

Phillips KR, et al. Griseofulvin significantly decreases serum salicylate concentrations. *Pediatr Infect Dis J.* 1993;12:350-352.

Aspirin (eg, *Bayer*)

Ibuprofen (eg, *Advil*)

SUMMARY: Ibuprofen appears to inhibit the antiplatelet effect of aspirin, and may reduce its cardioprotective effects.

RISK FACTORS: No specific risk factors are known.

RELATED DRUGS: Agents that do not appear to affect the antiplatelet effects of aspirin include diclofenac (eg, *Voltarin*), rofecoxib (*Vioxx*), and acetaminophen (eg, *Tylenol*). The effect of other NSAIDs and COX-2 inhibitors on the ability of aspirin to inhibit platelet aggregation is not established.

MANAGEMENT OPTIONS:

➡ ***Use Alternative.*** Based on current evidence, diclofenac, rofecoxib, and acetaminophen do not interfere with the antiplatelet effects of aspirin.

REFERENCES:

Catella-Lawson F, et al. Cyclooxygenase inhibitors and the antiplatelet effects of aspirin. *N Engl J Med.* 2001;345:1809-1817.

Rao GH, et al. Ibuprofen protects platelet cyclooxygenase from irreversible inhibition by aspirin. *Arteriosclerosis.* 1983;3:383-388.

Grennan DM, et al. The aspirin-ibuprofen interaction in rheumatoid arthritis. *Br J Clin Pharmacol.* 1979;8:497-503.

Aspirin

Intrauterine Contraceptive Devices (IUDs)

SUMMARY: Aspirin has been reported to decrease the efficacy of IUDs, but a causal relationship has not been established.

RISK FACTORS: No specific risk factors are known.

RELATED DRUGS: If this interaction is real, it would be expected to occur with other anti-inflammatory drugs as well such as nonsteroidal anti-inflammatory drugs and salicylates.

MANAGEMENT OPTIONS:

➡ *Circumvent/Minimize.* Although this interaction is not well documented, women using intrauterine contraceptive devices should consider using another form of contraception during short-term therapy with salicylates or other anti-inflammatory drugs. If the anti-inflammatory drug is used chronically, consider the possibility that the IUD failure rate may be increased somewhat when selecting a contraceptive method.

➡ *Monitor.* Since pregnancy is the potential outcome, monitoring guidelines are not applicable.

REFERENCES:

Buhler M, et al. Successive pregnancies in women fitted with intrauterine devices who take antiinflammatory drugs. *Lancet.* 1983;1:483.

Inkeles DM, et al. Unexpected pregnancy in a woman using an intrauterine device and receiving steroid therapy. *Ann Ophthalmol.* 1982;14:975.

Zerner J, et al. Failure of an intrauterine device concurrent with administration of corticosteroids. *Fertil Steril.* 1976;27:1467.

Aspirin 2

Methotrexate (eg, *Rheumatrex*)

SUMMARY: Case reports, limited pharmacokinetic and epidemiological reports, and animal studies all indicate that salicylates may enhance methotrexate toxicity.

RISK FACTORS:

➡ *Dosage Regimen.* The risk of adverse effects from this interaction is primarily in patients receiving antineoplastic doses of methotrexate rather than the lower doses used to treat rheumatoid arthritis, psoriasis, and related diseases.

RELATED DRUGS: All salicylates are likely to interact with methotrexate.

MANAGEMENT OPTIONS:

➡ *Avoid Unless Benefit Outweighs Risk.* Aspirin should generally be avoided in patients taking antineoplastic doses of methotrexate. The manufacturer of methotrexate also recommends that salicylates be avoided in patients receiving methotrexate. Remind patients receiving methotrexate of the many nonprescription mixtures that contain salicylates.

➡ *Monitor.* If the combination is used, anticipate that a reduction in methotrexate dosage may be required. Serum methotrexate determinations would be helpful, and also monitor for excessive methotrexate effect (eg, GI toxicity, stomatitis, bone marrow suppression, hepatotoxicity, infection).

REFERENCES:

Liegler DG, et al. The effect of organic acids on renal clearance of methotrexate in man. *Clin Pharmacol Ther.* 1969;10:849.

Taylor JR, et al. Effect of sodium salicylate and indomethacin on methotrexate-serum albumin binding. *Arch Dermatol.* 1977;113:588.

Aherne GW, et al. Prolongation and enhancement of serum methotrexate concentrations by probenecid. *BMJ.* 1978;1:1097.

Dixon RL, et al. Plasma protein binding of methotrexate and its displacement by various drugs. *Fed Proc.* 1965;24:454.

Dubin HV, et al. Liver disease associated with methotrexate treatment of psoriatic patients. *Arch Dermatol.* 1970;102:498.

Baker H. Intermittent high dose oral methotrexate therapy in psoriasis. *Br J Dermatol.* 1970;82:65.

Mandel MA. The synergistic effect of salicylates on methotrexate toxicity. *Plast Reconstr Surg.* 1976;57:733.

 Aspirin

Pentazocine (*Talwin*)

SUMMARY: A patient on chronic therapy with aspirin and large doses of pentazocine developed papillary necrosis, but a causal relationship between this drug combination and the papillary necrosis was not established.

RISK FACTORS: No specific risk factors are known.

RELATED DRUGS: The effect of salicylates other than aspirin combined with pentazocine is not established.

MANAGEMENT OPTIONS:

➥ *Monitor.* Until more information is available, be alert for evidence of renal papillary necrosis (eg, passing tissue via the urethra) in patients receiving large doses of pentazocine combined with aspirin.

REFERENCES:

Muhalwas KK, et al. Renal papillary necrosis caused by long-term ingestion of pentazocine and aspirin. *JAMA.* 1981;246:867.

 Aspirin

Prednisone (eg, *Meticorten*)

SUMMARY: Prednisone and other corticosteroids may enhance the elimination of salicylates markedly, resulting in subtherapeutic salicylate concentrations in some patients. Discontinuing corticosteroids during high-dose salicylate therapy may result in salicylate toxicity.

RISK FACTORS:

➥ *Dosage Regimen.* Patients taking large (antiarthritic) salicylate doses are at greater risk.

RELATED DRUGS: Salicylates other than aspirin also can be expected to interact similarly with corticosteroids.

MANAGEMENT OPTIONS:

➡ *Monitor.* Corticosteroids and salicylates are frequently administered together, and their concomitant use is not contraindicated. However, salicylate dose requirements may be higher in the presence of corticosteroids, and watch patients for salicylate intoxication if the corticosteroid dose is reduced. Keep in mind the possibility that concomitant therapy may increase the incidence or severity of GI ulceration.

REFERENCES:

Klinenberg JR, et al. Effect of corticosterolds on blood salicylate concentration. *JAMA*. 1965;194:601.

Elliott HC. Reduced adrenocortical steroid excretion rates in man following aspirin administration. *Metabolism*. 1962;11:1015.

Koren G, et al. Corticosteroids-salicylate interaction—a case of juvenile rheumatoid arthritis. *Ther Drug Monit*. 1987;9:177.

George CRP. Nonspecific enhancement of glomerular filtration by corticosteroids. *Lancet*. 1974;2:728.

Polak A, et al. Nonspecific enhancement of glomerular filtration by corticosteroids. *Lancet*. 1974;2:841.

Edelman J, et al. The effect of intra-articular steroids on plasma salicylate concentrations. *Br J Clin Pharmacol*. 1986;21:301.

Graham GG, et al. Patterns of plasma concentrations and urinary excretion of salicylate in rheumatoid arthritis. *Clin Pharmacol Ther*. 1977;22:410.

Aspirin

Probenecid (*Benemid*)

SUMMARY: Salicylates inhibit the uricosuric activity of probenecid, but they do not appear to affect the ability of probenecid to inhibit the renal elimination of penicillins.

RISK FACTORS:

➡ *Dosage Regimen.* Doses of salicylate that do not produce serum salicylate concentrations more than 5 mg/dL do not appear to affect probenecid uricosuria significantly. Thus, occasional analgesic doses of salicylate may be insufficient to interact with probenecid.

RELATED DRUGS: All salicylates probably interact with probenecid in a similar manner.

MANAGEMENT OPTIONS:

➡ *Circumvent/Minimize.* Avoid more than occasional small doses of salicylates in patients receiving probenecid as a uricosuric agent. Available evidence suggests that patients receiving probenecid to prolong serum penicillin levels do not have to avoid salicylates.

➡ *Monitor.* Monitor for reduced probenecid uricosuric effect if salicylates are given concurrently.

REFERENCES:

Pascale LR, et al. Inhibition of the uricosuric action of Benemid by salicylate. *J Lab Clin Med*. 1955;45:771.

Boger WP, et al. Probenecid and salicylates: the question of interaction in terms of penicillin excretion. *J Lab Clin Med*. 1955;45:478.

Regal, RE. Aspirin and uricosurics: interaction revisited. *Drug Intell Clin Pharm*. 1987;21:219.

Aspirin

Sulfinpyrazone (*Anturane*)

SUMMARY: Salicylates inhibit the uricosuric effect of sulfinpyrazone.

RISK FACTORS: No specific risk factors are known.

RELATED DRUGS: All salicylates probably interact with sulfinpyrazone in a similar manner.

MANAGEMENT OPTIONS:

➡ ***Circumvent/Minimize.*** Avoid more than occasional small doses of salicylates in patients receiving sulfinpyrazone.

➡ ***Monitor.*** Monitor for reduced uricosuric effect of sulfinpyrazone if salicylates are given concurrently.

REFERENCES:

Smith MJH, et al. The Salicylates. *A Critical Bibliographic Review.* New York: Interscience Publishers; 1966:86–90.

Oyer JH, et al. Suppression of salicylate-induced uricosuria by phenylbutazone. *Am J Med Sci.* 1966;251:1.

Yu TF, et al. Mutual suppression of the uricosuric effects of sulfinpyrazone and salicylate: a study in interactions between drugs. *J Clin Invest.* 1963;42:1330.

 Aspirin

Warfarin (eg, *Coumadin*)

SUMMARY: Aspirin (even in small doses) increases the risk of bleeding in anticoagulated patients by inhibiting platelet function and possibly by producing gastric erosions. Larger aspirin doses (eg, more than 3 g/day) may also enhance the hypoprothrombinemic response to warfarin. Nonetheless, the benefit of low-dose aspirin plus warfarin appears to outweigh the increased risk of bleeding in selected patients.

RISK FACTORS:

➡ ***Dosage Regimen.*** In most patients, more than 3 g/day of aspirin is likely to have an intrinsic hypoprothrombinemic effect that would be additive with that of oral anticoagulants; the aspirin dosage required for this effect varies from patient to patient.

RELATED DRUGS: *Nonacetylated salicylates* (eg, choline salicylate, magnesium salicylate, salsalate, sodium salicylate) are probably safer with oral anticoagulants than aspirin, since such salicylates have minimal effects on platelet function and the gastric mucosa. Enteric-coated aspirin tends to produce less gastric mucosal damage, but it would still be capable of increasing the hypoprothrombinemic response (if given in large doses) and inhibiting platelet function (in any dose).

MANAGEMENT OPTIONS:

➡ ***Avoid Unless Benefit Outweighs Risk.*** Combine aspirin with an oral anticoagulant only when used intentionally for additive anticoagulant effects. If the aspirin is being used as an analgesic or antipyretic, acetaminophen is probably safer to use with oral anticoagulants. If a salicylate is needed, nonacetylated salicylates are probably safer (see Related Drugs). Warn patients that many nonprescription products contain aspirin and advise them to read the ingredients carefully.

➡ *Monitor.* If aspirin is used with oral anticoagulants, note that the increased bleeding risk is usually not accompanied by an increase in the hypoprothrombinemic response, especially when small doses of aspirin are used. Thus, direct particular attention to early detection of bleeding, especially from the GI tract.

REFERENCES:

Chesbro JH, et al. Trial of combined warfarin plus dipyridamole or ASA therapy in prosthetic heart valve replacement: danger of ASA compared with dipyridamole. *Am J Cardiol.* 1983;51:1537.

Donaldson DR, et al. Assessment of the interaction of warfarin with aspirin and dipyridamole. *Thromb Haemost.* 1982;47:77.

Starr KJ, et al. Drug interactions in patients on long-term oral anticoagulant and antihypertensive adrenergic neuron-blocking drugs. *BMJ.* 1972;4:133.

Deckert FW. Ascorbic acid and warfarin. *JAMA.* 1973;223:440.

Udall JA. Drug interference with warfarin therapy. *Clin Med.* 1970;77:20.

Chignell CF, et al. Optical studies of drug-protein complexes. V. The interaction of phenylbutazone, flufenamic acid, and dicumarol with acetylsalicylic acid-treated human serum albumin. *Mol Pharmacol.* 1971;7:229.

Coldwell BB, et al. Effect of aspirin on the fate of bishydroxycoumarin in the rat. *J Pharm Pharmacol.* 1971;23:226.

Anon. Aspirin and gastrointestinal bleeding. *JAMA.* 1969;207:2430. Editorial.

Barrow MV, et al. Salicylate hypoprothrombinemia in rheumatoid arthritis with liver disease. *Arch Intern Med.* 1967;120:620.

Holmes EL. Pharmacology of the fenamates. IV. Toleration of normal human subjects. *Ann Phys Med (Suppl).* 1967;9:36.

O'Reilly RA, et al. Impact of aspirin and chlorthalidone on the pharmacodynamics of oral anticoagulant drugs in man. *Ann NY Acad Sci.* 1971;179:173.

Fausa O. Salicylate-induced hypoprothrombinemia: a report of four cases. *Acta Med Scand.* 1970;188:403.

Anon. Aspirin and bleeding. *JAMA.* 1971;218:89. Editorial.

O'Brien JR, et al. A comparison of an effect of different anti-inflammatory drugs on human platelets. *J Clin Pathol.* 1970;23:522.

Trunet P, et al. The role of iatrogenic disease in admissions to intensive care. *JAMA.* 1980;244:2617.

Hawthorne AB, et al. Aspirin-induced gastric mucosal damage: prevention by enteric-coating and relation to prostaglandin synthesis. *Br J Clin Pharmacol.* 1991;32:77.

Turpie AGG, et al. A comparison of aspirin with placebo in patients treated with warfarin after heart-valve replacement. *New Engl J Med.* 1993;329:524.

Hurlen M, et al. Comparison of bleeding complications of warfarin and warfarin plus acetylsalicylic acid: a study in 3166 outpatients. *J Int Med.* 1994;236:299.

Aspirin

Zafirlukast (*Accolate*)

SUMMARY: The manufacturer reports that aspirin can increase plasma concentrations of zafirlukast; adjustments in zafirlukast dose may be needed.

RISK FACTORS: No specific risk factors are known.

RELATED DRUGS: No information is available.

MANAGEMENT OPTIONS:

➡ *Monitor.* Monitor for altered zafirlukast effect if aspirin is initiated, discontinued, or changed in dosage. Adjust zafirlukast dose as needed.

REFERENCES:

Product information. Zafirlukast (*Accolate*). Zeneca Pharmaceuticals. 1997.

① Astemizole[†] (*Hismanal*)

AVOID **Erythromycin (eg, *E-Mycin*)**

SUMMARY: Preliminary reports indicate that erythromycin and astemizole administration can cause QT interval prolongation and arrhythmia.

RISK FACTORS: No specific risk factors are known.

RELATED DRUGS: Ketoconazole (*Nizoral*) and itraconazole (*Sporanox*) interact similarly in vitro. Troleandomycin (*TAO*) and clarithromycin (*Biaxin*) also may inhibit astemizole metabolism. Terfenadine (*Seldane*) is also known to interact with erythromycin.

MANAGEMENT OPTIONS:

➡ *AVOID COMBINATION.* It would be prudent to avoid giving the 2 drugs together. The use of sedating antihistamines or perhaps loratadine (*Claritin*) or cetirizine (*Zyrtec*) instead of astemizole would be preferred in patients taking erythromycin, ketoconazole, or itraconazole.

REFERENCES:

Gelb LN, ed. *FDA Medical Bull.* 1993;23:2.

Goss JE, et al. Torsades de pointes associated with astemizole (*Hismanal*) therapy. *Arch Intern Med.* 1993;153:2705.

Lavriisen K, et al. The interaction of ketoconazole, itraconazole and erythromycin with the in vitro metabolism of antihistamines in human liver microsomes. *Allergy.* 1993;48(Suppl.):34.

Snook J, et al. Torsades de pointes ventricular tachycardia associated with astemizole overdose. *Br J Clin Pract.* 1988;42:257.

Bishop R, et al. Prolonged Q-T interval following astemizole overdose. *Arch Emerg Med.* 1989;6:63.

† Not available in the US.

① Astemizole[†] (*Hismanal*)

AVOID **Fluvoxamine (*Luvox*)**

SUMMARY: Fluvoxamine appears to inhibit the enzyme that metabolizes astemizole, which theoretically could result in increased serum astemizole concentrations and cardiac arrhythmias; avoid the combination.

RISK FACTORS: No specific risk factors are known.

RELATED DRUGS: Terfenadine (*Seldane*) is also metabolized by CYP3A4 and can cause the same types of cardiac arrhythmias when combined with CYP3A4 inhibitors; thus, it may also interact adversely with fluvoxamine. Loratadine (*Claritin*) and cetirizine (*Zyrtec*) do not appear to produce cardiotoxicity when combined with CYP3A4 inhibitors.

MANAGEMENT OPTIONS:

➡ *AVOID COMBINATION.* Although this interaction is based largely upon theoretical considerations, avoid the combination of astemizole and fluvoxamine. The potential adverse effects of the interaction can be life-threatening, and astemizole is generally used for symptomatic relief of allergic disorders. Theoretically, loratadine would be a safer nonsedating antihistamine in the presence of fluvoxamine.

REFERENCES:

Fleishaker JC, et al. A pharmacokinetic and pharmacodynamic evaluation of the combined administration of alprazolam and fluvoxamine. *Eur J Clin Pharmacol*. 1994;46:35.

Product information. Fluvoxamine (*Luvox*). Solvay Pharmaceuticals. 1996.

† Not available in the US.

Astemizole† (*Hismanal*)
Ketoconazole (*Nizoral*) `AVOID`

SUMMARY: Ketoconazole administration can cause astemizole concentrations to increase and result in QT interval prolongation and arrhythmia.

RISK FACTORS: No specific risk factors are known.

RELATED DRUGS: Other antifungal agents (eg, miconazole [*Monistat*], itraconazole [*Sporanox*], fluconazole [*Diflucan*]) are likely to increase astemizole concentrations. Terfenadine (*Seldane*) concentrations have been noted to increase when it is administered with antifungal agents. Cetirizine (*Zyrtec*) and loratadine (*Claritin*) appear to be less likely to produce side effects when administered with ketoconazole.

MANAGEMENT OPTIONS:

➡ ***AVOID COMBINATION.*** It would be prudent to avoid giving the 2 drugs together. The use of sedating antihistamines or perhaps loratadine or cetirizine instead of astemizole would seem to be preferred in patients taking ketoconazole or other oral antifungal agents. If ketoconazole and astemizole are coadministered, monitor for cardiac arrhythmias.

REFERENCES:

Gelb LN, ed. *FDA Medical Bull*. 1993;23:2.

Lavriisen K, et al. The interaction of ketoconazole, itraconazole and erythromycin with the *in vitro* metabolism of antihistamines in human liver microsomes. *Allergy*. 1993;48(Suppl.):34.

Snook J, et al. Torsades de pointes ventricular tachycardia associated with astemizole overdose. *Br J Clin Pract*. 1988;42:257.

Bishop R, et al. Prolonged Q-T interval following astemizole overdose. *Arch Emerg Med*. 1989;6:63.

† Not available in the US.

Astemizole† (*Hismanal*)
Mibefradil (*Posicor*)

SUMMARY: Mibefradil is likely to increase astemizole serum concentrations; cardiac arrhythmias may result. Pending further information on this interaction, avoid the concomitant use of mibefradil and astemizole.

RISK FACTORS: No specific risk factors are known.

RELATED DRUGS: Mibefradil administration causes an accumulation of terfenadine resulting in prolonged QTc intervals. Other calcium channel blockers (eg, amlodipine [*Norvasc*], nifedipine [*Procardia*], nicardipine [*Cardene*]) would not be expected to change astemizole plasma concentrations. The metabolism of fexofenadine (*Al-*

legra), cetirizine (*Zyrtec*), and loratadine (*Claritin*) would be unlikely to be affected by mibefradil coadministration.

MANAGEMENT OPTIONS:

➡ ***Use Alternative.*** Because of the risk of a possibly serious arrhythmia, avoid the combination of mibefradil and astemizole (or terfenadine). Use available noninteracting antihistamines in patients receiving mibefradil.

REFERENCES:

Product information. Mibefradil (*Posicor*). Roche Laboratories, Inc. 1997.

† Not available in the US.

 Atenolol (*Tenormin*)

Dipyridamole (*Persantine*)

SUMMARY: Several patients developed bradycardia following the administration of dipyridamole and atenolol.

RISK FACTORS: No specific risk factors are known.

RELATED DRUGS: This interaction would be expected to occur with all beta blockers. A similar interaction would be expected with adenosine (*Adenocard*) and beta blockers.

MANAGEMENT OPTIONS:

➡ ***Circumvent/Minimize.*** Discontinuation of atenolol or other beta blockers before the administration of dipyridamole may be the most prudent approach.

➡ ***Monitor.*** Because of the potentially serious outcome of this interaction, carefully observe patients taking beta-adrenergic blockers or other drugs known to have negative chronotropic or dromotropic effects for signs of bradycardia following dipyridamole injections.

REFERENCES:

Roach PJ, et al. Asystole and bradycardia during dipyridamole stress testing in patients receiving beta blockers. *Int J Cardiol.* 1993;42:92.

Blumenthal MS, et al. Cardiac arrest during dipyridamole imaging. *Chest.* 1988;93:1103.

Picano E, et al. Safety of intravenous high-dose dipyridamole echocardiography. *Am J Cardiol.* 1992;70:252.

 Atenolol (*Tenormin*)

Valsartan (*Diovan*)

SUMMARY: A 40-year-old pregnant woman on valsartan and atenolol lost the fetus at 33 weeks gestation; it is possible that the drugs played a role in the fetal death.

RISK FACTORS: No specific risk factors are known.

RELATED DRUGS: Theoretically, other combinations of angiotensin-2 receptor antagonists and beta-blockers could also result in fetal compromise.

MANAGEMENT OPTIONS:

➡ *Avoid Unless Benefit Outweighs Risk.* If possible, avoid angiotensin-2 receptor antagonists and beta-blockers in pregnant women.

REFERENCES:

Briggs GG, et al. Fatal fetal outcome with the combined use of valsartan and atenolol. *Ann Pharmacother.* 2001;35:859.

Atevirdine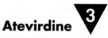
Fluconazole (*Diflucan*)

SUMMARY: Fluconazole administration causes an increase in the serum concentration of atevirdine; the clinical significance of this is unknown.

RISK FACTORS: No specific risk factors are known.

RELATED DRUGS: Other imidazole antifungal agents (eg, ketoconazole [eg, *Nizoral*], itraconazole [eg, *Sporanox*]) may interact in a similar manner with atevirdine.

MANAGEMENT OPTIONS:

➡ *Monitor.* Until further information is available, monitor patients receiving atevirdine who are prescribed fluconazole for increased atevirdine.

REFERENCES:

Borin MT, et al. The effect of fluconazole (FLU) on the pharmacokinetics of atevirdine mesylate (ATV) in HIV + patients. *Clin Pharmacol Ther.* 1994;55:193.

Atorvastatin (*Lipitor*)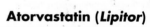
Clarithromycin (eg, *Biaxin*)

SUMMARY: Clarithromycin increases atorvastatin plasma concentrations; an increase in effect and possibly side effects may occur.

RISK FACTORS: No specific risk factors are known.

RELATED DRUGS: Erythromycin (eg, *E-Mycin*) is known to reduce the metabolism of atorvastatin. Azithromycin does not affect the metabolism of atorvastatin. Clarithromycin is likely to reduce the metabolism of lovastatin (eg, *Mevacor*) and simvastatin (*Zocor*) resulting in elevated plasma concentrations.

MANAGEMENT OPTIONS:

➡ *Circumvent/Minimize.* During treatment with clarithromycin, the dosing of atorvastatin could be withheld to avoid any potential adverse effects.

➡ *Monitor.* Monitoring for any evidence of atorvastatin side effects, such as myopathy, would be prudent during the coadministration of clarithromycin.

REFERENCES:

Amsden GW, et al. A study of the interaction potential of azithromycin and clarithromycin with atorvastatin in healthy volunteers. *J Clin Pharmacol.* 2002;42:442-447.

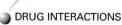

 Atorvastatin (*Lipitor*)

Clopidogrel (*Plavix*)

SUMMARY: Atorvastatin may inhibit the antiplatelet effects of clopidogrel, but it is not known if the therapeutic effect is reduced.

RISK FACTORS: No specific risk factors are known.

RELATED DRUGS: Since lovastatin (*Mevacor*) and simvastatin (*Zocor*), like atorvastatin, are metabolized by CYP3A4, theoretically they may also inhibit the conversion of clopidogrel to its active metabolite. Pravastatin (*Pravachol*) does not inhibit clopidogrel effect; theoretically, fluvastatin (*Lescol*) and rosuvastatin would not affect clopidogrel either, but clinical studies are needed for confirmation.

MANAGEMENT OPTIONS:

➡ *Consider Alternative.* Although data on this interaction are conflicting, it would be prudent to use alternatives to atorvastatin in patients receiving clopidogrel until more information is available. Because pravastatin (*Pravachol*) does not appear to significantly interfere with the antiplatelet effect of clopidogrel, it would be preferable to other statins in patients receiving clopidogrel.

➡ *Monitor.* If atorvastatin, lovastatin, or simvastatin is used in patients receiving clopidogrel, monitor platelet function and adjust clopidogrel dose as needed.

REFERENCES:

Clarke TA, et al. The metabolism of clopidogrel is catalyzed by human cytochrome P450 3A and is inhibited by atorvastatin. *Drug Metab Dispos.* 2003;31:53-59.

Lau WC, et al. Atorvastatin reduces the ability of clopidogrel to inhibit platelet aggregation: a new drug-drug interaction. *Circulation.* 2003;107:32-37.

Serebruany VL, et al. Statins do not affect platelet inhibition with clopidogrel during coronary stenting. *Atherosclerosis.* 2001;159:239-241.

 Atorvastatin (*Lipitor*)

Erythromycin (eg, *E-Mycin*)

SUMMARY: Erythromycin increases atorvastatin plasma concentrations; an increase in effect and possibly side effects may occur.

RISK FACTORS: No specific risk factors are known.

RELATED DRUGS: Clarithromycin (eg, *Biaxin*) is known to reduce the metabolism of atorvastatin. Azithromycin does not affect the metabolism of atorvastatin. Erythromycin is likely to reduce the metabolism of lovastatin (eg, *Mevacor*) and simvastatin (*Zocor*), resulting in elevated plasma concentrations.

MANAGEMENT OPTIONS:

➡ *Circumvent/Minimize.* During treatment with erythromycin, the dosing of atorvastatin could be withheld to avoid any potential adverse effects.

➡ ***Monitor.*** Monitoring for any evidence of atorvastatin side effects, such as myopathy, would be prudent during the coadministration of erythromycin.

REFERENCES:
Siedlik PH, et al. Erythromycin coadministration increases plasma atorvastatin concentrations. *J Clin Pharmacol.* 1999;39:501-504.

Atorvastatin (*Lipitor*)

Gemfibrozil (eg, *Lopid*)

SUMMARY: A patient on gemfibrozil developed rhabdomyolysis after starting atorvastatin therapy, but a causal relationship was not established.

RISK FACTORS: No specific risk factors are known.

RELATED DRUGS: Myopathy with or without rhabdomyolysis has also been reported following combined therapy with gemfibrozil and lovastatin (eg, *Mevacor*) and simvastatin (*Zocor*). Nonetheless, most of the cases have occurred with lovastatin or simvastatin, and it would appear that these 2 HMG-CoA reductase inhibitors are the most likely to interact adversely with gemfibrozil. Pravastatin (*Pravachol*) appears unlikely to interact adversely with gemfibrozil and limited evidence suggests that fluvastatin (eg, *Lescol*) is also usually safe in combination with gemfibrozil.

MANAGEMENT OPTIONS:

➡ ***Monitor.*** Alert patients receiving gemfibrozil with atorvastatin or another HMG-CoA reductase inhibitor for evidence of myopathy, such as muscle pain, muscle weakness, and darkened urine.

REFERENCES:
Duell PB, et al. Rhabdomyolysis after taking atorvastatin with gemfibrozil. *Am J Cardiol.* 1998;81:368-369.

Pierce LR, et al. Myopathy and rhabdomyolysis associated with lovastatin-gemfibrozil combination therapy. *JAMA.* 1990;264:71-75.

Tobert JA. Efficacy and long-term adverse effect pattern of lovastatin. *Am J Cardiol.* 1988;62:28J-34J.

Tal A, et al. Rhabdomyolysis associated with simvastatin-gemfibrozil therapy. *South Med J.* 1997;90:546-547.

Pogson GW, et al. Rhabdomyolysis and renal failure associated with cerivastatin-gemfibrozil combination therapy. *Am J Cardiol.* 1999;83:1146.

Wiklund O, et al. Pravastatin and gemfibrozil alone and in combination for treatment of hypercholesterolemia. *Am J Med.* 1993;94:13-20.

Athyros VG, et al. Safety and efficacy of long-term statin-fibrate combinations in patients with refractory familial combined hyperlipidemia. *Am J Cardiol.* 1997;80:608-613.

Pasternak RC, et al. Effect of combination therapy with lipid-reducing drugs in patients with coronary heart disease and "normal" cholesterol levels. *Ann Intern Med.* 1996;125:529-540.

Atorvastatin (eg, *Lipitor*)

Itraconazole (eg, *Sporanox*)

SUMMARY: Itraconazole administration increases the serum concentration of atorvastatin; increased toxicity (myopathy) could result.

RISK FACTORS: No specific risk factors are known.

RELATED DRUGS: Other antifungal drugs that inhibit CYP3A4 enzyme activities such as ketoconazole (*Nizoral*) or fluconazole (*Diflucan*) would be expected to have a similar effect on atorvastatin. Itraconazole inhibits the metabolism of lovastatin (*Mevacor*). Cerivastatin (*Baycol*) and simvastatin (*Zocor*) are metabolized by CYP3A4 and would probably be affected by itraconazole. Pravastatin (*Pravachol*) and fluvastatin (*Lescol*) may be less likely to interact with itraconazole. Terbinafine (*Lamisil*) may have limited effect on the metabolism of HMG-CoA reductase inhibitors.

MANAGEMENT OPTIONS:

➡ *Circumvent/Minimize.* Pravastatin or fluvastatin could be administered to patients receiving itraconazole. Terbinafine may have a limited effect on HMG-CoA reductase inhibitors, such as atorvastatin.

➡ *Monitor.* Monitor patients receiving atorvastatin and itraconazole for signs of myalgia and myopathy.

REFERENCES:

Kantola T, et al. Effect of itraconazole on the pharmacokinetics of atorvastatin. *Clin Pharmacol Ther.* 1998;64:58-65.

 Atorvastatin (eg, *Lipitor*)

Nelfinavir (*Viracept*)

SUMMARY: Nelfinavir administration increases atorvastatin concentrations moderately; some patients may experience increased side effects.

RISK FACTORS: No specific risk factors are known.

RELATED DRUGS: Other protease inhibitors such as ritonavir (*Norvir*), amprenavir (*Agenerase*), indinavir (*Crixivan*), and saquinavir (*Invirase*) would be expected to affect atorvastatin in a similar manner. The clearance of other statins that are metabolized by CYP3A4 would likely be reduced by nelfinavir. Lovastatin (*Mevacor*) and simvastatin (*Zocor*) may be affected to a greater degree than atorvastatin because of their greater susceptibility to CYP3A4 inhibitors.

MANAGEMENT OPTIONS:

➡ *Consider Alternative.* Because pravastatin (*Pravachol*) and fluvastatin (*Lescol*) are not metabolized by CYP3A4, consider using one of these agents in patients taking protease inhibitors.

➡ *Monitor.* Monitor patients taking atorvastatin and protease inhibitors for side effects including myopathy and myoglobinuria. It would be advisable to begin with a low dose of atorvastatin and slowly titrate the dose to the desired response.

REFERENCES:

Hsyu PH, et al. Pharmacokinetic interactions between nelfinavir and 3-hydroxy-3-methylglutaryl coenzyme A reductase inhibitors atorvastatin and simvastatin. *Antimicrob Agents Chemother.* 2001;45:3445-3450.

Atracurium (eg, *Tracrium*) ②

Gentamicin

SUMMARY: Aminoglycoside antibiotics like gentamicin potentiate the respiratory suppression produced by neuromuscular blockers.

RISK FACTORS:

➡ ***Concurrent Diseases.*** Patients with renal dysfunction are probably at greater risk.

➡ ***Dosage Regimen.*** Elevated aminoglycoside concentrations may lead to respiratory suppression.

RELATED DRUGS: Other aminoglycosides (eg, tobramycin [*Nebcin*]) also may produce enhanced neuromuscular blockade when administered in combination with neuromuscular blockers (eg, succinylcholine [*Anectine*], vecuronium [*Norcuron*]).

MANAGEMENT OPTIONS:

➡ ***Avoid Unless Benefit Outweighs Risk.*** Administer aminoglycoside antibiotics with extreme caution during surgery or in the immediate postoperative period.

➡ ***Monitor.*** Watch for respiratory depression; mechanical ventilation or treatment with anticholinesterase agents or calcium may be necessary.

REFERENCES:

Kronenfeld MA, et al. Recurrence of neuromuscular blockade after reversal of vecuronium in a patient receiving polymyxin/amikacin sternal irrigation. *Anesthesiology*. 1986;65:93-94.

Warner WA, et al. Neuromuscular blockade associated with gentamicin therapy. *JAMA*. 1971;215:1153-1154.

Wright EA, et al. Antibiotic-induced neuromuscular blockade. *Ann N Y Acad Sci*. 1971;183:358-368.

Levanen J, et al. Complete respiratory paralysis caused by a large dose of streptomycin and its treatment with calcium chloride. *Ann Clin Res*. 1975;7:47-49.

Lippmann M, et al. Neuromuscular blocking effects of tobramycin, gentamicin, and cefazolin. *Anesth Analg*. 1982;61:767-770.

Attapulgite (*Diasorb*) ▼③

Promazine (*Sparine*)

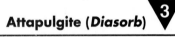

SUMMARY: Limited data indicate that attapulgite may reduce serum promazine concentrations.

RISK FACTORS: No specific risk factors are known.

RELATED DRUGS: The effect of attapulgite on other phenothiazines is not established, but consider the possibility that their absorption is also inhibited.

MANAGEMENT OPTIONS:

➡ ***Circumvent/Minimize.*** Although clinical evidence is very limited, it would be prudent to give phenothiazines 2 hours before or 6 hours after attapulgite.

➡ ***Monitor.*** Monitor for reduced phenothiazine effect if the combination is given.

REFERENCES:

Sorby DL, et al. Effects of adsorbents on drug absorption. II. Effect of an antidiarrhea mixture on promazine absorption. *J Pharm Sci*. 1966;55:504.

2   Azapropazone

Methotrexate (eg, *Rheumatrex*)

SUMMARY: A patient on chronic methotrexate developed evidence of methotrexate toxicity several days after starting azapropazone.

RISK FACTORS:

➡ **Concurrent Diseases.** Particular caution is suggested in patients with pre-existing renal impairment (who may be more susceptible to nonsteroidal anti-inflammatory drug [NSAID]-induced renal failure).

➡ **Dosage Regimen.** The risk of adverse effects from this interaction is primarily in patients receiving antineoplastic doses of methotrexate, rather than the lower doses used to treat rheumatoid arthritis, psoriasis, and related diseases.

RELATED DRUGS: Several other NSAIDs also have been shown to increase methotrexate serum concentrations although the magnitude varies depending upon which NSAID is used at what dose.

MANAGEMENT OPTIONS:

➡ **Avoid Unless Benefit Outweighs Risk.** Until more information is available on this interaction, it would be prudent to avoid azapropazone (as well as other NSAIDs) in patients receiving antineoplastic doses of methotrexate. Although decreasing the methotrexate dosage would be expected to reduce the likelihood of toxicity, the magnitude of the required reduction in methotrexate dosage has not been established. Rarely, low-dose methotrexate may interact adversely with a NSAID, as with the patient described above.

➡ **Monitor.** Many patients receiving methotrexate for rheumatoid arthritis will require a NSAID for symptomatic treatment. Closely monitor patients for evidence of increased methotrexate toxicity.

REFERENCES:

Aherne A, et al. Methotrexate kinetics in rheumatoid arthritis: is there an interaction with nonsteroidal antiinflammatory drugs? *J Rheumatol.* 1988;15:1356.

Furst DE, et al. Effect of aspirin and sulindac on methotrexate clearance. *J Pharm Sci.* 1990;79:782.

Dupuis LL, et al. Methotrexate-nonsteroidal antiinflammatory drug interaction in children with arthritis. *J Rheumatol.* 1990;17:1469.

Liegler DG, et al. The effect of organic acids on renal clearance of methotrexate in man. *Clin Pharmacol Ther.* 1969;10:849.

Skeith KJ, et al. Lack of significant interaction between low dose methotrexate and ibuprofen or flurbiprofen in patients with arthritis. *J Rheumatol.* 1990;17:1008.

Stewart CF, et al. Effect of aspirin (ASA) on the disposition of methotrexate (MTX) in patients with rheumatoid arthritis (RA). *Clin Pharmacol Ther.* 1990;47:139.

Taylor JR, et al. Effect of sodium salicylate and indomethacin on methotrexate-serum albumin binding. *Arch Dermatol.* 1977;113:588.

Tracy FS, et al. The effect of NSAIDS on methotrexate disposition in patients with rheumatoid arthritis. *Clin Pharmacol Ther.* 1990;47:138.

Daly HM, et al. Methotrexate toxicity precipitated by azapropazone. *Br J Dermatol.* 1986;114:733.

Azapropazone ②

Warfarin (eg, *Coumadin*)

SUMMARY: Azapropazone appeared to enhance the hypoprothrombinemic effect of warfarin markedly in one patient, but more study is needed to confirm this effect.

RISK FACTORS:

➡ *Concurrent Diseases.* Patients with peptic ulcer disease or a history of GI bleeding are probably at greater risk.

RELATED DRUGS: All NSAIDs inhibit platelet function, cause gastric erosions, and probably increase the risk of GI bleeding. Phenylbutazone (*Butazolidin*) markedly increases warfarin response. Some NSAIDs, however, such as ibuprofen (eg, *Advil*), naproxen (eg, *Naprosyn*), and diclofenac (*Voltaren*) may be less likely to increase oral anticoagulant-induced hypoprothrombinemia than other NSAIDs.

MANAGEMENT OPTIONS:

➡ *Avoid Unless Benefit Outweighs Risk.* Since all NSAIDs probably increase the risk of GI bleeding in patients on oral anticoagulants, use the combination only after careful consideration of the benefit vs risk. If a NSAID must be used with an oral anticoagulant it would be prudent to use NSAIDs that are unlikely to affect the hypoprothrombinemic response to oral anticoagulants (see Related Drugs). If the NSAID is being used as an analgesic or antipyretic, acetaminophen is probably safer to use with oral anticoagulants. Nonacetylated salicylates (eg, choline salicylate, magnesium salicylate, salsalate, sodium salicylate) are probably also safer with oral anticoagulants than NSAIDs, since such salicylates have minimal effects on platelet function and the gastric mucosa.

➡ *Monitor.* If any NSAID is used with an oral anticoagulant, monitor the prothrombin time carefully and watch for evidence of bleeding, especially from the GI tract.

REFERENCES:

McElnay JC, et al. Interaction between azapropazone and warfarin. *BMJ.* 1977;2:773.

Powell-Jackson PR. Interaction between azapropazone and warfarin. *BMJ.* 1977;1:1193.

Shorr RI, et al. Concurrent use of nonsteroidal anti-inflammatory drugs and oral anticoagulants places elderly persons at high risk for hemorrhagic peptic ulcer disease. *Arch Intern Med.* 1993;153:1665.

Azathioprine (*Imuran*)

Captopril (*Capoten*)

SUMMARY: Preliminary evidence indicates the likelihood of neutropenia may be greater with the combined use of captopril and azathioprine than with the use of either drug alone.

RISK FACTORS: No specific risk factors are known.

RELATED DRUGS: Given that azathioprine is converted to mercaptopurine in the body, one would expect mercaptopurine (6-MP) to interact with angiotensin-converting enzyme (ACE) inhibitors in a similar manner. Little is known regarding the combined use of azathioprine or mercaptopurine with ACE inhibitors other than captopril.

MANAGEMENT OPTIONS:

➡️ *Monitor.* Although evidence for an interaction between azathioprine and captopril is only preliminary, it would be prudent to monitor for laboratory and clinical evidence of bone marrow suppression in patients on both drugs.

REFERENCES:

Elijovisch F, et al. Captopril associated granulocytopenia in hypertension after renal transplantation. *Lancet*. 1980;1:927.

Edwards CRW, et al. Successful reintroduction of captopril following neutropenia. *Lancet*. 1981;1:723.

Case DB, et al. Successful low dose captopril rechallenge following drug-induced leukopenia. *Lancet*. 1981;1:1362.

Kirchertz EF, et al. Successful low dose captopril rechallenge following drug-induced leukopenia. *Lancet*. 1981;1:1363.

 Azathioprine (eg, *Imuran*)

Phenprocoumon[†]

SUMMARY: Two patients developed reduced phenprocoumon effect after azathioprine was started; monitor hypoprothrombinemic response.

RISK FACTORS: No specific risk factors are known.

RELATED DRUGS: Theoretically, azathioprine's active metabolite, mercaptopurine (6-MP), would also be expected to reduce phenprocoumon response. Both azathioprine and mercaptopurine have been reported to reduce the anticoagulant response to warfarin (eg, *Coumadin*).

MANAGEMENT OPTIONS:

➡️ *Monitor.* Monitor for altered phenprocoumon response if azathioprine is initiated, discontinued, or changed in dosage. Adjust phenprocoumon dose as needed.

REFERENCES:

Jeppesen U, et al. Clinically important interaction between azathioprine (*Imurel*) and phenprocoumon (*Marcoumar*). *Eur J Clin Pharmacol*. 1997;52:503-504.

† Not available in the United States.

Azathioprine (eg, *Imuran*)

Warfarin (eg, *Coumadin*)

SUMMARY: Azathioprine appeared to inhibit the hypoprothrombinemic response to warfarin in 1 patient; more information is needed to establish the clinical importance.

RISK FACTORS: No specific risk factors are known.

RELATED DRUGS: Mercaptopurine (6-MP) also has been reported to inhibit the hypoprothrombinemic response to warfarin.

MANAGEMENT OPTIONS:

➡️ *Monitor.* Monitor for altered oral anticoagulant effect if azathioprine is initiated, discontinued, or changed in dosage. Adjust the anticoagulant dose as needed.

REFERENCES:

Singleton JD, et al. Warfarin and azathioprine: an important drug interaction. *Am J Med*. 1992;92:217.

Benztropine (eg, *Cogentin*)

Haloperidol (eg, *Haldol*)

SUMMARY: Benztropine and other anticholinergics may inhibit the therapeutic response to neuroleptics; excess anticholinergic effects may occur.

RISK FACTORS: No specific risk factors are known.

RELATED DRUGS: Many combinations of antipsychotics and anticholinergics probably interact by 1 or more of the mechanisms described above. Trihexyphenidyl (*Artane*) apparently had a similar inhibitory effect on the therapeutic response to haloperidol in schizophrenic patients. However, there is also evidence that anticholinergics may reduce the GI absorption of chlorpromazine (eg, *Thorazine*). For example, trihexyphenidyl has been shown to reduce plasma chlorpromazine concentrations in schizophrenic patients, and orphenadrine (eg, *Norflex*) has been shown to reduce plasma concentrations and the pharmacologic response of chlorpromazine.

MANAGEMENT OPTIONS:

➡ *Circumvent/Minimize.* Do not use anticholinergics routinely in patients receiving neuroleptics. When the combination is needed, patients should take precautions to avoid heat stroke.

➡ *Monitor.* If the combination is used, be alert for evidence of reduced neuroleptic effects and for symptoms that may signal the onset of a dynamic ileus (eg, constipation, abdominal pain, distension).

REFERENCES:

Rivera-Calimlim L, et al. Clinical response and plasma levels: effect of dose, dosage schedules and drug interactions on plasma chlorpromazine levels. *Am J Psychiatry.* 1976;133:646-652.

Gershon S, et al. Interaction between some anticholinergic agents and phenothiazines. *Clin Pharmacol Ther.* 1965;6:749-756.

Alpert M, et al. Anticholinergic exacerbation of phenothiazine-induced extrapyramidal syndrome. *Am J Psychiatry.* 1976;133:1073-1075.

Rivera-Calimlim L. Chlorpromazine-trihexyphenidyl interaction. *Drug Ther.* 1976;6:196.

Singh MM, et al. Reversal of some therapeutic effects of an antipsychotic agent by an antiparkinsonisn drug. *J Nerv Ment Dis.* 1973;157:50-58.

Giordano J, et al. Fatal paralytic ileus complicating phenothiazine therapy. *South Med J.* 1975;68:351-353.

Warnes J, et al. A dynamic ileus during psychoactive medication: a report of three fatal and five severe cases. *Can Med Assoc J.* 1967;96:1112-1113.

Mann SC, et al. Psychotropic drugs, summer heat and humidity, and hyperpyrexia: a danger restated. *Am J Psychiatry.* 1978;135:1097-1100.

Hyperpyrexia from drug combinations. *JAMA.* 1973;225:1250.

Zelman S, et al. Heat stroke in phenothiazine-treated patients: a report of three fatalities. *Am J Psychiatry.* 1970;126:1787-1790.

Schaffer CB, et al. A case report of vomiting related to the interactions of antipsychotic and benztropine. *Am J Psychiatry.* 1981;138:833-835.

Rivera-Calimlim L, et al. Effects of mode of management on plasma chlorpromazine in psychiatric patients. *Clin Pharmacol Ther.* 1973;14:978-986.

Loga S, et al. Interactions of orphenadrine and phenobarbitone with chlorpromazine: plasma concentrations and effects in man. *Br J Clin Pharmacol.* 1975;2:197-208.

Bepridil (*Vascor*)

Digoxin (eg, *Lanoxin*)

SUMMARY: Bepridil increases digoxin serum concentrations; digoxin toxicity may result.

RISK FACTORS: No specific risk factors are known.

RELATED DRUGS: Verapamil (eg, *Calan*), diltiazem (eg, *Cardizem*), and nitrendipine (*Baypress*) appear to reduce digoxin elimination. Digitoxin (*Crystodigin*) is likely to be similarly affected.

MANAGEMENT OPTIONS:

➡ *Consider Alternative.* Nifedipine (eg, *Procardia*), isradipine (*DynaCirc*), nicardipine (eg, *Cardene*), felodipine (*Plendil*), and amlodipine (*Norvasc*) do not appear to increase digoxin concentrations.

➡ *Circumvent/Minimize.* Digoxin dosages may need to be reduced when bepridil is added to a patient stabilized on digoxin.

➡ *Monitor.* Monitor patients for evidence of increased serum digitalis effects (eg, bradycardia, heart block, GI upset, mental changes) in the presence of bepridil therapy.

REFERENCES:

Belz GG, et al. Digoxin and bepridil: pharmacokinetic and pharmacodynamic interactions. *Clin Pharmacol Ther.* 1986;39:65-71.

Kuhlmann J. Effects of nifedipine and diltiazem on plasma levels and renal excretion of beta-acetyldigoxin. *Clin Pharmacol Ther.* 1985;37:150-156.

Schwartz JB, et al. Effect of nifedipine on serum digoxin concentration and renal digoxin clearance. *Clin Pharmacol Ther.* 1984;36:19-24.

Belz GG, et al. Digoxin plasma concentrations and nifedipine. *Lancet.* 1981;1:844-845.

Hutt HJ, et al. Dose-dependence of the nifedipine/digoxin interaction? *Arch Toxicol Suppl.* 1986;9:209-212.

Rodin SM, et al. Comparative effects of verapamil and isradipine on steady-state digoxin kinetics. *Clin Pharmacol Ther.* 1988;43:668-672.

Debruyne D, et al. Nicardipine does not significantly affect serum digoxin concentrations at the steady state of patients with congestive heart failure. *Int J Clin Pharmacol Res.* 1989;9:15-19.

Kirch W, et al. The felodipine/digoxin interaction. A placebo-controlled study in patients with heart failure. *Br J Clin Pharmacol.* 1988;26:644P.

Schwartz JB. Effects of amlodipine on steady-state digoxin concentrations and renal digoxin clearance. *J Cardiovasc Pharmacol.* 1988;12:1-5.

Bethanechol (eg, *Urecholine*)

Tacrine (*Cognex*)

SUMMARY: Increased cholinergic effects may be seen when tacrine is combined with other cholinergic agents, like bethanechol.

RISK FACTORS: No specific risk factors are known.

RELATED DRUGS: Tacrine probably has additive effects with all cholinergic agents, including direct-acting cholinergics, as well as anticholinesterase agents, such as ambenonium (*Mytelase*), edrophonium (eg, *Tensilon*), neostigmine (eg, *Prostigmin*), and pyridostigmine (eg, *Mestinon*).

MANAGEMENT OPTIONS:

➡ *Monitor.* Monitor patients for excessive cholinergic response if tacrine is used with other cholinergic medications. Theoretically, it would be possible to reduce the dose of the cholinomimetic agent if tacrine is used concurrently without compromising the therapeutic response.

REFERENCES:

Taylor P. Agents acting at the neuromuscular junction and autonomic ganglia. In: Hardman JG, et al, eds. *Goodman and Gilman's The Pharmacological Basis of Therapeutics.* 9th ed. New York: Pergamon Press;1996;177–197.

Bezafibrate

Dicumarol

SUMMARY: A patient on dicumarol developed increased anticoagulant response and GI bleeding after bezafibrate was added to her therapy.

RISK FACTORS: No specific risk factors are known.

RELATED DRUGS: Both clofibrate (*Atromid-S*) and gemfibrozil (eg, *Lopid*) have been reported to increase dicumarol response. Bezafibrate has also been reported to increase the effect of warfarin (eg, *Coumadin*) and phenprocoumon.

MANAGEMENT OPTIONS:

➡ *Monitor.* Monitor patients receiving dicumarol or other anticoagulants for altered hypoprothrombinemic response if bezafibrate therapy is started, stopped, or changed in dosage.

REFERENCES:

Blum A, et al. Severe gastrointestinal bleeding induced by a probable hydroxycoumarin-bezafibrate interaction. *Isr J Med Sci.* 1992;28:47-49.

Beringer TR. Warfarin potentiation with bezafibrate. *Postgrad Med J.* 1997;73:657-658.

Bezafibrate

Warfarin (eg, *Coumadin*)

SUMMARY: Isolated cases of enhanced warfarin response have been reported in patients given bezafibrate concurrently.

RISK FACTORS: No specific risk factors are known.

RELATED DRUGS: Both clofibrate (*Atromid-S*) and gemfibrozil (eg, *Lopid*) have been reported to increase warfarin response. Bezafibrate has also been reported to increase the effect of dicumarol and phenprocoumon.

MANAGEMENT OPTIONS:

➡ *Monitor.* Monitor patients receiving warfarin or other anticoagulants for altered hypoprothrombinemic response if bezafibrate therapy is started, stopped, or changed in dosage.

REFERENCES:

Beringer TR. Warfarin potentiation with bezafibrate. *Postgrad Med J.* 1997;73:657-658.

Blum A, et al. Severe gastrointestinal bleeding induced by a probable hydroxycoumarin-bezafibrate interaction. *Isr J Med Sci.* 1992;28:47-49.

 ## Bismuth (eg, *Pepto-Bismol*)

Doxycycline (eg, *Vibramycin*)

SUMMARY: Bismuth can reduce the bioavailability of doxycycline significantly and could result in reduced antibacterial efficacy.

RISK FACTORS: No specific risk factors are known.

RELATED DRUGS: Tetracycline (*Actisite*) absorption is also affected by bismuth.

MANAGEMENT OPTIONS:

➡ *Use Alternative.* Patients taking tetracyclines for the treatment of infections should avoid bismuth. The use of doxycycline to prevent traveler's diarrhea should not include coadministration of bismuth.

REFERENCES:

Albert KS, et al. Decreased tetracycline bioavailability caused by a bismuth subsalicylate antidiarrheal mixture. *J Pharmaceut Sci.* 1979;68:586-588.

Ericsson CD, et al. Influence of subsalicylate bismuth on absorption of doxycycline. *JAMA.* 1982;247:2266-2267.

 ## Bismuth (eg, *Pepto-Bismol*)

Tetracycline (*Actisite*)

SUMMARY: Bismuth can reduce the bioavailability of tetracycline significantly and could result in reduced antibacterial efficacy.

RISK FACTORS: No specific risk factors are known.

RELATED DRUGS: Doxycycline (eg, *Vibramycin*) absorption is also affected by bismuth.

MANAGEMENT OPTIONS:

➡ *Use Alternative.* Patients taking tetracyclines for the treatment of infections should avoid bismuth. The use of doxycycline to prevent traveler's diarrhea should not include coadministration of bismuth.

REFERENCES:

Albert KS, et al. Decreased tetracycline bioavailability caused by a bismuth subsalicylate antidiarrheal mixture. *J Pharm Sci.* 1979;68:586-588.

 ## Bosentan (*Tracleer*)

Warfarin (eg, *Coumadin*)

SUMMARY: A patient on warfarin developed reduced anticoagulant effect after starting bosentan; monitor INR carefully in patients receiving the combination.

RISK FACTORS: No specific risk factors are known.

RELATED DRUGS: No information is available.

MANAGEMENT OPTIONS:

➡ *Monitor.* In patients receiving warfarin, be alert for alterations in INR if bosentan is started, stopped, or changed in dosage.

REFERENCES:

Murphey LM, et al. Bosentan and warfarin interaction. *Ann Pharmacother.* 2003;37:1028-1031.

Bromfenac

Lithium (eg, *Eskalith*)

SUMMARY: Because nonsteroidal anti-inflammatory drugs (NSAIDs) can increase lithium serum concentrations, bromfenac, theoretically, could also do so.

RISK FACTORS: No specific risk are factors known.

RELATED DRUGS: Other NSAIDs, except perhaps sulindac (eg, *Clinoril*), tend to increase lithium serum concentrations.

MANAGEMENT OPTIONS:

➡ *Monitor.* Be alert for evidence of lithium toxicity (eg, nausea, vomiting, diarrhea, anorexia, coarse tremor, slurred speech, vertigo, confusion, lethargy; in severe cases, seizures, stupor, coma, cardiovascular collapse). Adjust lithium dose as needed.

REFERENCES:

Product information. Bromfenac (*Duract*). Wyeth Laboratories, 1997.

Bromfenac

Phenytoin (eg, *Dilantin*)

SUMMARY: Study in healthy subjects found a substantial reduction in bromfenac plasma concentrations in the presence of phenytoin, but the clinical importance of this effect is not established.

RISK FACTORS: No specific risk factors are known.

RELATED DRUGS: Other enzyme inducers (eg, aminoglutethimide [*Cytadren*], barbiturates, carbamazepine [eg, *Tegretol*], griseofulvin, primidone [eg, *Mysoline*], rifabutin [*Mycobutin*], rifampin [eg, *Rifadin*], troglitazone [*Rezulin*]) may also reduce bromfenac plasma concentrations.

MANAGEMENT OPTIONS:

➡ *Monitor.* Monitor for reduced therapeutic effect of bromfenac if phenytoin is given concurrently. Adjust bromfenac dose as needed.

REFERENCES:

Gumbhir K, et al. Evaluation of pharmacokinetic interaction between bromfenac and phenytoin in healthy men. *J Clin Pharmacol.* 1997;37:160.

Product information. Bromfenac (*Duract*). Wyeth Laboratories, 1997.

Bromfenac

Warfarin (eg, *Coumadin*)

SUMMARY: Bromfenac does not appear to affect the hypoprothrombinemic response to warfarin, but cotherapy requires caution because of possible detrimental effects of bromfenac on gastric mucosa and platelet function.

RISK FACTORS:

➡ *Concurrent Diseases.* Patients with peptic ulcer disease or a history of GI bleeding are probably at greater risk for this interaction.

➡ *Dosage Regimen.* The risk of severe GI toxicity from bromfenac and other nonsteroidal anti-inflammatory drugs (NSAIDs) is directly related to the duration of NSAID therapy.

RELATED DRUGS: All NSAIDs inhibit platelet function, cause gastric erosions, and increase the risk of GI bleeding. Thus, any combination of an oral anticoagulant with an NSAID would theoretically increase the risk of bleeding.

MANAGEMENT OPTIONS:

➡ *Avoid Unless Benefit Outweighs Risk.* Because all NSAIDs increase the risk of GI bleeding in patients on oral anticoagulants, use the combination only after careful consideration of the benefit versus risk. If the NSAID is being used as an analgesic or antipyretic, acetaminophen (eg, *Tylenol*) is probably safer to use with oral anticoagulants. Nonacetylated salicylates (eg, choline salicylate [*Arthropan*], magnesium salicylate [eg, *Magan*], salsalate, sodium salicylate [eg, *Disalcid*]) also are probably safer with oral anticoagulants than standard NSAIDs since they have minimal effects on platelet function and the gastric mucosa.

➡ *Monitor.* Monitor the prothrombin time carefully and watch for evidence of bleeding, especially from the GI tract, if any NSAID is used with an oral anticoagulant.

REFERENCES:

Product information. Bromfenac (*Duract*). Wyeth Laboratories, 1997.

 Bromocriptine (*Parlodel*)

Erythromycin (eg, *E-Mycin*)

SUMMARY: Bromocriptine concentrations are markedly increased following erythromycin administration; the clinical significance is unknown.

RISK FACTORS: No specific risk factors are known.

RELATED DRUGS: Troleandomycin (*TAO*) and clarithromycin (*Biaxin*) may also inhibit the metabolism of bromocriptine.

MANAGEMENT OPTIONS:

➡ *Monitor.* Observe patients maintained on bromocriptine for bromocriptine toxicity (eg, hypotension, headache, nausea) during coadministration of erythromycin.

REFERENCES:

Nelson MV, et al. Pharmacokinetic evaluation of erythromycin and caffeine administered with bromocriptine in normal subjects. *Clin Pharmacol Ther.* 1990;47:694.

Bromocriptine (eg, *Parlodel*)

Isometheptene (eg, *Midrin*) `AVOID`

SUMMARY: A patient on bromocriptine developed hypertension and ventricular tachycardia after taking isometheptene; avoid the combination until additional data are available.

RISK FACTORS: No specific risk factors are known.

RELATED DRUGS: Assume that all sympathomimetics are capable of interacting adversely with bromocriptine.

MANAGEMENT OPTIONS:

➡ *AVOID COMBINATION.* Even though a causal relationship for this interaction has not been established conclusively, it would be prudent to avoid isometheptene (and other sympathomimetics) in patients receiving bromocriptine.

REFERENCES:

Kulig K, et al. Bromocriptine-associated headache: possible life-threatening sympathomimetic interaction. *Obstet Gynecol.* 1991;78:941.

Gittelman DK. Bromocriptine associated with postpartum hypertension, seizures, and pituitary hemorrhage. *Gen Hosp Psychiatry.* 1991;13:278.

Ruch A, et al. Postpartum myocardial infarction in a patient receiving bromocriptine. *Obstet Gynecol.* 1989;74:448.

Chan JC, et al. Postpartum hypertension, bromocriptine and phenylpropanolamine. *Drug Invest.* 1994;8:254.

Bromocriptine (*Parlodel*)

Thioridazine (eg, *Mellaril*)

SUMMARY: Phenothiazines probably inhibit the ability of bromocriptine to lower serum prolactin concentrations in patients with pituitary adenomas. Theoretically, bromocriptine should inhibit the antipsychotic effects of phenothiazines, but clinical evidence suggests that this may be uncommon.

RISK FACTORS: No specific risk factors are known.

RELATED DRUGS: It is likely that a similar interference with bromocriptine response would be seen with other phenothiazines and related neuroleptics such as haloperidol (eg, *Haldol*), chlorprothixene (*Taractan*), pimozide (*Orap*), thiothixene (eg, *Navane*), loxapine (eg, *Loxitane*), and molindone (*Moban*). Whether neuroleptics (eg, clozapine [eg, *Clozaril*]) that have less effect on serum prolactin concentrations would be less likely to interfere with the prolactin-lowering effect of bromocriptine is unknown.

MANAGEMENT OPTIONS:

➡ *Consider Alternative.* When possible, avoid the combined use of bromocriptine and neuroleptics.

➡ *Monitor.* When they are used concurrently, monitor the patient carefully for reduced effect of both drugs.

REFERENCES:

Robbins RJ, et al. Interactions between thioridazine and bromocriptine in a patient with a prolactin-secreting pituitary adenoma. *Am J Med.* 1984;76:921.

Langer G, et al. The prolactin response to neuroleptic drugs. A test of dopaminergic blockade: neuroendocrine studies in normal men. *J Clin Endocrinol Metab.* 1977;45:996.

Frye PE, et al. Bromocriptine associated with symptom exacerbation during neuroleptic treatment of schizoaffective schizophrenia. *J Clin Psychiatry.* 1982;43:252.

Kellner C, et al. Concurrent use of bromocriptine and fluphenazine. *J Clin Psychiatry.* 1985;46:455. Letter.

Ereshefsky L, et al. Clozapine: an atypical antipsychotic agent. *Clin Pharm.* 1989;8:691.

Perovich RM, et al. The behavioral toxicity of bromocriptine in patients with psychiatric illness. *J Clin Psychopharmacol.* 1989;9:417.

Bumetanide (eg, *Bumex*)

Indomethacin (eg, *Indocin*)

SUMMARY: Indomethacin administration reduces the diuretic and antihypertensive efficacy of bumetanide.

RISK FACTORS: No specific risk factors are known.

RELATED DRUGS: Prostaglandin inhibitors other than indomethacin (eg, other nonsteroidal anti-inflammatory drugs [NSAIDs]) may have a similar effect on bumetanide, but few data are available. However, aspirin may be less likely to interact with bumetanide. Furosemide (eg, *Lasix*) is also affected by indomethacin.

MANAGEMENT OPTIONS:

➥ *Consider Alternative.* Aspirin may be less likely than NSAIDs to interfere with the response to bumetanide and, thus, may be a possible substitute for indomethacin. Because furosemide also is affected by indomethacin, it is not a viable alternative.

➥ *Monitor.* Monitor for reduced diuretic and natriuretic response to bumetanide in the presence of indomethacin or other NSAIDs.

REFERENCES:

Brater DC, et al. Interaction studies with bumetanide and furosemide. Effects of probenecid and of indomethacin on response to bumetanide in man. *J Clin Pharmacol.* 1981;21(11-12 pt 2):647-653.

Brater DC, et al. Indomethacin and the response to butanimide. *Clin Pharmacol Ther.* 1980;27:421.

Kaufman J, et al. Bumetanide-induced diuresis and natriuresis: effect of prostaglandin synthetase inhibition. *J Clin Pharmacol.* 1981;21(11-12 pt 2):663-667.

Pedrinelli R, et al. Influence of indomethacin on the natriuretic and renin-stimulating effect of bumetanide in essential hypertension. *Clin Pharmacol Ther.* 1980;28:722-731.

Bunazosin

Enalapril (eg, *Vasotec*)

SUMMARY: Limited evidence suggests that patients receiving angiotensin-converting enzyme (ACE) inhibitors such as enalapril can have an exaggerated, first-dose hypotensive response to alpha-blockers such as bunazosin.

RISK FACTORS: No specific risk factors are known.

RELATED DRUGS: Theoretically, one would expect this interaction to occur with any combination of an ACE inhibitor (eg, benazepril [*Lotensin*], captopril [eg, *Capoten*], lisinopril [eg, *Prinivil*]) with alpha-blockers such as prazosin (eg, *Minipress*), terazosin (eg, *Hytrin*), doxazosin (eg, *Cardura*), and trimazosin.

MANAGEMENT OPTIONS:

➡ *Circumvent/Minimize.* In patients receiving ACE inhibitors, undertake initiation of therapy with bunazosin or other alpha-blockers with caution and with conservative doses. Taking the initial doses of the alpha-blocker at bedtime would be prudent.

➡ *Monitor.* Be alert for evidence of excessive hypotension.

REFERENCES:
Baba T, et al. Enhancement by an ACE inhibitor of first-dose hypotension caused by an alpha 1-blocker. *N Engl J Med.* 1990;322:1237.

Buspirone (*BuSpar*)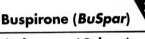

Citalopram (*Celexa*)

SUMMARY: A patient on excessive doses of buspirone and citalopram developed evidence of serotonin syndrome; the risk of this reaction in patients on therapeutic doses is not established.

RISK FACTORS:

➡ *Dosage Regimen.* Based on limited clinical data, it appears that large doses of one or both drugs increases the risk of interaction.

RELATED DRUGS: The effect of buspirone with other serotonin reuptake inhibitors is not established.

MANAGEMENT OPTIONS:

➡ *Monitor.* Be alert for evidence of serotonin syndrome. Serotonin syndrome can result in neurotoxicity (eg, myoclonus, tremors, rigidity, incoordination, restlessness, hyperreflexia, seizures, coma), psychiatric symptoms (eg, agitation, confusion, hypomania), and temperature regulation abnormalities (eg, fever, sweating). Fatalities have occurred.

REFERENCES:
Spigset O, et al. Combined serotonin syndrome and hyponatreamia caused by a citalopram-buspirone interaction. *Int Clin Psychopharmacol.* 1997;12:61.

Buspirone (*BuSpar*)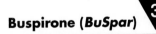

Diltiazem (*eg, Cardizem*)

SUMMARY: Diltiazem administration increases the concentration of buspirone; increased side effects could result in some patients.

RISK FACTORS: No specific risk factors are known.

RELATED DRUGS: Verapamil (eg, *Calan*) also produces an increase in buspirone concentrations. Although no data are available, dihydropyridine calcium channel blockers (eg, amlodipine [*Norvasc*], felodipine [*Plendil*], nifedipine [eg, *Procardia*]) would not be expected to interact with buspirone.

MANAGEMENT OPTIONS:

➡ *Consider Alternative.* Use of a dihydropyridine calcium channel blocker would probably avert this interaction. An alternative anxiolytic agent that does not undergo

CYP3A4 metabolism, such as diazepam (eg, *Valium*) or lorazepam (eg, *Ativan*), could be selected.

➡ *Monitor.* Monitor patients receiving the combination of buspirone and diltiazem for increased buspirone effects, such as sedation.

REFERENCES:

Lamberg TS, et al. Effects of verapamil and diltiazem on the pharmacokinetics and pharmacodynamics of buspirone. *Clin Pharmacol Ther.* 1998;63:640.

Buspirone (*BuSpar*)

Erythromycin (eg, *E-Mycin*)

SUMMARY: Erythromycin administration results in a large increase in buspirone concentrations; increased buspirone side effects are likely to result.

RISK FACTORS: No specific risk factors are known.

RELATED DRUGS: Other macrolide antibiotics that inhibit CYP3A4 such as clarithromycin (*Biaxin*) and troleandomycin (*TAO*) are likely to produce similar effects on buspirone pharmacokinetics. Noninhibiting macrolides include azithromycin (*Zithromax*) and dirithromycin (*Dynabac*). Other anxiolytics such as midazolam (*Versed*), alprazolam (eg, *Xanax*), and triazolam (eg, *Halcion*) are known to be inhibited by erythromycin. Anxiolytics not metabolized by CYP3A4 include lorazepam (eg, *Ativan*) and temazepam (eg, *Restoril*).

MANAGEMENT OPTIONS:

➡ *Consider Alternative.* Consider the use of a noninhibiting macrolide (see Related Drugs) for patients taking buspirone. Anxiolytics not metabolized by CYP3A4 (see Related Drugs) could be substituted for buspirone.

➡ *Monitor.* Monitor patients receiving buspirone for increased sedation if erythromycin is administered.

REFERENCES:

Kivisto KT, et al. Plasma buspirone concentrations are greatly increased by erythromycin and itraconazole. *Clin Pharmacol Ther.* 1997;62:348.

Buspirone (*BuSpar*)

Fluoxetine (*Prozac*)

SUMMARY: Isolated cases of reduced therapeutic response to buspirone or fluoxetine have been reported when the drugs were used together, and one patient on the combination developed a grand mal seizure. More study is needed to establish a causal relationship.

RISK FACTORS: No specific risk factors are known.

RELATED DRUGS: The effect of combining buspirone with other selective serotonin reuptake inhibitors is not established.

MANAGEMENT OPTIONS:

➡ *Monitor.* Until more information is available, monitor patients for altered response to either buspirone or fluoxetine when they are used together.

REFERENCES:

Bodkin JA, et al. Fluoxetine may antagonize the anxiolytic action of buspirone. *J Clin Psychopharmacol.* 1989;9:150. Letter.

Grady TA, et al. Seizure associated with fluoxetine and adjuvant buspirone therapy. *J Clin Psychopharmacol.* 1992;12:70. Letter.

Tanquary J, et al. Paradoxical reaction to buspirone augmentation of fluoxetine. *J Clin Psychopharmacol.* 1990;10:377. Letter.

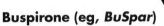

Buspirone (eg, *BuSpar*)

Grapefruit Juice

SUMMARY: Repeated doses of grapefruit juice markedly increase buspirone serum concentrations and also may enhance the subjective effect of buspirone.

RISK FACTORS: No specific risk factors are known.

RELATED DRUGS: Grapefruit juice also may increase the serum concentrations of benzodiazepines that are metabolized by CYP3A4 (eg, alprazolam [eg, *Xanax*], midazolam [eg, *Versed*], triazolam [eg, *Halcion*]), but only when the benzodiazepine is given orally.

MANAGEMENT OPTIONS:

➡ *Consider Alternative.* Orange juice does not inhibit CYP3A4 and would not be expected to interact with buspirone.

➡ *Circumvent/Minimize.* Advise patients to take buspirone at least 2 hours before or 6 to 8 hours after grapefruit juice.

➡ *Monitor.* If buspirone is taken with grapefruit juice, monitor for increased buspirone effect (eg, sedation, psychomotor impairment).

REFERENCES:

Lilja JJ, et al. Grapefruit juice substantially increases plasma concentrations of buspirone. *Clin Pharmacol Ther.* 1998;64:655–660.

Buspirone (eg, *BuSpar*)

Itraconazole (*Sporanox*)

SUMMARY: Itraconazole administration results in a large increase in buspirone concentrations; increased buspirone side effects are likely to result.

RISK FACTORS: No specific risk factors are known.

RELATED DRUGS: Other azole antifungals that inhibit CYP3A4 such as ketoconazole (eg, *Nizoral*) are likely to produce similar effects on buspirone pharmacokinetics. Non-inhibiting antifungals include terbinafine (*Lamisil*). Other anxiolytics such as midazolam (eg, *Versed*) and triazolam (eg, *Halcion*) are known to be inhibited by itraconazole. Anxiolytics not metabolized by CYP3A4 include lorazepam (eg, *Ativan*) and temazepam (eg, *Restoril*).

MANAGEMENT OPTIONS:

➡ *Consider Alternative.* Consider the use of a noninhibiting antifungal (see Related Drugs) for patients taking buspirone. Anxiolytics not metabolized by CYP3A4 (see Related Drugs) could be substituted for buspirone.

➡ *Monitor.* Monitor patients receiving buspirone for increased sedation if itraconazole is administered.

REFERENCES:

> Kivisto KT, et al. Plasma buspirone concentrations are greatly increased by erythromycin and itraconazole. *Clin Pharmacol Ther.* 1997;62:348-354.

Buspirone (eg, *BuSpar*)

Rifampin (eg, *Rifadin*)

SUMMARY: Rifampin markedly reduces the serum concentration of buspirone; loss of efficacy is likely to result.

RISK FACTORS: No specific risk factors are known.

RELATED DRUGS: No information is available.

MANAGEMENT OPTIONS:

➡ *Consider Alternative.* Because of the significant reduction in buspirone when administered with rifampin, consider an alternative antianxiety drug that is not metabolized by CYP3A4 (eg, lorazepam [eg, *Ativan*] or temazepam [eg, *Restoril*]).

➡ *Monitor.* Monitor patients taking buspirone for loss of efficacy following the coadministration of rifampin.

REFERENCES:

> Lamberg TS, et al. Concentrations and effects of buspirone are considerably reduced by rifampin. *Br J Clin Pharmacol.* 1998;45:381-385.

Buspirone (eg, *Buspar*)

Ritonavir (*Norvir*)

SUMMARY: Reduction of buspirone metabolism by ritonavir appears to have resulted in the development of Parkinson-like side effects.

RISK FACTORS: No specific risk factors are known.

RELATED DRUGS: Several other protease inhibitors, including indinavir (*Crixivan*), amprenavir (*Agenerase*), and saquinavir (eg, *Fortovase*) have been reported to inhibit the activity of CYP3A4. Other anxiolytics metabolized by CYP3A4 (eg, alprazolam [eg, *Xanax*], midazolam [eg, *Versed*]) may be affected in a similar manner by ritonavir.

MANAGEMENT OPTIONS:

➡ *Monitor.* Monitor patients receiving buspirone for evidence of elevated serum concentrations if ritonavir or other CYP3A4 inhibitors are coadministered.

REFERENCES:

> Clay PG, et al. Pseudo-Parkinson disease secondary to ritonavir-buspirone interaction. *Ann Pharmacother.* 2003;37:202-205.

Buspirone (eg, *BuSpar*)

Trazodone (eg, *Desyrel*)

SUMMARY: A patient on buspirone and trazodone developed myoclonic movements, possibly as a result of additive serotonergic effects; a causal relationship was not established.

RISK FACTORS: No specific risk factors are known.

RELATED DRUGS: No information is available.

MANAGEMENT OPTIONS:

➡ *Monitor.* Be alert for evidence of serotonin syndrome in patients receiving buspirone and trazodone. Serotonin syndrome can result in neurotoxicity (eg, myoclonus, tremors, rigidity, incoordination, hyperreflexia, seizures, coma), psychiatric symptoms (eg, agitation, confusion, hypomania, restlessness), and autonomic dysfunction (fever, sweating, tachycardia, hypertension).

REFERENCES:

Goldberg RJ, et al. Serotonin syndrome from trazodone and buspirone. *Psychosomatics.* 1992;33:235-236.

Sternbach H. The serotonin syndrome. *Am J Psychiatry.* 1991;148:705-713.

Buspirone (*BuSpar*)

Verapamil (eg, *Calan*)

SUMMARY: Verapamil administration increases the concentration of buspirone; increased side effects could result in some patients.

RISK FACTORS: No specific risk factors are known.

RELATED DRUGS: Diltiazem (eg, *Cardizem*) also produces an increase in buspirone concentrations. Although no data are available, dihydropyridine calcium channel blockers (eg, amlodipine [*Norvasc*], felodipine [*Plendil*], nifedipine [eg, *Procardia*]) would not be expected to interact with buspirone.

MANAGEMENT OPTIONS:

➡ *Consider Alternative.* Use of a dihydropyridine calcium channel blocker would probably avoid this interaction. An alternative anxiolytic agent that does not undergo CYP3A4 metabolism, such as diazepam (eg, *Valium*) or lorazepam (eg, *Ativan*), could be selected.

➡ *Monitor.* Monitor patients receiving the combination of buspirone and verapamil for increased buspirone effects such as sedation.

REFERENCES:

Lamberg TS, et al. Effects of verapamil and diltiazem on the pharmacokinetics and pharmacodynamics of buspirone. *Clin Pharmacol Ther.* 1998;63:640.

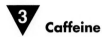

 Caffeine

Ciprofloxacin (*Cipro*)

SUMMARY: Ciprofloxacin increases caffeine concentrations and may enhance its side effects.

RISK FACTORS:

➡ **Dosage Regimen.** Ciprofloxacin doses of at least 250 mg twice daily can increase the risk of interaction.

RELATED DRUGS: Quinolones reported to inhibit caffeine metabolism include ciprofloxacin, enoxacin (*Penetrex*), norfloxacin (*Noroxin*), and pipemidic acid. Quinolones reported to have no effect on caffeine include ofloxacin (*Floxin*), lomefloxacin (*Maxaquin*), and rufloxacin.

MANAGEMENT OPTIONS:

➡ **Consider Alternative.** Ofloxacin or lomefloxacin could be used.

➡ **Circumvent/Minimize.** Patients who are taking ciprofloxacin should minimize their intake of caffeine.

➡ **Monitor.** Treatment with ciprofloxacin may cause significant increases in caffeine concentrations; advise patients of the potential for enhanced caffeine effects (eg, tachycardia, tremors, increased blood pressure).

REFERENCES:

Harder S, et al. 4-Quinolones inhibit biotransformation of caffeine. *Eur J Clin Pharmacol.* 1988;35:651.

Healy DP, et al. Interaction between oral ciprofloxacin and caffeine in normal volunteers. *Antimicrob Agents Chemother.* 1989;33:474.

Staib AH, et al. Gyrase inhibitors impair caffeine metabolism in man. *Methods Find Exp Clin Pharmacol.* 1987;9:193.

Stille W, et al. Decrease of caffeine elimination in man during coadministration of 4-quinolones. *J Antimicrob Chemother.* 1987;20:729.

Cesana M, et al. Effect of single doses of rufloxacin on the disposition of theophylline and caffeine after single administration. *Int J Clin Pharmacol Ther Toxicol.* 1991;29:133.

 Caffeine

Enoxacin (*Penetrex*)

SUMMARY: Enoxacin significantly increases caffeine serum concentrations and may increase caffeine side effects.

RISK FACTORS:

➡ **Dosage Regimen.** Increasing enoxacin doses from 100 to 400 mg twice daily can increase the risk of interaction.

RELATED DRUGS: Quinolones reported to inhibit caffeine metabolism include ciprofloxacin (*Cipro*), enoxacin (*Penetrex*), norfloxacin (*Noroxin*), and pipemidic acid. Quinolones reported to have no effect on caffeine include ofloxacin (*Floxin*), lomefloxacin (*Maxaquin*), and rufloxacin.

MANAGEMENT OPTIONS:

➡ **Consider Alternative.** Ofloxacin or lomefloxacin could be used.

➡ **Circumvent/Minimize.** Patients taking enoxacin should limit their intake of caffeine.

➡ *Monitor.* Treatment with enoxacin may cause significant increases in caffeine concentrations; advise patients of the potential for enhanced caffeine effects (eg, tachycardia, tremors, increased blood pressure).

REFERENCES:

Harder S, et al. 4-Quinolones inhibit biotransformation of caffeine. *Eur J Clin Pharmacol.* 1988;35:651.

Staib AH, et al. Gyrase inhibitors impair caffeine metabolism in man. *Methods Find Exp Clin Pharmacol.* 1987;9:193.

Peloquin CA, et al. Pharmacokinetics and clinical effects of caffeine alone and in combination with oral enoxacin. *Rev Infect Dis.* 1989;11 (Suppl. 5):S1095.

Cesana M, et al. Effect of single doses of rufloxacin on the disposition of theophylline and caffeine after single administration. *Int J Clin Pharmacol Ther Toxicol.* 1991;29:133.

Caffeine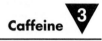

Fluconazole (*Diflucan*)

SUMMARY: Fluconazole increases the plasma concentration of caffeine.

RISK FACTORS:

➡ *Dosage Regimen.* High doses of fluconazole (more than 200 mg/day) can increase the risk of interaction.

RELATED DRUGS: Theoretically, other azole antifungal agents may interact in a similar manner with caffeine.

MANAGEMENT OPTIONS:

➡ *Monitor.* Be alert for increased caffeine effects such as tachycardia and nervousness.

REFERENCES:

Nix DE, et al. The effect of fluconazole on the pharmacokinetics of caffeine in young and elderly subjects. *Clin Pharmacol Ther.* 1992;51:183.

Caffeine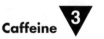

Methotrexate (eg, *Trexall*)

SUMMARY: Preliminary clinical evidence suggests that caffeine may inhibit the therapeutic effect of methotrexate in rheumatoid arthritis.

RISK FACTORS: No specific risk factors are known.

RELATED DRUGS: Theophylline also antagonizes adenosine and would be expected to interact with methotrexate in the same way as caffeine.

MANAGEMENT OPTIONS:

➡ *Circumvent/Minimize.* In patients with rheumatoid arthritis who do not respond adequately to methotrexate, it would be prudent to ask the patient about caffeine intake. If caffeine intake is high, a trial of reduced intake is recommended.

REFERENCES:

Nesher G, et al. Effect of caffeine consumption on efficacy of methotrexate in rheumatoid arthritis. *Arthritis Rheum.* 2003;48:571-572.

Caffeine

Norfloxacin (*Noroxin*)

SUMMARY: Norfloxacin increases caffeine serum concentrations; the clinical significance of these changes is probably limited.

RISK FACTORS:

➡ ***Dosage Regimen.*** Norfloxacin doses of greater than or equal to 800 mg twice daily can increase the risk of interaction.

RELATED DRUGS: Quinolones reported to inhibit caffeine metabolism included ciprofloxacin (*Cipro*), enoxacin (*Penetrex*), norfloxacin (*Noroxin*), and pipemidic acid. Quinolones having no effect on caffeine included ofloxacin (*Floxin*), lomefloxacin (*Maxaquin*), and rufloxacin.

MANAGEMENT OPTIONS:

➡ ***Consider Alternative.*** Ofloxacin or lomefloxacin could be used.

➡ ***Circumvent/Minimize.*** Patients taking norfloxacin should limit their intake of caffeinated beverages.

➡ ***Monitor.*** When high doses of norfloxacin (eg, greater than or equal to 800 mg twice daily) are administered, monitor patients for enhanced caffeine effects (eg, tachycardia, tremors, increased blood pressure).

REFERENCES:

Harder S, et al. 4-quinolones inhibit biotransformation of caffeine. *Eur J Clin Pharmacol.* 1988;35:651-656.

Carbo M, et al. Effect of quinolones on caffeine disposition. *Clin Pharmacol Ther.* 1989;45:234-240.

Cesana M, et al. Effect of single doses of rufloxacin on the disposition of theophylline and caffeine after single administration. *Int J Clin Pharmacol Ther Toxicol.* 1991;29:133-138.

Caffeine

Pipemidic Acid

SUMMARY: Pipemidic acid produces a large increase in caffeine serum concentrations and may increase caffeine side effects.

RISK FACTORS: No specific risk factors are known.

RELATED DRUGS: Quinolones reported to inhibit caffeine metabolism include ciprofloxacin (*Cipro*), enoxacin (*Penetrex*), norfloxacin (*Noroxin*), and pipemidic acid. Quinolones reported to have no effect on caffeine include ofloxacin (*Floxin*), lomefloxacin (*Maxaquin*), and rufloxacin.

MANAGEMENT OPTIONS:

➡ ***Consider Alternative.*** Ofloxacin or lomefloxacin could be used.

➡ ***Circumvent/Minimize.*** Patients taking pipemidic acid should limit their intake of caffeinated beverages.

➡ ***Monitor.*** When caffeine and pipemidic acid are administered, monitor patients for enhanced caffeine effects (eg, tachycardia, tremors, increased blood pressure).

REFERENCES:

Harder S, et al. 4-Quinolones inhibit biotransformation of caffeine. *Eur J Clin Pharmacol.* 1988;35:651.

Carbo M, et al. Effect of quinolones on caffeine disposition. *Clin Pharmacol Ther.* 1989;45:234.

Cesana M, et al. Effect of single doses of rufloxacin on the disposition of theophylline and caffeine after single administration. *Int J Clin Pharmacol Ther Toxicol.* 1991;29:133.

Calcium

Digoxin (eg, *Lanoxin*)

SUMMARY: Elevated calcium concentrations following parenteral administration have been associated with acute digoxin toxicity.

RISK FACTORS:

➡ ***Route of Administration.*** Administration of IV calcium can increase the risk of interaction.

RELATED DRUGS: A similar interaction would be expected with digitoxin.

MANAGEMENT OPTIONS:

➡ ***Circumvent/Minimize.*** Do not administer calcium IV to patients taking digoxin.

➡ ***Monitor.*** If calcium is administered IV, give slowly or in small amounts to avoid high serum calcium concentrations. Monitor patients for arrhythmias.

REFERENCES:

Schick D, et al. Current concepts of therapy with digitalis glycosides. Part II. *Am Heart J.* 1974;87:391.

Nola GT, et al. Assessment of the synergistic relationship between serum calcium and digitalis. *Am Heart J.* 1970;79:499.

Calcium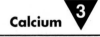

Thiazides

SUMMARY: The use of large doses of calcium with thiazides can result in the development of the milk-alkali syndrome.

RISK FACTORS:

➡ ***Dosage Regimen.*** Excessive doses of calcium appear to increase the risk of interaction.

RELATED DRUGS: No information is available.

MANAGEMENT OPTIONS:

➡ ***Circumvent/Minimize.*** Caution patients against excessive or prolonged self-administration of calcium, particularly if they are taking thiazides.

➡ ***Monitor.*** Monitor patients taking thiazides and calcium concurrently for evidence of hypercalcemia.

REFERENCES:

Gora ML, et al. Milk-alkali syndrome associated with use of chlorothiazide and calcium carbonate. *Clin Pharm.* 1989;8:227.

Hakim R, et al. Severe hypercalcemia associated with hydrochlorothiazide and calcium carbonate therapy. *Can Med Assoc J.* 1979;8:591.

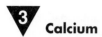

▼ Calcium

Verapamil (eg, *Calan*)

SUMMARY: Calcium administration may inhibit the activity of verapamil and other calcium channel blockers.

RISK FACTORS: No specific risk factors are known.

RELATED DRUGS: Calcium would be expected to reduce the effects of all calcium channel blockers.

MANAGEMENT OPTIONS:

➡ ***Monitor.*** Watch for evidence of reduced response, particularly hypotensive effects, when large doses of calcium products are given concurrently to patients receiving calcium channel blockers.

REFERENCES:

Bar-Or D, et al. Calcium and calciferol antagonise effect of verapamil in atrial fibrillation. *BMJ.* 1981;282:1585-1586.

Perkins CM. Serious verapamil poisoning: treatment with intravenous calcium gluconate. *BMJ.* 1978;2:1127.

Woie L, et al. Successful treatment of suicidal verapamil poisoning with calcium gluconate. *Eur Heart J.* 1981;2:239-242.

Salerno DM, et al. Intravenous verapamil for treatment of multifocal atrial tachycardia with and without calcium pretreatment. *Ann Intern Med.* 1987;107:623-628.

Schoen MD, et al. Clarification of the interaction between IV calcium chloride and IV verapamil. *Pharmacotherapy.* 1990;10:244.

O'Quinn SV, et al. Influence of calcium on the hemodynamic and antiischemic effects of nifedipine observed during treadmill exercise testing. *Pharmacotherapy.* 1990;10:247.

Wohns DH, et al. Influence of calcium administration on the short-term hemodynamic and anti-ischemic effects of nifedipine. *J Am Coll Cardiol.* 1991;18:1070-1076.

▼ Candesartan (*Atacand*)

Lithium (eg, *Eskalith*)

SUMMARY: A patient developed lithium toxicity after starting candesartan, but it is not known how often this combination would produce adverse consequences.

RISK FACTORS: No specific risk factors are known.

RELATED DRUGS: Both losartan (eg, *Cozaar*) and valsartan (*Diovan*) have also been reported to produce lithium toxicity, so it is possible that all angiotensin-II receptor antagonists interact with lithium. Angiotensin-converting enzyme inhibitors (ACEIs) have also been reported to cause lithium toxicity.

MANAGEMENT OPTIONS:

➡ ***Consider Alternative.*** In patients taking lithium, consider using alternatives to angiotensin II receptor antagonists such as candesartan. Note that ACEIs appear to interact with lithium in a similar manner, and may not be suitable as noninteracting alternatives.

➡ ***Monitor.*** If candesartan or other angiotensin II receptor antagonists are used concurrently with lithium, be alert for evidence of lithium toxicity (eg, nausea, vomiting, diarrhea, anorexia, coarse tremor, slurred speech, vertigo, confusion, lethargy; in severe cases, seizures, stupor, coma, cardiovascular collapse). Adjust lithium dose as needed.

REFERENCES:

Zwanzger P, et al. Lithium intoxication after administration of AT1 blockers. *J Clin Psychiatry.* 2001;62:208-209.

Blanche P, et al. Lithium intoxication in an elderly patient after combined treatment with losartan. *Eur J Clin Pharmacol.* 1997;52:501.

Leung M, et al. Potential drug interaction between lithium and valsartan. *J Clin Psychopharmacol.* 2000;20:392-393.

Captopril (*Capoten*)

Insulin

SUMMARY: Captopril and other angiotensin-converting enzyme (ACE) inhibitors appear to enhance insulin sensitivity. Nonetheless, ACE inhibitors are used intentionally in patients with diabetes and hypertension or heart failure.

RISK FACTORS: No specific risk factors are known.

RELATED DRUGS: While not all ACE inhibitors have been studied, one should assume that enalapril (eg, *Vasotec*), benazepril (*Lotensin*), fosinopril (*Monopril*), ramipril (*Altace*), quinapril (*Accupril*), trandolapril (*Mavik*), and moexipril (*Univasc*) may also affect glycemic control in patients with diabetes mellitus. Oral hypoglycemic agents including chlorpropamide (eg, *Diabinese*), tolbutamide (eg, *Orinase*), tolazamide (*Tolinase*), repaglinide (*Prandin*), metformin (*Glucophage*), glimepiride (*Amaryl*), glyburide (*DiaBeta*), and glipizide (eg, *Glucotrol*) should be expected to interact in a similar manner with ACE inhibitors.

MANAGEMENT OPTIONS:

➡ *Consider Alternative.* While data are limited, it appears that angiotensin II receptor inhibitors may not have the same effect on insulin sensitivity. Pending further clinical trials, the use of these agents (eg, losartan [*Cozaar*], candesartan [*Atacand*]) in patients with diabetes mellitus should be accompanied by blood glucose monitoring. Antihypertensive drugs from different classes could also be considered.

➡ *Monitor.* Monitor patients for altered hypoglycemic effect if ACE inhibitors therapy is initiated, discontinued, or changed in dose; adjust insulin and oral hypoglycemic doses as necessary.

REFERENCES:

Fogari R, et al. Comparative effects of lisinopril and losartan on insulin sensitivity in the treatment of non diabetic hypertensive patients. *Br J Clin Pharmacol.* 1998;46:467-471.

Paolisso G, et al. Lisinopril administration improves insulin action in aged patients with hypertension. *J Hum Hypertens.* 1995;9:541-546.

Rett K, et al. Role of angiotensin-converting enzyme inhibitors in early antihypertensive treatment in non-insulin dependent diabetes mellitus. *Postgrad Med J.* 1988;64(suppl 3):69-74.

Vuorinen-Markkola H, et al. Antihypertensive therapy with enalapril improves glucose storage and insulin sensitivity in hypertensive patients with non-insulin-dependent diabetes mellitus. *Metabolism.* 1995;44:85-89.

Arauz-Pacheco C, et al. Hypoglycemia induced by angiotensin-converting enzyme inhibitors in patients with non-insulin-dependent diabetes receiving sulfonylurea therapy. *Am J Med.* 1990;89:811-813.

Herings RM, et al. Hypoglycemia associated with use of inhibitors of angiotensin converting enzyme. *Lancet.* 1995;345:1195-1198.

Morris AD, et al. ACE inhibitor use is associated with hospitalization for severe hypoglycemia in patients with diabetes. *Diabetes Care.* 1997;20:1363.

Carbamazepine (eg, *Tegretol*)

Cimetidine (eg, *Tagamet*)

SUMMARY: Cimetidine may transiently increase plasma carbamazepine concentrations, but the effect appears to dissipate after 1 week of cimetidine therapy.

RISK FACTORS:

➡ ***Dosage Regimen.*** In most patients, clinically important inhibition of hepatic drug metabolism by cimetidine requires doses of at least 400 mg/day.

RELATED DRUGS: Ranitidine (eg, *Zantac*) does not appear to affect the elimination of single doses of carbamazepine. The effect of famotidine (eg, *Pepcid*) and nizatidine (*Axid*) on carbamazepine is unknown, but they would not be expected to interact.

MANAGEMENT OPTIONS:

➡ ***Consider Alternative.*** The use of ranitidine, famotidine, or nizatidine in place of cimetidine is likely to minimize the risk of carbamazepine toxicity.

➡ ***Monitor.*** Warn patients receiving carbamazepine of the possibility of side effects (eg, drowsiness, dizziness, nausea, vomiting, ataxia, headache, nystagmus, blurred vision) during the first few days of cimetidine therapy. Based upon current evidence, patients on chronic therapy with both cimetidine and carbamazepine do not appear to be at increased risk for adverse effects. Nevertheless, monitor patients for altered responses to carbamazepine if cimetidine is discontinued or changed in dosage.

REFERENCES:

Telerman-Toppet N, et al. Cimetidine interaction with carbamazepine. *Ann Intern Med.* 1981;94:544.

Webster LK, et al. Effect of cimetidine and ranitidine on carbamazepine and sodium valproate pharmacokinetics. *Eur J Clin Pharmacol.* 1984;27:341.

Dalton MJ, et al. The influence of cimetidine on single dose carbamazepine pharmacokinetics. *Clin Pharmacol Ther.* 1984;35:233.

MacPhee GJA, et al. Effects of cimetidine on carbamazepine auto-and hetero-induction in man. *Br J Clin Pharmacol.* 1984;18:411.

Sonne J, et al. Lack of interaction between cimetidine and carbamazepine. *Acta Neurol Scand.* 1983;68:253.

Levine M, et al. Differential effect of cimetidine on serum concentrations of carbamazepine and phenytoin. *Neurology.* 1985;35:562.

Dalton MJ, et al. Cimetidine and carbamazepine:a complex drug interaction. *Epilepsia.* 1986;27:553.

Dalton MJ, et al. Ranitidine does not alter single-dose carbamazepine pharmacokinetics in healthy adults. *Drug Intell Clin Pharm.* 1985;19:941.

Carbamazepine (eg, *Tegretol*)

Citalopram (*Celexa*)

SUMMARY: Isolated case reports suggest that carbamazepine reduces citalopram serum concentrations, but the clinical importance of this effect is not established.

RISK FACTORS: No specific risk factors are known.

RELATED DRUGS: The effect of carbamazepine on selective serotonin reuptake inhibitors other than citalopram is not established, but it is possible that their metabolism is affected by carbamazepine. The metabolism of carbamazepine may be inhibited by fluoxetine (*Prozac*) and fluvoxamine (*Luvox*), but paroxetine (*Paxil*) and sertraline (*Zoloft*) may be less likely to affect carbamazepine metabolism.

MANAGEMENT OPTIONS:

➠ *Monitor.* Monitor for reduced citalopram effect (eg, decreased effectiveness for indicated uses such as depression) if carbamazepine is given concurrently.

REFERENCES:

Lewis CF, et al. Dystonia associated with trazodone and sertraline. *J Clin Psychopharmacol.* 1997;17:64.

Carbamazepine (eg, *Tegretol*)

Clarithromycin (*Biaxin*)

SUMMARY: Clarithromycin administration appears to increase carbamazepine concentrations; carbamazepine toxicity could result.

RISK FACTORS: No specific risk factors are known.

RELATED DRUGS: Erythromycin and troleandomycin (*TAO*) are known to inhibit the metabolism of carbamazepine. Azithromycin (*Zithromax*) and dirithromycin (*Dynabac*) would be unlikely to decrease carbamazepine metabolism.

MANAGEMENT OPTIONS:

➠ *Consider Alternative.* Azithromycin does not appear to affect carbamazepine metabolism.

➠ *Monitor.* Until further information is available, carefully monitor patients maintained on carbamazepine for changing serum concentrations following the addition of clarithromycin.

REFERENCES:

Albani F, et al. Clarithromycin-carbamazepine interaction: a case report. *Epilepsia.* 1993;34:161.

Metz DC, et al. *Helicobacter pylori* gastritis therapy with omeprazole and clarithromycin increases serum carbamazepine levels. *Dig Dis Sci.* 1995;40:912.6

Carbamazepine (eg, *Tegretol*)

Clozapine (eg, *Clozaril*)

SUMMARY: Carbamazepine appears to considerably reduce clozapine plasma concentrations, but the clinical importance of this effect is not established.

RISK FACTORS: No specific risk factors are known.

RELATED DRUGS: Other enzyme-inducing anticonvulsants such as phenytoin (eg, *Dilantin*), primidone (eg, *Mysoline*), and barbiturates may have a similar effect.

MANAGEMENT OPTIONS:

➠ *Monitor.* Although more information is needed, monitor for altered clozapine response if carbamazepine therapy is initiated, discontinued, or changed in dosage.

REFERENCES:

Jerling M, et al. Fluvoxamine inhibition and carbamazepine induction of the metabolism of clozapine: evidence from a therapeutic drug monitoring service. *Ther Drug Monit.* 1994;16:368.

Tiihonen J, et al. Carbamazepine induced changes in plasma levels of neuroleptics. *Pharmacopsychiatry.* 1995;28:26.

Carbamazepine (eg, *Tegretol*)

Contraceptives, Oral (eg, *Ortho-Novum*)

SUMMARY: Carbamazepine and other enzyme-inducing anticonvulsants, such as barbiturates, phenytoin, and primidone, can inhibit the effect of oral contraceptives, resulting in menstrual irregularities and unplanned pregnancies.

RISK FACTORS:

➡ *Dosage Regimen.* Oral contraceptives with lower doses of hormones can increase the risk of interaction.

RELATED DRUGS:

MANAGEMENT OPTIONS:

➡ *Consider Alternative.* Consider an other means of contraception instead of, or in addition to, oral contraceptives when pregnancy is to be avoided in women receiving carbamazepine or other enzyme-inducing anticonvulsants such as phenobarbital (eg, *Solfoton*), phenytoin, and primidone (eg, *Mysoline*). Although an oral contraceptive with a higher estrogen content would be preferable for some women who are being treated with enzyme-inducing anticonvulsants, individualize based upon patient response (eg, lack of breakthrough bleeding).

➡ *Monitor.* Spotting or breakthrough bleeding in patients taking oral contraceptives and enzyme-inducing anticonvulsants could indicate that the drugs are interacting, although lack of breakthrough bleeding does not ensure contraceptive protection.

REFERENCES:

Rapport DJ, et al. Interactions between carbamazepine and birth control pills. *Psychosomatics.* 1989;30:462.

Kenyon IE. Unplanned pregnancy in an epileptic. *BMJ.* 1972;1:686.

Janz D, et al. Anti-epileptic drugs and failure of oral contraceptives. *Lancet.* 1974;1:1113.

Laengner H, et al. Antiepileptic drugs and failure of oral contraceptives. *Lancet.* 1974;2:600.

Coulam CG, et al. Do anticonvulsants reduce the efficacy of oral contraceptives? *Epilepsia.* 1979;20:519.

Haukkamaa M. Contraception by Norplant subdermal capsules is not reliable in epileptic patients on anticonvulsant treatment. *Contraception.* 1986;33:559.

McArthrur J. Oral contraceptives and epilepsy (Notes and Comments). *BMJ.* 1967;3:162.

Espir M, et al. Epilepsy and oral contraception. *BMJ.* 1969;1:294.

Crawford P, et al. The interaction of phenytoin and carbamazepine with combined oral contraceptive steroids. *Br J Clin Pharmacol.* 1990;30:892.

Crawford P, et al. The lack of effect on sodium valproate on the pharmacokinetics of oral contraceptive steroids. *Contraception.* 1986;33:23.

Mattson RH, et al. Use of oral contraceptives by women with epilepsy. *JAMA.* 1986;256:238.

Robertson YR, et al. Interactions between oral contraceptives and other drugs; a review. *Curr Med Res Opin.* 1976;3:647.

Carbamazepine (eg, *Tegretol*)

Cyclosporine (eg, *Neoral*)

SUMMARY: Carbamazepine can substantially reduce blood cyclosporine concentrations; adjustments in cyclosporine dosage may be required.

RISK FACTORS: No specific risk factors are known.

RELATED DRUGS: Other enzyme-inducing anticonvulsants such as phenobarbital, phenytoin (eg, *Dilantin*), and primidone (eg, *Mysoline*) appear to reduce blood cyclosporine concentrations, but in some cases valproic acid (eg, *Depakene*) was successfully substituted for carbamazepine without evidence of interaction. Tacrolimus (*Prograf*) probably is affected similarly by enzyme inducers.

MANAGEMENT OPTIONS:

➡ *Consider Alternative.* The interaction can be avoided (based upon limited clinical evidence) when valproic acid can be substituted for carbamazepine.

➡ *Monitor.* Be alert for evidence of altered cyclosporine effect if carbamazepine therapy is initiated or discontinued; monitor blood cyclosporine concentrations carefully.

REFERENCES:

Alvarez JS, et al. Effect of carbamazepine on cyclosporin blood level. *Nephron.* 1991;58:235.

Schofield OMV, et al. Cyclosporine A in psoriasis: interaction with carbamazepine. *Br J Dermatol.* 1990;122:425.

Lele P, et al. Cyclosporine and tegretol—another drug interaction. *Kidney Int.* 1985;27:344.

Hillebrand G, et al. Valproate for epilepsy in renal transplant recipients receiving cyclosporine. *Transplantation.* 1987;43:915.

Yee GC, et al. Pharmacokinetic drug interactions with cyclosporine (Part I). *Clin Pharmacokinet.* 1990;19:319.

Carbamazepine (eg, *Tegretol*)

Danazol (*Danocrine*)

SUMMARY: Danazol predictably increases serum carbamazepine concentrations substantially and induces carbamazepine toxicity (eg, dizziness, nausea, drowsiness, ataxia) in some patients receiving both drugs.

RISK FACTORS: No specific risk factors are known.

RELATED DRUGS: No information is available.

MANAGEMENT OPTIONS:

➡ *Avoid Unless Benefit Outweighs Risk.* If possible, avoid danazol in patients receiving carbamazepine.

➡ *Monitor.* Monitor patients on carbamazepine for evidence of carbamazepine toxicity for several weeks after danazol is initiated. Carbamazepine dosage may need to be reduced. Stopping danazol therapy may result in decreasing carbamazepine serum concentrations and response, necessitating an increase in carbamazepine dosage.

REFERENCES:

Kramer G, et al. Carbamazepine-danazol drug interaction: its mechanism examined by a stable isotope technique. *Ther Drug Monit.* 1986;8:387.

Zielinski JJ, et al. Clinically significant danazol-carbamazepine interaction. *Ther Drug Monit.* 1987;9:24.

② Carbamazepine (eg, *Tegretol*)

Diltiazem (*Cardizem*)

SUMMARY: Diltiazem increases carbamazepine serum concentrations, and frequently results in carbamazepine toxicity.

RISK FACTORS: No specific risk factors are known.

RELATED DRUGS: Verapamil can produce carbamazepine toxicity, but limited evidence suggests that nifedipine is less likely to do so. Felodipine undergoes extensive first-pass metabolism and is highly susceptible to enzyme induction; thus, it may be difficult to achieve therapeutic felodipine concentrations in the presence of carbamazepine. (Also see Carbamazepine/Verapamil and Carbamazepine/Felodipine monographs.)

MANAGEMENT OPTIONS:

➡ ***Avoid Unless Benefit Outweighs Risk.*** Given the high likelihood of carbamazepine toxicity with concurrent use and the possibility of reduced diltiazem effect, it would be best to avoid the combination if possible. (See Related Drugs section for possible alternative calcium channel blockers.)

➡ ***Monitor.*** If the combination is used, monitor for carbamazepine toxicity (eg, nausea, vomiting, dizziness, drowsiness, headache, diplopia, and confusion). Toxic symptoms are likely to occur within 2 to 3 days of starting diltiazem.

REFERENCES:

Brodie MJ, et al. Carbamazepine neurotoxicity precipitated by diltiazem. *BMJ.* 1986;292:1170.

Elmer M, et al. Elevated serum carbamazepine concentrations following diltiazem initiation. *Drug Intell Clin Pharm.* 1987;21:340.

Bahls F, et al. Interactions between calcium channel blockers and the anticonvulsants carbamazepine and phenytoin. *Neurol.* 1991;41:740.

Gadde K, et al. Diltiazem effect on carbamazepine levels in manic depression. *J Clin Psych.* 1990;10:378.

Ahmad S. Diltiazem-carbamazepine interaction. *Am Heart J.* 1990;120:1485.

③ Carbamazepine (eg, *Tegretol*)

Doxycycline (eg, *Vibramycin*)

SUMMARY: Doxycycline serum concentrations may be reduced by carbamazepine.

RISK FACTORS: No specific risk factors are known.

RELATED DRUGS: The effect of carbamazepine on other tetracyclines has not been established, but an interaction does not seem likely because they are largely excreted renally.

MANAGEMENT OPTIONS:

➠ *Monitor.* When carbamazepine and doxycycline are used concomitantly, be alert for a decreased clinical response to doxycycline.

REFERENCES:
Penttila O, et al. Interaction between doxycycline and some antiepileptic drugs. *BMJ.* 1974;2:470.

Carbamazepine (eg, *Tegretol*)

Erythromycin (eg, *E-Mycin*)

SUMMARY: Erythromycin markedly increases serum carbamazepine concentrations; numerous cases of carbamazepine toxicity have been reported in patients receiving both drugs.

RISK FACTORS: No specific risk factors are known.

RELATED DRUGS: Troleandomycin (*TAO*) and clarithromycin (*Biaxin*) also may produce carbamazepine toxicity. Azithromycin (*Zithromax*) and dirithromycin (*Dynabac*) would not be likely to cause carbamazepine toxicity.

MANAGEMENT OPTIONS:

➠ *Consider Alternative.* If possible, avoid erythromycin and troleandomycin in patients receiving carbamazepine. Azithromycin does not appear to affect carbamazepine.

➠ *Monitor.* If erythromycin is used in patients receiving carbamazepine, monitor for evidence of carbamazepine toxicity (eg, dizziness, drowsiness, nausea, vomiting, ataxia, headache, nystagmus, blurred vision), and reduce the dose of carbamazepine if necessary. Carbamazepine dosage may need to be increased when erythromycin is stopped.

REFERENCES:
Mesdjian E, et al. Carbamazepine intoxication due to triacetyloleandomycin administration in epileptic patients. *Epilepsia.* 1980;21:489.

Hedrick R, et al. Carbamazepine-erythromycin interaction leading to carbamazepine toxicity in four epileptic children. *Ther Drug Monit.* 1983;5:405.

Jaster PJ, et al. Erythromycin-carbamazepine interaction. *Neurology* 1986;36:594.

Goulden KJ, et al. Severe carbamazepine intoxication after coadministration of erythromycin. *J Pediatr.* 1986;109:135.

Berrettini WH. A case of erythromycin-induced carbamazepine toxicity. *J Clin Psychiatry.* 1986;47:147.

McNab AJ, et al. Heart block secondary to erythromycin-induced carbamazepine toxicity. *Pediatrics.* 1987;80:951.

Mitsch RA. Carbamazepine toxicity precipitated by intravenous erythromycin. *Drug Intell Clin Pharm.* 1989;23:878.

Wong YY, et al. Effect of erythromycin on carbamazepine kinetics. *Clin Pharmacol Ther.* 1983;33:460.

Carbamazepine (eg, *Tegretol*)

Felbamate (*Felbatol*)

SUMMARY: Felbamate modestly reduces plasma carbamazepine concentrations and increases plasma concentrations of carbamazepine-10,11-epoxide, the active metabolite of carbamazepine, resulting in signs of carbamazepine toxicity. Carbamazepine appears to decrease serum felbamate concentrations. The clinical importance of these changes is not established.

RISK FACTORS: No specific risk factors are known.

RELATED DRUGS: No information is available.

MANAGEMENT OPTIONS:

➥ ***Monitor.*** Serum concentrations of carbamazepine epoxide are not usually clinically available; therefore, patients need to be monitored for signs of carbamazepine toxicity that may occur concurrently with reductions in serum carbamazepine. Symptoms of carbamazepine toxicity include drowsiness, dizziness, nausea, vomiting, ataxia, headache, nystagmus, and blurred vision. It is not clear whether an alteration in felbamate dosage is needed when carbamazepine therapy is initiated or discontinued.

REFERENCES:

Graves NM, et al. Effects of felbamate on phenytoin and carbamazepine serum concentrations. *Epilepsia.* 1989;30:488.

Graves NM, et al. The effect of felbamate on the major metabolites of carbamazepine. *Pharmacotherapy.* 1989;9:196.

Albani F, et al. Effect of felbamate on plasma levels of carbamazepine and its metabolites. *Epilepsia* 1991;32:130.

Wilensky AJ, et al. Pharmacokinetics of W-544 (ADD03055) in epileptic patients. *Epilepsia.* 1985;26:602.

Wagner ML, et al. Discontinuation of phenytoin and carbamazepine in patients receiving felbamate. *Epilepsia.* 1991;32:398.

② **Carbamazepine (eg, *Tegretol*)**

Felodipine (*Plendil*)

SUMMARY: Felodipine bioavailability may be reduced dramatically in the presence of carbamazepine therapy.

RISK FACTORS: No specific risk factors are known.

RELATED DRUGS: Most calcium channel blockers have reduced bioavailability in the presence of enzyme inducers, but felodipine is probably one of the most markedly affected. Some calcium channel blockers (eg, diltiazem [eg, *Cardizem*] and verapamil [eg, *Calan*]) can produce carbamazepine toxicity. (Also see Carbamazepine/Diltiazem and Carbamazepine/Verapamil monographs.)

MANAGEMENT OPTIONS:

➥ ***Avoid Unless Benefit Outweighs Risk.*** Because it may prove difficult to achieve therapeutic felodipine concentrations in the presence of carbamazepine, even if the felodipine dose is increased, it may be prudent to avoid concurrent use when possible. Keep in mind that the metabolism of most, if not all, calcium channel blockers is enhanced by enzyme inducers, and some calcium channel blockers (eg, diltiazem, verapamil) regularly produce carbamazepine toxicity.

➡️ **Monitor.** If felodipine or another calcium channel blocker is used with carbamazepine, monitor for reduced calcium channel blocker response.

REFERENCES:
Capwell S, et al. Gross reduction in felodipine bioavailablility in patients taking anticonvulsants. *Br J Clin Pharmacol.* 1987;24:243P.

Carbamazepine (eg, *Tegretol*)

Fluconazole (*Diflucan*)

SUMMARY: Fluconazole administration may result in elevated carbamazepine concentrations with signs of toxicity.

RISK FACTORS:

➡️ **Dosage Regimen.** Fluconazole doses of 200 mg/day or higher have been noted to produce more profound inhibition of CYP3A4.

RELATED DRUGS: Ketoconazole (eg, *Nizoral*) and itraconazole (*Sporanox*) would be expected to inhibit carbamazepine metabolism. Fluconazole is known to inhibit the metabolism of phenytoin (eg, *Dilantin*), particularly when fluconazole doses exceed 200 mg/day.

MANAGEMENT OPTIONS:

➡️ **Consider Alternative.** Terbinafine (*Lamisil*) is an antifungal agent that does not affect the activity of CYP3A4. Depending on the indication for carbamazepine, an alternative such as gabapentin (*Neurontin*) could be considered.

➡️ **Monitor.** Carefully monitor patients stabilized on carbamazepine for increased carbamazepine concentrations and side effects (eg, sedation, lethargy) if fluconazole is added to their therapy.

REFERENCES:
Nair DR, et al. Potential fluconazole-carbamazepine toxicity. *Ann Phamacother.* 1999;33;790–92.

Carbamazepine (eg, *Tegretol*)

Fluoxetine (*Prozac*)

SUMMARY: Case reports describe carbamazepine toxicity, parkinsonism, and serotonin syndrome with concurrent use of fluoxetine, but data from pharmacokinetic studies are conflicting; one study found increased carbamazepine plasma concentrations, and another did not.

RISK FACTORS: No specific risk factors are known.

RELATED DRUGS: Fluvoxamine (*Luvox*) inhibits CYP3A4 and would be expected to inhibit carbamazepine metabolism. The effect of paroxetine (*Paxil*) and sertraline (*Zoloft*) on CYP3A4 is not established (but is being studied).

MANAGEMENT OPTIONS:

➡️ **Monitor.** Until additional information is available to resolve this interaction, monitor for altered carbamazepine response if fluoxetine is initiated, discontinued, or changed in dosage. Also be alert for evidence of parkinsonism or a serotonin syndrome in patients receiving the combination.

REFERENCES:

Pearson HJ. Interaction of fluoxetine with carbamazepine. *J Clin Psychiatry*. 1990;51:126.

Gernaat HBPE, et al. Fluoxetine and parkinsonism in patients taking carbamazepine. *Am J Psychiatry*. 1991;148:1604.

Dursun SM, et al. Toxic serotonin syndrome after fluoxetine plus carbamazepine. *Lancet*. 1993;342:442.

Grimsley SR, et al. Increased carbamazepine plasma concentrations after fluoxetine coadministration. *Clin Pharmacol Ther*. 1991;50:10.

Spina E, et al. Carbamazepine coadministration with fluoxetine or fluvoxamine. *Ther Drug Monit*. 1993;15:247.

Gidal BE, et al. Evaluation of the effect of fluoxetine on the formation of carbamazepine epoxide. *Ther Drug Monit*. 1993;15:405.

Carbamazepine (eg, *Tegretol*)

Fluvoxamine (*Luvox*)

SUMMARY: Case reports suggest that fluvoxamine can increase plasma carbamazepine concentrations to toxic levels, while one study in epileptic patients found no effect of fluvoxamine on carbamazepine. More study is needed to resolve these conflicting results.

RISK FACTORS: No specific risk factors are known.

RELATED DRUGS: Isolated reports suggest that fluoxetine (*Prozac*) and sertraline (*Zoloft*) may increase carbamazepine serum concentrations, but a causal relationship was not established. Preliminary evidence suggests that paroxetine (*Paxil*) does not affect carbamazepine plasma concentrations, but more study is needed.

MANAGEMENT OPTIONS:

➡ *Monitor.* Until additional information is available to resolve this interaction, monitor for altered carbamazepine response if fluvoxamine is initiated, discontinued, or changed in dosage.

REFERENCES:

Fritze J, et al. Interaction between carbamazepine and fluvoxamine. *Acta Psychiatr Scand*. 1991;84:583.

Spina E, et al. Carbamazepine coadministration with fluoxetine of fluvoxamine. *Ther Drug Monit*. 1993;15:247.

Carbamazepine (eg, *Tegretol*)

Grapefruit Juice

SUMMARY: Grapefruit juice may increase carbamazepine plasma concentrations; avoid grapefruit juice or monitor for evidence of carbamazepine toxicity.

RISK FACTORS: No specific risk factors are known.

RELATED DRUGS: No information is available.

MANAGEMENT OPTIONS:

➡ *Consider Alternative.* Orange juice is unlikely to affect the pharmacokinetics of carbamazepine.

➡ *Monitor.* If grapefruit juice is taken concurrently with carbamazepine, monitor for evidence of carbamazepine toxicity (eg, nausea, vomiting, dizziness, drowsiness, headache, diplopia, confusion). Adjust carbamazepine dosage as needed.

REFERENCES:

Bonin B, et al. Effect of grapefruit intake on carbamazepine bioavailability: a case report. *Thérapie.* 2001;56:69-71.

Garg SK, et al. Effect of grapefruit juice on carbamazepine bioavailability in patients with epilepsy. *Clin Pharmacol Ther.* 1998;64:286-288.

Carbamazepine (eg, *Tegretol*)

Haloperidol (eg, *Haldol*)

SUMMARY: Carbamazepine appears to decrease serum haloperidol concentrations and inhibit the response to haloperidol in some patients.

RISK FACTORS: No specific risk factors are known.

RELATED DRUGS: The effect of carbamazepine on other butyrophenones is not established.

MANAGEMENT OPTIONS:

➡ *Monitor.* Be alert for evidence of reduced haloperidol effect if carbamazepine is given concurrently.

REFERENCES:

Arana GW, et al. Does carbamazepine-induced reduction of plasma haloperidol levels worsen psychotic symptoms? *Am J Psychiatry.* 1986;143:650.

Jann MW, et al. Effects of carbamazepine on plasma haloperidol levels. *J Clin Psychopharmacol.* 1985;5:106.

Kidron R, et al. Carbamazepine-induced reduction of blood levels of haloperidol in chronic schizophrenia. *Biol Psychiatry.* 1985;20:219.

Forsman A, et al. Applied pharmacokinetics of haloperidol in man. *Curr Ther Res Clin Exp.* 1977;21:396.

Klein E, et al. Carbamazepine and haloperidol vs. placebo and haloperidol in excited psychoses; a controlled study. *Arch Gen Psychiatry.* 1984;41:165.

Kahn EM, et al. Change in haloperidol level due to carbamazepine: a complicating factor in combined medication for schizophrenia. *J Clin Psychopharmacol.* 1990;10:54.

Carbamazepine (eg, *Tegretol*)

Imipramine (eg, *Tofranil*)

SUMMARY: Preliminary evidence suggests that carbamazepine reduces serum concentrations of imipramine; other cyclic antidepressants probably are affected similarly.

RISK FACTORS: No specific risk factors are known.

RELATED DRUGS: Because cyclic antidepressants are metabolized primarily by the liver, one would expect most of them to be affected by carbamazepine. In one retrospective analysis, patients on concurrent carbamazepine therapy had significantly lower concentration/dose ratios of amitriptyline (eg, *Elavil*) (n = 10) and nortriptyline (eg, *Pamelor*) (n = 8) when compared with patients on monotherapy. In addition, carbamazepine increased the oral clearance of single doses of desipramine 30% in 6 normal volunteers. The effect of carbamazepine on other cyclic antidepressants is not known, but because most of them are extensively metabolized by the liver, they probably would also be affected by carbamazepine therapy.

MANAGEMENT OPTIONS:

➡ **Monitor.** Patients on chronic carbamazepine therapy may require larger than expected doses of cyclic and related antidepressants. Monitor patients for altered response to these antidepressants if carbamazepine therapy is started or stopped.

REFERENCES:

Moody JP, et al. Pharmacokinetic aspects of protriptyline plasma levels. *Eur J Clin Pharmacol.* 1977;11:51.

Brown CS, et al. Possible influence of carbamazepine on plasma imipramine concentration in children with attention-deficit hyperactivity disorder. *J Clin Psychopharmacol.* 1990;10:359.

De La Fuente JM. Carbamazepine-induced low plasma levels of tricyclic antidepressants. *J Clin Psychopharmacol.* 1991;12:67.

Spina E, et al. The effect of carbamazepine on the 2-hydroxylation of desipramine. *Psychopharmacology.* 1995;117:413.

Jerling M, et al. The use of therapeutic drug monitoring data to document kinetic drug interactions: an example with amitriptyline and nortriptyline. *Ther Drug Monit.* 1994;16:1.

Carbamazepine (eg, *Tegretol*)

Isoniazid (INH; eg, *Nydrazid*)

SUMMARY: Isoniazid appears to increase serum carbamazepine concentrations in most patients; symptoms of carbamazepine toxicity may occur. The interaction seems most likely to occur with INH doses of at least 200 mg/day, and carbamazepine toxicity may occur within the first day or two of INH therapy.

RISK FACTORS:

➡ **Dosage Regimen.** INH doses higher than 200 mg/day can increase the risk of interaction.

RELATED DRUGS: No information is available.

MANAGEMENT OPTIONS:

➡ **Monitor.** Isoniazid is likely to reduce the dosage requirements for carbamazepine in a majority of patients. Watch for symptoms of carbamazepine toxicity (dizziness, drowsiness, nausea, vomiting, ataxia, headache, nystagmus, blurred vision), and monitor serum carbamazepine concentrations if possible. Monitor for evidence of reduced serum carbamazepine concentrations when INH is discontinued or reduced in dosage.

REFERENCES:

Block SH. Carbamazepine-isoniazid interaction. *Pediatrics.* 1982;69:494.

Valsalan VC, et al. Carbamazepine intoxication caused with isoniazid. *BMJ.* 1982;285:261.

Wright JM, et al. Isoniazid-induced carbamazepine toxicity and vice versa. *N Engl J Med.* 1982;307:1325.

Carbamazepine (eg, *Tegretol*)

Isotretinoin (*Accutane*)

SUMMARY: In one patient, isotretinoin decreased the area under the concentration-time curve (AUC) of carbamazepine and carbamazepine epoxide, the active metabolite of carbamazepine. The clinical importance of this effect is unknown.

RISK FACTORS: No specific risk factors are known.

RELATED DRUGS: No information is available.

MANAGEMENT OPTIONS:

➡ *Monitor.* Be alert for evidence of a reduced response to carbamazepine if isotretinoin is given concurrently. Until the clinical significance of this interaction is determined, monitor plasma concentrations of carbamazepine more frequently when the 2 drugs are given concurrently.

REFERENCES:

Marsden JR. Effect of isotretinoin on carbamazepine pharmacokinetics. *Br J Dermatol.* 1988;119:403.

Carbamazepine (eg, *Tegretol*)

Ketoconazole (eg, *Nizoral*)

SUMMARY: The administration of ketoconazole to patients stabilized on carbamazepine may increase carbamazepine concentrations; toxicity could result.

RISK FACTORS: No specific risk factors are known.

RELATED DRUGS: Other antifungal agents that are known to inhibit CYP3A4 (eg, itraconazole [*Sporanox*], fluconazole [*Diflucan*]) would be expected to increase carbamazepine concentrations in a similar manner.

MANAGEMENT OPTIONS:

➡ *Consider Alternative.* Consider the use of an alternative antifungal agent such as terbinafine (*Lamisil*) that does not inhibit CYP3A4 activity.

➡ *Circumvent/Minimize.* Adjust the carbamazepine dosage to maintain therapeutic concentrations when ketoconazole is coadministered.

➡ *Monitor.* Monitor patients receiving carbamazepine and ketoconazole for increased carbamazepine concentrations and possible toxicity. Consider the potential for reduced ketoconazole efficacy.

REFERENCES:

Spina E, et al. Elevation of plasma carbamazepine concentrations by ketoconazole in patients with epilepsy. *Ther Drug Monit.* 1997;19:535.

Carbamazepine (eg, *Tegretol*)

Lamotrigine (*Lamictal*)

SUMMARY: Lamotrigine may increase the carbamazepine epoxide to carbamazepine ratio and result in signs of carbamazepine toxicity. Carbamazepine reduces the concentrations of lamotrigine. The clinical importance of these changes in not established.

RISK FACTORS: No specific risk factors are known.

RELATED DRUGS: No information is available.

MANAGEMENT OPTIONS:

➡ *Monitor.* Serum concentrations of carbamazepine epoxide usually are not clinically available; therefore, patients need to be monitored for signs of carbamazepine toxicity that may occur concurrent with reductions in serum carbamazepine. Symptoms of carbamazepine toxicity include drowsiness, dizziness, nausea, vomiting, ataxia, headache, nystagmus, and blurred vision. Doses of carbamazepine may need to be reduced. It is not clear whether an alteration in lamotrigine dosage is needed when carbamazepine therapy is initiated or discontinued.

REFERENCES:

Warner T, et al. Lamotrigine induced carbamazepine toxicity: an interaction with carbamazepine-10,11-epoxide. *Epilepsy Res.* 1992;11:147.

Graves N, et al. Effect of lamotrigine on the carbamazepine epoxide concentrations. *Epilepsia.* 1991;32(Suppl. 3):13.

Pisani F, et al. Single dose pharmacokinetics of carbamazepine-10,11-epoxide in patients on lamotrigine monotherapy. *Epilepsy Res.* 1994;19:245.

Jawad S, et al. Lamotrigine: single dose pharmacokinetics and initial 1 week experience in refractory epilepsy. *Epilepsy Res.* 1987;1:194.

 Carbamazepine (eg, *Tegretol*)

Lithium (eg, *Eskalith*)

SUMMARY: Several cases of neurotoxicity (in the absence of toxic serum lithium concentrations) have been reported in patients receiving lithium and carbamazepine, but the combination has been used to advantage in some manic patients. Lithium reverses carbamazepine-induced leukopenia but additive antithyroidal effects can occur.

RISK FACTORS: No specific risk factors are known.

RELATED DRUGS: No information is available.

MANAGEMENT OPTIONS:

➡ ***Monitor.*** Be alert for evidence of lithium toxicity when carbamazepine is given concurrently. It is not yet established whether plasma lithium concentrations are useful in monitoring this interaction since the carbamazepine might increase the effect of lithium without increasing plasma lithium concentrations.

REFERENCES:

Ghose K. Effect of carbamazepine in polyuria associated with lithium therapy. *Pharmacopsychiatria.* 1978;11:241.

Chaudhry RP, et al. Lithium and carbamazepine interaction: possible neurotoxicity. *J Clin Psychiatry.* 1983;44:30.

Lipinski JF, et al. Possible synergistic action between carbamazepine and lithium carbonate in the treatment of three acutely manic patients. *Am J Psychiatry.* 1982;139:948.

Laird KL, et al. The use of carbamazepine and lithium in controlling a case of chronic rapid cycling. *Pharmacotherapy.* 1987;7:130.

Kramlinger KG, et al. Addition of lithium carbonate to carbamazepine: hematological and thyroid effects. *Am J Psychiatry.* 1990;147:5.

 Carbamazepine (eg, *Tegretol*)

Mebendazole (eg, *Vermox*)

SUMMARY: Carbamazepine decreases plasma mebendazole concentrations. This may be most important when large oral doses of mebendazole are used for the treatment of *Echinococcus multilocularis* or *Echinococcus granulosus* (hydatid disease).

RISK FACTORS: No specific risk factors are known.

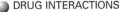

RELATED DRUGS: Theoretically, carbamazepine could affect thiabendazole (*Mintezol*) in a similar manner.

MANAGEMENT OPTIONS:

➡ *Consider Alternative.* No special precautions appear necessary during cotherapy with carbamazepine in patients receiving mebendazole to treat intestinal helminths. However, in patients receiving mebendazole for tissue-dwelling organisms, avoid enzyme-inducing drugs if possible. If carbamazepine is being used for seizures in such patients, valproic acid could be considered as an alternative to carbamazepine, because it does not appear to reduce plasma mebendazole concentrations.

➡ *Monitor.* If carbamazepine is used with mebendazole (for tissue-dwelling organisms), monitor for reduced mebendazole effect.

REFERENCES:

Luder PJ, et al. Treatment of hydatid disease with high oral doses of mebendazole. Long-term follow-up of plasma mebendazole levels and drug interactions. *Eur J Clin Pharmacol.* 1986;31:443.

Witassek F, et al. Chemotherapy of larval echinococcus with mebendazole: microsomal liver function and cholestasis as determinants of plasma drug level. *Eur J Clin Pharmacol.* 1983;25:85.

Bekhti A, et al. A correlation between serum mebendazole concentrations and the aminopyrine breath test. Implications in the treatment of hydatid disease. *Br J Clin Pharmacol* 1986;21:223.

Carbamazepine (eg, *Tegretol*)
Methadone (eg, *Dolophine*)

SUMMARY: Carbamazepine may decrease serum methadone concentrations, thereby increasing symptoms associated with narcotic withdrawal.

RISK FACTORS: No specific risk factors are known.

RELATED DRUGS: Other enzyme-inducing drugs (eg, barbiturates, phenytoin [eg, *Dilantin*]) may interact similarly.

MANAGEMENT OPTIONS:

➡ *Monitor.* Patients receiving enzyme inducers such as carbamazepine may require larger doses of methadone than patients who are not on enzyme inducers. Observe for symptoms of methadone withdrawal such as lacrimation, rhinorrhea, sweating, restlessness, insomnia, and piloerection.

REFERENCES:

Bell J, et al. The use of serum methadone levels in patients receiving methadone maintenance. *Clin Pharmacol Ther.* 1988;43:623.

Carbamazepine (eg, *Tegretol*)
Methylphenidate (eg, *Ritalin*)

SUMMARY: Isolated cases suggest that carbamazepine may reduce methylphenidate's effect in attention deficit disorders.

RISK FACTORS: No specific risk factors are known.

RELATED DRUGS: No information is available.

MANAGEMENT OPTIONS:

➡ *Monitor.* Watch for evidence of reduced methylphenidate response if carbamazepine is given concurrently. Substantially increasing the methylphenidate dose to overcome the interaction may be necessary.

REFERENCES:

Behar D, et al. Extreme reduction of methylphenidate levels by carbamazepine. *J Am Acad Child Adolesc Psychiatry.* 1998;37:1128.

Schaller JL, et al. Carbamazepine and methylphenidate in ADHD. *J Am Acad Child Adolesc Psychiatry.* 1999;38:112.

 Carbamazepine (eg, *Tegretol*)

Metronidazole (eg, *Flagyl*)

SUMMARY: Metronidazole may increase carbamazepine plasma concentrations resulting in symptoms of toxicity (eg, dizziness, nausea, diplopia).

RISK FACTORS: No specific risk factors are known.

RELATED DRUGS: No information is available.

MANAGEMENT OPTIONS:

➡ *Monitor.* Until more definitive studies of this interaction are available, monitor patients receiving carbamazepine for altered response and plasma concentrations if metronidazole therapy is initiated or discontinued.

REFERENCES:

Patterson BD. Possible interaction between metronidazole and carbamazepine. *Ann Pharmacother.* 1994;28:1303.

 Carbamazepine (eg, *Tegretol*)

Midazolam (*Versed*)

SUMMARY: Carbamazepine markedly reduces the effect of oral midazolam, but parenteral midazolam is likely to be less affected.

RISK FACTORS:

➡ *Route of Administration.* Because the majority of the interaction is likely caused by increased presystemic metabolism of oral midazolam by the gut wall and liver, parenteral midazolam is likely to be much less affected.

RELATED DRUGS: Triazolam (eg, *Halcion*) and alprazolam (eg, *Xanax*) and to some extent diazepam (eg, *Valium*) also are metabolized by CYP3A4 and would be expected to interact with enzyme inducers in a manner similar to midazolam.

MANAGEMENT OPTIONS:

➡ *Consider Alternative.* When midazolam is used orally as a sedative-hypnotic (as it is in several countries) patients receiving enzyme inducers such as carbamazepine are unlikely to respond unless very large doses of midazolam are used. Thus, it may be preferable to use alternative sedative-hypnotics in such patients.

➥ *Monitor.* Although parenteral midazolam is likely to be much less affected, monitor for inadequate midazolam effect and increase its dose if needed.

REFERENCES:
Backman JT, et al. Concentrations and effects of oral midazolam are greatly reduced in patients treated with carbamazepine or phenytoin. *Epilepsia.* 1996;37:253.

Carbamazepine (eg, *Tegretol*)
Omeprazole (*Prilosec*)

SUMMARY: Omeprazole may increase carbamazepine plasma concentrations; however, studies are conflicting.

RISK FACTORS: No specific risk factors are known.

RELATED DRUGS: The effect of lansoprazole (*Prevacid*) on carbamazepine is not established; in general, lansoprazole has little effect on drug metabolizing enzymes.

MANAGEMENT OPTIONS:

➥ *Monitor.* Until additional information is available, monitor for altered carbamazepine response if omeprazole is initiated, discontinued, or changed in dosage. Carbamazepine toxicity can result in dizziness, drowsiness, headache, diplopia, nausea, and vomiting.

REFERENCES:
Naidu MUR, et al. Effect of multiple dose omeprazole on the pharmacokinetics of carbamazepine. *Drug Invest.* 1994;7:8.

Bottiger Y, et al. No effect on plasma carbamazepine concentration with concomitant omeprazole treatment. *Clin Drug Invest.* 1995;9:180.

Carbamazepine (eg, *Tegretol*)
Phenytoin (eg, *Dilantin*)

SUMMARY: Combined use of phenytoin and carbamazepine may decrease the serum concentrations of both drugs. In some patients, however, phenytoin concentrations may increase or stay the same when carbamazepine is added.

RISK FACTORS: No specific risk factors are known.

RELATED DRUGS: No information is available.

MANAGEMENT OPTIONS:

➥ *Monitor.* During coadministration of phenytoin and carbamazepine, serum concentrations of carbamazepine and phenytoin could decrease or phenytoin serum concentrations could increase. Monitor plasma concentrations of both phenytoin and carbamazepine during dosage changes. Also clinically monitor patients to determine if a change of dosage of either drug is required.

REFERENCES:
Christiansen J, et al. Influence of phenobarbital and diphenylhydantoin on plasma carbamazepine levels in patients with epilepsy. *Acta Neurol Scand.* 1973;49:543.

Hansen JM, et al. Carbamazepine-induced acceleration of diphenylhydantoin and warfarin metabolism in man. *Clin Pharmacol Ther.* 1971;12:539.

Cereghino JJ, et al. The efficacy of carbamazepine combinations in epilepsy. *Clin Pharmacol Ther.* 1975;18:733.

Rane A, et al. Kinetics of carbamazepine and its 10,11-epoxide metabolite in children. *Clin Pharmacol Ther.* 1976;19:276.

Windorfer A. Drug interaction during anticonvulsive therapy. *Int J Clin Pharmacol.* 1976;14:236.

Levy RH, et al. Pharmacokinetics of carbamazepine in normal man. *Clin Pharmacol Ther.* 1977;17:657.

Zielinski JJ, et al. Dual effects of carbamazepine-phenytoin interaction. *Ther Drug Monit.* 1987;9:21.

Brown TR, et al. Carbamazepine increases phenytoin serum concentrations and reduces phenytoin clearance. *Neurology.* 1988;38:1146.

Carbamazepine (eg, *Tegretol*)

Propoxyphene (eg, *Darvon-N*)

SUMMARY: Propoxyphene markedly increases plasma carbamazepine concentrations; carbamazepine toxicity is likely to occur in most patients receiving both drugs.

RISK FACTORS: No specific risk factors are known.

RELATED DRUGS: Other analgesics have not been shown to interact with carbamazepine.

MANAGEMENT OPTIONS:

➡ *Use Alternative.* Use analgesics other than propoxyphene in patients receiving carbamazepine.

REFERENCES:

Dam M, et al. Interaction of propoxyphene with carbamazepine. *Lancet.* 1977;2:509.

Hansen BS, et al. Influence of dextropropoxyphene on steady state serum levels and protein binding of three antiepileptic drugs in man. *Acta Neurol Scand.* 1980;61:357.

Yu YL, et al. Interaction between carbamazepine and dextropropoxyphene. *Postgrad Med J.* 1986;62:231.

Kubacka RT, et al. Carbamazepine-propoxyphene interaction. *Clin Pharm.* 1983;2:104.

Carbamazepine (eg, *Tegretol*)

Risperidone (*Risperdal*)

SUMMARY: Carbamazepine appears to reduce risperidone plasma concentrations; adjustment of risperidone dose may be needed.

RISK FACTORS: No specific risk factors are known.

RELATED DRUGS: No information is available.

MANAGEMENT OPTIONS: Be alert for evidence of altered risperidone effect if carbamazepine is initiated, discontinued, or changed in dosage.

REFERENCES:

Takahashi H, et al. Development of parkinsonian symptoms after discontinuation of carbamazepine in patients concurrently treated with risperidone: two case reports. *Clin Neuropharmacol.* 2001;24:358-360.

Spina E, et al. Plasma concentrations of risperidone and 9-hydroxyrisperidone: effect of comedication with carbamazepine or valproate. *Ther Drug Monit.* 2000;22:481-485.

Carbamazepine (eg, *Tegretol*)

Ritonavir (eg, *Norvir*)

SUMMARY: Ritonavir administration appears to increase carbamazepine concentrations; carbamazepine toxicity may result.

RISK FACTORS: No specific risk factors are known.

RELATED DRUGS: Nelfinavir (*Viracept*), saquinavir (eg, *Invirase*), and indinavir (*Crixivan*) also inhibit CYP3A4 and may reduce carbamazepine metabolism to some degree.

MANAGEMENT OPTIONS:

➡ *Monitor.* Monitor patients stabilized on carbamazepine for altered serum concentrations and signs of carbamazepine toxicity if ritonavir is started or discontinued. Also, be alert for reduced antiviral response in patients taking ritonavir and carbamazepine.

REFERENCES:

Mateu-de Antonio J, et al. Ritonavir-induced carbamazepine toxicity. *Ann Pharmacother.* 2001;35:125.

Carbamazepine (eg, *Tegretol*)

Theophylline (eg, *Theolair*)

SUMMARY: Carbamazepine may reduce serum theophylline concentrations, thus increasing theophylline dosage requirements.

RISK FACTORS: No specific risk factors are known.

RELATED DRUGS: No information is available.

MANAGEMENT OPTIONS:

➡ *Monitor.* Be alert for evidence of altered theophylline serum levels when carbamazepine is initiated, discontinued, or changed in dosage.

REFERENCES:

Rosenberry KR, et al. Reduced theophylline half-life induced by carbamazepine therapy. *J Pediatr.* 1983;102:472.

Phenytoin-theophylline-quinidine interactions. *N Engl J Med.* 1983;308:724.

Carbamazepine (eg, *Tegretol*)

Thyroid

SUMMARY: Carbamazepine appears to increase the elimination of thyroid and may increase the requirements for thyroid in hypothyroid patients.

RISK FACTORS: No specific risk factors are known.

RELATED DRUGS: Other enzyme inducers (eg, phenytoin, rifampin) also appear to interact similarly.

MANAGEMENT OPTIONS:

➡ *Monitor.* If carbamazepine therapy is initiated or discontinued in hypothyroid patients receiving thyroid replacement therapy, be alert for clinical and laboratory evidence of altered circulating thyroid concentrations. Adjust thyroid dosage as needed.

REFERENCES:

Blackshear JL, et al. Thyroxine replacement requirements in hypothyroid patients receiving phenytoin. *Ann Intern Med.* 1983;99:341.

Isley WL. Effect of rifampin therapy on thyroid function tests in a hypothyroid patient on replacement L-thyroxine. *Ann Intern Med.* 1987;107:517.

Connell JM, et al. Changes in circulating thyroid hormones during short-term hepatic enzyme induction with carbamazepine. *Eur J Clin Pharmacol.* 1984;26:453.

Cathro DM, et al. Sub-normal serum thyroxine levels associated with carbamazepine and valproic acid treatment. *Nebr Med J.* 1985;70:235.

Roy-Byrne PP, et al. Carbamazepine and thyroid function in affectively ill patients. Clinical and theoretical implications. *Arch Gen Psychiatry.* 1984;41:1150.

Joffe RT, et al. The effects of carbamazepine on the thyrotropin response to thyrotropin-releasing hormone. *Psychiatry Res.* 1984;12:161.

Aanderud S, et al. The influence of carbamazepine on thyroid hormones and thyroxine binding globulin in hypothyroid patients substituted with thyroxine. *Clin Endocrinol.* 1981;15:247.

Carbamazepine (eg, *Tegretol*)

Troleandomycin (*TAO*)

SUMMARY: Troleandomycin may increase plasma carbamazepine concentrations; carbamazepine toxicity has occurred in some patients receiving both drugs.

RISK FACTORS: No specific risk factors are known.

RELATED DRUGS: Erythromycin (eg, *E-Mycin*) and clarithromycin (*Biaxin*) appear to inhibit carbamazepine metabolism. Azithromycin (*Zithromax*) and dirithromycin (*Dynabac*) would be unlikely to interact with carbamazepine.

MANAGEMENT OPTIONS:

➡ *Consider Alternative.* Avoid concomitant use of troleandomycin and carbamazepine if possible. Azithromycin does not appear to alter carbamazepine metabolism.

➡ *Monitor.* When both drugs are used, monitor for evidence of carbamazepine toxicity (dizziness, drowsiness, nausea, vomiting, ataxia, headache, nystagmus, blurred vision), and measure plasma carbamazepine concentrations as needed. Monitor for evidence of reduced serum carbamazepine concentrations when troleandomycin is discontinued or reduced in dosage.

REFERENCES:

Dravet C, et al. Interaction between carbamazepine and triacetyloleandomycin. *Lancet.* 1977;2:810.

Mesdjian E, et al. Carbamazepine intoxication due to triacetyloleandomycin administration in epileptic patients. *Epilepsia.* 1980;21:489.

Carbamazepine (eg, *Tegretol*)

Valproic Acid (eg, *Depakene*)

SUMMARY: Valproic acid can increase, decrease, or have no effect on carbamazepine serum concentrations. Plasma concentrations of carbamazepine-epoxide, the active metabolite, also can increase. Carbamazepine decreases plasma concentrations of valproic acid and larger doses of valproic acid are required to maintain therapeutic steady-state concentrations.

RISK FACTORS: No specific risk factors are known.

RELATED DRUGS: No information is available.

MANAGEMENT OPTIONS:

➠ *Monitor.* The unpredictability of the effect of valproic acid on total carbamazepine plasma concentrations and carbamazepine-epoxide (which is not routinely monitored) makes interpretation of carbamazepine plasma concentrations difficult when the 2 drugs are used concurrently. Carbamazepine-epoxide contributes significantly to the therapeutic and, possibly, the toxic effects of carbamazepine. Monitor patients for symptoms of carbamazepine toxicity and measure serum carbamazepine concentrations. Symptoms of carbamazepine toxicity include drowsiness, dizziness, nausea, vomiting, ataxia, headache, nystagmus, and blurred vision. Monitor for a decreased therapeutic response to carbamazepine when valproic acid is discontinued or reduced in dosage. An increase in valproic acid dose may be needed if carbamazepine is added. Monitor for evidence of valproic acid toxicity if carbamazepine is discontinued or reduced in dosage.

REFERENCES:

Acid DJ, et al. Sodium valproate in the treatment of intractable seizure disorders; a clinical and electroencephalographic study. *Neurology.* 1978;28:152.

Kondo T, et al. The effects of phenytoin and carbamazepine on serum concentrations of mono-unsaturated metabolites of valproic acid. *Br J Clin Pharmacol.* 1990;29:116-19.

Jann MW, et al. Increased valproate serum concentrations upon carbamazepine cessation. *Epilepsia.* 1988;29:578.

Wilder BJ, et al. Valproic acid: interaction with other anticonvulsant drugs. *Neurology.* 1978;28:892.

Rambeck B, et al. Valproic acid-induced carbamazepine-10,11-epoxide toxicity in children and adolescents. *Eur Neurol.* 1990;30:79.

Ramsey RE, et al. Carbamazepine metabolism in humans: effect of concurrent anticonvulsant therapy. *Ther Drug Monit.* 1990;12:235.

Carbamazepine (eg, *Tegretol*)

Verapamil (eg, *Calan*)

SUMMARY: Verapamil increases carbamazepine serum concentrations, and frequently results in carbamazepine toxicity.

RISK FACTORS: No specific risk factors are known.

RELATED DRUGS: Diltiazem also can produce carbamazepine toxicity, but limited evidence suggests that nifedipine is less likely to do so. Felodipine (*Plendil*) undergoes extensive first-pass metabolism and is highly susceptible to enzyme induction; thus, it may be difficult to achieve therapeutic felodipine concentrations in the presence of carbamazepine. (Also see Carbamazepine/Diltiazem and Carbamazepine/Felodipine monographs.)

MANAGEMENT OPTIONS:

➠ *Avoid Unless Benefit Outweighs Risk.* Given the high likelihood of carbamazepine toxicity with concurrent use and the possibility of reduced verapamil effect, it would be best to avoid the combination if possible. (See Related Drugs section for possible alternative calcium channel blockers.)

➠ *Monitor.* If the combination is used, monitor for carbamazepine toxicity (eg, nausea, vomiting, dizziness, drowsiness, headache, diplopia, and confusion). Toxic symptoms are likely to occur within 2 to 3 days of starting the verapamil.

REFERENCES:

Macphee GJ, et al. Verapamil potentiates carbamazepine neurotoxicity: a clinically important inhibitory interaction. *Lancet.* 1986;1:700.

Price WA. Verapamil-carbamazepine neurotoxicity. *J Clin Psych.* 1988;49:80.

Beattie B, et al. Verapamil-induced carbamazepine neurotoxicity. *Eur Neurol.* 1988;28:104.

Bahls F, et al. Interactions between calcium channel blockers and the anticonvulsants carbamazepine and phenytoin. *Neurol.* 1991;41:740.

 Carbamazepine (eg, *Tegretol*)

Warfarin (eg, *Coumadin*)

SUMMARY: Carbamazepine inhibits the hypoprothrombinemic response to oral anticoagulants; adjustments in anticoagulant dosage may be required during cotherapy.

RISK FACTORS: No specific risk factors are known.

RELATED DRUGS: Oral anticoagulants other than warfarin are likely to be similarly affected by carbamazepine.

MANAGEMENT OPTIONS:

➠ *Monitor.* Monitor patients taking oral anticoagulants for altered hypoprothrombinemic response to warfarin if carbamazepine therapy is initiated, discontinued, or changed in dosage; adjust the anticoagulant dose as needed.

REFERENCES:

Hansen JM, et al. Carbamazepine-induced acceleration of diphenylhydantoin and warfarin metabolism in man. *Clin Pharmacol Ther.* 1971;12:539.

Kendall AG, et al. Warfarin-carbamazepine interaction. *Ann Intern Med.* 1981;94:280.

Massey EW. Effect of carbamazepine on coumadin metabolism. *Ann Neurol.* 1983;13:691.

 Carbamazepine (*Tegretol*)

Ziprasidone (*Geodon*)

SUMMARY: Carbamazepine moderately reduces ziprasidone serum concentrations, but the clinical importance of this effect is not established.

RISK FACTORS: No specific risk factors are known.

RELATED DRUGS: Other anticonvulsants such as phenytoin (eg, *Dilantin*), primidone (*Mysoline*), and phenobarbital (eg, *Solfoton*) increase CYP3A4 activity, and would be expected to reduce ziprasidone effect.

MANAGEMENT OPTIONS:

➥ *Monitor.* Monitor for reduced ziprasidone efficacy if carbamazepine is used concurrently. Adjustment of ziprasidone dose may be needed if carbamazepine therapy is initiated, discontinued, or changed in dosage.

REFERENCES:

Miceli JJ, et al. The effect of carbamazepine on the steady-state pharmacokinetics of ziprasidone in healthy volunteers. *Br J Clin Pharmacol.* 2000;49 (suppl 1):65S-70S.

Carbenicillin (*Geocillin*)

Gentamicin (eg, *Garamycin*)

SUMMARY: Carbenicillin and some penicillins inactivate gentamicin and other aminoglycosides in vitro and, in certain patients with severe renal dysfunction, in vivo. The effect of the aminoglycoside can be reduced.

RISK FACTORS:

➥ *Route of Administration.* In vitro mixing of the antibiotics before administration can increase the risk of interaction.

➥ *Concurrent Diseases.* Patients with severe renal dysfunction are at increased risk.

➥ *Assay Delay.* Delay in aminoglycoside assay when penicillin is present in serum can increase the risk of interaction.

RELATED DRUGS: Other extended spectrum penicillins are likely to inactivate some aminoglycosides.

MANAGEMENT OPTIONS:

➥ *Consider Alternative.* Choose an alternative antibiotic for the aminoglycoside or penicillin. Amikacin and netilmicin may be less likely than other aminoglycosides to interact with extended-spectrum penicillins; however, observe the same precautions with all combinations of aminoglycosides and extended-spectrum penicillins.

➥ *Circumvent/Minimize.* Avoid mixing antibiotics in vitro (eg, in the same IV bag or line).

➥ *Monitor.* If the antibiotics must be coadministered, monitor serum gentamicin (or other aminoglycoside) concentrations for evidence of the interaction (note potential for in vitro serum inactivation) and doses adjusted accordingly.

REFERENCES:

Riff LJ, et al. Laboratory and clinical conditions for gentamicin inactivation by carbenicillin. *Arch Intern Med.* 1972;130:887.

McLaughlin JE, et al. Clinical and laboratory evidence for inactivation of gentamicin by carbenicillin. *Lancet.* 1971;1:261.

Ervin FR, et al. Inactivation of gentamicin by penicillins in patients with renal failure. *Antimicrob Agents Chemother.* 1976;9:1004.

Weibert RT, et al. Carbenicillin-gentamicin interaction in acute renal failure. *Am J Hosp Pharm.* 1977;34:1137.

Davies M, et al. Interactions of carbenicillin and ticarcillin with gentamicin. *Antimicrob Agents Chemother.* 1975;7:431.

Henderson JL, et al. *In vitro* inactivation of gentamicin, tobramycin, and netilmicin by carbenicillin, azlocillin, or mezlocillin. *Am J Hosp Pharm.* 1981;38:1167.

Matzke GR, et al. Effect of ticarcillin on gentamicin and tobramycin pharmacokinetics in a patient with end-stage renal disease. *Pharmacotherapy*. 1984;4:158.

Halstenson CE, et al. Effect of concomitant administration of piperacillin on the disposition of netilmicin and tobramycin in patients with end-stage renal disease. *Antimicrob Agents Chemother*. 1990;34:128.

Uber WE, et al. *In vivo* inactivation of tobramycin by piperacillin. *DICP, Ann Pharmacother*. 1991;25:357.

Halstenson CE, et al. Effect of concomitant administration of piperacillin on the dispositions of isepanicin and gentamicin in patients with end-stage renal disease. *Antimicrob Agents Chemother*. 1992;36:1832.

Carbenicillin (*Geocillin*)

Methotrexate

SUMMARY: Administration of carbenicillin and other penicillins may increase methotrexate serum concentrations and may potentiate methotrexate toxicity.

RISK FACTORS: No specific risk factors are known.

RELATED DRUGS: Other penicillins administered in large doses could have similar effects on methotrexate.

MANAGEMENT OPTIONS:

➡ *Monitor.* Monitor patients for evidence of enhanced methotrexate effect and possible toxicity (eg, mucositis, leukopenia) when large doses of carbenicillin or other penicillins are given concurrently.

REFERENCES:

Gibson DL, et al. Midyear Clinical Meeting Abstracts. American Society of Hospital Pharmacists. New Orleans; 1981:305 Dec 6–10.

Dean R, et al. Possible methotrexate-mezlocillin interaction. *Am J Pediatr Hematol Oncol*. 1992;141:88.

Mayall B, et al. Neutropenia due to low-dose methotrexate therapy for psoriasis and rheumatoid arthritis may be fatal. *Med J Aust*. 1991;155:480.

Carbenicillin (*Geocillin*)

Tobramycin (eg, *Nebcin*)

SUMMARY: Carbenicillin and some other penicillins inactivate tobramycin and other aminoglycosides in vitro and, in certain patients with severe renal dysfunction, in vivo. the effect of the aminoglycoside can be reduced.

RISK FACTORS:

➡ *Route of Administration.* In vitro mixing of the antibiotics before administration can increase the risk of interaction.

➡ *Concurrent Diseases.* Patients with severe renal dysfunction are at increased risk.

➡ *Assay Delay.* Delay in aminoglycoside assay when penicillin is present in serum can increase the risk of interaction.

RELATED DRUGS: Other extended spectrum penicillins (eg, ticarcillin, piperacillin) are likely to inactivate some aminoglycosides (eg, gentamicin). Amikacin (eg, *Amikin*) and netilmicin (*Netromycin*) may be less likely to interact with extended spectrum penicillins.

MANAGEMENT OPTIONS:

➡ *Consider Alternative.* Choose an alternative antibiotic for the aminoglycoside or the penicillin. Amikacin and netilmicin may be less likely than other aminoglycosides to interact with extended spectrum penicillins; however, observe the same precautions with all combinations of aminoglycosides and extended spectrum penicillins.

➡ *Circumvent/Minimize.* Avoid mixing antibiotics in vitro (eg, in the same IV bag or line).

➡ *Monitor.* If the antibiotics must be coadministered, evaluations of serum tobramycin (or other aminoglycoside) concentrations should consider the possibility of the interaction (note potential) for in vitro serum inactivational and adjust doses accordingly.

REFERENCES:

Riff LJ, et al. Laboratory and clinical conditions for gentamicin inactivation by carbenicillin. *Arch Intern Med.* 1972;130:887.

McLaughlin JE, et al. Clinical and laboratory evidence for inactivation of gentamicin by carbenicillin. *Lancet.* 1971;1:261.

Ervin FR, et al. Inactivation of gentamicin by penicillins in patients with renal failure. *Antimicrob Agents Chemother.* 1976;9:1004.

Weibert RT, et al. Carbenicillin-gentamicin interaction in acute renal failure. *Am J Hosp Pharm.* 1977;34:1137.

Davies M, et al. Interactions of carbenicillin and ticarcillin with gentamicin. *Antimicrob Agents Chemother.* 1975;7:431.

Henderson JL, et al. In vitro inactivation of gentamicin, tobramycin, and netilmicin by carbenicillin, azlocillin, or mezlocillin. *Am J Hosp Pharm.* 1981;38:1167.

Matzke GR, et al. Effect of ticarcillin on gentamicin and tobramycin pharmacokinetics in a patient with end-stage renal disease. *Pharmacotherapy.* 1984;4:158.

Halstenson CE, et al. Effect of concomitant administration of piperacillin on the disposition of netilmicin and tobramycin in patients with end-stage renal disease. *Antimicrob Agents Chemother.* 1990;34:128.

Uber WE, et al. In vivo inactivation of tobramycin by piperacillin. *DICP. Ann Pharmacother.* 1991;25:357.

Halstenson CE, et al. Effect of concomitant administration of piperacillin on the disposition of isepanicin and gentamicin in patients with end-stage renal disease. *Antimicrob Agents Chemother.* 1992;36:1832.

Carbenoxolone

Chlorthalidone (eg, *Hygroton*)

SUMMARY: Severe hypokalemia may result from the coadministration of carbenoxolone and chlorthalidone.

RISK FACTORS: No specific risk factors are known.

RELATED DRUGS: The combination of carbenoxolone with other potassium-wasting diuretics such as furosemide (eg, *Lasix*), bumetanide (eg, *Bumex*), metolazone (eg, *Zaroxolyn*), or thiazides would most likely produce a similar effect, especially in the absence of potassium supplementation.

MANAGEMENT OPTIONS:

➡ *Monitor.* Closely monitor the potassium status of patients receiving carbenoxolone and a potassium-wasting. Potassium supplementation may be necessary.

REFERENCES:

Descamps C. Rhabdomyolysis and acute tubular necrosis associated with carbenoxolone and diuretic treatment. *BMJ.* 1977;1:272.

Carboplatin (*Paraplatin*)

Gentamicin (eg, *Garamycin*)

SUMMARY: The combination of carboplatin and aminoglycoside antibiotics causes more hearing loss than would be expected with either agent alone.

RISK FACTORS: No specific risk factors are known.

RELATED DRUGS: It is likely that other aminoglycosides such as amikacin (eg, *Amikin*), kanamycin (eg, *Kantrex*), netilmicin (*Netromycin*), streptomycin, and tobramycin (eg, *Nebcin*) also may result in additive ototoxicity with carboplatin.

MANAGEMENT OPTIONS:

➡ *Consider Alternative.* Consider alternatives to aminoglycosides in patients receiving high doses of carboplatin.

➡ *Monitor.* If aminoglycosides are used, be alert for evidence of ototoxicity.

REFERENCES:

Lee EJ, et al. Phase I and pharmacokinetic trial of carboplatin in refractory adult leukemia. *J Natl Cancer Inst.* 1988;80:131-35.

Carisoprodol (eg, *Soma*)

Oxycodone (eg, *Oxycontin*)

SUMMARY: A patient on oxycodone became unconscious after adding an excessive dose of carisoprodol.

RISK FACTORS: No specific risk factors are known.

RELATED DRUGS: Carisoprodol should be expected to increase the CNS depression of opiates other than oxycodone as well.

MANAGEMENT OPTIONS:

➡ *Monitor.* Use carisoprodol and oxycodone (or other opiates) concomitantly only with careful monitoring for excessive CNS depression.

REFERENCES:

Reeves RR, et al. Possible dangerous interaction of *Oxycontin* and carisoprodol. *Am Fam Physician.* 2003;67:2273.

Carmustine (eg, *BiCNU*)

Cimetidine (eg, *Tagamet*)

SUMMARY: Epidemiological evidence indicates that cimetidine increases the myelotoxicity of carmustine.

RISK FACTORS: No specific risk factors are known.

RELATED DRUGS: Little is known regarding the effect of cimetidine on the myelosuppressive effect of other cytotoxic drugs, but be alert for such effects. Isolated reports indicate that chloramphenicol (eg, *Chloromycetin*) and phenytoin (eg, *Dilantin*) may be more myelosuppressive in the presence of cimetidine. A similar interaction has been reported with lomustine (*CeeNu*), another nitrosourea. Severe myelosuppression developed in a 55-year-old man receiving lomustine and cimetidine and resolved rapidly upon discontinuation of cimetidine. Myelosuppression from subsequent doses of lomustine, after the cimetidine had been discontinued, was less severe. The effect of other H_2-receptor antagonists such as famotidine (eg, *Pepcid*), nizatidine (eg, *Axid*), and ranitidine (eg, *Zantac*) on carmustine is not established; theoretically, they may be less likely to interact.

MANAGEMENT OPTIONS:

➡ *Consider Alternative.* Other H_2-receptor antagonists theoretically would be less likely to interact.

➡ *Monitor.* Until more is known regarding the incidence and magnitude of this potential interaction, monitor carefully for evidence of excessive bone marrow suppression when cimetidine is used concurrently with carmustine or other myelosuppressive drugs.

REFERENCES:

Selker RG, et al. Bone-marrow depression with cimetidine plus carmustine. *N Engl J Med.* 1978;299:834.

Volkin RL, et al. Potentiation of carmustine-cranial irradiation-induced myelosuppression by cimetidine. *Arch Intern Med.* 1982;142:243-245.

Farber BF, et al. Rapid development of aplastic anemia after intravenous chloramphenicol and cimetidine therapy. *South Med J.* 1981;74:1257-1258.

Sazie E, et al. Severe granulocytopenia with cimetidine and phenytoin. *Ann Intern Med.* 1980;93:151-152.

Al-Kawas FH, et al. Cimetidine and agranulocytosis. *Ann Intern Med.* 1979;90:992-993.

Hess WA, et al. Combination of lomustine and cimetidine in the treatment of a patient with malignant glioblastoma: a case report. *Cancer Treat Rep.* 1985;69:733.

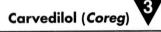

Carvedilol (*Coreg*)

Digoxin (eg, *Lanoxin*)

SUMMARY: Carvedilol appears to modestly increase digoxin concentrations. Some patients may require a reduction in digoxin dose to avoid toxicity.

RISK FACTORS: No specific risk factors are known.

RELATED DRUGS: It is possible that carvedilol would have a similar effect on digitoxin concentrations. No other beta-blockers have been identified as inhibitors of p-glycoprotein transporters.

MANAGEMENT OPTIONS:

➡ *Monitor.* Check digoxin concentrations in patients whenever carvedilol is added or deleted from drug regimens. Watch for signs of digoxin toxicity, including arrhythmias, anorexia, nausea, or visual changes.

REFERENCES:

Takara K, et al. Interaction of digoxin with antihypertensive drugs via MDR1. *Life Sci.* 2002;70:1491-1500.

Kakumoto M, et al. Effects of carvedilol on MDR1-mediated multidrug resistance: comparison with verapamil. *Cancer Sci.* 2003;94:81-86.

De Mey C, et al. Carvedilol increases the systemic bioavailability of oral digoxin. *Br J Clin Pharmacol.* 1990;29:486-490.

Grunden JW, et al. Augmented digoxin concentrations with carvedilol dosing in mild-moderate heart failure. *Am J Ther.* 1994;1:157-161.

Wermeling DP, et al. Effects of long-term oral carvedilol on the steady-state pharmacokinetics of oral digoxin in patients with mild to moderate hypertension. *Pharmacotherapy.* 1994;14:600-606.

Ratnapalan S, et al. Digoxin-carvedilol interactions in children. *J Pediatr.* 2003;142:572-574.

Carvedilol (*Coreg*)

Fluoxetine (eg, *Prozac*)

SUMMARY: Fluoxetine increases the plasma concentrations of carvedilol; the clinical significance is unknown, but increased cardiovascular effects such as hypotension or bradycardia may result.

RISK FACTORS: Extensive metabolizers of CYP2D6 will be affected to a greater degree than poor CYP2D6 metabolizers.

RELATED DRUGS: Paroxetine (*Paxil*) is also a potent inhibitor of CYP2D6 and would be likely to affect carvedilol in a similar manner. Fluoxetine may also inhibit the metabolism of other beta-blockers that are metabolized by CYP2D6, including metoprolol (eg, *Lopressor*), propranolol (eg, *Inderal*), and timolol (eg, *Blocadren*).

MANAGEMENT OPTIONS:

➡ *Consider Alternative.* Other SSRI antidepressants such as citalopram (*Celexa*) or nefazodone (*Serzone*) do not inhibit CYP2D6 and would be less likely to alter carvedilol plasma concentrations. If not treating heart failure, a beta-blocker that does not undergo CYP2D6 metabolism, such as atenolol (eg, *Tenormin*), could be considered.

➡ *Monitor.* Watch for increased alpha- or beta-blocking effects if carvedilol is coadministered with fluoxetine.

REFERENCES:

Graff DW, et al. Effect of fluoxetine on carvedilol stereo-specific pharmacokinetics in patients with heart failure. *Clin Pharmacol Ther*. 1999;65:148.

Cefamandole (*Mandol*)

Ethanol (Ethyl Alcohol)

SUMMARY: Cefamandole and some other cephalosporins may cause a disulfiram-like reaction when administered with ethanol.

RISK FACTORS: No specific risk factors are known.

RELATED DRUGS: Cefoperazone, cefotetan, and moxalactam also produce disulfiram reactions following alcohol ingestion.

MANAGEMENT OPTIONS:

➡ *Circumvent/Minimize.* Counsel patients to avoid alcohol while taking the cephalosporins noted and for 2 to 3 days after discontinuing the cephalosporin.

➡ *Monitor.* If ethanol is administered to a patient taking cefamandole or other cephalosporins, be alert for flushing, nausea, headache, or tachycardia.

REFERENCES:

Neu HC, et al. Interaction between moxalactam and alcohol. *Lancet*. 1980;1:1422.

Portier H, et al. Interaction between cephalosporins and alcohol. *Lancet*. 1980;2:263.

Drummer S, et al. Antabuse-like effect of beta-lactam antibiotics. *N Engl J Med*. 1980;303:1417-1418.

Elenbaas RM, et al. On the disulfiram-like activity of moxalactam. *Clin Pharmacol Ther*. 1982;32:347-355.

Buening MK, et al. Disulfiram-like reaction to beta-lactams. *JAMA*. 1981;245:2027.

Kline SS, et al. Cefotetan-induced disulfiram-type reactions and hypoprothrombinemia. *Antimicrob Agents Chemother*. 1987;31:1328-1331.

Cefpodoxime Proxetil (*Vantin*)

Ranitidine (eg, *Zantac*)

SUMMARY: Serum concentrations of cefpodoxime proxetil are reduced by coadministration of agents that increase gastric pH; antibiotic efficacy may be reduced.

RISK FACTORS: No specific risk factors are known.

RELATED DRUGS: Cefuroxime axetil concentrations are reduced by ranitidine. Cefetamet pivoxil and cefixime (*Suprax*) appear to be unaffected by concurrent ranitidine administration. Other H_2-receptor antagonists [eg, cimetidine (eg, *Tagamet*), nizatidine (*Axid*)], antacids, and proton pump inhibitors [eg, omeprazole (*Prilosec*), lansoprazole (*Prevacid*)] would be expected to have similar effects.

MANAGEMENT OPTIONS:

➡ *Consider Alternative.* Cefetamet pivoxil pharmacokinetics were not affected by *Maalox* or ranitidine administration; similarly, cefixime pharmacokinetics were unaffected by antacids. Pending determination of the clinical importance of the changes in serum concentrations, patients receiving cefpodoxime proxetil or cefuroxime axetil should avoid agents that increase gastric pH.

➡ *Monitor.* If the drugs are used together, watch for diminished antibiotic effect.

REFERENCES:

Hughes GS, et al. The effects of gastric pH and food on the pharmacokinetics of a new oral cephalosporin, cefpodoxime proxetil. *Clin Pharmacol Ther*. 1989;46:674.

Sommers DEK, et al. Influence of food and reduced gastric acidity on the bioavailability of bacampicillin and cefuroxime axetil. *Br J Clin Pharmacol*. 1984;18:535.

Blouin RA, et al. Influence of antacid and ranitidine on the pharmacokinetics of oral cefetamet pivoxil. *Antimicrob Agents Chemother*. 1990;34:1744.

Petitjean O, et al. Study of a possible pharmacokinetic interaction between cefixime and two antacids. *Presse Med*. 1989;18:1596.

Saathoff N, et al. Pharmacokinetics of cefpodoxime proxetil and interactions with an antacid and an H_2-receptor antagonist. *Antimicrob Agents Chemother*. 1992;36:796.

Ceftazidime (*Fortaz*)

Chloramphenicol (eg, *Chloromycetin*)

SUMMARY: Chloramphenicol may inhibit the antibacterial activity of ceftazidime.

RISK FACTORS: No specific risk factors are known.

RELATED DRUGS: Other cephalosporins or antibiotics that inhibit bacterial cell wall synthesis also may be inhibited.

MANAGEMENT OPTIONS:

➡ *Consider Alternative.* Although definitive data are unavailable regarding the interaction of bactericidal and bacteriostatic antibiotics, it would be appropriate to avoid such combinations until they are proven to be without harm.

➡ **Monitor.** If chloramphenicol is used with a cephalosporin, carefully monitor the patient for continuing signs and symptoms of an interaction.

REFERENCES:

French, et al. Antagonism of ceftazidime by chloramphenicol *in vitro* and *in vivo* during treatment of gram negative meningitis. *BMJ.* 1985;291:636.

 Cefuroxime (eg, *Ceftin*)

Ranitidine (eg, *Zantac*)

SUMMARY: Serum concentrations of cefpodoxime proxetil and cefuroxime axetil are reduced by coadministration of agents that increase gastric pH; antibiotic efficacy may be reduced.

RISK FACTORS: No specific risk factors are known.

RELATED DRUGS: Cefpodoxime concentrations are reduced following ranitidine administration. Cefetamet pivoxil and cefixime (*Suprax*) appear to be unaffected by ranitidine coadministration. Other H_2-receptor antagonists (eg, cimetidine [eg, *Tagamet*], famotidine [eg, *Pepcid*], nizatidine [*Axid*]), antacids, and proton pump inhibitors (eg, omeprazole [*Prilosec*], lansoprazole [*Prevacid*]) are expected to have similar effects.

MANAGEMENT OPTIONS:

➡ **Consider Alternative.** Cefetamet pivoxil pharmacokinetics were not affected by *Maalox* or ranitidine administration; similarly, cefixime (*Suprax*) pharmacokinetics were unaffected by antacids. Pending determination of the clinical importance of the changes in serum concentrations, patients receiving cefpodoxime proxetil or cefuroxime axetil should avoid agents that increase gastric pH.

➡ **Monitor.** If the drugs are used together, watch for diminished antibiotic effect.

REFERENCES:

Hughes GS, et al. The effects of gastric pH and food on the pharmacokinetics of a new oral cephalosporin, cefpodoxime proxetil. *Clin Pharmacol Ther.* 1989;46:674-685.

Sommers DK, et al. Influence of food and reduced gastric acidity on the bioavailability of bacampicillin and cefuroxime axetil. *Br J Clin Pharmacol.* 1984;18:535-539.

Saathoff N, et al. Pharmacokinetics of cefpodoxime proxetil and interactions with an antacid and an H_2 receptor antagonist. *Antimicrob Agents Chemother.* 1992;36:796-800.

Blouin RA, et al. Influence of antacid and ranitidine on the pharmacokinetics of oral cefetamet pivoxil. *Antimicrob Agents Chemother.* 1990;34:1744-1748.

Petitjean O, et al. Pharmacokinetic interaction of cefixime and 2 antacids. Preliminary results [in French]. *Presse Med.* 1989;18:1596-1598.

 Charcoal

Digoxin (eg, *Lanoxin*)

SUMMARY: Activated charcoal significantly reduces digoxin serum concentrations, and apparently to a lesser extent, digitoxin (*Crystodigin*) serum concentrations.

RISK FACTORS: No specific risk factors are known.

RELATED DRUGS: Digitalis concentrations are also reduced by charcoal coadministration, but to an apparently lesser extent than digoxin.

MANAGEMENT OPTIONS:

➡ *Avoid Unless Benefit Outweighs Risk.* Do not administer activated charcoal to patients taking digoxin because loss of the therapeutic effect of digoxin is likely. This combination might be beneficial in patients with digitalis glycoside intoxication.

➡ *Monitor.* Watch patients taking digoxin or digitoxin for reduced glycoside concentrations if charcoal is coadministered.

REFERENCES:

Neuvonen, PJ et al. Effects of resins and activated charcoal on the absorption of digoxin, carbamazepine and furosemide. *Br J Clin Pharmacol.* 1988;25:229.

Reissell P, et al. Effect of administration of activated charcoal and fibre on absorption, excretion and steady blood levels of digoxin and digitoxin. Evidence for intestinal secretion of the glycosides. *Acta Med Scand Suppl.* 1982; 668:88.

Neuvonen, PJ et al. Reduction of absorption of digoxin, phenytoin and aspirin by activated charcoal in man. *Eur J Clin Pharmacol.* 1978;13:213.

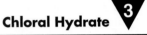

Chloral Hydrate

Ethanol (Ethyl Alcohol)

SUMMARY: Ethanol and chloral hydrate have at least additive CNS-depressant effects; combined use may be dangerous in patients performing tasks requiring alertness.

RISK FACTORS: No specific risk factors are known.

RELATED DRUGS: Alcohol would be expected to increase the CNS depression of all sedative-hypnotic drugs.

MANAGEMENT OPTIONS:

➡ *Circumvent/Minimize.* Warn patients taking chloral hydrate of the combined CNS depressant activity with ethanol. Patients with cardiovascular disease who are taking chloral hydrate should be careful about ingesting ethanol because the tachycardia and hypotension associated with the vasodilation reaction could adversely affect their disease.

➡ *Monitor.* If the combination is used, monitor for excessive CNS depression, flushing, headache, and tachycardia.

REFERENCES:

Kaplan HL, et al. Chloral hydrate and alcohol metabolism in human subjects. *J Forensic Sci.* 1967;12:295.

Freeman J, et al. Reactions of chloral hydrate and ethanol with alcohol dehydrogenase from human liver. *Fed Proc.* 1970;29:275.

Gessner PK, et al. A study of the interaction of the hypnotic effects and of the toxic effects of chloral hydrate and ethanol. *J Pharmacol Exp Ther.* 1970;174:247.

Sellers EM, et al. Interaction of chloral hydrate and ethanol in man. I. Metabolism. *Clin Pharmacol Ther.* 1972;13:37.

Chapman AH. Reaction to alcohol and chloral hydrate (Questions and Answers). *JAMA.* 1958;167:273.

Sellers EM, et al. Interaction of chloral hydrate and ethanol in man. II. Hemodynamics and performance. *Clin Pharmacol Ther.* 1972;13:50.

▼ Chloral Hydrate

Warfarin (eg, *Coumadin*)

SUMMARY: Chloral hydrate may produce a transient increase in the hypoprothrombinemic response to warfarin.

RISK FACTORS: No specific risk factors are known.

RELATED DRUGS: Alternative sedative/hypnotic drugs unlikely to interact with oral anticoagulants include flurazepam (eg, *Dalmane*), chlordiazepoxide (eg, *Librium*), diazepam (eg, *Valium*), or diphenhydramine (eg, *Benadryl*). Barbiturates would not be suitable alternatives, because they can enhance oral anticoagulant metabolism.

MANAGEMENT OPTIONS:

➤ *Consider Alternative.* Even though the interaction between chloral hydrate and warfarin usually does not cause adverse effects, it is preferable to use hypnotic drugs that do not appear to interact with anticoagulants, such as flurazepam or diazepam.

➤ *Monitor.* When chloral hydrate is given to a patient receiving an oral anticoagulant, monitor the patient for excessive hypoprothrombinemia during the first several days of chloral hydrate therapy. However, long-term coadministration of the 2 drugs probably does not increase the hazard of bleeding significantly.

REFERENCES:

Sellers EM, et al. Potentiation of warfarin-induced hypoprothrombinemia by chloral hydrate. *N Engl J Med.* 1970;283:827.

Weiner M. Species differences in the effect of chloral hydrate on coumarin anticoagulants. *Ann NY Acad Sci.* 1971;179:226.

Sellers EM, et al. Kinetics and clinical importance of displacement of warfarin from albumin by acidic drugs. *Ann NY Acad Sci.* 1971;179:213.

Boston Collaborative Drug Surveillance Program. Interaction between chloral hydrate and warfarin. *N Engl J Med.* 1972;286:53.

Udall JA. Warfarin-chloral hydrate interaction: pharmacological activity and clinical significance. *Ann Intern Med.* 1974;81:341.

Griner PF, et al. Chloral hydrate and warfarin interaction: clinical significance? *Ann Intern Med.* 1971;74:540.

Udall JA. Chloral hydrate and warfarin therapy. *Ann Intern Med.* 1971;75:141.

Beliles RP, et al. Interaction of bishydroxycoumarin with chloral hydrate and trichloroethyl phosphate. *Toxicol Appl Pharmacol.* 974;27:225.

Udall JA. Drug interference with warfarin therapy. *Clin Med.* 1970;77:20.

Cucinell SA, et al. The effect of chloral hydrate on bishydroxycoumarin metabolism. *JAMA.* 1966;197:366.

Robinson DS, et al. Interaction of commonly prescribed drugs and warfarin. *Ann Intern Med.* 1970;72:853.

MacDonald MG, et al. The effects of phenobarbital, chloral betaine, and glutethimide administration of warfarin plasma levels and hypoprothrombinemic responses in man. *Clin Pharmacol Ther.* 1969;10:80.

Rickles FR, et al. Chloral hydrate and warfarin. *N Engl J Med.* 1972;286:611.

Anon. Chloral hydrate and oral anticoagulants. *Lancet.* 1972;1:524.

Udall JA. Clinical implications of warfarin interactions with five sedatives. *Am J Cardiol.* 1975;35:67.

Galinsky RE, et al. "Post hoc" and hypoprothrombinemia. *Ann Intern Med.* 1975;83:286.

Chloramphenicol (eg, *Chloromycetin*)

Chlorpropamide (eg, *Diabinese*)

SUMMARY: Chloramphenicol may increase the hypoglycemic effects of chlorpropamide.

RISK FACTORS: No specific risk factors are known.

RELATED DRUGS: Chloramphenicol has been reported to increase the half-life of tolbutamide. The effect of chloramphenicol on other oral antidiabetics is unknown.

MANAGEMENT OPTIONS:

➡ *Monitor.* Monitor patients receiving tolbutamide or chlorpropamide who receive chloramphenicol concurrently for hypoglycemia.

REFERENCES:

Petitpierre B, et al. Behavior of chlorpropamide in renal insufficiency and under the effect of associated drug therapy. *Int J Clin Pharmacol Ther Toxicol.* 1972;6:120.

Christensen LK, et al. Inhibition of drug metabolism by chloramphenicol. *Lancet.* 1969;2:1397.

Petitpierre B, et al. Chlorpropamide and chloramphenicol. *Lancet.* 1970;1:789.

Brunova E, et al. Interaction of tolbutamide and chloramphenicol in diabetic patients. *Int J Clin Pharmacol.* 1977;15:7.

Chloramphenicol (eg, *Chloromycetin*)

Dicumarol

SUMMARY: Chloramphenicol may enhance the hypoprothrombinemic response to dicumarol and possibly other oral anticoagulants.

RISK FACTORS:

➡ *Diet/Food.* Dietary deficiency of vitamin K can increase the risk of interaction.

RELATED DRUGS: Although the effect of chloramphenicol on the metabolism of warfarin (eg, *Coumadin*) and other oral anticoagulants has not been established, theoretical considerations suggest that it would be similar to the effect on dicumarol. Warfarin would be expected to interact similarly with chloramphenicol because chloramphenicol is known to inhibit CYP2C9, the enzyme primarily responsible for warfarin metabolism.

MANAGEMENT OPTIONS:

➡ *Use Alternative.* Avoid concomitant use of chloramphenicol and dicumarol. Warfarin may not be an acceptable alternative anticoagulant.

REFERENCES:

Christensen LK, et al. Inhibition of drug metabolism by chloramphenicol. *Lancet.* 1969;2:1397.

O'Reilly RA, et al. Determinants of the response to oral anticoagulant drugs in man. *Pharmacol Rev* 1970;22:35.

Koch-Weser J, et al. Drug interactions with coumarin anticoagulants (First of two parts). *N Engl J Med.* 1971;285:487.

Koch-Weser J, et al. Drug interactions with coumarin anticoagulants (Second of two parts). *N Engl J Med.* 1971;285:547.

Finegold SM. Interaction of antimicrobial therapy and intestinal flora. *Am J Clin Nutr.* 1970;23:1466.

Kippel AP, et al. Hypoprothrombinemia secondary to antibiotic therapy and manifested by massive gastrointestinal hemorrhage. Report of three cases. *Arch Surg.* 1968;96:266.

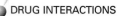

Loeliger EA, et al. The biological disappearance rate of prothrombin and factors VII, IX and X from plasma in hypothyroidism, hyperthyroidism and during fever. *Thromb Diath Haemorrh*. 1964;10:267.

Ansell JE, et al. The spectrum of vitamin K deficiency. *JAMA*. 1977;238:40.

Chloramphenicol (eg, *Chloromycetin*)

Penicillin G

SUMMARY: Chloramphenicol may inhibit the antibacterial activity of penicillins.

RISK FACTORS: No specific risk factors are known.

RELATED DRUGS: Other bactericidal antibiotics could interact with chloramphenicol in a similar manner.

MANAGEMENT OPTIONS:

➡ *Consider Alternative.* Avoid the use of chloramphenicol and penicillins except where the combination has been demonstrated to be beneficial.

➡ *Circumvent/Minimize.* Be sure that adequate amounts of each agent are being given and, if possible, begin administration of the penicillin a few hours or more before the chloramphenicol.

➡ *Monitor.* Observe patients for failure of antibiotic efficacy when the 2 agents are coadministered.

REFERENCES:

Garrod LP. Causes of failure in antibiotic treatment. *BMJ*. 1972;4:441.

De Ritis F, et al. Chloramphenicol combined with ampicillin in treatment of typhoid. *BMJ*. 1972;4:17.

Wallace JF, et al. Studies on the pathogenesis of meningitis. VI. Antagonism between penicillin and chloramphenicol in experimental pneumococcal meningitis. *J Lab Clin Med*. 1967;70:408.

Jawetz E. The use of combinations of antimicrobial drugs. *Ann Rev Pharmacol*. 1968;8:151.

Mills J, et al. Clinical use of antimicrobials. In: Katzung BG. Basic and Clinical Pharmacology. 4th ed. Los Altos: Lange Medical Publications; 1989;624–29.

Chloramphenicol (eg, *Chloromycetin*)

Phenobarbital

SUMMARY: Chloramphenicol can increase serum barbiturate concentrations, and barbiturates can reduce chloramphenicol concentrations.

RISK FACTORS: No specific risk factors are known.

RELATED DRUGS: Other barbiturates may be similarly affected by chloramphenicol and could reduce chloramphenicol concentrations as well.

MANAGEMENT OPTIONS:

➡ *Circumvent/Minimize.* Increased chloramphenicol dosage may be needed in some patients.

➡ *Monitor.* In patients receiving phenobarbital (and possibly other barbiturates), watch for evidence of reduced chloramphenicol effect. Also be alert for evidence of increased effect of phenobarbital (and possibly other barbiturates) when chloramphenicol is given concurrently.

REFERENCES:

Koup JR, et al. Interaction of chloramphenicol with phenytoin and phenobarbital. Case report. *Clin Pharmacol Ther.* 1978;24:571.

Bloxham RA, et al. Chloramphenicol and phenobarbitone. A drug interaction. *Arch Dis Child.* 1979;54:76.

Chloramphenicol (eg, *Chloromycetin*)

Phenytoin (eg, *Dilantin*)

SUMMARY: Chloramphenicol predictably increases serum phenytoin concentrations; symptoms of phenytoin toxicity have occurred. Phenytoin also may affect serum chloramphenicol concentrations, but results have been conflicting.

RISK FACTORS: No specific risk factors are known.

RELATED DRUGS: No information is available.

MANAGEMENT OPTIONS:

➡ *Consider Alternative.* If possible, avoid chloramphenicol use in patients receiving phenytoin.

➡ *Monitor.* Watch patients who receive both phenytoin and chloramphenicol closely for signs of phenytoin toxicity (eg, nystagmus, lethargy, ataxia, rash).

REFERENCES:

Ballek RE, et al. Inhibition of diphenylhydantoin metabolism by chloramphenicol. *Lancet.* 1973;1:150.

Rose JQ, et al. Intoxication caused by interaction of chloramphenicol and phenytoin. *JAMA.* 1977;237:2630.

Koup JR, et al. Interaction of chloramphenicol with phenytoin and phenobarbital. Case report. *Clin Pharmacol Ther.* 1978;24:571.

Saltiel MS, et al. Phenytoin-chloramphenicol interaction. *Drug Intel Clin Pharm* 1980;14:221.

Greenlaw CW. Chloramphenicol-phenytoin drug interaction. *Drug Intell Clin Pharm* 1979;13:609.

Harper JM, et al. Phenytoin-chloramphenicol interaction: a retrospective study. *Drug Intel Clin Pharm.* 1970;13:425.

Powell DA, et al. Interactions among chloramphenicol, phenytoin, and phenobarbital in a pediatric patient. *J Pediatr.* 1981;98:1001.

Krasinski K, et al. Pharmacologic interactions among chloramphenicol, phenytoin and phenobarbital. *Pediatr Infect Dis.* 1982;1:232.

Chloramphenicol (eg, *Chloromycetin*)

Rifampin (eg, *Rifadin*)

SUMMARY: Rifampin can reduce chloramphenicol concentrations, potentially reducing its antibacterial efficacy.

RISK FACTORS: No specific risk factors are known.

RELATED DRUGS: No information is available.

MANAGEMENT OPTIONS:

➡ *Consider Alternative.* If possible, avoid rifampin use in patients receiving chloramphenicol.

➥ **Monitor.** Monitor chloramphenicol concentrations when rifampin is coadminis-tered.

REFERENCES:
Prober CG. Effect of rifampin on chloramphenicol levels. *N Engl J Med.* 1985;312:788.
Kelly HW, et al. Interaction of chloramphenicol and rifampin. *J Pediatr.* 1988;12:817.

Chlordiazepoxide (eg, *Librium*)

Ketoconazole (eg, *Nizoral*)

SUMMARY: Ketoconazole increases chlordiazepoxide concentrations, but the degree to which chlordiazepoxide adverse effects are increased is not established.

RISK FACTORS: No specific risk factors are known.

RELATED DRUGS: Other antifungal agents (eg, itraconazole [*Sporanox*], fluconazole [*Diflucan*]) are likely to increase chlordiazepoxide concentrations. Ketoconazole also inhibits the metabolism of alprazolam (eg, *Xanax*), midazolam (*Versed*), and triazolam (*Halcion*).

MANAGEMENT OPTIONS:

➥ **Monitor.** Observe patients on chronic chlordiazepoxide who receive ketoconazole for increased sedation.

REFERENCES:
Brown MW, et al. Effect of ketoconazole on hepatic oxidative drug metabolism. *Clin Pharmacol Ther.* 1985;37:290.

Chlormethiazole

Cimetidine (eg, *Tagamet*)

SUMMARY: Cimetidine increases chlormethiazole (a sedative-hypnotic with anticonvulsant effects available in Europe) serum concentrations and may increase its pharmacologic effect. Study in patients is needed to establish the clinical significance of this interaction.

RISK FACTORS: No specific risk factors are known.

RELATED DRUGS: Ranitidine (eg, *Zantac*) does not appear to affect the pharmacokinetics of chlormethiazole; the effect of famotidine (eg, *Pepcid*) and nizatidine (*Axid*) on chlormethiazole is not established, but an interaction would not be expected.

MANAGEMENT OPTIONS:

➥ **Consider Alternative.** Ranitidine may be preferable to cimetidine in this situation because it does not appear to interact with chlormethiazole.

➥ **Monitor.** If the combination is used, be alert for altered chlormethiazole response (eg, sedation, respiratory depression) if cimetidine is initiated, discontinued, or changed in dosage.

REFERENCES:
Shaw G, et al. Cimetidine impairs the elimination of chlormethiazole. *Eur J Clin Pharmacol.* 1981;21:83.

Chloroquine (eg, *Aralen*)

Chlorpromazine (eg, *Thorazine*)

SUMMARY: Chlorpromazine concentrations are increased by chloroquine and other antimalarial agents; the clinical significance of these changes is unknown.

RISK FACTORS: No specific risk factors are known.

RELATED DRUGS: Other phenothiazines may be similarly affected by chloroquine and other antimalarials.

MANAGEMENT OPTIONS:

➡ *Monitor.* Monitor patients maintained on chlorpromazine for increased neuroleptic effects if antimalarial agents are prescribed.

REFERENCES:

Makanjuola ROA, et al. Effects of antimalarial agents on plasma levels of chlorpromazine and its metabolites in schizophrenic patients. *Trop Geogr Med.* 1988;40:31.

Chloroquine (eg, *Aralen*)

Cyclosporine (eg, *Neoral*)

SUMMARY: Patients stabilized on cyclosporine may develop elevated cyclosporine concentrations following the addition of chloroquine. Signs and symptoms of cyclosporine toxicity may accompany the interaction.

RISK FACTORS: No specific risk factors are known.

RELATED DRUGS: Tacrolimus (*Prograf*) may be affected similarly by coadministered chloroquine.

MANAGEMENT OPTIONS:

➡ *Circumvent/Minimize.* Cyclosporine dosages may require reduction during concomitant chloroquine treatment.

➡ *Monitor.* Carefully observe patients taking cyclosporine for increased cyclosporine concentrations if chloroquine is coadministered.

REFERENCES:

Finielz P, et al. Interaction between cyclosporin and chloroquine. *Nephron.* 1993;65:333.

Nampoory MRN, et al. Drug interaction of chloroquine with ciclosporin. *Nephron.* 1992;62:108.

Chloroquine (eg, *Aralen*)

Methotrexate

SUMMARY: Methotrexate concentrations are reduced by chloroquine coadministration; the clinical significance is unknown but some patients could experience reduced methotrexate efficacy.

RISK FACTORS: No specific risk factors are known.

RELATED DRUGS: Hydroxychloroquine (eg, *Plaquenil*) may affect methotrexate in a similar manner.

MANAGEMENT OPTIONS:

➥ **Monitor.** Until more information is available, monitor patients receiving methotrexate for loss of efficacy during chloroquine coadministration.

REFERENCES:

Seidman P, et al. Chloroquine reduces the bioavailability of methotrexate in patients with rheumatoid arthritis. *Arthritis Rheum.* 1994;37:830.

Chloroquine (eg, *Aralen*)

Praziquantel (*Biltricide*)

SUMMARY: Chloroquine administration reduces the plasma concentration of praziquantel; loss of efficacy could occur.

RISK FACTORS: No specific risk factors are known.

RELATED DRUGS: Hydroxychloroquine (eg, *Plaquenil*) could affect praziquantel in a similar manner.

MANAGEMENT OPTIONS:

➥ **Monitor.** Until more information is available, monitor patients taking praziquantel for reduced plasma concentrations and possible loss of efficacy if they receive chloroquine concurrently.

REFERENCES:

Masimirembwa CM, et al. The effect of chloroquine on the pharmacokinetics and metabolism of praziquantel in rats and in humans. *Biopharm Drug Dispos.* 1994;15:33.

Chlorpromazine (eg, *Thorazine*)

Cigarette Smoking

SUMMARY: Preliminary evidence indicates that cigarette smokers have less drowsiness and hypotension from chlorpromazine than nonsmokers, but the clinical importance of these findings is unclear.

RISK FACTORS: No specific risk factors are known.

RELATED DRUGS: Little is known regarding the effect of cigarette smoking on the response of other phenothiazines or neuroleptics. It is possible that some of them are similarly affected by cigarette smoking.

MANAGEMENT OPTIONS:

➥ **Monitor.** Be alert for evidence of increased neuroleptic dosage requirements in cigarette smokers and for reduced neuroleptic dosage requirements in patients who stop cigarette smoking.

REFERENCES:

Swett C Jr. Drowsiness due to chlorpromazine in relation to cigarette smoking. *Arch Gen Psychiatry.* 1974;31:211.

Swett C Jr, et al. Hypotension due to chlorpromazine: relation to cigarette smoking, blood pressure and dosage. *Arch Gen Psychiatry.* 1977;34:661.

Panguck EJ, et al. Cigarette smoking and chlorpromazine disposition and actions. *Clin Pharmacol Ther.* 1982;31:533.

Stimmel GL, et al. Chlorpromazine plasma levels, adverse effects, and tobacco smoking: case report. *J Clin Psychiatry.* 1983;44:420.

Chlorpromazine (eg, *Thorazine*)

Clonidine (eg, *Catapres*)

SUMMARY: Isolated cases of severe hypotensive episodes or delirium have been reported following the concurrent use of clonidine and chlorpromazine, but a causal relationship has not been established.

RISK FACTORS: No specific risk factors are known.

RELATED DRUGS: Other antipsychotics also may interact with clonidine. The combined use of clonidine and fluphenazine (eg, *Prolixin*) was associated with delirium (eg, confusion, disorientation, agitation) in a 33-year-old man, but a causal relationship was not established. Additionally, the combined use of haloperidol and clonidine was associated with a case of hypotension. Although little is known regarding the effect of centrally acting alpha-agonists other than clonidine such as guanabenz (*Wytensin*) and guanfacine (eg, *Tenex*), consider the possibility that they interact with neuroleptic drugs until clinical information is available.

MANAGEMENT OPTIONS:

➥ *Monitor.* Watch for additive hypotensive effects when clonidine and neuroleptics are used concurrently, especially when the neuroleptic is initiated in a patient with impaired cardiac function.

REFERENCES:

Gruncillo RJ, et al. Severe hypotension associated with concurrent clonidine and antipsychotic medication. *Am J Psychiatry.* 1985;142:274.

McEvoy GK, ed. AHFS Drug Information 89. Bethesda, MD: American Society of Hospital Pharmacists; 1995:1189.

Allen RM, et al. Delirium associated with combined fluphenazine-clonidine therapy. *J Clin Psychiatry.* 1979;40:236.

Chlorpromazine (eg, *Thorazine*)

Epinephrine (eg, *Adrenalin*)

SUMMARY: Chlorpromazine, and possibly some other phenothiazines, may reverse the pressor response of epinephrine.

RISK FACTORS: No specific risk factors are known.

RELATED DRUGS: Neuroleptics such as thioridazine (eg, *Mellaril*) and clozapine (eg, *Clozaril*) could theoretically interact with epinephrine similarly, but other neuroleptics with a low incidence of postural hypotension may have less effect on alpha-adrenergic receptors and may be less likely to affect epinephrine response (eg, fluphenazine [eg, *Prolixin*], trifluoperazine [eg, *Stelazine*], haloperidol [eg, *Haldol*], loxapine [eg, *Loxitane*], molindone [*Moban*], and pimozide [*Orap*]).

MANAGEMENT OPTIONS:

➥ *Consider Alternative.* It has been suggested that in neuroleptic-treated patients with hypotension, alpha-adrenergic agonists with little beta-adrenergic activity (eg, phenylephrine [eg, *Neo-Synephrine*], levarterenol [*Levophed*]) would be more effective in increasing the blood pressure than epinephrine.

➡ *Monitor.* Monitor the blood pressure when epinephrine is given to hypotensive patients receiving neuroleptics, particularly chlorpromazine, thioridazine, or clozapine.

REFERENCES:

Foster CA. Chlorpromazine: a study of its action on the circulation in man. *Lancet.* 1954;2:614.

Yagiela JA, et al. Drug interaction and vasoconstrictors used in local anesthetic solutions. *Oral Surg Oral Med Oral Pathol.* 1985;59:565.

Lear E, et al. A clinical study of mechanisms of action of chlorpromazine. *JAMA.* 1957;163:30.

Gonzales, ER. Catecholamine selection for vasopressor-dependent patients. *Clin Pharm.* 1988;7:493.

Alexander CS. Epinephrine not contraindicated in cardiac arrest attributed to phenothiazine. *JAMA.* 1976;236:405.

Chlorpromazine (eg, *Thorazine*)

Ethanol (Ethyl Alcohol)

SUMMARY: Patients receiving antipsychotic doses of chlorpromazine are probably more sensitive to the adverse effects of ethanol on psychomotor skills and behavior. Thioridazine may be less likely to induce this effect with ethanol, but the effects of other neuroleptics have not been well studied. More study also is needed to assess the ability of ethanol to induce extrapyramidal reactions in patients on neuroleptics.

RISK FACTORS: No specific risk factors are known.

RELATED DRUGS: Thioridazine (eg, *Mellaril*) may be less likely to add to the detrimental effects of ethanol on psychomotor skills. One would expect neuroleptics other than chlorpromazine to add to the psychomotor impairment of alcohol, but there may be differences in degree with different phenothiazines.

MANAGEMENT OPTIONS:

➡ *Circumvent/Minimize.* Patients receiving neuroleptics (especially large doses) should be aware that ethanol ingestion can impair motor performance and driving ability. The possibility that ethanol might precipitate extrapyramidal reactions in certain susceptible patients receiving neuroleptics is another reason to limit ethanol intake.

➡ *Monitor.* Be alert for evidence of excessive CNS depression if ethanol and phenothiazines are used together.

REFERENCES:

Milner G, et al. Alcohol, thioridazine and chlorpromazine effects on skills related to driving behaviour. *Br J Psychiatry.* 1971;118:351.

Zirkle GA, et al. Effects of chlorpromazine and alcohol on coordination and judgment. *JAMA.* 1959;168:1496.

Saario I. Psychomotor skills during subacute treatment with thioridazine and bromazepam, and their combined effects with alcohol. *Ann Clin Res.* 1976;8:117.

Lutz EG. Neuroleptic-induced akathisia and dystonia triggered by alcohol. *JAMA.* 1976;236:2422.

Chlorpromazine (eg, *Thorazine*)

Guanethidine (*Ismelin*)

SUMMARY: Phenothiazines may inhibit the antihypertensive response to guanethidine.

RISK FACTORS: No specific risk factors are known.

RELATED DRUGS: Guanadrel (*Hylorel*) is pharmacologically similar to guanethidine and also may be inhibited by phenothiazines.

MANAGEMENT OPTIONS:

➡ *Consider Alternative.* Consider using an antihypertensive agent other than guanethidine (or drugs related to guanethidine such as guanadrel). Keep in mind that the intrinsic hypotensive effect of phenothiazines might enhance the effect of antihypertensives other than guanethidine or guanadrel.

➡ *Monitor.* If the combination is used, monitor blood pressure for evidence of the interaction. If guanethidine antagonism is noted, consider increasing the guanethidine dose, or using an alternative antihypertensive agent.

REFERENCES:

Day MD, et al. Antagonism of guanethidine and betrylium by various agents. *Lancet.* 1962;2:1282.

Ober KF, et al. Drug interactions with guanethidine. *Clin Pharmacol Ther.* 1973;14:190.

Tuck D, et al. Drug interactions: effect of chlorpromazine on the uptake of monoamines into adrenergic neurons in man. *Lancet.* 1972;2:492..

Reports of Suspected Adverse Reactions to Drugs. 1970, No. 700201-056-00101.

Lahti RA, et al. The tricyclic antidepressants: inhibition of norepinephrine uptake as related to potentiation of norepinephrine and clinical efficacy. *Biochem Pharmacol.* 1971;20:482.

Fann WE, et al. Chlorpromazine reversal of the antihypertensive action of guanethidine. *Lancet.* 1971;2:436.

Janowsky DS, et al. Antagonism of guanethidine by chlorpromazine. *Am J Psychiatry.* 1973;130:808.

Chlorpromazine (eg, *Thorazine*)

Levodopa (eg, *Larodopa*)

SUMMARY: Phenothiazines and related neuroleptic agents may inhibit the antiparkinsonian effect of levodopa.

RISK FACTORS: No specific risk factors are known.

RELATED DRUGS: Levodopa also probably is inhibited by butyrophenones (eg, haloperidol [eg, *Haldol*]) and other neuroleptics.

MANAGEMENT OPTIONS:

➡ *Avoid Unless Benefit Outweighs Risk.* If possible, avoid administration of phenothiazines and other neuroleptics to patients receiving levodopa.

➡ *Monitor.* Monitor patients for reduced levodopa effect if phenothiazines are used.

REFERENCES:

Mims RB, et al. Inhibition of L-dopa-induced growth hormone stimulation by pyridoxine and chlorpromazine. *J Clin Endocrinol Metab.* 1975;40:256.

Yaryura-Tobias JA, et al. Action of L-dopa in a drug-induced extrapyramidalism. *Dis Nerv Syst.* 1970;31:60.

Yahr MD, et al. Drug therapy of parkinsonism. *N Engl J Med.* 1972;287:20.

Campbell JB. Long-term treatment of Parkinson's disease with levodopa. *Neurology.* 1970;20:18.

▼ Chlorpromazine (eg, *Thorazine*)

Lithium (eg, *Eskalith*)

SUMMARY: Combined use of lithium and chlorpromazine may lower serum concentrations of both drugs. Rare cases of severe neurotoxicity have been reported in acute manic patients receiving lithium and phenothiazines, especially thioridazine.

RISK FACTORS:

➡ *Concurrent Diseases.* Patients with acute manic symptoms appear to be more likely to manifest neurotoxicity with the concurrent use of lithium and phenothiazines.

RELATED DRUGS: Consider the possibility that lithium interacts with other phenothiazines (especially thioridazine). The combined use of haloperidol and lithium has been implicated in the production of severe neurotoxic symptoms.

MANAGEMENT OPTIONS:

➡ *Monitor.* Monitor patients for neurotoxicity (eg, delirium, seizures, encephalopathy) with the concurrent use of lithium and phenothiazines (especially thioridazine) in patients with acute manic symptoms. Chronic therapy with these combinations appears less likely to result in an adverse interaction. Although the clinical importance of the pharmacokinetic interactions of phenothiazine and lithium is not well established, be alert for evidence of reduced phenothiazine response in the presence of lithium therapy.

REFERENCES:

Zall H, et al. Lithium carbonate: a clinical study. *Am J Psychiatry.* 1968;125:549.

Crammer JL, et al. Blood levels and management of lithium treatment. *BMJ.* 1974;3:650.

Kerzner B, et al. Lithium and chlorpromazine (CPZ) interaction. *Clin Pharmacol Ther.* 1976;19:109.

Sletten I, et al. The effect of chlorpromazine on lithium excretion in psychiatric subjects. *Curr Ther Res.* 1966;8:441.

Strayhorn JM, et al. Severe neurotoxicity despite "therapeutic" serum lithium levels. *Dis Nerv Syst.* 1977;38:107.

Rivera-Calimlim L, et al. Effect of lithium on plasma chlorpromazine levels. *Clin Pharmacol Ther.* 1978;23:451.

Ghadirian AM, et al. Neurological side effects of lithium: organic brain syndrome, seizures, extrapyramidal side effects, and EEG changes. *Compr Psychiatry.* 1981;21:327.

Spring S, et al. New data on lithium and haloperidol incompatibility. *Am J Psychiatry.* 1981;138:818.

Kamlana SH, et al. Lithium: some drug interactions. *Practitioner.* 1980;224:1291.

Addonizio G. Rapid induction of extrapyramidal side effects with combined use of lithium and neuroleptics. *J Clin Psychopharmacol.* 1985;5:296.

Yassa R. A case of lithium-chlorpromazine interaction. *J Clin Psychiatry.* 1986;47:90.

Bailine SH, et al. Neurotoxicity induced by combined lithium-thioridazine treatment. *Biol Psychiatry.* 1986;21:834.

Miller F, et al. Lithium-neuroleptic neurotoxicity in the elderly bipolar patient. *J Clin Psychopharmacol.* 1986;6:176.

Addonizio G, et al. Rapid induction of extrapyramidal side effects with combined use of lithium and neuroleptics. *J Clin Psychopharmacol.* 1985;5:296.

Pakes GE. Lithium toxicity with neuroleptics withdrawal. *Lancet.* 1979;2:701.

Yassa R. A case of lithium-chlorpromazine interaction. *J Clin Psychiatry.* 1986;47:90.

Chlorpromazine (eg, *Thorazine*)

Meperidine (eg, *Demerol*)

SUMMARY: The combination of chlorpromazine and meperidine may result in hypotension and excessive CNS depression.

RISK FACTORS: No specific risk factors are known.

RELATED DRUGS: Whether other combinations of neuroleptics and narcotic analgesics would produce similar effects is unknown, but, in general, expect enhanced respiratory depression and hypotension with such combinations.

MANAGEMENT OPTIONS:

➡ *Monitor.* Be alert for evidence of excessive CNS depression, hypotension, and respiratory depression when meperidine and chlorpromazine are used concurrently. Until more information is available, caution is advised for other combinations of neuroleptics and narcotic analgesics.

REFERENCES:

Stambaugh JE, et al. Drug interaction: meperidine and chlorpromazine, a toxic combination. *J Clin Pharmacol.* 1981;21:140.

Swett C, et al. Hypotension due to chlorpromazine. *Arch Gen Psychiatry.* 1977;34:661.

Chlorpromazine (eg, *Thorazine*)

Orphenadrine (eg, *Norflex*)

SUMMARY: The combination of orphenadrine and chlorpromazine may result in lower serum chlorpromazine concentrations and excessive anticholinergic effects. Also, a patient on chlorpromazine and orphenadrine developed hypoglycemia; the clinical importance of this effect is unclear.

RISK FACTORS: No specific risk factors are known.

RELATED DRUGS: The effect of orphenadrine combined with other phenothiazines is not established. There was no mention of adverse effects caused by drug interaction in 6 patients who were receiving orphenadrine and fluphenazine (eg, *Prolixin*).

MANAGEMENT OPTIONS:

➡ *Monitor.* In patients on concomitant neuroleptics and orphenadrine, be alert for evidence of excessive anticholinergic effects (especially ileus), reduced neuroleptic plasma concentrations, or hypoglycemia.

REFERENCES:

Loga S, et al. Interactions of orphenadrine and phenobarbitone with chlorpromazine: plasma concentrations and effects in man. *Br J Clin Pharmacol.* 1975;2:197.

Fleming P, et al. Levodopa in drug-induced extrapyramidal disorders. *Lancet.* 1970;2:1186.

Buckle RM, et al. Hypoglycaemic coma occurring during treatment with chlorpromazine and orphenadrine. *BMJ.* 1967;4:599.

Chlorpromazine (eg, *Thorazine*)

Phenobarbital

SUMMARY: Barbiturates may reduce some chlorpromazine concentrations, but the degree to which the therapeutic response to chlorpromazine is reduced is not established.

RISK FACTORS: No specific risk factors are known.

RELATED DRUGS: The effect of barbiturates on other neuroleptics is not established, but be aware of a possible reduction in the antipsychotic effect. There is also some evidence that thioridazine (eg, *Mellaril*) may reduce serum phenobarbital concentrations. One patient undergoing withdrawal from barbiturates and methaqualone developed fatal hyperthermia after he was given haloperidol (eg, *Haldol*). It was proposed that the tendency of sedative-hypnotic withdrawal to produce hyperpyrexia was markedly enhanced by the ability of the haloperidol to interfere with thermoregulation.

MANAGEMENT OPTIONS:

➡ *Monitor.* It does not seem necessary to avoid concomitant use of neuroleptics and barbiturates, but monitor patients for evidence of a reduced effect of either drug if the combination is used.

REFERENCES:

Forrest FM, et al. Modification of chlorpromazine metabolism by some other drugs frequently administered to psychiatric patients. *Biol Psychiatry.* 1970;2:53.

Curry SH, et al. Factors affecting chlorpromazine plasma levels in psychiatric patients. *Arch Gen Psychiatry.* 1970;22:209.

Loga S et, al. Interactions of orphenadrine and phenobarbitone with chlorpromazine: plasma concentrations and effects in a man. *Br J Clin Pharmacol.* 1975;2:197.

Gay PE, et al. Interaction between phenobarbital and thioridazine. *Neurology.* 1983;33:1631.

Greenblatt DJ, et al. Fatal hyperthermia following haloperidol therapy of sedative-hypnotic withdrawal. *J Clin Psychiatry.* 1978;39:673.

Chlorpromazine (eg, *Thorazine*)

Propranolol (eg, *Inderal*)

SUMMARY: Propranolol and some beta blockers and neuroleptics such as chlorpromazine can increase the plasma concentrations of each other, resulting in accentuated pharmacologic responses of both drugs.

RISK FACTORS: No specific risk factors are known.

RELATED DRUGS: Thiothixene and thioridazine concentrations increase in patients treated with propranolol, while propranolol appears to have little effect on haloperidol concentrations. While other pairs of beta blockers and neuroleptics may interact in a similar manner, the interaction may not occur with beta blockers excreted primarily by the kidneys, such as atenolol (eg, *Tenormin*) and nadolol (eg, *Corgard*).

MANAGEMENT OPTIONS:

➡ *Consider Alternative.* The use of beta blockers (eg, nadolol) that are renally eliminated may lessen the magnitude of this interaction.

➥ *Monitor.* Monitor patients receiving neuroleptics and beta blockers for enhanced effects of both drugs. The dosage of one or both drugs may require reduction.

REFERENCES:

Alvarez-Mena SC, et al. Phenothiazine-induced abnormalities. *JAMA.* 1973;224:1730.

Peet M, et al. Propranolol in schizophrenia. II. Clinical and biochemical aspects of combining propranolol with chlorpromazine. *Br J Psychiatry.* 1981;139:112.

Arita M, et al. Effects of phenothiazine and propranolol on ECG. The effects of propranolol on the electrocardiographic abnormalities induced by phenothiazine derivatives. *Jpn Circ J.* 1970;34:391.

Greendyke RM, et al. Plasma propranolol levels and their effect on plasma thioridazine and haloperidol concentrations. *J Clin Psychopharmacol.* 1987;7:178.

Silver JM, et al. Elevation of thioridazine plasma levels by propranolol. *Am J Psychiatry.* 1986;143:1290.

Vestal RE, et al. Inhibition of propranolol metabolism by chlorpromazine. *Clin Pharmacol Ther.* 1979;25:19.

Peet M, et al. Pharmacokinetic interaction between propranolol and chlorpromazine in schizophrenic patients. *Lancet.* 1980;2:978.

Miller FA. Adverse effects of combined propranolol and chlorpromazine therapy. *Am J Psychiatry.* 1982;139:1198.

Chlorpromazine (eg, *Thorazine*)

Trazodone (eg, *Desyrel*)

SUMMARY: Isolated case reports suggest that concurrent therapy with trazodone and neuroleptics such as chlorpromazine may produce an additive hypotension.

RISK FACTORS: No specific risk factors are known.

RELATED DRUGS: Trifluoperazine (eg, *Stelazine*) appears to interact similarly.

MANAGEMENT OPTIONS:

➥ *Monitor.* Monitor patients for hypotension if trazodone and neuroleptics are used concurrently.

REFERENCES:

Asayesh K, et al. Combination of trazodone and phenothiazines; a possible additive hypotensive effect. *Can J Psychiatry.* 1986;31:857.

Chlorpropamide (eg, *Diabinese*)

Clofibrate (*Atromid-S*)

SUMMARY: Clofibrate may enhance the effects of oral hypoglycemic drugs in some patients.

RISK FACTORS: No specific risk factors are known.

RELATED DRUGS: Other sulfonylureas may be similarly affected by clofibrate.

MANAGEMENT OPTIONS:

➥ *Monitor.* Closely monitor patients treated with clofibrate and chlorpropamide or other sulfonylureas for hypoglycemia. This caution would apply especially when clofibrate is started or stopped in patients stabilized on a sulfonylurea.

REFERENCES:

Petitpierre B, et al. Behavior of chlorpropamide in renal insufficiency and under the effect of associated drug therapy. *Int J Clin Pharmacol Ther Toxicol.* 1972;6:120.

Daubresse JC, et al. Potentiation of hypoglycemic effect of sulfonylureas by clofibrate. *N Engl J Med.* 1976;294:613..

Ferrari C, et al. Potentiation of hypoglycemic response to intravenous tolbutamide by clofibrate. *N Engl J Med.* 1976;294:613.

Albert M, et al. Vascular symptomatic relief during administration of ethylchlorophenoxyisobutyrate (clofibrate). *Metabolism.* 1969;18:635.

Daubresse JC, et al. Clofibrate and diabetes control in patients treated with oral hypoglycaemic agents. *Br J Clin Pharmacol.* 1979;7:599.

Jain AK, et al. Potentiation of hypoglycemic effect of sulfonylureas by halofenate. *N Engl J Med.* 1975;239:1283.

Chlorpropamide (eg, *Diabinese*)

Erythromycin (eg, *E-Mycin*)

SUMMARY: A patient developed severe hepatic toxicity during the coadministration of erythromycin ethylsuccinate and chlorpropamide.

RISK FACTORS: No specific risk factors are known.

RELATED DRUGS: No information is available.

MANAGEMENT OPTIONS:

➡ *Monitor.* Until more information is available on this potential interaction, monitor patients taking chlorpropamide and erythromycin for changes in hypoglycemic control and hepatotoxicity.

REFERENCES:
Geubel AP, et al. Prolonged cholestasis and disappearance of interlobular bile ducts following chlorpropamide and erythromycin ethylsuccinate: case of drug interaction? *Liver.* 1988;8:350.

Chlorpropamide (eg, *Diabinese*)

AVOID Ethanol (Ethyl Alcohol)

SUMMARY: Excessive ethanol intake may lead to altered glycemic control, most commonly hypoglycemia. An "*Antabuse*"-like reaction may occur in patients taking sulfonylureas.

RISK FACTORS: No specific risk factors are known.

RELATED DRUGS: Excessive ethanol may produce hypoglycemia in patients taking insulin or other oral hypoglycemic agents. Prolonged heavy intake of ethanol markedly decreases the half-life of tolbutamide, probably by inducing hepatic enzymes. Ethanol ingestion may contribute to lactic acidosis in patients receiving phenformin.

MANAGEMENT OPTIONS:

➡ *AVOID COMBINATION.* Because an "*Antabuse* reaction" may occur following ethanol ingestion in patients receiving sulfonylureas, inform patients of this possibility when therapy is initiated. Avoid ingestion of moderate to large amounts of ethanol by patients on antidiabetic drugs because of the possible adverse effects of alcohol on diabetic control.

REFERENCES:
Arky RA, et al. Irreversible hypoglycemia, a complication of alcohol and insulin. *JAMA.* 1968;206:575.

Hartling SG, et al. Interaction of ethanol and glipizide in humans. *Diabetes Care.* 1987;10:263.

Kater RMH, et al. Increased rate tolbutamide metabolism in alcoholic patients. *JAMA.* 1969;207:363.

Johnson HK, et al. Relationship of alcohol and hyperlactatemia in diabetic subjects treated with phenformin. *Am J Med.* 1968;45:98.

Kreisberg RA, et al. Hyperlacticacidemia in man: ethanol-phenformin synergism. *J Clin Endocrinol.* 1972;34:29.

Carulli N, et al. Alcohol-drugs interaction in man: alcohol and tolbutamide. *Eur J Clin Invest.* 1971;1:421.

Baruh S, et al. Fasting hypoglycemia. *Med Clin North Am.* 1973;57:1441.

Yamamoto LT. Diabetes insipidus and drinking alcohol. *N Engl J Med.* 1976;294:55.

Sotaniemi EA, et al. Half-life of intravenous tolbutamide in the serum of patients in medical wards. *Ann Clin Res.* 1974;6:146.

Assad MM, et al. Studies on the biochemical aspects of the "disulfiram like" reaction induced by oral hypoglycemics. *Eur Pharmacol.* 1976;35:301.

Wardle EN, et al. Alcohol and glibenclamide. *BMJ.* 1971;3:309.

Cholestyramine (eg, *Questran*)

Diclofenac (eg, *Voltaren*)

SUMMARY: Single dose studies in healthy subjects suggest that cholestyramine substantially reduces the bioavailability of diclofenac; reduced diclofenac effect may occur.

RISK FACTORS: No specific risk factors are known.

RELATED DRUGS: Cholestyramine also reduces the serum concentrations of other nonsteroidal anti-inflammatory drugs such as ketoprofen (eg, *Orudis*), piroxicam (eg, *Feldene*), and tenoxicam. Colestipol (*Colestid*) also appears to inhibit the absorption of diclofenac, but to a somewhat lesser extent.

MANAGEMENT OPTIONS:

➡ *Consider Alternative.* Colestipol appears to reduce diclofenac absorption to a lesser extent than cholestyramine, but it still would be prudent to give the diclofenac 2 hours before or 6 hours after the colestipol.

➡ *Circumvent/Minimize.* Giving diclofenac 2 hours before or 6 hours after the cholestyramine would be expected to optimize the absorption of the diclofenac. Nonetheless, because diclofenac undergoes enterohepatic circulation, reduced diclofenac plasma concentrations may occur even if dosing of the drugs is separated.

➡ *Monitor.* Monitor patients for reduced diclofenac effect, regardless of how far apart the doses are separated.

REFERENCES:
Al-balla SR, et al. The effects of cholestyramine and colestipol on the absorption of diclofenac in man. *Int J Clin Pharmacol Ther.* 1994;32;441.

Cholestyramine (eg, *Questran*)

Digoxin (*Lanoxin*)

SUMMARY: Cholestyramine appears to reduce the serum concentrations of digoxin and digitoxin (*Crystodigin*), but the clinical impact in chronically treated patients has not been adequately assessed.

RISK FACTORS: No specific risk factors are known.

RELATED DRUGS: Digitoxin concentrations and pharmacologic activity were reduced after cholestyramine coadministration. Colestipol (*Colestid*) also has been noted to reduce digitalis glycoside concentrations.

MANAGEMENT OPTIONS:

➡ *Monitor.* Until more is known about this interaction, monitor patients on digitalis glycosides for underdigitalization when cholestyramine is coadministered. Giving the digitalis product at least 2 hours before the cholestyramine may lessen the magnitude of the interaction.

REFERENCES:

Brown DD, et al. A steady-state evaluation of the effects of propantheline bromide and cholestyramine on the bioavailability of digoxin when administered as tablets or capsules. *J Clin Pharmacol.* 1985;25:360.

Caldwell JH, et al. Interruption of the enterohepatic circulation of digitoxin by cholestyramine. *J Clin Invest.* 1971;50:2638.

Hall WH, et al. Effect of cholestyramine on digoxin absorption and excretion in man. *Am J Cardiol.* 1977;39:213.

Brown DD, et al. Decreased bioavailability of digoxin due to hypocholesterolemic interventions. *Circulation.* 1978;58:164.

Pieroni RE, et al. Use of cholestyramine resin in digitoxin toxicity. *JAMA.* 1981;245:1939.

Neuvonen PJ, et al. Effects of resins and activated charcoal on the absorption of digoxin, carbamazepine and furosemide. *Br J Clin Pharmacol.* 1988;25:229.

Cholestyramine (eg, *Questran*)

Furosemide (eg, *Lasix*)

SUMMARY: Study in healthy subjects suggests that cholestyramine markedly reduces the bioavailability and diuretic response of furosemide.

RISK FACTORS: No specific risk factors are known.

RELATED DRUGS: Colestipol (*Colestid*) also substantially reduces the bioavailability of furosemide. The effect of cholestyramine and colestipol on other loop diuretics is not established.

MANAGEMENT OPTIONS:

➡ *Circumvent/Minimize.* Although the ability to circumvent the interaction by separating doses of furosemide from cholestyramine has not been systematically studied, giving furosemide 2 hours before or 6 hours after the cholestyramine would be expected to minimize the interaction.

➡ *Monitor.* Monitor patients for altered furosemide response if cholestyramine therapy is initiated, discontinued, changed in dosage, or if the interval between doses of the 2 drugs is changed.

REFERENCES:

Neuvonen PJ, et al. Effects of resins and activated charcoal on the absorption of digoxin, carbamazepine and furosemide. *Br J Clin Pharmacol.* 1988;25:229.

Cholestyramine (eg, *Questran*)

Hydrocortisone (eg, *Hycort*)

SUMMARY: Cholestyramine may lower plasma concentrations of oral hydrocortisone, possibly reducing its therapeutic effect.

RISK FACTORS: No specific risk factors are known.

RELATED DRUGS: The effect of cholestyramine on other corticosteroids is not established, but because corticosteroids are closely related structurally, it is possible that cholestyramine affects their absorption as well. Colestipol (*Colestid*) probably interacts with corticosteroids in a manner similar to cholestyramine, but evidence is lacking.

MANAGEMENT OPTIONS:

➡ *Circumvent/Minimize.* Separate doses of oral hydrocortisone (and other corticosteroids) from cholestyramine as much as possible to minimize their mixing in the GI tract. Theoretically, giving the corticosteroid 2 hours before or 6 hours after the cholestyramine would optimize corticosteroid absorption. It also would be prudent to maintain a constant interval between the doses of corticosteroids and cholestyramine to minimize fluctuation of any interaction that does occur.

➡ *Monitor.* Monitor patients for evidence of reduced corticosteroid response and increase the dose as needed when these drugs are used concurrently.

REFERENCES:
Johansson C, et al. Interaction by cholestyramine on the uptake of hydrocortisone in the GI tract. *Acta Med Scand.* 1978;204:509.

Cholestyramine (eg, *Questran*)

Imipramine (eg, *Tofranil*)

SUMMARY: Cholestyramine may produce a modest reduction in imipramine plasma concentrations, but the clinical importance of this effect is not established.

RISK FACTORS: No specific risk factors are known.

RELATED DRUGS: Little is known about the effect of cholestyramine on antidepressants other than imipramine, but consider the possibility of reduced antidepressant plasma concentrations if cholestyramine is taken concurrently. Theoretically, the binding resin colestipol (*Colestid*) also may interact with tricyclic antidepressants (TCAs).

MANAGEMENT OPTIONS:

➡ *Circumvent/Minimize.* Although the ability to circumvent the interaction by separating doses of imipramine before cholestyramine has not been systematically studied, giving imipramine 2 hours before or 6 hours after the cholestyramine would be expected to minimize the interaction.

➥ **Monitor.** Monitor patients for altered TCA effect if cholestyramine is initiated, discontinued, or changed in dosage; adjust antidepressant dose as needed.

REFERENCES:

Spina E, et al. Decreased plasma concentrations of imipramine and desipramine following cholestyramine intake in depressed patients. *Ther Drug Monit.* 1994;16:432.

 Cholestyramine (eg, *Questran*)

Methotrexate

SUMMARY: Preliminary evidence indicates that cholestyramine binds methotrexate in the gut and thus may reduce serum methotrexate concentrations. The degree to which this effect reduces the therapeutic response to methotrexate is not established.

RISK FACTORS: No specific risk factors are known.

RELATED DRUGS: The effect of colestipol (*Colestid*) on methotrexate is unknown, but it may be similar to that of cholestyramine.

MANAGEMENT OPTIONS:

➥ **Circumvent/Minimize.** Until clinical studies are performed, it would be prudent to separate oral doses of methotrexate from cholestyramine as much as possible.

➥ **Monitor.** Be alert for altered response to oral or parenteral methotrexate when cholestyramine is given concurrently.

REFERENCES:

Erttmann R, et al. Effect of oral cholestyramine on elimination of highdose methotrexate. *J Cancer Res Clin Oncol.* 1985;110:48.

Ellman MH, et al. Benefit of G-CSF for methotrexate-induced neutropenia in rheumatoid arthritis. *Am J Med.* 1992;92:337.

McAnena OJ, et al. Alteration of methotrexate metabolism in rats by administration of an elemental liquid diet. *Cancer.* 1987;59:1091.

 Cholestyramine (eg, *Questran*)

Metronidazole (eg, *Flagyl*)

SUMMARY: Cholestyramine administration reduced the bioavailability of metronidazole in a single-dose study of healthy subjects.

RISK FACTORS: No specific risk factors are known.

RELATED DRUGS: Colestipol (*Colestid*) might affect metronidazole in a similar manner.

MANAGEMENT OPTIONS:

➥ **Circumvent/Minimize.** Advise patients to separate taking metronidazole from doses of cholestyramine as much as possible and take at least 2 hours before the cholestyramine.

➥ **Monitor.** If metronidazole and bile acid binding resins are coadministered, watch for reduced metronidazole efficacy.

REFERENCES:

Molokhia AM, et al. Effect of oral coadministration of some adsorbing drugs on the bioavailability of metronidazole. *Drug Dev Ind Pharm.* 1987;13:1229.

Cholestyramine (eg, *Questran*)

Piroxicam (eg, *Feldene*)

SUMMARY: Cholestyramine enhanced the elimination of piroxicam in one study, but the clinical importance of this effect is unknown.

RISK FACTORS: No specific risk factors are known.

RELATED DRUGS: The elimination of IV tenoxicam, a nonsteroidal anti-inflammatory drug (NSAID) related to piroxicam, also was enhanced by cholestyramine in this study. Although little is known regarding the effect of cholestyramine on other NSAIDs, it would not be surprising to find that some of them also interact. The effect of another binding resin, colestipol (*Colestid*), on the pharmacokinetics of piroxicam or other NSAIDs is not established, but some evidence suggests that colestipol binds drugs less avidly than cholestyramine.

MANAGEMENT OPTIONS:

➡ *Circumvent/Minimize.* Separate the doses of piroxicam and cholestyramine as much as possible.

➡ *Monitor.* Monitor the patient for inadequate piroxicam response. If an inadequate piroxicam response appears to be related to the use of cholestyramine, consider the use of an alternative hypolipidemic agent or NSAID therapy.

REFERENCES:

Meinertz T, et al. Interruption of the enterohepatic circulation of phenprocoumon by cholestyramine. *Clin Pharmacol Ther.* 1977;21:731.

Jahnchen E, et al. Enhanced elimination of warfarin during treatment with cholestyramine. *Br J Clin Pharmacol.* 1978;5:437.

Guentert TW, et al. Accelerated elimination of tenoxicam and piroxicam by cholestyramine. *Clin Pharmacol Ther.* 1988;43:179.

Cholestyramine (eg, *Questran*)

Pravastatin (*Pravachol*)

SUMMARY: Cholestyramine can inhibit the bioavailability of pravastatin, but this effect appears to be more than offset by the additive lipid-lowering effect of concurrent therapy.

RISK FACTORS: No specific risk factors are known.

RELATED DRUGS: Colestipol affects pravastatin similarly. Although little is known regarding the effect of bile acid binding resins on the absorption of other HMG-CoA reductase inhibitors such as lovastatin (*Mevacor*), simvastatin (*Zocor*), or fluvastatin (*Lescol*), they may be similarly affected.

MANAGEMENT OPTIONS:

➡ *Circumvent/Minimize.* Cholestyramine or colestipol-induced reduction in pravastatin bioavailability probably is minimized by giving the cholestyramine or colestipol with meals and the pravastatin at bedtime. Other dosing schedules also may be suitable, but it would be best to avoid giving bile acid binding resins at the same time as pravastatin or other HMG-CoA reductase inhibitors.

➡ **Monitor.** Monitor patients for reduced pravastatin effect if cholestyramine is also given.

REFERENCES:

Pan HY, et al. Pharmacokinetics and pharmacodynamics of pravastatin alone and with cholestyramine in hypercholesterolemia. *Clin Pharmacol Ther.* 1990;48:201.

Pan HY. Clinical pharmacology of pravastatin, a selective inhibitor of HMG-CoA reductase. *Eur J Clin Pharmacol.* 1991;40:S15.

 Cholestyramine (eg, *Questran*)

Thyroid

SUMMARY: Cholestyramine may reduce serum thyroid concentrations in patients receiving thyroid replacement therapy.

RISK FACTORS: No specific risk factors are known.

RELATED DRUGS: Until more information is available, assume that the absorption of all thyroid preparations can be reduced by cholestyramine administration. Although the effect of colestipol (*Colestid*) on thyroid absorption is not established, assume that it also interacts until proved otherwise.

MANAGEMENT OPTIONS:

➡ **Circumvent/Minimize.** The available evidence suggests that at least 4 to 5 hours should elapse between administration of cholestyramine and thyroid. Also, try to maintain a relatively constant interval between doses of the 2 drugs.

➡ **Monitor.** Even with the above precautions, monitor for altered thyroid response (eg, serum thyroid-stimulating hormone concentrations) when cholestyramine is initiated, discontinued, changed in dosage, or when the interval between doses of the 2 drugs is changed for more than a few days.

REFERENCES:

Northcutt RC, et al. The influence of cholestyramine on thyroxine absorption. *JAMA.* 1969;208:1857.

 Cholestyramine (eg, *Questran*)

Valproic Acid (eg, *Depakene*)

SUMMARY: Cholestyramine inhibits the GI absorption of valproic acid, but it is not known how often this would result in a clinically important reduction in valproic acid effect.

RISK FACTORS: No specific risk factors are known.

RELATED DRUGS: Theoretically, one would expect colestipol (*Colestid*) also to inhibit the absorption of valproic acid.

MANAGEMENT OPTIONS:

➡ **Circumvent/Minimize.** Although the magnitude of the interaction appears small in most people, it would be prudent to take valproic acid at least 2 hours before or 6 hours after cholestyramine, and maintain a relatively constant interval between administration of the 2 drugs.

➡ *Monitor.* Even if the doses of the drugs are separated appropriately, it would be prudent to monitor for reduced effect, especially in the first few weeks of combined therapy.

REFERENCES:

Malloy MJ, et al. Effect of cholestyramine resin on single dose valproate pharmacokinetics. *Int J Clin Pharmacol Ther.* 1996;34:208.

Cholestyramine (eg, *Questran*)

Warfarin (eg, *Coumadin*)

SUMMARY: Cholestyramine may inhibit the hypoprothrombinemic response to warfarin, phenprocoumon, and possibly other oral anticoagulants; colestipol (*Colestid*) might be less likely to interact.

RISK FACTORS: No specific risk factors are known.

RELATED DRUGS: Phenprocoumon interacts similarly. Some evidence suggests that colestipol (*Colestid*) is less likely than cholestyramine to interact with warfarin or phenprocoumon.,

MANAGEMENT OPTIONS:

➡ *Consider Alternative.* Consider hypolipidemic therapy, but keep in mind that other agents also may interact with oral anticoagulants (eg, clofibrate [*Atromid-S*], gemfibrozil [eg, *Lopid*], and lovastatin [*Mevacor*]).

➡ *Circumvent/Minimize.* Giving the anticoagulant at least 2 hours before or 6 hours after the binding resin probably minimizes the impairment of oral anticoagulant absorption. However, any anticoagulant that undergoes enterohepatic circulation (eg, warfarin, phenprocoumon) may be affected by cholestyramine therapy even if the doses are separated. The binding resin and the oral anticoagulant should consistently be given the same number of hours apart so that any interaction that does occur will be relatively consistent from day to day.

➡ *Monitor.* Monitor patients for altered response to oral anticoagulants if a binding resin is initiated, discontinued, changed in dosage, or if the interval between the resin and the anticoagulant is changed.

REFERENCES:

Meinertz T, et al. Interruption of the enterohepatic circulation of phenprocoumon by cholestyramine. *Clin Pharmacol Ther.* 1977;21:731.

Jahnchen E, et al. Enhanced elimination of warfarin during treatment with cholestyramine. *Br J Clin Pharmacol.* 1978;5:437.

Robinson DS, et al. Interaction of warfarin and nonsystemic gastrointestinal drugs. *Clin Pharmacol Ther.* 1971;12:491.

Gross L, et al. Hypoprothrombinemia and hemorrhage associated with cholestyramine therapy. *Ann Intern Med.* 1970;72:95.

Harvengt C, et al. Effect of colestipol, a new bile acid sequestrant, on the absorption of phenprocoumon in man. *Eur J Clin Pharmacol.* 1973;6:19.

Product information. Colestipol (*Colestid*). Upjohn Company. 1993.

Cigarette Smoking

AVOID Contraceptives, Oral (eg, *Ortho-Novum*)

SUMMARY: Smoking increases the risk of oral contraceptive-induced adverse cardiovascular events.

RISK FACTORS:

➡ **Dosage Regimen.** Smoking more than 15 cigarettes/day places women at greater risk.

➡ **Effects of Age.** Women older than 35 years of age are at greater risk.

MANAGEMENT OPTIONS:

➡ **AVOID COMBINATION.** Encourage women taking oral contraceptives not to smoke; if they continue to smoke, consider suggesting an alternative form of contraception.

REFERENCES:

Goldbaum GM, et al. The relative impact of smoking and oral contraceptive use on women in the United States. *JAMA.* 1987;258:1339.

Fredricksen H, et al. Thromboembolism, oral contraceptives and cigarettes. *Public Health Rep.* 1970;85:197.

Product information. (*Ovulen*). Searle Laboratories. 1984.

Crawford FE, et al. Oral contraceptive steroid plasma concentrations in smokers and nonsmokers. *BMJ.* 1981;282:1829.

Cigarette Smoking

Insulin

SUMMARY: Cigarette smoking may increase glucose concentrations and decrease response to insulin administration.

RISK FACTORS: No specific risk factors are known.

RELATED DRUGS: No information is available.

MANAGEMENT OPTIONS:

➡ **Monitor.** Inform patients that a change in smoking habits may change the response to insulin.

REFERENCES:

Madsbad S, et al. Influence of smoking on insulin requirement and metabolic status in diabetes mellitus. *Diabetes Care.* 1980;3:41.

Klemp P, et al. Smoking reduces insulin absorption from subcutaneous tissue. *BMJ.* 1982;284:237.

Cigarette Smoking

Quinine

SUMMARY: Cigarette smokers have lower quinine serum concentrations than nonsmokers; clinical efficacy could be reduced.

RISK FACTORS: No specific risk factors are known.

RELATED DRUGS: No information is available.

MANAGEMENT OPTIONS:

➡ *Circumvent/Minimize.* Smokers requiring quinine therapy for malaria may need increased quinine doses to achieve a cure.

➡ *Monitor.* Consider measurement of plasma quinine concentrations in smokers to ensure therapeutic plasma concentrations are attained.

REFERENCES:
Wanwimolruk S, et al. Cigarette smoking enhances the elimination of quinine. *Br J Clin Pharmacol.* 1993;36:610.

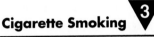

Cigarette Smoking

Tacrine (*Cognex*)

SUMMARY: Cigarette smoking appears to reduce tacrine plasma concentrations markedly and may increase tacrine dosage requirements.

RISK FACTORS: No specific risk factors are known.

RELATED DRUGS: No information is available.

MANAGEMENT OPTIONS:

➡ *Monitor.* Monitor tacrine response, and keep in mind that smokers are likely to have higher tacrine dosage requirements than nonsmokers.

REFERENCES:
Welty D, et al. The effect of smoking on the pharmacokinetics and metabolism of Cognex in healthy volunteers. *Pharm Res.* 1993;10:S334.

Product information. Tacrine (*Cognex*). Parke-Davis. 1993.

Watkins PB, et al. Hepatotoxic effects of tacrine administration in patients with Alzheimer's disease. *JAMA.* 1994;271:992.

Winker MA. Tacrine for Alzheimer's disease: which patient, what dose? *JAMA.* 1994;271:1023. Editorial.

Cigarette Smoking

Theophylline (eg, *Theolair*)

SUMMARY: Cigarette smoking increases the elimination of theophylline, thus increasing theophylline dosage requirements.

RISK FACTORS: No specific risk factors are known.

RELATED DRUGS: No information is available.

MANAGEMENT OPTIONS:

➡ *Monitor.* Monitor theophylline response and serum concentrations. Keep in mind that smokers require considerably larger maintenance dosages of theophylline than nonsmokers in order to achieve adequate serum theophylline levels.

REFERENCES:
Jenne J, et al. Decreased theophylline half-life in cigarette smokers. *Life Sci.* 1975;17:195.

Jusko WJ, et al. Enhanced biotransformation of theophylline in marihuana and tobacco smokers. *Clin Pharmacol Ther.* 1978;24:405-410.

Pfeifer HJ, et al. Clinical toxicity of theophylline in relation to cigarette smoking. A report from the Boston Collaborative Drug Surveillance. *Chest.* 1978;73:455-459.

Hunt SN, et al. Effect of smoking on theophylline disposition. *Clin Pharmacol Ther*. 1976;19:546-551.

Powell JR, et al. The influence of cigarette smoking and sex on theophylline disposition. *Am Rev Respir Dis*. 1977;116:17-23.

Cigarette Smoking

Thioridazine (eg, *Mellaril*)

SUMMARY: Cigarette smokers tend to have lower plasma concentrations of thioridazine and may require larger doses to achieve adequate therapeutic response.

RISK FACTORS: No specific risk factors are known.

RELATED DRUGS: Some evidence suggests that cigarette smoking may also reduce chlorpromazine (eg, *Thorazine*) effect, but little is known regarding the effect of smoking on other phenothiazines. Some other antipsychotics, such as clozapine (eg, *Clozaril*) and olanzapine (*Zyprexa*), are metabolized by CYP1A2 and would also be expected to be affected by cigarette smoking.

MANAGEMENT OPTIONS:

➡ *Monitor.* Be alert for evidence of increased thioridazine dosage requirements in patients who smoke cigarettes. Other phenothiazines and neuroleptics may be similarly affected.

REFERENCES:

Berecz R, et al. Thioridazine steady-state plasma concentrations are influenced by tobacco smoking and CYP2D6, but not by the CYP2C9 genotype. *Eur J Clin Pharmacol*. 2003;59:45-50.

Cimetidine (eg, *Tagamet*)

Cisapride†

SUMMARY: Cimetidine substantially increased the bioavailability of cisapride in healthy subjects, but the clinical importance of the interaction is not established.

RISK FACTORS: No specific risk factors are known.

RELATED DRUGS: The effect of other H_2-receptor antagonists, such as ranitidine (eg, *Zantac*), famotidine (eg, *Pepcid*), and nizatidine (eg, *Axid*), on cisapride pharmacokinetics is not established; theoretically, they would be less likely to affect cisapride metabolism than cimetidine.

MANAGEMENT OPTIONS:

➡ *Consider Alternative.* Although there is little evidence to suggest that the combination is dangerous, given the potential severity of the adverse interaction it would be prudent to use an alternative to cimetidine, such as ranitidine, famotidine, or nizatidine.

➡ *Monitor.* If the combination is used, monitor for evidence of ventricular arrhythmias (eg, fainting, palpitations).

REFERENCES:

Kirch W, et al. Cisapride-cimetidine interaction: enhanced cisapride bioavailability and accelerated cimetidine absorption. *Ther Drug Monit*. 1989;11:411-414.

Galmiche P, et al. Combined therapy with cisapride and cimetidine in severe reflux oesophagitis: a double blind controlled trial. *Gut*. 1988;29:675-681.

† Available only through an investigational limited access program.

Cimetidine (eg, *Tagamet*)

Citalopram (*Celexa*)

SUMMARY: Cimetidine appears to moderately increase citalopram serum concentrations, but it is not known how often this would result in adverse outcomes.

RISK FACTORS: No specific risk factors are known.

RELATED DRUGS: Famotidine (eg, *Pepcid*), nizatidine (eg, *Axid*), and ranitidine (eg, *Zantac*) are theoretically unlikely to interact with citalopram, but clinical studies are needed for confirmation. Theoretically, omeprazole (eg, *Prilosec*) could interact with citalopram because of its ability to inhibit CYP2C19.

MANAGEMENT OPTIONS:

➡ ***Consider Alternative.*** Consider using an alternative H$_2$-receptor antagonist such as famotidine, nizatidine, or ranitidine.

➡ ***Monitor.*** If the combination is used, monitor for altered citalopram effect if cimetidine is initiated, discontinued, or changed in dosage; adjust citalopram dose as needed.

REFERENCES:

Priskorn M, et al. Pharmacokinetic interaction study of citalopram and cimetidine in healthy subjects. *Eur J Clin Pharmacol*. 1997;52:241-242.

Cimetidine (eg, *Tagamet*)

Clozapine (eg, *Clozaril*)

SUMMARY: A patient receiving clozapine developed increased serum clozapine concentrations and evidence of clozapine toxicity after starting cimetidine. Although this reaction was probably caused by an interaction between cimetidine and clozapine, the frequency and magnitude of this interaction is not established.

RISK FACTORS:

➡ ***Dosage Regimen.*** In most patients, clinically important inhibition of hepatic drug metabolism by cimetidine requires doses of 400 mg/day or more.

RELATED DRUGS: Based on this case, it appears that ranitidine would be preferable to cimetidine in patients receiving clozapine. Theoretically, famotidine (eg, *Pepcid*) and nizatidine (eg, *Axid*) also would be unlikely to interact with clozapine.

MANAGEMENT OPTIONS:

➡ ***Consider Alternative.*** Until more information is available, avoid the use of cimetidine in patients receiving clozapine. Theoretically, famotidine and nizatidine would be unlikely to interact and can be considered as alternatives.

➡ **Monitor.** If the combination is used, monitor for altered clozapine effect if cimetidine is initiated, discontinued, or changed in dosage. Adjust clozapine dosage as needed.

REFERENCES:

Szymanski S, et al. A case report of cimetidine-induced clozapine toxicity. *J Clin Psychiatry.* 1991;52:21-22.

Cimetidine (eg, *Tagamet*)

Desipramine (eg, *Norpramin*)

SUMMARY: Limited clinical evidence suggests that cimetidine increases serum desipramine concentrations. Given the proven effect of cimetidine on tricyclic antidepressants closely related to desipramine, it seems likely that desipramine is affected similarly.

RISK FACTORS:

➡ **Dosage Regimen.** In most patients, clinically important inhibition of hepatic drug metabolism by cimetidine requires doses 400 mg/day or higher.

RELATED DRUGS: Theoretically, ranitidine (eg, *Zantac*), famotidine (eg, *Pepcid*), and probably nizatidine (*Axid*) would be less likely to interact with desipramine. Other clinical studies suggest that cimetidine also inhibits the elimination of other tricyclic antidepressants such as imipramine (eg, *Tofranil*) and nortriptyline (eg, *Pamelor*). Little clinical information is available on the effect of cimetidine on tricyclics such as amitriptyline (eg, *Elavil*), amoxapine (eg, *Asendin*), protriptyline, trimipramine (*Surmontil*), maprotiline (eg, *Ludiomil*), or trazodone (eg, *Desyrel*). However, theoretical considerations would indicate that their elimination also might be reduced by cimetidine therapy.

MANAGEMENT OPTIONS:

➡ **Consider Alternative.** Consider using an alternative to cimetidine. Ranitidine, famotidine, and probably nizatidine are less likely to interact.

➡ **Monitor.** Until more information is available, be alert or altered desipramine effect if cimetidine therapy is initiated, discontinued, or changed in dosage.

REFERENCES:

Miller DD, et al. Cimetidine-imipramine interaction: a case report. *Am J Psychiatry.* 1983;140:351.

Cimetidine (eg, *Tagamet*)

Diazepam (eg, *Valium*)

SUMMARY: Plasma levels of diazepam and several other benzodiazepines or their active metabolites can be increased by cimetidine, but the frequency of adverse effects associated with increased benzodiazepine concentration is unknown.

RISK FACTORS:

➡ **Dosage Regimen.** In most patients, clinically important inhibition of hepatic drug metabolism by cimetidine requires doses 400 mg/day or higher.

➡ **Effects of Age.** The elderly can be more susceptible to the sedative effects of benzodiazepines.

RELATED DRUGS: Because clorazepate (eg, *Tranxene*), halazepam (*Paxipam*), and prazepam are metabolized to active desmethyldiazepam, they probably also interact with cimetidine. Clonazepam (eg, *Klonopin*) and flurazepam (eg, *Dalmane*) undergo oxidative metabolism in the liver, and their elimination would be expected to be reduced by cimetidine. Cimetidine also reduces plasma clearance of chlordiazepoxide (eg, *Librium*), desmethyldiazepam, and probably also alprazolam (eg, *Xanax*) and triazolam (*Halcion*). The pharmacokinetics of benzodiazepines that undergo glucuronide conjugation, such as lorazepam (eg, *Ativan*), oxazepam (eg, *Serax*), and temazepam (eg, *Restoril*), do not appear to be affected by cimetidine therapy. Ranitidine (eg, *Zantac*) appears to be less likely to interact with benzodiazepines than cimetidine; famotidine (eg, *Pepcid*) and probably nizatidine (*Axid*) also appear unlikely to interact.

MANAGEMENT OPTIONS:

➡ **Consider Alternative.** Consider using an alternative to cimetidine. Ranitidine, famotidine, and probably nizatidine appear less likely to interact.

➡ **Monitor.** Watch patients receiving benzodiazepines that undergo oxidative metabolism for evidence of altered benzodiazepine response when cimetidine is initiated, discontinued, or changed in dosage.

REFERENCES:

Greenblatt DJ, et al. Clinical importance of the interaction of diazepam and cimetidine. *N Engl J Med.* 1984;310:1639.

Klotz U, et al. Delayed clearance of diazepam due to cimetidine. *N Engl J Med.* 1980;302:1012.

Desmond PV, et al. Cimetidine impairs elimination of chlordiazepoxide (*Librium*) in man. *Ann Intern Med.* 1980;93:266.

Klotz U, et al. Elevation of steady-state diazepam levels by cimetidine. *Clin Pharmacol Ther.* 1981;30:513.

Patwardhan RV, et al. Lack of tolerance and rapid recovery of cimetidine-inhibited chlordiazepoxide (*Librium*) elimination. *Gastroenterology.* 1981;81:547.

Ruffalo RL, et al. Cimetidine-benzodiazepine drug interaction. *Am J Hosp Pharm.* 1981;38:1365.

Gough PA, et al. Influence of cimetidine on oral diazepam elimination with measurement of subsequent cognitive change. *Br J Clin Pharmacol.* 1982;14:739.

Greenblatt DJ, et al. The diazepam-cimetidine interaction: is it clinically important? *Clin Pharmacol Ther.* 1984;35:245.

Greenblatt DJ, et al. Old age, cimetidine, and disposition of alprazolam and triazolam. *Clin Pharmacol Ther.* 1983;33:253.

Klotz U, et al. Influence of cimetidine on the pharmacokinetics of desmethyldiazepam and oxazepam. *Eur J Clin Pharmacol.* 1980;18:517.

Patwardhan RV, et al. Cimetidine spares the glucuronidation of lorazepam and oxazepam. *Gastroenterology.* 1970;79:912.

Cimetidine (eg, *Tagamet*)

Diltiazem (eg, *Cardizem*)

SUMMARY: Cimetidine can increase the serum concentration of diltiazem; excessive diltiazem effects may be seen.

RISK FACTORS: No specific risk factors are known.

RELATED DRUGS: Cimetidine also increases the concentrations of nifedipine (eg, *Procardia*), nisoldipine (*Sular*), nitrendipine, and verapamil (eg, *Calan*). Other H$_2$-receptor antagonists, such as ranitidine (eg, *Zantac*), famotidine (eg, *Pepcid*), and nizatidine (*Axid*), would be less likely to affect diltiazem concentrations.

MANAGEMENT OPTIONS:

➡ *Consider Alternative.* Ranitidine 150 mg twice daily does not appear to affect diltiazem concentrations. Nizatidine and famotidine also would be unlikely to affect diltiazem pharmacokinetics.

➡ *Monitor.* Monitor patients receiving diltiazem carefully (eg, bradycardia, hypotension) when cimetidine is added or deleted from their drug regimen.

REFERENCES:

Winship LC, et al. The effect of ranitidine and cimetidine on singledose diltiazem pharmacokinetics. *Pharmacotherapy.* 1985;5:16.

Cimetidine (eg, *Tagamet*)

Dofetilide (*Tikosyn*)

SUMMARY: Cimetidine increases the concentration and effect of dofetilide; toxicity may result.

RISK FACTORS: No specific risk factors are known.

RELATED DRUGS: As noted above, ranitidine 150 mg twice daily had no effect on dofetilide. Effects of other H₂-receptor antagonists (eg, famotidine [eg, *Pepcid*], nizatidine [*Axid*]) on dofetilide elimination are unknown, but would likely be limited. Omeprazole (*Prilosec*) and an antacid (eg, *Maalox*) had no effect on dofetilide concentrations or pharmacodynamic effects.

MANAGEMENT OPTIONS:

➡ *Circumvent/Minimize.* Patients receiving dofetilide should avoid using cimetidine, even in *otc* doses. Ranitidine would appear to be a safe alternative at doses of no more than 150 mg twice daily.

➡ *Monitor.* Monitor patients carefully for increased QTc intervals if they take dofetilide with cimetidine.

REFERENCES:

Walker DK, et al. Significance of metabolism in the disposition and action of the antidysrhythmic drug, dofetilide. In vitro studies and correlation with in vivo date. *Drug Metab Dispos.* 1996;24(4):447-55.

Abel S, et al. Effect of cimetidine and ranitidine on pharmacokinetics and pharmacodynamics of a single dose of dofetilide. *Br J Clin Pharmacol.* 2000;49(1):64-71.

Vincent J, et al. Cimetidine inhibits renal elimination of dofetilide without altering QTc activity on multiple dosing. *Clin Pharmacol Ther.* 1998;63:210.

Vincent J, et al. Concurrent administration of omeprazole and antacid does not alter the pharmacokinetics and pharmacodynamics of dofetilide in healthy subjects. *Clin Pharmacol Ther.* 1996;59:182.

Cimetidine (eg, *Tagamet*)

Doxepin (eg, *Sinequan*)

SUMMARY: Cimetidine substantially increased serum concentrations of doxepin in healthy subjects, but it is not known how often this results in doxepin toxicity.

RISK FACTORS:

➡ *Dosage Regimen.* In most patients, clinically important inhibition of hepatic drug metabolism by cimetidine requires doses 400 mg/day or higher.

RELATED DRUGS: Ranitidine does not appear to interact with doxepin. In 6 healthy men, ranitidine (eg, *Zantac*) 150 mg twice daily had no effect on steady-state plasma doxepin concentrations. Theoretically, famotidine (eg, *Pepcid*) and nizatidine (*Axid*) also would be unlikely to affect doxepin metabolism. Other clinical studies suggest that cimetidine also inhibits the elimination of other tricyclic antidepressants (TCAs) such as imipramine (eg, *Tofranil*), desipramine (eg, *Norpramin*), and nortriptyline (eg, *Pamelor*). Little clinical information is available on the effect of cimetidine on TCAs such as amitriptyline (eg, *Elavil*), amoxapine (eg, *Asendin*), protriptyline (eg, *Vivactil*), trimipramine (*Surmontil*), maprotiline (eg, *Ludiomil*), or trazodone (eg, *Desyrel*). However, theoretical considerations would indicate that their elimination also might be reduced by cimetidine therapy.

MANAGEMENT OPTIONS:

➥ *Consider Alternative.* Consider using an alternative to cimetidine, such as ranitidine, famotidine, or nizatidine.

➥ *Circumvent/Minimize.* In patients who are already receiving cimetidine and are about to begin a course of therapy with doxepin, consider using conservative doxepin doses until the patient's response to therapy can be evaluated.

➥ *Monitor.* In patients stabilized on doxepin who are then given cimetidine, be alert for evidence of doxepin toxicity (eg, severe dry mouth, blurred vision, urinary retention, tachycardia, constipation, postural hypotension). If cimetidine is discontinued or its dose substantially reduced in a patient stabilized on both doxepin and cimetidine, monitor the patient for an inadequate response to the doxepin.

REFERENCES:
Sutherland DL, et al. The influence of cimetidine versus ranitidine on doxepin pharmacokinetics. *Eur J Clin Pharmacol.* 1987;32:159.

Smedley HM. Malignant breast change in man given two drugs associated with breast hyperplasia. *Lancet.* 1981;2:638.

Cimetidine (eg, *Tagamet*)

Femoxetine

SUMMARY: Preliminary study in healthy subjects suggests that cimetidine markedly increases femoxetine serum concentrations, but an increase in adverse effects was not observed.

RISK FACTORS: No specific risk factors are known.

RELATED DRUGS: The effect of H_2-receptor antagonists other than cimetidine on femoxetine pharmacokinetics is unknown; theoretically, famotidine (eg, *Pepcid*), nizatidine (*Axid*), and ranitidine (eg, *Zantac*) would not be expected to interact.

MANAGEMENT OPTIONS:

➥ *Consider Alternative.* Theoretically, other H_2-receptor antagonists such as ranitidine, famotidine, or nizatidine would be less likely to interact with femoxetine; thus, their use may be preferred over cimetidine until more information is available on this interaction.

➥ *Monitor.* Patients receiving cimetidine may have lower dosage requirements for femoxetine. However, the results of this study suggest that femoxetine has little dosedependent toxicity. Nonetheless, it would be prudent to monitor for alter-

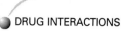

ations in therapeutic and toxic effects of femoxetine if cimetidine is initiated, discontinued, or changed in dosage.

REFERENCES:

Schmidt J et al. Femoxetine and cimetidine: interaction in healthy volunteers. *Eur J Clin Pharmacol.* 1986;31:299.

 Cimetidine (eg, *Tagamet*)

Flecainide (eg, *Tambocor*)

SUMMARY: Cimetidine increases the plasma concentration of flecainide, but the clinical importance of this effect is not established.

RISK FACTORS:

➡ ***Concurrent Diseases.*** Patients with renal failure are more likely to experience this interaction.

RELATED DRUGS: Ranitidine (eg, *Zantac*), famotidine (eg, *Pepcid*), and nizatidine (*Axid*) are less likely to interact with flecainide because they have little or no effect on hepatic metabolism.

MANAGEMENT OPTIONS:

➡ ***Monitor.*** Monitor patients stabilized on flecainide (particularly those with renal disease) for increased flecainide effect if cimetidine is added to their therapy.

REFERENCES:

Tjamdra-Maga TB, et al. Altered pharmacokinetics of oral flecainide by cimetidine. *Br J Clin Pharmacol.* 1986;22:108.

 Cimetidine (eg, *Tagamet*)

Imipramine (eg, *Tofranil*)

SUMMARY: Cimetidine can increase serum concentrations of imipramine substantially leading to imipramine toxicity in some patients.

RISK FACTORS:

➡ ***Dosage Regimen.*** In most patients, clinically important inhibition of hepatic drug metabolism by cimetidine requires doses of 400 mg/day or higher.

RELATED DRUGS: Ranitidine (eg, *Zantac*) does not appear to affect imipramine metabolism or pharmacokinetics. Theoretically, it is unlikely that famotidine (eg, *Pepcid*) and nizatidine (*Axid*) will interact with imipramine because these H_2-receptor antagonists have little effect on drug metabolism. Cimetidine also may increase serum concentrations of desipramine (eg, *Norpramin*), doxepin (eg, *Sinequan*), and nortriptyline (eg, *Pamelor*).

MANAGEMENT OPTIONS:

➡ ***Consider Alternative.*** Consider using an alternative to cimetidine (eg, ranitidine, famotidine, nizatidine).

➡ *Circumvent/Minimize.* In patients who are already receiving cimetidine and are about to begin a course of therapy with imipramine, consider using conservative imipramine doses until the patient's response to therapy can be evaluated.

➡ *Monitor.* In patients stabilized on imipramine who are then given cimetidine, be alert for evidence of imipramine toxicity (eg, severe dry mouth, blurred vision, urinary retention, tachycardia, constipation, and postural hypotension). If cimetidine is discontinued or its dose substantially reduced in a patient stabilized on both imipramine and cimetidine, monitor the patient for an inadequate response to the cyclic antidepressant.

REFERENCES:

Abernethy DR, et al. Imipramine-cimetidine interaction: impairment of clearance and enhanced bioavailability. *Clin Pharmacol Ther.* 1983;33:237.

Henauer SA, et al. Cimetidine interaction with imipramine and nortriptyline. *Clin Pharmacol Ther.* 1984;35:183.

Miller DD, et al. Cimetidine-imipramine interaction: a case report. *Am J Psychiatry.* 1983;140:351.

Shapiro PA. Cimetidine-imipramine interaction: case report and comments. *Am J Psychiatry.* 1984;141:152.

Wells BG, et al. The effect of ranitidine and cimetidine on imipramine disposition. *Eur J Clin Pharmacol.* 1986;31:285.

Spine E, et al. Differential effects of cimetidine and ranitidine on imipramine demethylation and desmethylimipramine hydroxylation by human liver microsomes. *Eur J Clin Pharmacol.* 1986;30:239.

Cimetidine (eg, *Tagamet*)

Ketoconazole (eg, *Nizoral*)

SUMMARY: Cimetidine administration reduces ketoconazole concentrations.

RISK FACTORS: No specific risk factors are known.

RELATED DRUGS: Other oral imidazole antifungal agents (eg, fluconazole [*Diflucan*]) may be affected similarly by cimetidine administration. Other H_2-receptor antagonists (eg, ranitidine [eg, *Zantac*], famotidine [eg, *Pepcid*], nizatidine [*Axid*]) and proton pump inhibitors would be expected to reduce ketoconazole absorption.

MANAGEMENT OPTIONS:

➡ *Circumvent/Minimize.* Several recommendations have been made to avoid this interaction in patients with elevated gastric pH. The product information for ketoconazole suggests that each ketoconazole tablet should be dissolved in 4 mL of an aqueous solution of 0.2 N hydrochloric acid with the resulting mixture ingested with a straw (to avoid contact with teeth) and followed by a glass of water. Others suggest that an easier and equally effective method is to give 2 capsules of glutamic acid hydrochloride 15 minutes before the ketoconazole.

➡ *Monitor.* Until more is known about this interaction, be alert for evidence of reduced ketoconazole effect when cimetidine or other agents that increase gastric pH are coadministered.

REFERENCES:

Van Der Meet JWM, et al. The influence of gastric acidity on the bioavailability of ketoconazole. *J Antimicrob Chemother.* 1980;6:552.

Lelawongs P, et al. Effect of food and gastric acidity on absorption of orally administered ketoconazole. *Clin Pharm.* 1988;7:228.

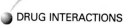
Product information. Ketoconazole (*Nizoral*). Janssen. 1993.

Blum RA, et al. Effect of increased gastric pH on the relative bioavailability of fluconazole and ketoconazole. *Pharm Res.* 1990;7:S52.

Cimetidine (eg, *Tagamet*)

Lidocaine (eg, *Xylocaine*)

SUMMARY: Cimetidine modestly increases lidocaine serum concentrations, but it is not known how often this would cause lidocaine toxicity.

RISK FACTORS: No specific risk factors are known.

RELATED DRUGS: Ranitidine (eg, *Zantac*) may be a good alternative to cimetidine because it has minimal effect on lidocaine disposition. For similar reasons, it is unlikely that famotidine (eg, *Pepcid*) and nizatidine (*Axid*) would interact with lidocaine.

MANAGEMENT OPTIONS:

➥ *Consider Alternative.* Ranitidine, famotidine, or nizatidine would be less likely to interact with lidocaine.

➥ *Monitor.* Monitor patients for lidocaine toxicity when cimetidine and lidocaine are given concurrently.

REFERENCES:

Wing LMH, et al. Lidocaine disposition: sex differences and effects of cimetidine. *Clin Pharmacol Ther.* 1984;35:695.

Jackson JE, et al. Effects of histamine-2 receptor blockade on lidocaine kinetics. *Clin Pharmacol Ther.* 1985;37:544.

Bauer LA, et al. Cimetidine-induced decrease in lidocaine metabolism. *Am Heart J.* 1984;108:413.

Feely J, et al. Increased toxicity and reduced clearance of lidocaine by cimetidine. *Ann Intern Med.* 1982;96:592.

Knapp AB, et al. The cimetidine-lidocaine interaction. *Ann Intern Med.* 1983;98:174.

Feely J, et al. Reduction of liver blood flow and propranolol metabolism by cimetidine. *N Engl J Med.* 1981;304:692.

Jackson JE, et al. The effects of H₂-blockers on lidocaine disposition. *Clin Pharmacol Ther.* 1983;33:255.

Powell JR, et al. Lack of cimetidine-lidocaine interaction in patients with suspected myocardial infarction. *Drug Intell Clin Pharm.* 1983;17:445.

Powell JR, et al. Effect of duration of lidocaine infusion and route of cimetidine administration on lidocaine pharmacokinetics. *Clin Pharm.* 1986;5:993.

Bauer LA, et al. Influence of long-term infusion on lidocaine kinetics. *Clin Pharmacol Ther.* 1982;31:433.

Cimetidine (eg, *Tagamet*)

Melphalan (*Alkeran*)

SUMMARY: Cimetidine administration appears to reduce the serum concentrations of melphalan, but the clinical importance of this effect is not established.

RISK FACTORS: No specific risk factors are known.

RELATED DRUGS: Other inhibitors of gastric acid secretion also may reduce the serum concentrations of melphalan, but little clinical information is available.

MANAGEMENT OPTIONS:

➡ *Monitor.* Until further information is available, monitor patients treated with melphalan and cimetidine for reduced melphalan activity.

REFERENCES:

Sviland L, et al. Interaction of cimetidine with oral melphalan. *Cancer Chemother Pharmacol.* 1987;20:173

Cimetidine (eg, *Tagamet*)

Meperidine (eg, *Demerol*)

SUMMARY: Cimetidine may increase the effect of meperidine and possibly other narcotic analgesics; morphine may be less likely to interact than other narcotics.

RISK FACTORS: No specific risk factors are known.

RELATED DRUGS: In vitro studies also indicate that cimetidine may inhibit the hepatic microsomal metabolism of meperidine and fentanyl. Morphine disposition was not affected by cimetidine pretreatment in 7 healthy men, probably because morphine undergoes glucuronidation, a metabolic process little affected by cimetidine. Cimetidine may inhibit some of the cardiovascular effects of histamine, which is released in response to administration of narcotic analgesics. Pharmacodynamic interactions between cimetidine and narcotic analgesics are also possible but not well studied. Ranitidine (eg, *Zantac*) is probably less likely to interact than cimetidine and thus may be preferable in patients receiving meperidine. Theoretically, famotidine (eg, *Pepcid*) and nizatidine (*Axid*) also would be less likely to interact than cimetidine.

MANAGEMENT OPTIONS:

➡ *Consider Alternative.* Ranitidine may be preferable in patients receiving meperidine, as it is less likely to interact.

➡ *Monitor.* Until these interactions are better described, be alert for evidence of enhanced respiratory and CNS depression during combined therapy with cimetidine and narcotic analgesics.

REFERENCES:

Guay DRP, et al. Cimetidine alters pethidine disposition in man. *Br J Clin Pharmacol.* 1984;18:907.

Guay DRP, et al. Ranitidine does not alter pethidine disposition in man. *Br J Clin Pharmacol.* 1985;20:55.

Fine A, et al. Potentially lethal interaction of cimetidine and morphine. *Can Med Assoc J.* 1981;124:1434.

Lam AM, et al. Cimetidine and prolonged post-operative somnolence. *Can Anaesth Soc J.* 1981;28:450.

Knodell RG, et al. Drug metabolism by rat and human hepatic microsomes in response to interaction with H_2-receptor antagonists. *Gastroenterology.* 1982;82:84.

Lee HR, et al. Effect of histamine H_2-receptors on fentanyl metabolism. *Pharmacologist.* 1982;24:145.

Mojaverian P, et al. Cimetidine does not alter morphine disposition in man. *Br J Clin Pharmacol.* 1982;14:309.

Cimetidine (eg, *Tagamet*)

Metformin (*Glucophage*)

SUMMARY: Cimetidine administration increases metformin plasma concentrations; an increase in therapeutic effect or toxicity may occur.

RISK FACTORS:

➡ **Concurrent Diseases.** Patients with reduced renal function may be at an increased risk of elevated metformin concentrations during cimetidine administration.

RELATED DRUGS: Other drugs that may compete with metformin for secretion at the renal tubular organic cation system (eg, procainamide [eg, *Ponestyl*], trimethoprim [eg, *Proloprim*]) could result in a similar effect on metformin elimination. While no data are available, other acid suppressive agents [eg, famotidine (eg, *Pepcid*)] may be less likely to affect metformin renal elimination.

MANAGEMENT OPTIONS:

➡ **Consider Alternative.** Consider the use of an alternative H_2-antagonist such as famotidine in patients taking metformin. The effect of proton pump inhibitors such as omeprazole (*Prilosec*) on the renal tubular secretion of metformin is unknown.

➡ **Monitor.** Monitor patients taking metformin for lactic acidosis (eg, hyperventilation, tachycardia, nausea) if cimetidine is administered.

REFERENCES:

Somogyi A, et al. Reduction of metformin renal tubular secretion by cimetidine in man. *Br J Clin Pharmacol*. 1987;23:545.

Cimetidine (eg, *Tagamet*)

Moricizine (*Ethmozine*)

SUMMARY: In a single-dose study in healthy subjects, cimetidine significantly increased moricizine serum concentrations.

RISK FACTORS: No specific risk factors are known.

RELATED DRUGS: Theoretically, other H_2-receptor antagonists such as ranitidine (eg, *Zantac*), famotidine (eg, *Pepcid*), and nizatidine (*Axid*), would be less likely to interact with moricizine.

MANAGEMENT OPTIONS:

➡ **Monitor.** Monitor patients taking moricizine for increased moricizine concentrations and increased cardiovascular effects if cimetidine is added.

REFERENCES:

Biollaz J, et al. Cimetidine inhibition of moricizine metabolism. *Clin Pharmacol Ther*. 1985;37:665.

Cimetidine (eg, *Tagamet*)

Nicotine (eg, *Nicorette*)

SUMMARY: Cimetidine increases blood nicotine concentrations and may reduce the amount of nicotine gum or patches needed.

RISK FACTORS: No specific risk factors are known.

RELATED DRUGS: Ranitidine may reduce nicotine clearance as mentioned above. The effect of famotidine (eg, *Pepcid*) and nizatidine (*Axid*) on nicotine elimination is unknown, but one would expect them to interact minimally as does ranitidine.

MANAGEMENT OPTIONS:

➡ *Circumvent/Minimize.* Patients on cimetidine therapy may not need to use as much nicotine gum or nicotine patches as those not on cimetidine. For smokers, it is possible that cimetidine therapy would allow a reduction in the number of cigarettes smoked while maintaining the same blood nicotine concentrations.

➡ *Monitor.* Be alert for evidence of excessive nicotine response.

REFERENCES:

Bendayan R, et al. Effect of cimetidine and ranitidine on the hepatic and renal elimination of nicotine in humans. *Eur J Clin Pharmacol*. 1990;38:165.

Cimetidine (eg, *Tagamet*)

Nifedipine (eg, *Procardia*)

SUMMARY: Cimetidine can increase the serum concentration of nifedipine; excessive nifedipine effects can occur.

RISK FACTORS: No specific risk factors are known.

RELATED DRUGS: Ranitidine (eg, *Zantac*) appears to have a smaller effect on nifedipine serum concentrations but may increase nifedipine AUC 13% to 48%. If confirmed, other H_2-receptor antagonists (eg, famotidine [eg, *Pepcid*] and nizatidine [*Axid*]), omeprazole (*Prilosec*), and lansoprazole (*Prevacid*) would be expected to have a similar effect. Increased nifedipine effects (eg, headache, hypotension) could occur. Cimetidine also increases the concentrations of diltiazem (eg, *Cardizem*), nisoldipine (*Sular*), nitrendipine, and verapamil (eg, *Calan*).

MANAGEMENT OPTIONS:

➡ *Monitor.* Carefully monitor patients receiving nifedipine when cimetidine or other drugs that alter gastric pH are added or deleted from their drug regimen.

REFERENCES:

Kirch W, et al. Einflub von cimetidine und ranitidin auf pharmakokinetic und antihypertensive effekt von nifedipin. *Dtsch Med Wochenschr*. 1983;108:1757.

Renwick AG, et al. Factors affecting the pharmacokinetics of nifedipine. *Eur J Clin Pharmacol*. 1987;32:351.

Smith SR, et al. Ranitidine and cimetidine; drug interactions with single and steady-state nifedipine administration. *Br J Clin Pharmacol*. 1987;23:311.

Adams LJ, et al. Effect of ranitidine on bioavailability of nifedipine. *Gastroenterology*. 1986;90:1320.

Kirch W, et al. Ranitidine increases bioavailability of nifedipine. *Clin Pharmacol Ther*. 1985;37:204.

Schwartz JB, et al. Effect of cimetidine or ranitidine administration of nifedipine pharmacokinetics and pharmacodynamics. *Clin Pharmacol Ther*. 1988;43:673.

Khan A, et al. The pharmacokinetics and pharmacodynamics of nifedipine at steady state during concomitant administration of cimetidine or high dose ranitidine. *Br J Clin Pharmacol*. 1991;32:519.

Cimetidine (eg, *Tagamet*)

Nimodipine (*Nimotop*)

SUMMARY: Cimetidine can increase the serum concentration of nimodipine; the clinical significance of this interaction is unknown.

RISK FACTORS: No specific risk factors are known.

RELATED DRUGS: Cimetidine also increases the concentrations of diltiazem (eg, *Cardizem*), nisoldipine (*Sular*), nifedipine (eg, *Procardia*), and verapamil (eg, *Calan*). Ranitidine (eg, *Zantac*) 300 mg/day for 5 days produced no change in the pharmacokinetics of nimodipine. Other drugs that increase gastric pH (eg, omeprazole [*Prilosec*]) may affect nimodipine similarly.

MANAGEMENT OPTIONS:

➡ *Monitor.* Monitor patients receiving nimodipine for excessive effects (eg, headache, hypotension) when cimetidine is added or deleted from their drug regimen.

REFERENCES:

Muck W, et al. Influence of the H2-receptor antagonists cimetidine and ranitidine on the pharmacokinetics of nimodipine in healthy volunteers. *Eur J Clin Pharmacol*. 1992;42:325.

Cimetidine (eg, *Tagamet*)

Nisoldipine (*Sular*)

SUMMARY: Cimetidine can increase the serum concentration of nisoldipine; excessive nisoldipine effects may be seen.

RISK FACTORS:

➡ *Route of Administration.* Oral administration of nisoldipine increases the likelihood of this interaction.

RELATED DRUGS: Cimetidine also increases the concentrations of diltiazem (eg, *Cardizem*), nifedipine (eg, *Procardia*), nitrendipine, and verapamil (eg, *Calan*). Other drugs that increase gastric pH (eg, famotidine [eg, *Pepcid*], nizatidine [*Axid*], ranitidine [eg, *Zantac*], omeprazole [*Prilosec*]) may affect nisoldipine in a similar manner.

MANAGEMENT OPTIONS:

➡ *Monitor.* Carefully monitor patients receiving nisoldipine for altered hypotensive effects when cimetidine or other drugs that alter gastric pH are added or deleted from their drug regimen.

REFERENCES:

van Harten J, et al. Pharmacokinetics and hemodynamic effects of nisoldipine and its interaction with cimetidine. *Clin Pharmacol Ther*. 1988;43:332.

Cimetidine (eg, *Tagamet*)

Nitrendipine (*Baypress*)

SUMMARY: Cimetidine can increase the serum concentration of nitrendipine; excessive nitrendipine effects may be seen.

RISK FACTORS: No specific risk factors are known.

RELATED DRUGS: Cimetidine also increases the concentrations of diltiazem (eg, *Cardizem*), nisoldipine (*Sular*), nifedipine (eg, *Procardia*), and verapamil (eg, *Calan*). Ranitidine (eg, *Zantac*) 300 mg/day for 1 week increased the AUC of nitrendipine 50% without changing its hemodynamic effects. Other drugs that increase gastric pH (eg, famotidine [eg, *Pepcid*], nizatidine [*Axid*], omeprazole [*Prilosec*]) may affect nitrendipine in a similar manner.

MANAGEMENT OPTIONS:

➡ *Monitor.* Carefully monitor patients receiving nitrendipine for altered hypotensive effects when cimetidine or other drugs that increase gastric pH are added or deleted from their drug regimen.

REFERENCES:

Halabi A, et al. Influence of ranitidine on kinetics of nitrendipine and on noninvasive hemodynamic parameters. *Ther Drug Monit.* 1990;12:303.

Soons PA, et al. Grapefruit juice and cimetidine inhibit stereoselective metabolism of nitrendipine in humans. *Clin Pharmacol Ther.* 1991;50:394.

Cimetidine (eg, *Tagamet*)

Nortriptyline (eg, *Pamelor*)

SUMMARY: Limited clinical evidence suggests that cimetidine increases serum nortriptyline concentrations; given the proven effect of cimetidine on tricyclic antidepressants closely related to nortriptyline, it seems likely that nortriptyline is affected similarly.

RISK FACTORS:

➡ *Dosage Regimen.* In most patients, clinically important inhibition of hepatic drug metabolism by cimetidine requires doses 400 mg/day or higher.

RELATED DRUGS: The evidence suggests that ranitidine (eg, *Zantac*) is unlikely to interact with cyclic antidepressants. Theoretically, it is unlikely that famotidine (eg, *Pepcid*) and nizatidine (*Axid*) will interact with cyclic antidepressants because these H₂-receptor antagonists have little effect on drug metabolism. Cimetidine also may increase serum concentrations of desipramine (eg, *Norpramin*), doxepin (eg, *Sinequan*), imipramine (eg, *Tofranil*), and protriptyline (eg, *Vivactil*).

MANAGEMENT OPTIONS:

➡ *Consider Alternative.* Consider using an alternative to cimetidine (eg, ranitidine, nizatidine, famotidine).

➡ *Circumvent/Minimize.* In patients who are already receiving cimetidine and are about to begin a course of therapy with nortriptyline, consider using conservative nortriptyline doses until the patient's response to therapy can be evaluated.

➡️ *Monitor.* In patients stabilized on nortriptyline who are then given cimetidine, be alert for evidence of nortriptyline toxicity (eg, severe dry mouth, blurred vision, urinary retention, tachycardia, constipation, postural hypotension). If cimetidine is discontinued or its dose substantially reduced in a patient stabilized on both nortriptyline and cimetidine, monitor the patient for an inadequate nortriptyline response.

REFERENCES:
Miller DD, et al. Cimetidine's effect on steady-state serum nortriptyline concentrations. *Drug Intell Clin Pharm.* 1983;17:904.

Henauer SA, et al. Cimetidine interaction with imipramine and nortriptyline. *Clin Pharmacol Ther.* 1984;35:183.

 Cimetidine (eg, *Tagamet*)

Paroxetine (*Paxil*)

SUMMARY: Preliminary evidence suggests that cimetidine substantially increases paroxetine serum concentrations, but the clinical importance of the interaction is not established.

RISK FACTORS: No specific risk factors are known.

RELATED DRUGS: The effect of ranitidine (eg, *Zantac*), famotidine (eg, *Pepcid*), and nizatidine (*Axid*) on paroxetine pharmacokinetics is unknown; theoretically they would not be expected to interact.

MANAGEMENT OPTIONS:

➡️ *Consider Alternative.* Theoretically, other H_2-receptor antagonists, such as ranitidine, famotidine, and nizatidine, would be less likely to interact with paroxetine; thus their use may be preferred over cimetidine until more information is available on this interaction.

➡️ *Monitor.* Monitor patients for alterations in therapeutic and toxic effects of paroxetine if cimetidine is initiated, discontinued, or changed in dosage. Patients receiving cimetidine may require lower doses of paroxetine. However, determining whether to adjust the dose of paroxetine and by how much may not be easy, because the degree to which paroxetine produces dose-dependent adverse effects is not well established.

REFERENCES:
Greb WH, et al. The effect of liver enzyme inhibition by cimetidine and enzyme induction by phenobarbitone on the pharmacokinetics of paroxetine. *Acta Psychiatr Scand.* 1989;80(Suppl. 350):95.

Bannister SJ, et al. Evaluation of the potential for interactions of paroxetine with diazepam, cimetidine, warfarin, and digoxin. *Acta Psychiatr Scand.* 1989;80(Suppl. 350):102.

Cimetidine (eg, *Tagamet*)

Phenytoin (eg, *Dilantin*)

SUMMARY: Cimetidine increases serum phenytoin concentrations; phenytoin intoxication occurs in some patients. Ranitidine may increase serum phenytoin concentrations in some patients, but the data are limited.

RISK FACTORS:

➡ **Dosage Regimen.** Cimetidine doses of 400 mg/day may increase serum phenytoin slightly, but larger cimetidine doses can produce greater increases.

RELATED DRUGS: Ranitidine (eg, *Zantac*), famotidine (eg, *Pepcid*), and nizatidine (*Axid*) do not appear to affect phenytoin metabolism. Case reports have suggested that ranitidine may increase serum phenytoin concentrations, but the cases were complicated by other confounding variables.

MANAGEMENT OPTIONS:

➡ **Consider Alternative.** Ranitidine, famotidine, and nizatidine would be preferable to cimetidine in most patients receiving phenytoin.

➡ **Monitor.** Be alert for evidence of phenytoin toxicity (eg, nystagmus, ataxia, confusion) when cimetidine is given concurrently. In a patient well stabilized on both drugs, discontinuation of cimetidine may result in inadequate serum phenytoin concentrations.

REFERENCES:

Levine M, et al. Differential effect of cimetidine on serum concentrations of carbamazepine and phenytoin. *Neurology*. 1985;35:562.

Hetzel DJ, et al. Cimetidine interaction with phenytoin. *BMJ*. 1981;282:1512.

Neuvonen PJ, et al. Cimetidine-phenytoin interaction: effect on serum phenytoin concentration and antipyrine test. *Eur J Clin Pharmacol*. 1981;21:215.

Algozzine GJ, et al. Decreased clearance of phenytoin with cimetidine. *Ann Intern Med*. 1981;95:244.

Bartle WR, et al. Dose-dependent effect of cimetidine on phenytoin kinetics. *Clin Pharmacol Ther*. 1983;33:649.

Salem RB, et al. Effect of cimetidine on phenytoin serum levels. *Epilepsia*. 1983;24:284.

Iteogu MO, et al. Effect of cimetidine on single-dose phenytoin kinetics. *Clin Pharm*. 1983;2:302.

Phillips P, Hansky J. Phenytoin toxicity secondary to cimetidine administration. *Med J Aust*. 1984;141:602.

Watts RW, et al. Lack of interaction between ranitidine and phenytoin. *Br J Clin Pharmacol*. 1983;15:499.

Sambol NC, et al. Influence of famotidine (Fam) and cimetidine (Cim) on the disposition of phenytoin (Phe) and indocyanine green (ICG). *Clin Pharmacol Ther*. 1986;39:225.

Bramhall D, et al. Possible interaction of ranitidine with phenytoin. *Drug Intell Clin Pharm*. 1988;22:979.

Tse CST, et al. Phenytoin concentration elevation subsequent to ranitidine administration. *Ann Pharmacother*. 1993;27:1448.

Tse CST, et al. Phenytoin and ranitidine interaction. *Ann Intern Med*. 1994;120:892.

Cimetidine (eg, *Tagamet*)

Praziquantel (*Biltricide*)

SUMMARY: Cimetidine increases praziquantel concentrations; the clinical significance of these changes are unknown, but toxicity is possible.

RISK FACTORS: No specific risk factors are known.

RELATED DRUGS: Other H_2-receptor antagonists, such as ranitidine (eg, *Zantac*), famotidine (eg, *Pepcid*), and nizatidine (*Axid*), would be unlikely to affect the metabolism of praziquantel.

MANAGEMENT OPTIONS:

➡ ***Consider Alternative.*** In patients not receiving anticonvulsants, an alternative H_2-receptor antagonist (eg, ranitidine, famotidine, nizatidine) probably would avoid the interaction.

➡ ***Monitor.*** Monitor patients who receive cimetidine and praziquantel for increased praziquantel plasma concentrations and potential toxicity (eg, headache, nausea, dizziness).

REFERENCES:

Dachman WD, et al. Cimetidine-induced rise in praziquantel levels in a patient with neurocysticercosis being treated with anticonvulsants. *J Infect Dis.* 1994;169:689.

Metwally A, et al. Effect of cimetidine, bicarbonate and glucose on the bioavailability of different formulations of praziquantel. *Arzneimittelforschung.* 1995;45:460.

Cimetidine (eg, *Tagamet*)

Procainamide (eg, *Pronestyl*)

SUMMARY: Cimetidine may increase procainamide serum concentrations significantly; procainamide toxicity from this interaction has been reported.

RISK FACTORS:

➡ ***Concurrent Diseases.*** Patients with renal dysfunction are at particular risk.

RELATED DRUGS: Ranitidine (eg, *Zantac*) produces a small increase in procainamide concentrations; famotidine (eg, *Pepcid*) appears to have no effect. Theoretically, nizatidine (*Axid*) is unlikely to interact. Although no data exist, proton pump inhibitors (eg, omeprazole [*Prilosec*]) would be unlikely to alter procainamide clearance.

MANAGEMENT OPTIONS:

➡ ***Consider Alternative.*** Famotidine or nizatidine use would likely avoid the interaction.

➡ ***Monitor.*** Be alert for evidence of enhanced procainamide and NAPA response (eg, wide QRS, QT interval) in the presence of cimetidine therapy. A reduction in procainamide dose may be necessary.

REFERENCES:

Somogyi A, et al. Cimetidine-procainamide pharmacokinetic interaction in man: evidence of competition for tubular secretion of basic drugs. *Eur J Clin Pharmacol.* 1983;25:339.

Drayer DE, et al. Cumulation of N-acetylprocainamide, an active metabolite of procainamide, in patients with impaired renal function. *Clin Pharmacol Ther.* 1977;22:63.

Reidenberg MM, et al. Aging and renal clearance of procainamide and acetylprocainamide. *Clin Pharmacol Ther.* 1980;28:732.

Higbee MD, et al. Procainamide-cimetidine interaction: a potential toxic interaction in the elderly. *J Am Geriatr Soc.* 1984;32:162.

Christain CW Jr, et al. Cimetidine inhibits renal procainamide clearance. *Clin Pharmacol Ther.* 1984;36:221.

Lai MY, et al. Dose dependent effect of cimetidine on procainamide disposition in man. *Int J Clin Pharmacol Ther Toxicol.* 1988;26:118.

Bauer LA, et al. Procainamide-cimetidine drug interaction in elderly male patients. *J Am Geriatr Soc.* 1990;38:467.

Cimetidine (eg, *Tagamet*)

Propafenone (*Rythmol*)

SUMMARY: Cimetidine significantly increased propafenone concentration in 8 of 12 subjects stabilized on propafenone.

RISK FACTORS: No specific risk factors are known.

RELATED DRUGS: The effects of other H_2-receptor antagonists on propafenone are unknown; ranitidine (eg, *Zantac*), nizatidine (*Axid*), and famotidine (eg, *Pepcid*) would be expected to have little effect on propafenone.

MANAGEMENT OPTIONS:

➡ *Monitor.* Until further information is available, carefully observe patients maintained on propafenone for increased propafenone response if cimetidine is added or for a reduced response if cimetidine is removed from their drug regimen.

REFERENCES:

Pritchett ELC, et al. Pharmacokinetic and pharmacodynamic interactions of propafenone and cimetidine. *J Clin Pharmacol.* 1988;28:619.

Cimetidine (eg, *Tagamet*)

Propranolol (eg, *Inderal*)

SUMMARY: Propranolol and other plasma concentrations of beta blockers that undergo significant hepatic metabolism (eg, metoprolol, labetalol) may be increased by cimetidine therapy.

RISK FACTORS: No specific risk factors are known.

RELATED DRUGS: Metoprolol (eg, *Lopressor*) pharmacokinetics (100 mg single dose) were not affected by cimetidine in one study, but cimetidine substantially increased plasma concentrations of metoprolol 100 mg twice daily for 7 days in other studies. The bioavailability of labetalol (eg, *Normodyne*) was increased 55% to 80% without significant change in systemic clearance after the administration of cimetidine 1.6 g/day for 3 days, while the bioavailability of dilevalol increased 11% and the area under the concentration-time curve (AUC) increased 20% following cimetidine 1.2 g/day. The renal clearance of pindolol (eg, *Visken*) was reduced approximately 30% and its AUC increased approximately 45% with cimetidine 400 mg twice daily coadministration. Atenolol (eg, *Tenormin*), penbutolol (*Levatol*), and nadolol (eg, *Corgard*) appear to be affected minimally by cimetidine therapy. Ranitidine (eg, *Zantac*) does not affect propranolol concentrations. Famotidine (eg, *Pepcid*) and nizatidine (*Axid*) would be unlikely to affect propranolol concentrations.

MANAGEMENT OPTIONS:

➡ *Consider Alternative.* Atenolol or nadolol could be administered instead of hepatically metabolized beta blockers. Ranitidine, famotidine, nizatidine, antacids, or sucralfate (eg, *Carafate*) also may be suitable alternatives to cimetidine, although beta blocker doses probably should be separated from antacids or sucralfate to minimize the possibility of impaired absorption of the beta blocker.

➡ *Monitor.* Be alert for evidence of altered response to propranolol, labetalol, and possibly other beta blockers when cimetidine therapy is initiated or discontinued.

REFERENCES:

Duchin KL, et al. Comparison of kinetic interaction of nadolol and propranolol with cimetidine. *Am Heart J.* 1984;108(Part 2):1084.

Spahn H, et al. Penbutolol pharmacokinetics: the influence of concomitant administration of cimetidine. *Eur J Clin Pharmacol.* 1986;29:555.

Mutschler E, et al. The interaction between H$_2$-receptor antagonists and beta-adrenoceptor blockers. *Br J Clin Pharmacol.* 1984;17:51S.

Kirch W, et al. Interaction of metoprolol, propranolol and atenolol with concurrent administration of cimetidine. *Klin Wochenschr.* 1982;60:1401.

Tomonori T, et al. The influence of diltiazem versus cimetidine on propranolol metabolism. *J Clin Pharmacol.* 1992;32:1099.

Reimann IW, et al. Cimetidine increases steady plasma levels of propranolol. *Br J Clin Pharmacol.* 1981;12:785.

Houtzagers JJR, et al. The effect of pretreatment with cimetidine on the bioavailability and disposition of atenolol and metoprolol. *Br J Clin Pharmacol.* 1982;14:67.

Daneshmend TK, et al. Cimetidine and bioavailability of labetalol. *Lancet.* 1981;1:565.

Daneshmend TK, et al. The effects of enzyme induction and enzyme inhibition of labetalol pharmacokinetics. *Br J Clin Pharmacol.* 1984;18:393.

Donn KH, et al. Stereoselectivity of cimetidine inhibition of propranolol oral clearance. *Clin Pharmacol Ther.* 1988;43:283.

Toon S, et al. The racemic metoprolol H2-antagonist interaction. *Clin Pharmacol Ther.* 1988;43:283.

Somogyi AA, et al. Stereoselective inhibition of pindolol renal clearance by cimetidine in humans. *Clin Pharmacol Ther.* 1992;51:379.

Cimetidine (eg, *Tagamet*)

Quinidine (eg, *Quinora*)

SUMMARY: Cimetidine coadministration elevates quinidine serum concentrations; watch for evidence of quinidine toxicity.

RISK FACTORS: No specific risk factors are known.

RELATED DRUGS: While ranitidine (eg, *Zantac*) would not be expected to alter quinidine metabolism, a case of ventricular bigeminy during quinidine and ranitidine coadministration has been reported.

MANAGEMENT OPTIONS:

➡ *Consider Alternative.* Other H$_2$-receptor antagonists, such as ranitidine, famotidine (eg, *Pepcid*), and nizatidine (*Axid*), are probably less likely to interact with quinidine than cimetidine.

➡ *Monitor.* Be alert for evidence of altered quinidine response when cimetidine is started or stopped. Serum quinidine determinations would be useful if the interaction is suspected.

REFERENCES:

Polish LB, et al. Digitoxin-quinidine interaction: potentiation during administration of cimetidine. *South Med J.* 1981;74:633-634.

Farringer JA, et al. Cimetidine-quinidine interaction. *Clin Pharm.* 1984;3:81-83.

Kolb KW, et al. The effect of cimetidine on urinary pH and quinidine clearance. American Society of Hospital Pharmacists Midyear Clinical Meeting; December, 1982.

Hardy BG, et al. Effect of cimetidine on the pharmacokinetics and pharmacodynamics of quinidine. *Am J Cardiol*. 1983;52:172-175.

MacKichan JJ, et al. Effect of cimetidine on quinidine bioavailability. *Biopharm Drug Dispos*. 1989;10:121-125.

Hardy BG, et al. Lack of effect of cimetidine on the metabolism of quinidine: effect on renal clearance. *Int J Clin Pharmacol Ther Toxicol*. 1988;26:388-391.

Iliopoulou A, et al. Quinidine-ranitidine adverse reaction. *Eur Heart J*. 1986;7:360.

Cimetidine (eg, *Tagamet*)

Tacrine (*Cognex*)

SUMMARY: Cimetidine substantially increases tacrine plasma concentrations, but the degree to which it increases tacrine adverse effects is not established.

RISK FACTORS:

➡ ***Dosage Regimen.*** In most patients, clinically important inhibition of hepatic drug metabolism by cimetidine requires doses of 400 mg/day or higher.

RELATED DRUGS: The effect of ranitidine (eg, *Zantac*), famotidine (eg, *Pepcid*), and nizatidine (*Axid*) on tacrine metabolism is not established, but an interaction would not be expected.

MANAGEMENT OPTIONS:

➡ ***Consider Alternative.*** Until the clinical importance of the cimetidine-tacrine interaction is established, consider using alternative H₂-receptor antagonists such as ranitidine, famotidine, or nizatidine.

➡ ***Monitor.*** If cimetidine and tacrine are used concurrently, monitor for excessive cholinergic response (eg, nausea, vomiting, anorexia, diarrhea, abdominal pain) and adjust tacrine dosage as needed.

REFERENCES:

de Vries TM, et al. Effect of cimetidine and low-dose quinidine on tacrine pharmacokinetics in humans. *Pharm Res*. 1993;10:S337.

Product information. Tacrine (*Cognex*). Parke-Davis. 1993.

Madden S, et al. An investigation into the formation of stable, proteinreactive and cytotoxic metabolites from tacrine in vitro. Studies with human and rat liver microsomes. *Biochem Pharmacol*. 1993;46:13.

Spaldin V, et al. The effect of enzyme inhibition on the metabolism and activation of tacrine by human liver microsomes. *Br J Clin Pharmacol*. 1994;38:15.

Cimetidine (eg, *Tagamet*)

Theophylline (eg, *Theolair*)

SUMMARY: Cimetidine increases serum theophylline concentrations, resulting in symptoms of theophylline toxicity in some patients.

RISK FACTORS:

➡ ***Dosage Regimen.*** The magnitude of this interaction increases as the dose of cimetidine increases.

➡ ***Habits.*** Cimetidine may have a greater effect in smokers and other patients with high basal theophylline clearance.

RELATED DRUGS: H$_2$-receptor antagonists other than cimetidine, such as famotidine (eg, *Pepcid*), nizatidine (*Axid*), and ranitidine (eg, *Zantac*), are unlikely to affect theophylline pharmacokinetics.

MANAGEMENT OPTIONS:

➧ *Consider Alternative.* Ranitidine does not appear to affect theophylline disposition and thus would be preferable to cimetidine in patients receiving theophylline. Famotidine and nizatidine are also unlikely to interact with theophylline.

➧ *Monitor.* If cimetidine is used with theophylline, monitor for altered theophylline response if cimetidine therapy is initiated, discontinued, or changed in dosage; the dose of theophylline may need to be adjusted. In a patient already receiving cimetidine, initial doses of theophylline should be conservative until the dosage requirement is determined. Serum theophylline determinations would be useful in following this interaction.

REFERENCES:

Grygiel JJ, et al. Differential effects of cimetidine on theophylline metabolic pathways. *Eur J Clin Pharmacol.* 1984;265:335.

Jackson JE, et al. Cimetidine decreases theophylline clearance. *Am Rev Respir Dis.* 1981;23:615.

Reitberg DP, et al. Alteration of theophylline clearance and half-life by cimetidine in normal volunteers. *Ann Intern Med.* 1981;95:582.

Roberts RK, et al. Cimetidine impairs the elimination of theophylline and antipyrine. *Gastroenterology.* 1981;81:19.

Schwartz JI, et al. Impact of cimetidine on the pharmacokinetics of theophylline. *Clin Pharm.* 1982;1:534.

Lalonde RL, et al. The effects of cimetidine on theophylline pharmacokinetics at steady state. *Chest.* 1983;2:221.

Kelly JF, et al. The effect of cimetidine on theophylline metabolism in the elderly. *Clin Pharmacol Ther.* 1982;31:238.

Fenje PC, et al. Interaction of cimetidine and theophylline in two infants. *Can Med Assoc J.* 1982;126:1178.

Cluxton RJ, et al. Cimetidine-theophylline interaction. *Ann Intern Med.* 1982;96:684.

Jackson JE, et al. More on cimetidine-theophylline interaction. *Drug Intell Clin Pharm.* 1981;15:809.

Hendeles L, et al. The interaction of cimetidine and theophylline. *Drug Intell Clin Pharm.* 1981;15:808.

Weinberger MM, et al. Decreased theophylline clearance due to cimetidine. *N Engl J Med.* 1981;304:672.

Campbell MA, et al. Cimetidine decreases theophylline clearance. *Ann intern Med.* 1981;95:68.

Lofgren RP, et al. Cimetidine and theophylline. *Ann Intern Med.* 1982;96:378.

Bauman JH, et al. Cimetidine-theophylline interaction: report of four patients. *Ann Allergy.* 1982;48:100.

Anderson JR, et al. A fatal case of theophylline intoxication. *Arch Intern Med.* 1983;143:559.

Boehning W, et al. Effect of cimetidine and ranitidine on plasma theophylline in patients with chronic obstructive airways disease treated with theophylline and corticosteroids. *Eur J Clin Pharmacol.* 1990;38:43.

Lin JH, et al. Comparative effect of famotidine and cimetidine on the pharmacokinetics of theophylline in normal volunteers. *Br J Clin Pharmacol.* 1987;24:669.

Cimetidine (eg, *Tagamet*)

Tolbutamide (eg, *Orinase*)

SUMMARY: Tolbutamide, glipizide, and glyburide serum concentrations may be increased by cimetidine. Cimetidine may have independent effects on serum glucose.

RISK FACTORS: No specific risk factors are known.

RELATED DRUGS: Ranitidine (eg, *Zantac*) does not alter tolbutamide pharmacokinetics. The effect of famotidine (eg, *Pepcid*) and nizatidine (*Axid*) on sulfonylureas is unknown, but they may interact if increased gastric pH is involved in the observed changes with cimetidine and ranitidine. Glipizide and glyburide interact similarly with cimetidine. Sucralfate (*Carafate*) produced a significant but small (8%) reduction in the chlorpropamide AUC in healthy subjects.

MANAGEMENT OPTIONS:

➡ *Consider Alternative.* Sucralfate may be a good alternative therapy for the treatment of ulcer disease in diabetics because it appears unlikely to alter glycemic control to a clinically significant degree.

➡ *Monitor.* Observe diabetics stabilized on any hypoglycemic therapy in whom H$_2$-receptor antagonist therapy is initiated or discontinued for altered glycemic responses.

REFERENCES:

Catt EW, et al. Inhibition of tolbutamide elimination by cimetidine but not ranitidine. *J Clin Pharmacol.* 1986;26:372.

Stockley C, et al. Lack of inhibition of tolbutamide hydroxylation by cimetidine in man. *Eur J Clin Pharmacol.* 1986;31:235.

Dey NG, et al. The effect of cimetidine on tolbutamide kinetics. *Br J Clin Pharmacol.* 1983;16:438.

Feely J, et al. Potentiation of the hypoglycemic response to glipizide in diabetic patients by histamine H$_2$-receptor antagonists. *Br J Clin Pharmacol.* 1993;35:321.

Kubacka RT, et al. The paradoxical effect of cimetidine and ranitidine on glibenclamide pharmacokinetics and pharmacodynamics. *Br J Clin Pharmacol.* 1987;23:743.

Letendre PW, et al. Effect of sucralfate on the absorption and pharmacokinetics of chlorpropamide. *J Clin Pharmacol.* 1986;26:622.

Adebayo GI, et al. Lack of efficacy of cimetidine and ranitidine as inhibitors of tolbutamide metabolism. *Eur J Clin Pharmacol.* 1988;34:653.

Lahtela JT, et al. The effect of liver microsomal enzyme inducing and inhibiting drugs on insulin mediated glucose metabolism in man. *Br J Clin Pharmacol.* 1986;21:19.

Toon S, et al. Effects of cimetidine, ranitidine and omeprazole on tolbutamide pharmacokinetics. *J Pharm Pharmacol.* 1995;47:85.

Cimetidine (eg, *Tagamet*)

Verapamil (eg, *Calan*)

SUMMARY: Cimetidine can increase the serum concentration of verapamil; excessive verapamil effects may be seen.

RISK FACTORS: No specific risk factors are known.

RELATED DRUGS: Cimetidine also increases the concentrations of diltiazem (eg, *Cardizem*), nisoldipine (*Sular*), nifedipine (eg, *Procardia*), and nitrendipine. Ranitidine (eg, *Zantac*), famotidine (eg, *Pepcid*), and nizatidine (*Axid*) would not be expected to alter verapamil metabolism.

MANAGEMENT OPTIONS:

➡ *Consider Alternative.* Although data is limited, other H$_2$-receptor antagonists (eg, ranitidine, famotidine, nizatidine) would be unlikely to inhibit the metabolism of verapamil.

➡️ *Monitor.* Carefully monitor patients receiving verapamil for signs of toxicity (eg, hypotension, bradycardia, heart block) when cimetidine is added to their drug regimen.

REFERENCES:

Smith MS, et al. Influence of cimetidine on verapamil kinetics and dynamics. *Clin Pharmacol Ther.* 1984;36:551.

Wing LMH, et al. Verapamil disposition—effects of sulphinpyrazone and cimetidine. *Br J Clin Pharmacol.* 1985;19:385.

Abernethy DR, et al. Lack of interaction between verapamil and cimetidine. *Clin Pharmacol Ther.* 1985;38:342.

Loi C-M, et al. Effect of cimetidine on verapamil disposition. *Clin Pharmacol Ther.* 1985;37:654.

Mikus G, et al. Interaction of verapamil and cimetidine: stereochemical aspects of drug metabolism, drug disposition and drug action. *J Pharmacol Exper Ther.* 1990;253:1042.

 Cimetidine (eg, *Tagamet*)

Warfarin (eg, *Coumadin*)

SUMMARY: Cimetidine may increase the hypoprothrombinemic response to oral anticoagulants; the effect is usually modest, but bleeding has occurred in some patients receiving both drugs.

RISK FACTORS:

➡️ *Dosage Regimen.* The interaction between cimetidine and warfarin is dose related. For example, cimetidine doses of 800 mg nightly tend to affect warfarin less than larger doses given at least 2 times daily, and 400 mg/day of cimetidine may be insufficient to produce clinically significant effects on warfarin in some patients.

RELATED DRUGS: Ranitidine (eg, *Zantac*), famotidine (eg, *Pepcid*), and probably nizatidine (*Axid*) are unlikely to affect the hypoprothrombinemic response to warfarin., Phenprocoumon does not appear to be affected by cimetidine. Omeprazole (*Prilosec*), at least in doses of 20 mg/day, appears to produce a small increase in the hypoprothrombinemic response of warfarin. Cimetidine also inhibits the metabolism of acenocoumarol and possibly other oral anticoagulants with the exception of phenprocoumon, which undergoes glucuronide conjugation. Cimetidine does not appear to affect glucuronidation of drugs in the liver.

MANAGEMENT OPTIONS:

➡️ *Use Alternative.* Use ranitidine, famotidine, or nizatidine instead of cimetidine in patients receiving oral anticoagulants. If cimetidine is used, monitor for altered oral anticoagulant effect if cimetidine is initiated, discontinued, or changed in dosage. Adjust the anticoagulant dose as needed.

REFERENCES:

Burnham D, et al. Effects of low cimetidine doses on steady-state warfarin pharmacokinetics and prothrombin time. *J Clin Pharmacol.* 1989;29:862.

Hunt BA, et al. Stereoselective alterations in the pharmacokinetics of warfarin enantiomers with two cimetidine dose regimens. *Pharmacotherapy.* 1989;9:184.

Toon S, et al. The warfarin-cimetidine interaction: stereochemical considerations. *Br J Clin Pharmacol.* 1986;21:245-246.

Choonara IA, et al. Stereoselective interaction between the R enantiomer of warfarin and cimetidine. *Br J Clin Pharmacol.* 1986;21:271-277.

Niopas I, et al. Further insight into the stereoselective interaction between warfarin and cimetidine in man. *Br J Clin Pharmacol.* 1991;32:508-511.

Flind AC. Cimetidine and oral anticoagulants. *BMJ.* 1978;2:1367.

Serlin MJ, et al. Cimetidine: interaction with oral anticoagulants in man. *Lancet.* 1979;2:317-319.

Puurunen J, et al. Effect of cimetidine on microsomal drug metabolism in man. *Eur J Clin Pharmacol.* 1980;18:185-187.

Kerley B, et al. Cimetidine potentiation of warfarin action. *Can Med Assoc J.* 1982;126:116.

Silver BA, et al. Cimetidine potentiation of the hypoprothrombinemic effect of warfarin. *Ann Intern Med.* 1979;90:348-349.

Hetzel D, et al. Cimetidine interaction with warfarin. *Lancet.* 1979;2:639.

Serlin MJ, et al. Lack of effect of ranitidine on warfarin action. *Br J Clin Pharmacol.* 1981;12:791-794.

O'Reilly RA. Comparative interaction of cimetidine and ranitidine with racemic warfarin in man. *Fed Proc.* 1983;42:1175.

Harenberg J, et al. Lack of effect of cimetidine on action of phenprocoumon. *Eur J Clin Pharmacol.* 1982;23:365-367.

Kroon C, et al. Interaction between single dose acenocoumarol and cimetidine or pentobarbitone: validation of a single dose model to predict interactions in steady state. *Br J Clin Pharmacol.* 1990;29:643P.

Ciprofloxacin (*Cipro*)

Clozapine (*Clozaril*)

SUMMARY: Ciprofloxacin administration increases clozapine concentrations; some patients may develop clozapine-induced adverse effects.

RISK FACTORS: No specific risk factors are known.

RELATED DRUGS: Other quinolones known to inhibit CYP1A2 (eg, enoxacin [*Penetrex*]) may increase clozapine concentrations in a similar manner. Ciprofloxacin also may increase the concentrations of olanzapine (eg, *Zyprexa*), a psychotropic agent that also is metabolized by CYP1A2.

MANAGEMENT OPTIONS:

➡ *Consider Alternative.* For patients taking clozapine, consider a quinolone that does not inhibit CYP1A2 (eg, ofloxacin [*Floxin*], lomefloxacin [*Maxaquin*]).

➡ *Monitor.* Monitor patients stabilized on clozapine for increased side effects if ciprofloxacin is coadministered.

REFERENCES:

Raaska K, et al. Ciprofloxacin increases serum clozapine and N-desmethylclozapine: a study in patients with schizophrenia. *Eur J Clin Pharmacol.* 2000;56:585-589.

Markowitz JS, et al. Fluoroquinolone inhibition of clozapine metabolism. *Am J Psychiatry.* 1997;154:881.

Ciprofloxacin (*Cipro*)

Diazepam (eg, *Valium*)

SUMMARY: The plasma concentrations of diazepam are increased by ciprofloxacin; the clinical significance of this interaction is unknown.

RISK FACTORS: No specific risk factors are known.

RELATED DRUGS: Other quinolones also may inhibit the metabolism of diazepam or compete with it at the GABA receptor. Other benzodiazepines may be inhibited by ciprofloxacin.

MANAGEMENT OPTIONS:

➥ **Monitor.** Patients stabilized on diazepam may experience increased plasma concentrations if ciprofloxacin is administered. Observe patients for any increased or prolonged diazepam effects (eg, sedation, ataxia).

REFERENCES:

Kamali F, et al. The influence of steady-state ciprofloxacin on the pharmacokinetics and pharmacodynamics of a single dose of diazepam in healthy volunteers. *Eur J Clin Pharmacol.* 1993;44:365.

Ciprofloxacin (*Cipro*)

Didanosine (*Videx*)

SUMMARY: The buffers contained in didanosine markedly reduce the plasma concentrations of ciprofloxacin and will likely reduce the efficacy of ciprofloxacin.

RISK FACTORS: No specific risk factors are known.

RELATED DRUGS: Other orally administered quinolones also would be expected to interact with didanosine. Drugs containing magnesium or aluminum will likely interact with ciprofloxacin in a similar manner.

MANAGEMENT OPTIONS:

➥ **Circumvent/Minimize.** To avoid this interaction, take ciprofloxacin at least 2 hours before didanosine. Ciprofloxacin administration up to 6 hours after the didanosine will probably not avoid the interaction because of the persistence of aluminum and magnesium in the gut.

➥ **Monitor.** Monitor patient response to ciprofloxacin if this combination is administered.

REFERENCES:

Sahai J, et al. Cations in the didanosine tablet reduce ciprofloxacin bioavailability. *Clin Pharmacol Ther.* 1993;53:292.

Nix DE, et al. Effects of aluminum and magnesium antacids and ranitidine on the absorption of ciprofloxacin. *Clin Pharmacol Ther.* 1989;46:700.

Ciprofloxacin (*Cipro*)

Food

SUMMARY: The administration of ciprofloxacin with milk or yogurt reduces ciprofloxacin concentrations; the clinical significance is unknown but could result in therapeutic failure in some patients.

RISK FACTORS: No specific risk factors are known.

RELATED DRUGS: Lomefloxacin (*Maxaquin*) and temafloxacin pharmacokinetics were not affected significantly by administration with meals. Additionally, ofloxacin (*Floxin*) appears to be similarly unaffected. Some of the other quinolones may be similarly affected.

MANAGEMENT OPTIONS:

➥ **Consider Alternative.** Lomefloxacin, ofloxacin, or temafloxacin could be considered for use instead of ciprofloxacin.

➡ *Circumvent/Minimize.* Counsel patients to avoid taking ciprofloxacin with milk or yogurt.

➡ *Monitor.* Watch for decreased quinolone efficacy if administered with milk or high calcium foods. Quinolone administration with foods not high in calcium appears to be acceptable.

REFERENCES:
Neuvonen PJ, et al. Interference of diary products with the absorption of ciprofloxacin. *Clin Pharmacol Ther.* 1991;50:498.

Frost RW, et al. Ciprofloxacin pharmacokinetics after a standard or high-fat/high-calcium breakfast. *J Clin Pharmacol.* 1989;29:953.

Hooper WD, et al. Effect of food on absorption of lomefloxacin. *Antimicrob Agents Chemother.* 1990;34:1797.

Mack G, et al. Effects of enzyme supplementation on oral absorption of ciprofloxacin in patients with cystic fibrosis. *Antimicrob Agents Chemother.* 1991;35:1484.

Noer BL, et al. The effect of enteral feedings on ciprofloxacin pharmacokinetics. *Pharmacotherapy.* 1990;10:58.

Piccolo ML, et al. Effect of coadministration of a nutritional supplement on ciprofloxacin absorption. *Am J Hosp Pharm.* 1994;51:2697.

Yuk JH, et al. Relative bioavailability in healthy volunteers of ciprofloxacin administered through a nasogastric tube with and without enteral feedings. *Antimicrob Agents Chemother.* 1989;33:1118.

Granneman GR, et al. The effect of food on the bioavailability of temafloxacin. *Clin Pharmacokinet.* 1992;22(Suppl. 1):48.

Lehto P, et al. Different effects of products containing metal ions on the absorption of lomefloxacin. *Clin Pharmacol Ther.* 1994;56:477.

Ciprofloxacin (*Cipro*)

Foscarnet (*Foscavir*)

SUMMARY: The combination of ciprofloxacin and foscarnet has resulted in tonic-clonic seizure activity in 2 patients; the potential significance of this purported interaction requires additional study.

RISK FACTORS: No specific risk factors are known.

RELATED DRUGS: Other quinolones potentially could produce a similar interaction with foscarnet.

MANAGEMENT OPTIONS:

➡ *Monitor.* Until further evidence of this purported interaction is available, monitor patients receiving foscarnet and ciprofloxacin for seizure activity.

REFERENCES:
Fan-Havard P, et al. Concurrent use of foscarnet and ciprofloxacin may increase the propensity for seizures. *Ann Pharmacother.* 1994;28:869.

Ciprofloxacin (*Cipro*)

Iron

SUMMARY: The administration of iron salts with ciprofloxacin lowers the antibiotic serum concentration and may lead to therapeutic failure.

RISK FACTORS: No specific risk factors are known.

RELATED DRUGS: Other quinolones, including norfloxacin (*Noroxin*), have been reported to be affected similarly by iron. Ofloxacin (*Floxin*) absorption may be less affected by iron.

MANAGEMENT OPTIONS:

➠ *Consider Alternative.* Patients taking ciprofloxacin (and probably other quinolones) should not take oral iron salts concurrently because serum ciprofloxacin concentrations may be subtherapeutic. Ofloxacin absorption may be less affected by iron.

➠ *Circumvent/Minimize.* IV iron or IV ciprofloxacin doses could be considered to avoid the interaction. If ciprofloxacin is administered orally, give it at least 2 hours before any oral iron product.

➠ *Monitor.* If the drugs are used together, watch for lessened antibiotic effect.

REFERENCES:

Polk RE, et al. Effect of ferrous sulfate and multivitamins with zinc on absorption of ciprofloxacin in normal volunteers. *Antimicrob Agents Chemother*. 1989;33:1841.

Le Pennec, MP, et al. Possible interaction of ciprofloxacin with ferrous sulfate. *J Antimicrob Chemother*. 1990;25:184.

Brouwers JRBJ, et al. Decreased ciprofloxacin absorption with concomitant administration of ferrous fumarate. Pharmaceut Weekly. *Sci Ed*. 1990;12:182.

Akerele JO, et al. Influence of oral co-administered metallic drugs on ofloxacin pharmacokinetics. *J Antimicrob Chemother*. 1991;28:87.

Kara M, et al. Clinical and chemical interactions between iron preparations and ciprofloxacin. *Br J Clin Pharmacol*. 1991;31:257.

Campbell NCR, et al. Norfloxacin interactions with antacids and minerals. *Br J Clin Pharmacol*. 1992;33:115.

Lehto P, et al. The effect of ferrous sulphate on the absorption of norfloxacin, ciprofloxacin and ofloxacin. *Br J Clin Pharmacol*. 1994;37:82.

Ciprofloxacin (*Cipro*)

Metoprolol (eg, *Lopressor*)

SUMMARY: Ciprofloxacin increases the concentration of metoprolol enantiomers; the greatest effect is on the enantiomer with the least beta-blocking activity.

RISK FACTORS: No specific risk factors are known.

RELATED DRUGS: Quinolones reported to inhibit drug metabolism include ciprofloxacin, enoxacin (*Penetrex*), norfloxacin (*Noroxin*), pipemidic acid, and pefloxacin. These quinolones also may inhibit metoprolol metabolism. Other beta blockers (eg, propranolol [eg, *Inderal*]) may be affected similarly by ciprofloxacin administration.

MANAGEMENT OPTIONS:

➠ *Monitor.* Because patients stabilized on oral metoprolol might experience increased beta blockade during ciprofloxacin coadministration, monitor for bradycardia, heart failure, or prolonged atrioventricular conduction.

REFERENCES:

Waite NM, et al. Disposition of the (+) and (−) isomers of metoprolol following ciprofloxacin treatment. *Pharmacotherapy*. 1990;10:236.

Ciprofloxacin (*Cipro*)

Pentoxifylline (eg, *Trental*)

SUMMARY: Ciprofloxacin increases pentoxifylline plasma concentrations and may increase adverse effects.

RISK FACTORS: No specific risk factors are known.

RELATED DRUGS: Other quinolones that inhibit metabolism (eg, enoxacin [*Penetrex*], norfloxacin [*Noroxin*], pipemidic acid, pefloxacin) would be expected to produce a similar reaction.

MANAGEMENT OPTIONS:

➥ *Monitor.* Monitor patients taking pentoxifylline for increased pentoxifylline effects and side effects (eg, flushing, nausea, headache) if ciprofloxacin is administered.

REFERENCES:

Cleary JD, et al. Ciprofloxacin (CIPRO) and pentoxifylline (PTF): a clinically significant drug interaction. *Pharmacotherapy.* 1992;12:259.

Ciprofloxacin (*Cipro*)

Phenytoin (eg, *Dilantin*)

SUMMARY: Preliminary evidence suggests that ciprofloxacin administration may elevate plasma phenytoin concentrations modestly.

RISK FACTORS: No specific risk factors are known.

RELATED DRUGS: Other quinolones that inhibit metabolism (eg, enoxacin [*Penetrex*], norfloxacin [*Noroxin*], pipemidic acid, pefloxacin) would be expected to produce a similar reaction.

MANAGEMENT OPTIONS:

➥ *Monitor.* Until further data are available, monitor patients for phenytoin toxicity (eg, nystagmus, ataxia, confusion, dizziness, slurred speech, involuntary muscular movements) when ciprofloxacin is started. Serum phenytoin determinations may also be useful. When ciprofloxacin therapy is stopped in the presence of phenytoin therapy, monitor the patient for a reduced phenytoin effect.

REFERENCES:

Schroeder D, et al. Effect of ciprofloxacin on serum phenytoin concentrations in epileptic patients. *Pharmacotherapy.* 1991;11:276.

Hull RL. Possible phenytoin-ciprofloxacin interaction. *Ann Pharmacother.* 1993;27:1283.

Job ML, et al. Effect of ciprofloxacin on the pharmacokinetics of multiple-dose phenytoin serum concentrations. *Ther Drug Monit.* 1994;16:427.

Ciprofloxacin (*Cipro*)

Ropinirole (*Requip*)

SUMMARY: Ropinirole concentrations are increased during coadministration of ciprofloxacin; increased side effects may result.

RISK FACTORS: No specific risk factors are known.

RELATED DRUGS: Some quinolone antibiotics [eg, enoxacin (*Penetrex*) or pefloxacin] may also increase ropinirole concentrations. Ofloxacin (*Floxin*) and lomefloxacin (*Maxaquin*) may be less likely to interact.

MANAGEMENT OPTIONS:

➡ **Consider Alternative.** The use of ofloxacin or lomefloxacin instead of ciprofloxacin would probably avoid any significant increase in ropinirole concentrations.

➡ **Monitor.** Monitor patients taking ropinirole who are administered ciprofloxacin for increased ropinirole effects and side effects including nausea, dizziness, and syncope.

REFERENCES:

Product information. Ropinirole (*Requip*). SmithKline Beecham Pharmaceuticals. 1997.

Ciprofloxacin (*Cipro*)

Sucralfate (eg, *Carafate*)

SUMMARY: The administration of sucralfate markedly reduced ciprofloxacin serum concentrations; loss of antibiotic effect may occur.

RISK FACTORS: No specific risk factors are known.

RELATED DRUGS: Sucralfate inhibits the absorption of fleroxacin, norfloxacin (*Noroxin*), and ofloxacin (*Floxin*). Antacids containing aluminum also inhibit ciprofloxacin absorption.

MANAGEMENT OPTIONS:

➡ **Consider Alternative.** If dosage separation is not possible, consider an alternative to sucralfate (eg, H_2-receptor antagonist, omeprazole, but not an antacid).

➡ **Circumvent/Minimize.** Avoid the coadministration of ciprofloxacin and sucralfate if possible. Administer ciprofloxacin several hours before sucralfate or 6 hours after.

➡ **Monitor.** If sucralfate and a quinolone are coadministered, monitor the patient for reduced antibiotic efficacy.

REFERENCES:

Nix DE, et al. The effect of sucralfate pretreatment on the pharmacokinetics of ciprofloxacin. *Pharmacotherapy.* 1989;9:377.

Yuk JH, et al. Ciprofloxacin levels when receiving sucralfate. *JAMA.* 1989;262:901.

Brouwers JRBJ, et al. Important reduction of ciprofloxacin absorption by sucralfate and magnesium citrate solution. *Drug Invest.* 1990;2:197.

Garrelts JC, et al. Sucralfate significantly reduces ciprofloxacin concentrations in serum. *Antimicrob Agents Chemother.* 1990;34:931.

Van Slooten AD, et al. Combined use of ciprofloxacin and sucralfate. *DICP, Ann Pharmacother.* 1991;25:578.

Ciprofloxacin (*Cipro*)

Theophylline (eg, *Theolair*)

SUMMARY: Ciprofloxacin increases the serum concentration of theophylline and can induce theophylline toxicity.

RISK FACTORS:

➡ ***Dosage Regimen.*** High doses of ciprofloxacin place one at greater risk.

RELATED DRUGS: Quinolones reported to inhibit the metabolism of drugs include enoxacin (*Penetrex*), norfloxacin (*Noroxin*), pipemidic acid, and pefloxacin.

MANAGEMENT OPTIONS:

➡ ***Consider Alternative.*** Quinolones reported to produce no or minor changes in theophylline kinetics include fleroxacin, flosequinan, lomefloxacin (*Maxaquin*), ofloxacin (*Floxin*), rufloxacin, sparfloxacin (*Zagam*), and temafloxacin.

➡ ***Monitor.*** Monitor patients maintained on theophylline for increased serum theophylline concentrations and signs of toxicity (eg, palpitations, tachycardia, nausea, tremor) during coadministration of ciprofloxacin.

REFERENCES:

Nix DE, et al. Effect of multiple dose oral ciprofloxacin on the pharmacokinetics of theophylline and indocyanine green. *J Antimicrob Chemother.* 1987;19:263.

Wijnands WJA, et al. The influence of quinolone derivatives on theophylline clearance. *Br J Clin Pharmacol.* 1986;22:677.

Schwartz J, et al. Impact of ciprofloxacin on theophylline clearance and steady-state concentrations in serum. *Antimicrob Agents Chemother.* 1988;32:75.

Bachmann KA, et al. Predicting the ciprofloxacin-theophylline interaction from single plasma theophylline measurements. *Br J Clin Pharmacol.* 1988;26:191.

Prince RA, et al. Effect of quinolone antimicrobials on theophylline pharmacokinetics. *J Clin Pharmacol.* 1989;29:650.

Karki SD, et al. Seizure with ciprofloxacin and theophylline combined therapy. *DICP, Ann Pharmacother.* 1990;24:595.

Wijnands WJA, et al. Steady-state kinetics of the quinolone derivatives ofloxacin, enoxacin, ciprofloxacin, and pefloxacin during maintenance treatment with theophylline. *Drugs.* 1987;34(Suppl. 1):159.

Loi CM, et al. Individual and combined effects of cimetidine and ciprofloxacin on theophylline metabolism in male nonsmokers. *Br J Clin Pharmacol.* 1993;36:195.

Bader MB. Role of ciprofloxacin in fatal seizures. *Chest.* 1992;101:883.

Batty KT, et al. The effect of ciprofloxacin on theophylline pharmacokinetics in healthy subjects. *Br J Clin Pharmacol.* 1995;39:305.

Ciprofloxacin (*Cipro*)

Warfarin (eg, *Coumadin*)

SUMMARY: Several cases of enhanced hypoprothrombinemic responses to warfarin have been associated with ciprofloxacin administration, but prospective trials have not supported this observation.

RISK FACTORS:

➡ ***Concurrent Diseases.*** Fever may enhance the catabolism of clotting factors thus enhancing the oral anticoagulant effect.

RELATED DRUGS: Norfloxacin (*Noroxin*) and ofloxacin (*Floxin*) have been noted to increase INRs in a few case reports.

MANAGEMENT OPTIONS:

➡ *Consider Alternative.* Consider using an antibiotic other than ciprofloxacin to avoid the potential interaction.

➡ *Monitor.* In patients receiving oral anticoagulants, monitor for altered hypopro-thrombinemic response when ciprofloxacin is initiated or discontinued and adjust the anticoagulant dose as needed.

REFERENCES:

Kamada AK. Possible interaction between ciprofloxacin and warfarin. *DICP, Ann Pharmacother.* 1990;24:27.

Mott FE, et al. Ciprofloxacin and warfarin. *Ann Intern Med.* 1989;111:542.

Renzi R, et al. Ciprofloxacin interaction with sodium warfarin: a potentially dangerous side effect. *Am J Emerg Med.* 1991;9:551.

Dugoni-Kramer BM. Ciprofloxacin-warfarin interaction. *DICP, Ann Pharmacother.* 1991;25:1397.

Johnson KC, et al. Drug interaction. *J Fam Pract.* 1991;33:338.

Rindone JP, et al. Hypoprothrombinemic effect of warfarin not influenced by ciprofloxacin. *Clin Pharm.* 1991;10:136.

Loclinger EA, et al. The biological disappearance rate of prothrombin and factors VII, IX and X from plasma in hypothyroidism, hyperthyroidism and during fever. *Thromb Diath Haemorrh.* 1964;10:267.

Linville D, et al. Ciprofloxacin and warfarin interaction. *Am J Med.* 1991;90:765.

▼3 Ciprofloxacin (*Cipro*)

Zinc

SUMMARY: The administration of multivitamins with zinc may reduce the serum concentration of ciprofloxacin; however the clinical significance appears to be minimal.

RISK FACTORS: No specific risk factors are known.

RELATED DRUGS: The absorption of other quinolones (eg, norfloxacin [*Noroxin*], enoxacin [*Penetrex*]) is likely to be reduced by zinc.

MANAGEMENT OPTIONS:

➡ *Circumvent/Minimize.* Patients taking ciprofloxacin, and probably other quinolone antibiotics, should avoid the coadministration of oral multivitamins containing zinc. If the drugs are used together, administer the ciprofloxacin at least 2 hours before the zinc.

➡ *Monitor.* Watch for antibiotic failure when zinc and a quinolone are coadministered.

REFERENCES:

Polk RE, et al. Effect of ferrous sulfate and multivitamins with zinc on absorption of ciprofloxacin in normal volunteers. *Antimicrob Agents Chemother.* 1989;33:1841.

Cisapride† (eg, *Propulsid*) ②
Clarithromycin (*Biaxin*)

SUMMARY: Clarithromycin may increase cisapride concentrations leading to toxicity including cardiac arrhythmias.

RISK FACTORS:

➡ *Concurrent Diseases.* Preexisting cardiovascular disease or an electrolyte imbalance may increase the risk of the interaction.

RELATED DRUGS: Ketoconazole (eg, *Nizoral*) can increase cisapride concentrations. Troleandomycin (*TAO*) and erythromycin (eg, *E-Mycin*) also may inhibit cisapride metabolism. Azithromycin (*Zithromax*) and dirithromycin (*Dynabac*) would not be expected to inhibit cisapride metabolism.

MANAGEMENT OPTIONS:

➡ *Avoid Unless Benefit Outweighs Risk.* Patients who are receiving cisapride and require clarithromycin should have their cisapride temporarily discontinued. Metoclopramide (eg, *Reglan*) or an H_2-receptor antagonist could be considered as a substitute for cisapride.

➡ *Monitor.* If cisapride is used with clarithromycin, monitor patient for arrhythmias and prolonged QT intervals.

REFERENCES:

Product information. Cisapride (*Propulsid*). Janssen Pharmaceutica. 1995.

† Available only through an investigational limited access program.

Cisapride† (eg, *Propulsid*) ②
Erythromycin (eg, *E-Mycin*)

SUMMARY: Erythromycin may increase cisapride concentrations leading to toxicity including cardiac arrhythmias.

RISK FACTORS:

➡ *Concurrent Diseases.* Preexisting cardiovascular disease or electrolyte imbalance may increase the risk of the interaction.

RELATED DRUGS: Ketoconazole (eg, *Nizoral*) can increase cisapride concentrations. Troleandomycin (*TAO*) and clarithromycin (*Biaxin*) also may inhibit cisapride metabolism.

MANAGEMENT OPTIONS:

➡ *Avoid Unless Benefit Outweighs Risk.* Patients who are receiving cisapride and require erythromycin should have their cisapride temporarily discontinued. Consider metoclopramide (eg, *Reglan*) or an H_2-receptor antagonist as a substitute for cisapride.

➡ *Monitor.* If cisapride is used with erythromycin, monitor patient for arrhythmias and prolonged QT intervals.

REFERENCES:

Product information. Cisapride (*Propulsid*). Janssen Pharmaceutica. 1998.

† Available only through an investigational limited access program.

Cisapride† (*Propulsid*)

Grapefruit Juice

SUMMARY: A single glass of grapefruit juice moderately increased cisapride plasma concentrations; although the risk of this combination is not known, grapefruit juice would be best avoided in patients on cisapride.

RISK FACTORS: No specific risk factors are known.

RELATED DRUGS: No information is available.

MANAGEMENT OPTIONS:

➥ *Use Alternative.* Orange juice is unlikely to interact with cisapride.

➥ *Monitor.* If grapefruit juice is used in a patient on cisapride, monitor for cardiac arrhythmias and prolonged QT intervals.

REFERENCES:

Offman EM, et al. Red wine-cisapride interaction: comparison with grapefruit juice. *Clin Pharmacol Ther.* 2001;70:17.

† Available only through an investigational limited access program.

 ## Cisapride† (eg, *Propulsid*)

Indinavir (*Crixivan*)

SUMMARY: Indinavir is likely to increase cisapride serum concentrations potentially resulting in adverse effects including cardiac arrhythmias. Until further information is available, avoid the concomitant use of indinavir and cisapride.

RISK FACTORS: No specific risk factors are known.

RELATED DRUGS: Ritonavir (*Norvir*) would be likely to inhibit the metabolism of cisapride in a similar manner. Delavirdine (*Rescriptor*) is a CYP3A4 inhibitor and also may affect cisapride's metabolism. While no data are available, other antiviral agents such as saquinavir (*Fortovase*) or famciclovir (*Valtrex*) may be less likely to interact with cisapride. The metabolism of metoclopramide (eg, *Reglan*) would be unlikely to be affected by indinavir coadministration.

MANAGEMENT OPTIONS:

➥ *Use Alternative.* Avoid the combination of indinavir and cisapride because of the risk of a possibly serious arrhythmia. Nonintegrated alternatives are available and consider in patients requiring a prokinetic agent and an antiviral agent.

REFERENCES:

Product information. Cisapride (*Propulsid*). Janssen Pharmaceutica. 1998.

† Available only through an investigational limited access program.

Cisapride† (eg, *Propulsid*)

Itraconazole (*Sporanox*)

SUMMARY: Itraconazole may increase cisapride concentrations and lead to toxicity including arrhythmias.

RISK FACTORS:

➡ **Concurrent Diseases.** Preexisting cardiovascular disease or electrolyte imbalance may increase the risk of the interaction.

RELATED DRUGS: In vitro studies have shown ketoconazole (eg, *Nizoral*) and miconazole could interact with cisapride in a similar manner. Fluconazole (*Diflucan*) appears to produce less in vitro inhibition, but caution is warranted if this agent is administered (especially at high doses) with cisapride, particularly in patients with other risk factors for arrhythmias (eg, hypokalemia, cardiovascular disease, antiarrhythmic drug therapy). Itraconazole would not be expected to alter the elimination of metoclopramide (eg, *Reglan*).

MANAGEMENT OPTIONS:

➡ **Avoid Unless Benefit Outweighs Risk.** Patients who are receiving cisapride and require itraconazole should have their cisapride temporarily discontinued. The use of H₂-receptor antagonists or proton pump inhibitors is not recommended because they reduce the absorption of oral antifungal agents. Metoclopramide therapy could be considered as a substitute for cisapride.

➡ **Monitor.** Pending further information on this interaction, the manufacturer recommends avoiding the concomitant use of itraconazole and cisapride. If they are coadministered, monitor patients carefully for arrhythmias and prolonged QT intervals.

REFERENCES:

Product information. Cisapride (*Propulsid*). Janssen Pharmaceutica. 1998.

† Available only through an investigational limited access program.

Cisapride†

Ketoconazole (eg, *Nizoral*)

SUMMARY: Ketoconazole increases cisapride concentrations and may lead to toxicity, including arrhythmias.

RISK FACTORS:

➡ **Concurrent Diseases.** Pre-existing cardiovascular disease or electrolyte imbalance may increase the risk of the interaction.

RELATED DRUGS: Other antifungal inhibitors of CYP3A4 (eg, itraconazole [*Sporanox*], fluconazole [*Diflucan*], miconazole are likely to increase cisapride concentrations. Ketoconazole would not be expected to alter the elimination of metoclopramide (eg, *Reglan*).

MANAGEMENT OPTIONS:

➡ **Avoid Unless Benefit Outweighs Risk.** Until further information on this interaction is available, the manufacturer recommends avoiding the concomitant use of ketoconazole and cisapride. The use of H₂-receptor antagonists or proton pump inhibitors (omeprazole [*Prilosec*], lansoprazole [*Prevacid*]) is not recommended because they may reduce the absorption of some oral antifungal agents. Metoclopramide therapy could be considered as a substitute for cisapride.

➡ **Monitor.** Monitor patients who are receiving cisapride, particularly in patients with other risk factors for arrhythmias, and require ketoconazole for arrhythmias and prolonged QT intervals.

REFERENCES:

Product Information. Cisapride (*Propulsid*). Janssen Pharmaceutica. 1998.

† Available only through an investigational limited access program.

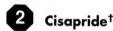 **Cisapride†**

Mibefradil (*Posicor*)

SUMMARY: Mibefradil is likely to increase cisapride serum concentrations, potentially resulting in adverse effects including cardiac arrhythmias. Pending further information on this interaction, avoid the concomitant use of mibefradil and cisapride.

RISK FACTORS: No specific risk factors are known.

RELATED DRUGS: Other calcium channel blockers [eg, amlodipine (*Norvasc*), nifedipine (eg, *Procardia*), nicardipine (eg, *Cardene*)] would not be expected to change cisapride plasma concentrations. The metabolism of metoclopramide (eg, *Reglan*) would be unlikely to be affected by mibefradil coadministration.

MANAGEMENT OPTIONS:

➡ **Use Alternative.** Avoid the combination of mibefradil and cisapride because of a possibly serious arrhythmia. Noninteracting alternatives are available and consider in patients requiring a prokinetic agent and a calcium channel blocker.

REFERENCES:

Product information. Mibefradil (*Posicor*). Roche Laboratories, Inc. 1997.

† Available only through an investigational limited access program.

 Cisapride†

Miconazole

SUMMARY: IV miconazole may increase cisapride concentrations and lead to toxicity including arrhythmias.

RISK FACTORS:

➡ **Concurrent Diseases.** Preexisting cardiovascular disease or electrolyte imbalance may increase the risk of the interaction.

RELATED DRUGS: Other antifungal agents that inhibit CYP3A4 (eg, ketoconazole [eg, *Nizoral*], itraconazole [*Sporanox*], fluconazole [*Diflucan*]) are likely to increase cisapride concentrations. Miconazole would not be expected to alter the elimination of metoclopramide (eg, *Reglan*).

MANAGEMENT OPTIONS:

➡ **Avoid Unless Benefit Outweighs Risk.** Until further information on this interaction is available, the manufacturer recommends avoiding the concomitant use of miconazole and cisapride. Patients who are receiving cisapride and require miconazole should have their cisapride temporarily discontinued. Metoclopramide therapy could be considered as a substitute for cisapride.

➡ *Monitor.* If a patient requires both cisapride and miconazole, monitor for cardiac arrhythmias and prolonged QT intervals.

REFERENCES:

Product information. Cisapride (*Propulsid*). Janssen Pharmaceutica. 1998.

† Available only through an investigational limited access program.

Cisapride†
Nefazodone (*Serzone*)

SUMMARY: Nefazodone is likely to increase cisapride serum concentrations potentially resulting in adverse effects including cardiac arrhythmias. Until further information is available, avoid the concomitant use of nefazodone and cisapride.

RISK FACTORS: No specific risk factors are known.

RELATED DRUGS: While no data are available, other antidepressants including fluoxetine (*Prozac*), paroxetine (*Paxil*), and sertraline (*Zoloft*) would not be likely to affect the metabolism of cisapride. The metabolism of metoclopramide (eg, *Reglan*) would be unlikely to be affected by concomitant nefazodone administration.

MANAGEMENT OPTIONS:

➡ *Use Alternative.* Because of the risk of a possibly serious arrhythmia, avoid the combination of nefazodone and cisapride. Noninteracting alternatives are available and should be considered in patients requiring a prokinetic agent and an antidepressant.

REFERENCES:

Product information. Cisapride (*Propulsid*). Janssen Pharmaceutica. 1998.

† Available only through an investigational limited access program.

Cisapride† (eg, *Propulsid*)
Ritonavir (*Norvir*)

SUMMARY: Ritonavir is likely to increase cisapride serum concentrations, potentially resulting in adverse effects including cardiac arrhythmias. Until further information is available, avoid the concomitant use of ritonavir and cisapride.

RISK FACTORS: No specific risk factors are known.

RELATED DRUGS: Indinavir (*Crixivan*) would likely inhibit the metabolism of cisapride in a similar manner. Delavirdine (*Rescriptor*) is a CYP3A4 inhibitor and also may affect cisapride's metabolism. While no data are available, other antiviral agents such as saquinavir (*Fortovase*) or famciclovir (*Valtrex*) may be less likely to interact with cisapride. The metabolism of metoclopramide (eg, *Reglan*) would be unlikely to be affected by ritonavir coadministration.

MANAGEMENT OPTIONS:

➡ *Use Alternative.* Because of the risk of a possibly serious arrhythmia, avoid the combination of ritonavir and cisapride. Noninteracting alternatives are available and consider in patients requiring a prokinetic agent and an antiviral agent.

REFERENCES:

Product information. Cisapride (*Propulsid*). Janssen Pharmaceutica. 1998.

† Available only through an investigational limited access program.

Cisapride† (eg, *Propulsid*)

Simvastatin (*Zocor*)

SUMMARY: In healthy subjects, simvastatin slightly increased cisapride plasma concentrations, and cisapride moderately decreased simvastatin acid plasma concentrations; the clinical importance of these changes is not established.

RISK FACTORS: No specific risk factors are known.

RELATED DRUGS: Theoretically, pravastatin (*Pravachol*) and fluvastatin (*Lescol*) would be less likely to increase cisapride plasma concentrations, but clinical data are lacking. Lovastatin (*Mevacor*) has drug interactions similar to simvastatin, and would be expected to interact similarly with cisapride.

MANAGEMENT OPTIONS:

➡ *Consider Alternative.* Consider using an alternative to one of the drugs (see Related Drugs).

➡ *Monitor.* In patients receiving both drugs, monitor for a reduced cholesterol lowering effect of simvastatin and for evidence of cisapride toxicity (eg, syncope, palpitations).

REFERENCES:

Simard C, et al. Study of the drug-drug interaction between simvastatin and cisapride in man. *Eur J Clin Pharmacol.* 2001;57:229.

† Available only through an investigational limited access program.

② Cisapride† (eg, *Propulsid*)

Troleandomycin (*TAO*)

SUMMARY: Troleandomycin may increase cisapride concentrations and lead to toxicity including arrhythmias.

RISK FACTORS:

➡ *Concurrent Diseases.* Preexisting cardiovascular disease or electrolyte imbalance may increase the risk of the interaction.

RELATED DRUGS: Erythromycin (eg, *E-Mycin*) and clarithromycin (*Biaxin*) also may inhibit cisapride metabolism.

MANAGEMENT OPTIONS:

➡ *Avoid Unless Benefit Outweighs Risk.* Patients who are receiving cisapride and require troleandomycin should have their cisapride temporarily discontinued. Consider metoclopramide (eg, *Reglan*) or an H$_2$-receptor antagonist as a substitute for cisapride. Azithromycin (*Zithromax*) could be substituted for troleandomycin (*TAO*).

➡ *Monitor.* If cisapride is used with troleandomycin, monitor patients for arrhythmias and prolonged QT intervals.

REFERENCES:

Product information. Cisapride (*Propulsid*). Janssen Pharmaceutica. 1998.

† Available only through an investigational limited access program.

Cisplatin (eg, *Platinol-AQ*)

Diazoxide (*Hyperstat*)

SUMMARY: A patient developed nephrotoxicity following combined use of cisplatin and a potent combination of antihypertensive drugs, but a causal relationship was not established.

RISK FACTORS: No specific risk factors are known.

RELATED DRUGS: Theoretically, any potent hypotensive drug regimen could increase cisplatin or carboplatin nephrotoxicity.

MANAGEMENT OPTIONS:

➡ *Monitor.* Monitor renal function if potent antihypertensive drugs are used with cisplatin.

REFERENCES:

Markman M, et al. Nephrotoxicity with cisplatin and antihypertensive medications. *Ann Intern Med.* 1982;96:257.

Cisplatin (eg, *Platinol-AQ*)

Ethacrynic Acid (*Edecrin*)

SUMMARY: Severe ototoxicity has been noted in animals given cisplatin and ethacrynic acid.

RISK FACTORS: No specific risk factors are known.

RELATED DRUGS: Furosemide (eg, *Lasix*) and bumetanide (eg, *Bumex*) appear to be less ototoxic than ethacrynic acid and might be less likely to cause ototoxicity when combined with cisplatin.

MANAGEMENT OPTIONS:

➡ *Avoid Unless Benefit Outweighs Risk.* Avoid concurrent use of ethacrynic acid and cisplatin if possible.

➡ *Monitor.* If any loop diuretic is used with cisplatin, monitor the patient carefully for ototoxicity.

REFERENCES:

Komune S, et al. Potentiating effects of cisplatin and ethacrynic acid in ototoxicity. *Arch Otolaryngol.* 1981;107:594.

Cisplatin (eg, *Platinol-AQ*)

Gentamicin (eg, *Garamycin*)

SUMMARY: Cisplatin may enhance the nephrotoxicity of aminoglycosides like gentamicin, but the clinical importance is not established.

RISK FACTORS:

➡ *Concurrent Diseases.* Renal dysfunction places one at particular risk for the interaction.

RELATED DRUGS: Other aminoglycosides may increase the risk of nephrotoxicity with cisplatin. Carboplatin may interact in a similar manner with aminoglycosides.

MANAGEMENT OPTIONS:

➡ *Consider Alternative.* Select an antibiotic other than an aminoglycoside.

➡ *Monitor.* Observe patients receiving the combination for renal dysfunction or hypomagnesemia.

REFERENCES:

Dentino M, et al. Long term effect of cis-diaminedichloride platinum (CDDP) on renal functions and structure in man. *Cancer.* 1978;41:1274.

Cisplatin (eg, *Platinol-AQ*)

Phenytoin (eg, *Dilantin*)

SUMMARY: Phenytoin levels may be decreased by antineoplastic drugs like cisplatin, which may result in increased seizure activity or increased phenytoin dosage requirement.

RISK FACTORS: No specific risk factors are known.

RELATED DRUGS: A 46-year-old man receiving chronic phenytoin experienced increased seizure activity associated with subtherapeutic phenytoin levels following chemotherapy with methotrexate, vinblastine, and carmustine. In another case, a pharmacokinetic study of IV phenytoin was performed in a 10-year-old boy with acute lymphocytic leukemia being treated with prednisone, vincristine, methotrexate, leucovorin, and mercaptopurine. The clearance of phenytoin was more than doubled on the seventh day after starting chemotherapy. Plasma protein binding of phenytoin was unchanged.

MANAGEMENT OPTIONS:

➡ *Circumvent/Minimize.* Case reports suggest that phenytoin levels will begin to return to normal 2 to 3 weeks following chemotherapy. If a patient had required a dosage increase to maintain a therapeutic level following chemotherapy, it would be important to anticipate this and reduce the dosage accordingly to prevent phenytoin toxicity from developing.

➡ *Monitor.* Monitor patient phenytoin levels 2 to 3 days after a dose of chemotherapy. If the phenytoin concentration has decreased significantly, adjust the phenytoin dosage and monitor phenytoin concentrations weekly.

REFERENCES:

Grossman SA, et al. Decreased phenytoin levels in patients receiving chemotherapy. *Am J Med.* 1989;87:505.

Bollini P, et al. Decreased phenytoin level during antineoplastic therapy: a case report. *Epilepsia.* 1983;24:75.

Neef C, et al. An interaction between cytostatic and anticonvulsant drugs. *Clin Pharmacol Ther.* 1988;43:372.

Sylvester RK, et al. Impaired phenytoin bioavailability secondary to cisplatinum, vinblastine, and bleomycin. *Ther Drug Monit.* 1984;6:302.

Dofferhoff ASM, et al. Decreased phenytoin level after carboplatin treatment. *Am J Med.* 1990;89:247.

Jarosinski PF, et al. Altered phenytoin clearance during intensive chemotherapy for acute lymphoblastic leukemia. *J Pediatr.* 1988;112:996.

Fincham RW, et al. Decreased phenytoin levels in antineoplastic therapy. *Ther Drug Monit.* 1979;1:277.

Citalopram (*Celexa*)
Moclobemide

SUMMARY: Combined overdose of citalopram and moclobemide has resulted in fatal serotonin syndrome, but the danger of combining therapeutic doses of the 2 drugs is not known.

RISK FACTORS:

➡ *Dosage Regimen.* The observed reactions occurred in overdose situations.

RELATED DRUGS: In a preliminary report on the use of therapeutic moclobemide doses with another SSRI, fluoxetine (eg, *Prozac*), no unexpected side effect occurred. Little is known regarding the effect of moclobemide combined with SSRIs other than citalopram or fluoxetine.

MANAGEMENT OPTIONS:

➡ *Avoid Unless Benefit Outweighs Risk.* Although it is possible that the danger of concomitant use of citalopram and moclobemide is restricted to overdoses, the lack of safety data at therapeutic doses dictates extreme caution in using this combination.

➡ *Monitor.* It would be prudent to carefully monitor and use conservative dosing in patients given the combination.

REFERENCES:

Neuvonen PJ, et al. Five fatal cases of serotonin syndrome after moclobemide-citalopram or moclobemide-clomipramine overdoses. *Lancet.* 1993;342:1419.

Beasley CM, et al. Possible monoamine oxidase inhibitor-serotonin reuptake inhibitor interaction: fluoxetine clinical data and preclinical findings. *J Clin Psychopharmacol.* 1993;13:312-320.

Graber MA, et al. Sertraline-phenelzine drug interaction: a serotonin syndrome reaction. *Ann Pharmacother.* 1994;28:732-735.

Dingemanse J, et al. Pharmacodynamic and pharmacokinetic interactions between fluoxetine and moclobemide. *Clin Pharmacol Ther.* 1993;53:178.

Clarithromycin (*Biaxin*)

Colchicine

SUMMARY: Severe colchicine toxicity can occur in patients concomitantly receiving clarithromycin.

RISK FACTORS: No specific risk factors are known.

RELATED DRUGS: Erythromycin is also known to reduce colchicine elimination; troleando-mycin (*TAO*) would be expected to interact in a similar manner.

MANAGEMENT OPTIONS:

➡ *Consider Alternative.* The macrolide antibiotics azithromycin (*Zithromax*) and dirithro-mycin (*Dynabac*) do not reduce CYP3A4 activity and should be considered for use in patients receiving colchicine. A nonsteroidal anti-inflammatory agent could be substituted for colchicine during clarithromycin administration.

➡ *Monitor.* Carefully monitor patients taking colchicine for evidence of toxicity (fever, diarrhea, abdominal pain) if any CYP3A4 inhibitor is coadministered.

REFERENCES:

Dogukan A, et al. Acute fatal colchicine intoxication in a patient on continuous ambulatory peritoneal dialysis (CAPD). Possible role of clarithromycin administration. *Clin Nephrol.* 2001;55:181-182.

Severe colchicine-macrolide interactions. *Prescrire Int.* 2003;12:18-19.

 Clarithromycin (*Biaxin*)

Cyclosporine (eg, *Neoral*)

SUMMARY: Cyclosporine concentrations are likely to be increased by clarithromycin coadministration; toxic cyclosporine concentrations and renal toxicity may result.

RISK FACTORS:

➡ *Concomitant Diseases.* Renal dysfunction can increase the risk of interaction.

RELATED DRUGS: Erythromycin (eg, *E-Mycin*) and, to a lesser extent, josamycin and rox-ithromycin, have been noted to increase cyclosporine concentrations; azithromycin (*Zithromax*) and dirithromycin (*Dynabac*) would be unlikely to inhibit cyclosporine metabolism. Tacrolimus (*Prograf*) is similarly affected by macrolide administration.

MANAGEMENT OPTIONS:

➡ *Monitor.* Carefully monitor cyclosporine concentrations in patients stabilized on cyclosporine and adjust doses as required during clarithromycin administration.

REFERENCES:

Neu HC. The development of macrolides: clarithromycin in perspective. *J Antimicrob Chemother.* 1991;27(suppl. A):1-9.

Ferrari SL, et al. The interaction between clarithromycin and cyclosporine in kidney transplant recipients. *Transplantation.* 1994;58:725-727.

Harnett JD, et al. Erythromycin-cyclosporine interaction in renal transplant recipients. *Transplantation.* 1987;43:316-318.

Kreft-Jais C, et al. Effect of josamycin on plasma cyclosporine levels. *Eur J Clin Pharmacol.* 1987;32:327-328.

Billaud EM, et al. Interaction between roxithromycin and cyclosporin in heart transplant patients. *Clin Pharmacokinet.* 1990;19:499-502.

Clarithromycin (eg, *Biaxin*)

Digoxin (eg, *Lanoxin*)

SUMMARY: Clarithromycin administration increases the plasma concentration of digoxin; digoxin toxicity including nausea, malaise, visual changes, and arrhythmias may occur.

RISK FACTORS: No specific risk factors are known.

RELATED DRUGS: Digitoxin[†] would likely be affected in a similar manner by clarithromycin. Erythromycin also increases digoxin plasma concentrations. There is little data on the effect of other macrolides on digoxin.

MANAGEMENT OPTIONS:

➥ *Consider Alternative.* Select an antibiotic known to have no effect on digoxin concentrations in patients receiving chronic digoxin therapy. If azithromycin (*Zithromax*) or dirithromycin (*Dynabac*) are used, monitor for changes in digoxin concentrations.

➥ *Monitor.* In patients receiving digoxin, monitor for changes in digoxin concentrations when clarithromycin is added or removed from the drug regimen.

REFERENCES:

Xu H, et al. Clarithromycin-induced digoxin toxicity: a case report and review of the literature. *Conn Med.* 2001;65:527-529.

Zapater P, et al. A prospective study of the clarithromycin-digoxin interaction in elderly patients. *J Antimicrob Chemother.* 2002;50:601-606.

Tanaka H, et al. Effect of clarithromycin on steady-state digoxin concentrations. *Ann Pharmacother.* 2003;37:178-181.

Nordt SP, et al. Clarithromycin induced digoxin toxicity. *J Accid Emerg Med.* 1998;15:194-195.

Juurlink DN, et al. Drug-drug interactions among elderly patients hospitalized for drug toxicity. *JAMA.* 2003;289:1652-1658.

† Not available in the United States.

Clarithromycin (*Biaxin*)

Ergotamine (*Ergomar*)

SUMMARY: The coadministration of clarithromycin and ergotamine may result in ergotism, including hypertension and ischemia.

RISK FACTORS: No specific risk factors are known.

RELATED DRUGS: Erythromycin (eg, *E-Mycin*) also has been reported to cause ergotamine toxicity. Although no data are available, azithromycin (*Zithromax*) or dirithromycin (*Dynabac*) would be unlikely to inhibit the metabolism of ergotamine.

MANAGEMENT OPTIONS:

➥ *Use Alternative.* The use of macrolides such as azithromycin or dirithromycin that do not inhibit drug metabolism is preferable in patients with migraine headaches who require ergotamine for acute migraine attacks.

REFERENCES:

Horowitz RS, et al. Clinical ergotism with lingual ischemia induced by clarithromycin-ergotamine interaction. *Arch Intern Med.* 1996;156:456-458.

Ghali R, et al. Erythromycin-associated ergotamine intoxication: arteriographic and electrophysiologic analysis of a rare cause of severe ischemia of the lower extremities and associated ischemic neuropathy. *Ann Vasc Surg.* 1993;7:291-296.

Clarithromycin (*Biaxin*)

Indinavir (*Crixivan*)

SUMMARY: Clarithromycin can increase indinavir serum concentrations possibly resulting in toxicity. Indinavir increased clarithromycin concentrations; the clinical significance of these changes is unknown.

RISK FACTORS: No specific risk factors are known.

RELATED DRUGS: Clarithromycin produces a small increase in ritonavir (*Norvir*) serum concentrations that are unlikely to produce toxicity. Ritonavir significantly increased clarithromycin concentrations. Other macrolides (eg, erythromycin [eg, *E-Mycin*], troleandomycin [*TAO*]) are likely to affect indinavir in a similar manner. Dirithromycin (*Dynabac*) and azithromycin (*Zithromax*) would not be likely to inhibit indinavir metabolism.

MANAGEMENT OPTIONS:

➥ *Circumvent/Minimize.* The dose of indinavir may require reduction during administration of clarithromycin or certain other macrolides.

➥ *Monitor.* Monitor patients for possible indinavir toxicity (eg, nausea, vomiting, headache).

REFERENCES:
   Product information. Indinavir (*Crixivan*). Merck and Company, Inc. 1996.

 Clarithromycin (*Biaxin*)

Itraconazole (*Sporanox*)

SUMMARY: Itraconazole concentrations are nearly doubled during clarithromycin coadministration; an increase in itraconazole side effects is possible.

RISK FACTORS:

➥ *Route of Administration.* Oral administration of clarithromycin is likely to produce a greater effect on itraconazole concentrations than IV dosing.

RELATED DRUGS: It is possible that other macrolide antibiotics (eg, erythromycin [eg, *E-Mycin*]) could alter itraconazole pharmacokinetics in a similar manner. Macrolide antibiotics that have little effect on CYP3A4 activity include azithromycin (*Zithromax*) or dirithromycin (*Dynabac*).

MANAGEMENT OPTIONS:

➥ *Consider Alternative.* Consider macrolide antibiotics that have little effect on CYP3A4 activity (see Related Drugs) for patients taking itraconazole.

➥ *Monitor.* Observe patients receiving both drugs for increased itraconazole side effects (eg, nausea, vomiting, headache) during the coadministration of clarithromycin.

REFERENCES:
   Hardin TC, et al. Evaluation of the pharmacokinetic interaction between itraconazole and clarithromycin following chronic oral dosing in HIV-infected patients. *Pharmacotherapy.* 1997;17:52.

Clarithromycin (*Biaxin*)

Midazolam (eg, *Versed*)

SUMMARY: Clarithromycin administration increases midazolam serum concentrations and accentuates its pharmacologic effects.

RISK FACTORS:

➡ **Route of Administration.** The oral administration of midazolam increases the risk of this interaction.

RELATED DRUGS: Erythromycin (eg, *E-Mycin*) and roxithromycin have been reported to inhibit the metabolism of midazolam. Azithromycin (*Zithromax*) does not appear to significantly affect midazolam metabolism, and dirithromycin (*Dynabac*) would not be expected to inhibit midazolam metabolism. Clarithromycin is likely to reduce the metabolism of other benzodiazepines such as diazepam (eg, *Valium*), which are metabolized by CYP3A4; however, temazepam (eg, *Restoril*) which is metabolized by conjugation, is expected to interact. Other benzodiazepines (eg, lorazepam [eg, *Ativan*], oxazepam [eg, *Serax*]) that are eliminated by CYP3A4 are unlikely to be affected by clarithromycin.

MANAGEMENT OPTIONS:

➡ **Use Alternative.** The risk of prolonged sedation during the concomitant use of midazolam and clarithromycin suggests avoiding the combination. Azithromycin (*Zithromax*) does not appear to significantly affect midazolam metabolism. Temazepam is metabolized by conjugation and is expected to be affected by clarithromycin.

REFERENCES:

Yeates RA, et al. Interaction between midazolam and clarithromycin: comparison with azithromycin. *Int J Clin Pharmacol Ther*. 1996;34:400.

Clarithromycin (eg, *Biaxin*)

Pimozide (*Orap*)

SUMMARY: Elevated pimozide concentrations and cardiac arrhythmias may occur if pimozide and clarithromycin are coadministered.

RISK FACTORS: No specific risk factors are known.

RELATED DRUGS: Erythromycin (eg, *E-Mycin*) and troleandomycin (*TAO*) would likely produce similar increases in pimozide plasma concentrations. Azithromycin and dirithromycin do not inhibit CYP3A4 activity and would not be expected to reduce pimozide metabolism.

MANAGEMENT OPTIONS:

➡ **Use Alternative.** Patients receiving pimozide should not be administered clarithromycin or erythromycin. Azithromycin or dirithromycin are suitable alternatives.

➡ *Monitor.* If clarithromycin, troleandomycin, or erythromycin is coadministered with pimozide, monitor the ECG for evidence of QTc prolongation.

REFERENCES:

Desta Z, et al. Effect of clarithromycin on the pharmacokinetics and pharmacodynamics of pimozide in healthy poor and extensive metabolizers of cytochrome P450 2D6 (CYP2D6). *Clin Pharmacol Ther.* 1999;65:10-20.

Product Information. Pimozide (*Orap*). Gate Pharmaceuticals. 1999.

Desta Z, et al. In vitro inhibition of pimozide N-dealkylation by selective serotonin reuptake inhibitors and azithromycin. *J Clin Psychopharmacol.* 2002;22:162-168.

Flockhart DA, et al. Studies on the mechanism of a fatal clarithromycin-pimozide interaction in a patient with tourette syndrome. *J Clin Psychopharmacol.* 2000;20:317-324.

Clarithromycin (*Biaxin*)

Prednisone (eg, *Deltasone*)

SUMMARY: The coadministration of clarithromycin and prednisone may lead to elevated prednisone concentrations and altered mental function.

RISK FACTORS: No specific risk factors are known.

RELATED DRUGS: Erythromycin (eg, *E-Mycin*) and troleandomycin (*TAO*) are likely to inhibit the metabolism of prednisone and prednisolone. Methylprednisolone (eg, *Medrol*) is also a substrate for CYP3A4 and may interact with these macrolides in a similar manner. Azithromycin (*Zithromax*) and dirithromycin (*Dynabac*) do not inhibit CYP3A4 activity and are not expected to interact with corticosteroids.

MANAGEMENT OPTIONS:

➡ *Consider Alternative.* Consider azithromycin or dirithromycin for patients taking corticosteroids who require macrolide antibiotics.

➡ *Monitor.* Observe patients receiving prednisone and CYP3A4-inhibiting macrolides for evidence of excessive steroid effects, including changing mental function, glucose intolerance, and muscle weakness.

REFERENCES:

Finkenbine R, et al. Case of mania due to prednisone-clarithromycin interaction. *Can J Psychiatry.* 1997;42:778.

Finkenbine RD, et al. Case of psychosis due to prednisone-clarithromycin interaction. *Gen Hosp Psychiatry.* 1998;20:325-326.

Clarithromycin (*Biaxin*)

AVOID Rifabutin (*Mycobutin*)

SUMMARY: Clarithromycin increases the plasma concentrations of rifabutin and increases its toxicity. Rifabutin reduces the concentration of clarithromycin and may result in a loss of efficacy. Avoid the combination.

RISK FACTORS: No specific risk factors are known.

RELATED DRUGS: Troleandomycin and erythromycin would be expected to interact in a similar manner with rifabutin. Azithromycin (*Zithromax*) does not increase rifabutin concentrations but increased adverse effects have been reported during coadministration of rifabutin and azithromycin. The effect of the coadministration of dirithromycin (*Dynabac*) and rifabutin is unknown but should be avoided pending trial outcomes. Rifampin also induces the metabolism of clarithromycin.

MANAGEMENT OPTIONS:

➡ *AVOID COMBINATION.* Because of the risk of increased toxicity and potential loss of efficacy, avoid the combination of clarithromycin and rifabutin.

REFERENCES:

Jordan MK, et al. Effects of fluconazole and clarithromycin on rifabutin and 25-*O*-desacetylrifabutin pharmacokinetics. *Antimicrob Agents Chemother*. 2000.44:2170-2172.

Hafner R, et al. Tolerance and pharmacokinetic interactions of rifabutin and clarithromycin in human immunodeficiency virus-infected volunteers. *Antimicrob Agents Chemother*. 1998;42:631-639.

Apseloff G, et al. Comparison of azithromycin and clarithromycin in their interactions with rifabutin in healthy volunteers. *J Clin Pharmacol*. 1998;38:830-835.

Griffith DE, et al. Adverse events associated with high-dose rifabutin in macrolide-containing regimens for the treatment of *Mycobacterium avium* complex lung disease. *Clin Infect Dis*. 1995;21:594-598.

Benson CA, et al. Clarithromycin or rifabutin alone or in combination for primary prophylaxis of *Mycobacterium avium* complex disease in patients with AIDS: a randomized, double-blind, placebo-controlled trial. *J Infect Dis*. 2000;181:1289-1297.

Lowe SH, et al. Uveitis during treatment of disseminated *Mycobacterium avium*-intracellulare complex infection with the combination of rifabutin, clarithromycin and ethambutol. *Neth J Med*. 1996;48:211-215.

Wallace RJ, et al. Reduced serum levels of clarithromycin in patients treated with multidrug regimens including rifampin or rifabutin for *Mycobacterium avium-M. intracellulare* infection. *J Infect Dis*. 1995;171:747-750.

Hafner R, et al. Tolerance and pharmacokinetic interactions of rifabutin and azithromycin. *Antimicrob Agents Chemother*. 2001;45:1572-1577.

Clarithromycin (*Biaxin*)

Rifampin (eg, *Rifadin*)

SUMMARY: Rifampin reduces the plasma concentrations of clarithromycin. Loss of antimicrobial activity may result.

RISK FACTORS: No specific risk factors are known.

RELATED DRUGS: Erythromycin may be affected in a similar manner by rifampin coadministration. Rifabutin also increases the metabolism of clarithromycin.

MANAGEMENT OPTIONS:

➡ *Consider Alternative.* Azithromycin (*Zithromax*) is not metabolized by CYP3A4 and may offer an alternative to clarithromycin in patients receiving rifampin.

➡ *Monitor.* If rifampin is coadministered to patients taking clarithromycin or erythromycin, monitor for the potential loss of antibiotic efficacy.

REFERENCES:

Wallace RJ, et al. Reduced serum levels of clarithromycin in patients treated with multidrug regimens including rifampin or rifabutin for *Mycobacterium avium-M. intracellulare* infection. *J Infect Dis*. 1995;171:747-750.

Clarithromycin (*Biaxin*)

Simvastatin (*Zocor*)

SUMMARY: Clarithromycin administration can increase simvastatin concentrations; myalgia and rhabdomyolysis may result.

RISK FACTORS: No specific risk factors are known.

RELATED DRUGS: Erythromycin (eg, *E-Mycin*) and troleandomycin (*TAO*) are expected to affect simvastatin metabolism in a similar manner. Lovastatin (eg, *Mevacor*) also appears to be very sensitive to CYP3A4 inhibitors. Cerivastatin and atorvastatin (*Lipitor*) also are metabolized by CYP3A4.

MANAGEMENT OPTIONS:

➥ *Use Alternative.* A macrolide that does not inhibit CYP3A4, such as azithromycin (*Zithromax*) or dirithromycin (*Dynabac*), is preferred in patients taking HMG-CoA reductase inhibitors. Pravastatin (*Pravachol*) and fluvastatin (*Lescol*) are not metabolized by CYP3A4 and are safer alternatives for patients requiring drugs that inhibit the enzyme.

➥ *Circumvent/Minimize.* If the clarithromycin is going to be used for a short course of therapy, discontinue the simvastatin during clarithromycin therapy. The simvastatin could be restarted several days after completion of the clarithromycin therapy.

➥ *Monitor.* Monitor patients taking HMG-CoA reductase inhibitors for muscle pain or weakness.

REFERENCES:

Lee AJ, et al. Rhabdomyolysis secondary to a drug interaction between simvastatin and clarithromycin. *Ann Pharmacother*. 2001;35:26-31.

 Clarithromycin (*Biaxin*)

Tacrolimus (*Prograf*)

SUMMARY: Tacrolimus concentrations may increase during clarithromycin administration; nephrotoxicity could result.

RISK FACTORS: No specific risk factors are known.

RELATED DRUGS: Erythromycin (eg, *E-Mycin*) also has been reported to increase tacrolimus concentrations. Troleandomycin (*TAO*) is expected to affect tacrolimus in a similar manner. Azithromycin (*Zithromax*) and dirithromycin (*Dynabac*) are unlikely to increase tacrolimus concentrations. Clarithromycin is expected to affect cyclosporine (eg, *Neoral*) in a similar manner.

MANAGEMENT OPTIONS:

➥ *Monitor.* Until more information is available, carefully monitor patients receiving tacrolimus for decreasing renal function and increasing tacrolimus serum concentrations following the addition of clarithromycin.

REFERENCES:

Wolter K, et al. Interaction between FK 506 and clarithromycin in a renal transplant patient. *Eur J Clin Pharmacol*. 1994;47:207-208.

Shaeffer MS, et al. Interaction between FK506 and erythromycin. *Ann Pharmacother*. 1994;28:280-281.

Clarithromycin (eg, *Biaxin*)

Terfenadine†

SUMMARY: Clarithromycin appears to increase terfenadine and terfenadine carboxylate plasma concentrations. Cardiac arrhythmias could result from elevated terfenadine concentrations.

RISK FACTORS: No specific risk factors are known.

RELATED DRUGS: Erythromycin (eg, *E-Mycin*) and troleandomycin (*TAO*) have been reported to inhibit the metabolism of terfenadine. Azithromycin (*Zithromax*) and dirithromycin (*Dynabac*) are unlikely to increase terfenadine concentrations. Astemizole is likely to be similarly affected by clarithromycin.

MANAGEMENT OPTIONS:

➡ **Use Alternative.** Astemizole may not be a safe alternative to terfenadine because it has been associated with arrhythmias when administered with drugs that inhibit its metabolism. The use of sedating antihistamines, loratadine (*Claritin*), fexofenadine (*Allegra*), or cetirizine (*Zyrtec*), may be preferable in patients who require antihistamine therapy during clarithromycin treatment. Azithromycin may be substituted for clarithromycin in some cases.

➡ **Monitor.** Monitor patients taking clarithromycin and terfenadine for changes in cardiac conduction.

REFERENCES:

Honig P, et al. Comparison of the effect of the macrolide antibiotics erythromycin, clarithromycin and azithromycin on terfenadine steadystate pharmacokinetics and electrocardiographic parameters. *Drug Invest.* 1994;7:148.

† Not available in the US.

Clarithromycin (eg, *Biaxin*)

Triazolam (*Halcion*)

SUMMARY: Clarithromycin administration can increase triazolam plasma concentrations and pharmacologic effects.

RISK FACTORS: No specific risk factors are known.

RELATED DRUGS: Erythromycin (eg, *E-Mycin*) and troleandomycin (*TAO*) are known to inhibit triazolam metabolism. Azithromycin (*Zithromax*) does not alter triazolam metabolism.

MANAGEMENT OPTIONS:

➡ **Consider Alternative.** Consider azithromycin as an alternative for patients taking triazolam. A benzodiazepine that is not metabolized by CYP3A4 (eg, temazepam [*Restoril*], lorazepam [*Ativan*]) could be considered for administration when patients are taking clarithromycin.

➡ **Monitor.** If clarithromycin is administered to patients taking triazolam, monitor for increased CNS effects.

REFERENCES:

Greenblatt DJ, et al. Inhibition of triazolam clearance by macrolide antimicrobial agents: in vitro correlates and dynamic consequences. *Clin Pharmacol Ther.* 1998;64:278-285.

Clarithromycin (eg, *Biaxin*)

Warfarin (eg, *Coumadin*)

SUMMARY: Clarithromycin appears to increase the anticoagulant effect of warfarin.

RISK FACTORS: No specific risk factors are known.

RELATED DRUGS: Erythromycin has been reported to reduce the metabolism of warfarin. The metabolism of acenocoumarol also appears to be inhibited by clarithromycin administration.

MANAGEMENT OPTIONS:

➡ ***Consider Alternative.*** Consider a macrolide antibiotic that does not inhibit metabolism (eg, azithromycin [*Zithromax*]). Note that while cases of azithromycin-induced enhanced warfarin response have been noted, no definitive studies have confirmed this effect.

➡ ***Monitor.*** Monitor INRs for patients stabilized on warfarin therapy during clarithromycin therapy. Check the INR after 3 to 5 days of clarithromycin administration for evidence of increased response.

REFERENCES:

Recker MW, et al. Potential interaction between clarithromycin and warfarin. *Ann Pharmacother.* 1997;31:996-998.

Oberg KC. Delayed elevation of international normalized ratio with concurrent clarithromycin and warfarin therapy. *Pharmacotherapy.* 1998;18:386-391.

Clinafloxacin[†]

Theophylline (eg, *Theolair*)

SUMMARY: A case report noted an apparent increase in theophylline concentration following the addition of clinafloxacin therapy.

RISK FACTORS: No specific risk factors are known.

RELATED DRUGS: Other quinolones known to inhibit the metabolism of theophylline include ciprofloxacin (*Cipro*), enoxacin (*Penetrex*), norfloxacin (*Noroxin*), pipemidic acid, and pefloxacin. Quinolones reported to produce no or minor changes in theophylline pharmacokinetics include fleroxacin, flosequinan, lomefloxacin (*Maxaquin*), ofloxacin (*Floxin*), rufloxacin, sparfloxacin (*Zagam*), and temafloxacin. (Also, see Ciprofloxacin/Theophylline; Enoxacin/Theophylline; Norfloxacin/Theophylline; Pefloxacin/Theophylline monographs.)

MANAGEMENT OPTIONS:

➡ ***Consider Alternative.*** Consider using a quinolone reported to produce no or minor changes in theophylline pharmacokinetics (eg, fleroxacin, flosequinan, lomefloxacin, ofloxacin, rufloxacin, sparfloxacin, temafloxacin).

➡ **Monitor.** Monitor patients maintained on theophylline for increased serum theophylline concentrations and signs of toxicity (eg, palpitations, tachycardia, nausea, tremor) during coadministration of clinafloxacin.

REFERENCES:

Matuschka PR, et al. Clinafloxacin-theophylline drug interaction. *Ann Pharmacother.* 1995;29:378-380.

† Not available in the US.

Clobazam (*Frisium*)

Phenytoin (eg, *Dilantin*)

SUMMARY: Case reports suggest that clobazam addition to phenytoin can lead to clinically obvious phenytoin toxicity in patients who have been taking maximum tolerated phenytoin doses.

RISK FACTORS: No specific risk factors are known.

RELATED DRUGS: No information is available.

MANAGEMENT OPTIONS:

➡ **Monitor.** Be alert for signs of increased phenytoin concentrations when clobazam is initiated, especially in patients maintained at high therapeutic phenytoin concentrations.

REFERENCES:

Zifkin, et al. Phenytoin toxicity due to interaction with clobazam. *Neurology.* 1991;41:313.

Clofibrate (*Atromid-S*)

Furosemide (eg, *Lasix*)

SUMMARY: Furosemide and clofibrate effects may be enhanced in patients with hypoalbuminemia who receive both agents.

RISK FACTORS:

➡ **Concurrent Diseases.** Risk appears higher in nephrotic syndrome or other disorders resulting in hypoalbuminemia.

RELATED DRUGS: It is not known whether other fibric acids such as gemfibrozil (eg, *Lopid*) would interact with furosemide, nor is it known whether loop diuretics other than furosemide would interact with clofibrate.

MANAGEMENT OPTIONS:

➡ **Consider Alternative.** In patients with hypoalbuminemia who are receiving furosemide, consider using hypolipidemic agents other than clofibrate.

➡ **Circumvent/Minimize.** If furosemide and clofibrate are used concurrently in patients with hypoalbuminemia, consider using conservative doses of 1 or both drugs until patient response is determined.

➡ *Monitor.* If furosemide and clofibrate are used concurrently in patients with hypo-albuminemia, monitor for evidence of myopathy (eg, muscle pain, weakness) and for excessive diuretic effect.

REFERENCES:

Bridgman JF, et al. Complications during clofibrate treatment of nephrotic-syndrome hyperlipoprotein-emia. *Lancet.* 1972;2:506.

Prandota J, et al. Furosemide binding to human albumin and plasma of nephrotic children. *Clin Pharmacol Ther.* 1975;17:159.

Clofibrate (*Atromid-S*)

Rifampin (eg, *Rifadin*)

SUMMARY: Clofibrate serum concentrations can be reduced by rifampin.

RISK FACTORS: No specific risk factors are known.

RELATED DRUGS: No information is available.

MANAGEMENT OPTIONS:

➡ *Circumvent/Minimize.* An increased dose of clofibrate may be necessary during rifampin coadministration.

➡ *Monitor.* When rifampin therapy is prolonged in patients on clofibrate, monitor serum lipid levels to detect inhibition of clofibrate effect.

REFERENCES:

Houin G, et al. Clofibrate and enzymatic induction in man. *Int J Clin Pharmacol.* 1978;16:150.

Clofibrate (*Atromid-S*)

Warfarin (eg, *Coumadin*)

SUMMARY: Clofibrate increases the hypoprothrombinemic effect of warfarin and probably other oral anticoagulants; serious bleeding episodes have occurred in some patients receiving warfarin and clofibrate.

RISK FACTORS: No specific risk factors are known.

RELATED DRUGS: Gemfibrozil (eg, *Lopid*), lovastatin (*Mevacor*), and simvastatin (*Zocor*) may increase the effect of oral anticoagulants while cholestyramine (eg, *Questran*) and colestipol (*Colestid*) may reduce their effect.

MANAGEMENT OPTIONS:

➡ *Avoid Unless Benefit Outweighs Risk.* Avoid concomitant therapy with clofibrate and oral anticoagulants if possible. If oral anticoagulant therapy is begun in a patient receiving clofibrate, anticoagulant doses probably should be conservative until the maintenance dose is established.

➡ *Monitor.* Monitor for altered oral anticoagulant effect if clofibrate is initiated, discontinued, or changed in dosage.

REFERENCES:

Starr KJ, et al. Drug interactions in patients on long term oral anticoagulant and antihypertensive adrenergic neuron-blocking drugs. *BMJ.* 1972;4:133.

Udall JA. Drug interference with warfarin therapy. *Clin Med.* 1970;77:20.

Solomon RB, et al. Massive hemorrhage and death during treatment with clofibrate and warfarin. *NY State J Med.* 1973;73:2002.

Eastham RD. Warfarin dosage influenced by clofibrate plus age. *Lancet.* 1973;1:1450.

Oliver MF, et al. Effect of Atromid and ethyl chlorophenoxyisobutyrate on anticoagulant requirements. *Lancet.* 1963;1:143.

Schrogie JJ, et al. The anticoagulant response to bishydroxycoumarin II: the effect of D-thyroxine, clofibrate, and norethandrolone. *Clin Pharmacol Ther.* 1967;8:70.

Hunninghake DB, et al. Drug interactions with warfarin. *Arch Intern Med.* 1968;121:349.

Pond SM, et al. The effects of allopurinol and clofibrate on the elimination of coumarin anticoagulants in man. *Aust NZ J Med.* 1975;5:324.

Corrigan JJ, et al. Coagulopathy associated with vitamin E ingestion. *JAMA.* 1974;230:1300.

Williams JRB, et al. Effect of concomitantly administered drugs on the control of long term anticoagulant therapy. *Q J Med.* 1976;45:63.

Bjornsson TD, et al. Interaction of clofibrate with warfarin: studies using radiolabeled vitamin K. *Clin Pharmacol Ther.* 1977;21:99.

Bjornsson TD, et al. Clofibrate displaces warfarin from plasma proteins in man: an example of a pure displacement interaction. *J Pharmacol Exp Ther.* 1979;210:316.

Roberts SD, et al. Effect of Atromid on requirements of warfarin. *J Atheroscler Res.* 1963;3:655.

Bjornsson TD, et al. Interaction of clofibrate with warfarin: effect of clofibrate on the disposition of the optical enantiomorphs of warfarin. *J Pharmacokinet Biopharm.* 1977;5:495.

Clomipramine (eg, *Anafranil*)

Fluvoxamine (*Luvox*)

SUMMARY: Fluvoxamine substantially increased clomipramine serum concentrations in 1 patient, probably by inhibition of clomipramine metabolism; adjustments in clomipramine dosage may be needed.

RISK FACTORS: No specific risk factors are known.

RELATED DRUGS: Other combinations of tricyclic antidepressants and selective serotonin reuptake inhibitors also may interact (see Desipramine-Fluoxetine monograph and Index).

MANAGEMENT OPTIONS:

➡ ***Monitor.*** Monitor for evidence of excessive clomipramine effect if fluvoxamine is given concurrently; adjust the clomipramine dosage as needed.

REFERENCES:

Oesterheld J, et al. Grapefruit juice and clomipramine: shifting metabolic ratios. *J Clin Psychopharmacol.* 1997;17:62.

Clomipramine (eg, *Anafranil*)

Grapefruit Juice

SUMMARY: Grapefruit juice increased clomipramine serum concentrations in 2 patients, probably by inhibition of clomipramine metabolism; adjustments in clomipramine dosage may be needed.

RISK FACTORS: No specific risk factors are known.

RELATED DRUGS: The effect of grapefruit juice on other tricyclic antidepressants is not established.

MANAGEMENT OPTIONS:

➡ *Monitor.* Monitor for evidence of excessive clomipramine effect if it is taken with grapefruit juice; adjust the clomipramine dosage as needed.

REFERENCES:

Oesterheld J, et al. Grapefruit juice and clomipramine: shifting metabolic ratios. *J Clin Psychopharmacol.* 1997;17:62.

Clomipramine (eg, *Anafranil*)

Ibuprofen (eg, *Motrin*)

SUMMARY: The combined use of clomipramine with ibuprofen (or other nonsteroidal anti-inflammatory drugs [NSAIDs]) appears to increase the risk of upper GI bleeding.

RISK FACTORS: No specific risk factors are known.

RELATED DRUGS: Assume that all other drugs that inhibit serotonin reuptake (eg, citalopram [*Effexor*], fluoxetine [*Prozac*], fluvoxamine [*Luvox*], nefazodone [*Serzone*], paroxetine [*Paxil*], sertraline [*Zoloft*], and venlafaxine [*Effexor*]) would interact with all NSAIDs (eg, diclofenac [*Voltaren*], diflunisal [*Dolobid*], etodolac [*Lodine*], fenoprofen [*Nalfon*], flurbiprofen [*Ansaid*], ibuprofen [*Motrin*], indomethacin [*Indocin*], ketoprofen [*Orudis*], ketorolac [*Toradol*], meclofenamate [*Meclomen*], mefenamic acid [*Ponstel*], meloxicam [*Mobic*], nabumetone [*Relafen*], naproxen [*Aleve*], oxaprozin [*Daypro*], piroxicam [*Feldene*], sulindac [*Clinoril*], tolmetin [*Tolectin*]).

MANAGEMENT OPTIONS:

➡ *Consider Alternative.* Consider using a non-NSAID analgesic such as acetaminophen (eg, *Tylenol*). If an NSAID is needed, consider a nonacetylated salicylate such as choline magnesium trisalicylate (*Trilisate*), salsalate (*Disalcid*), or magnesium salicylate (*Doan's*) since these products have minimal effects on platelets and the gastric mucosa. It is not known whether COX-2 inhibitors such as celecoxib (*Celebrex*), rofecoxib (*Vioxx*), or valdecoxib (*Bextra*) would be less likely to cause GI bleeding with clomipramine. Antidepressants with less effect on serotonin may reduce the risk of GI bleeding when combined with NSAIDs.

➡ *Monitor.* Patients receiving both a clomipramine and an NSAID should be alert for evidence of GI bleeding.

REFERENCES:

Dalton SO, et al. Use of selective serotonin reuptake inhibitors and risk of upper gastrointestinal tract bleeding. *Arch Intern Med.* 2003;163:59-64.

de Abajo FJ, et al. Association between selective serotonin reuptake inhibitors and upper gastrointestinal bleeding: population based case-control study. *BMJ.* 1999;319:1106-1109.

Clomipramine (eg, *Anafranil*)

Moclobemide

SUMMARY: The combination of moclobemide and clomipramine (in overdose) has been associated with fatal serotonin syndrome and (in therapeutic doses) with nonfatal serotonin syndrome. Moclobemide generally should not be given with clomipramine or with other tricyclic antidepressants (TCAs) that inhibit serotonin reuptake (eg, amitriptyline, imipramine, trazodone) or with selective serotonin reuptake inhibitors (SSRIs).

RISK FACTORS: No specific risk factors are known.

RELATED DRUGS: Other antidepressants that inhibit serotonin reuptake such as SSRIs, amitriptyline (eg, *Elavil*), imipramine (eg, *Tofranil*), and trazodone (eg, *Desyrel*) also would be expected to interact adversely with moclobemide.

MANAGEMENT OPTIONS:

➡ ***Avoid Unless Benefit Outweighs Risk.*** Avoid combined use of moclobemide and clomipramine. Also avoid other TCAs that can inhibit serotonin uptake (eg, amitriptyline, imipramine, trazodone) in patients taking moclobemide unless additional data prove that they are safe. SSRIs probably also should be avoided with moclobemide, although some combinations may be safe. If a patient develops serotonin syndrome from one of these interactions, intensive supportive therapy is needed to treat convulsions, hyperthermia, and cardiorespiratory problems. Some also have recommended the use of methysergide (a serotonin antagonist) and dantrolene (for muscle rigidity and hyperpyrexia).

➡ ***Monitor.*** If the combination is used, be alert for evidence of serotonin syndrome which can result in neurologic findings (eg, dizziness, tremor, myoclonus, rigidity, seizures, incoordination, coma), psychiatric symptoms (eg, agitation, confusion, hypomania), and disorders of temperature regulation (eg, fever, sweating, shivering); severe cases can be fatal.

REFERENCES:

Neuvonen PJ, et al. Five fatal cases of serotonin syndrome after moclobemide-citalopram or moclobemide-clomipramine overdoses. *Lancet.* 1993;342:1419.

Spigset O, et al. Serotonin syndrome caused by a moclobemide-clomipramine interaction. *BMJ.* 1993;306:248.

Clomipramine (eg, *Anafranil*)

Phenelzine (*Nardil*) `AVOID`

SUMMARY: Avoid clomipramine and imipramine in patients receiving phenelzine or other nonselective monoamine oxidase inhibitors (MAOIs).

RISK FACTORS: No specific risk factors are known.

RELATED DRUGS: Other antidepressants that inhibit serotonin reuptake such as amitriptyline (eg, *Elavil*), imipramine (eg, *Tofranil*), and trazodone (eg, *Desyrel*) would be expected to interact adversely with nonselective MAOIs, including tranylcypromine (*Parnate*), and isocarboxazid. Other TCAs also may interact with MAOIs, but some TCAs and nonselective MAOIs can be given together safely if the following precautions are observed: 1) avoid large doses, 2) give the drugs orally, 3) avoid clomipramine and imipramine, and 4) monitor the patient closely.

MANAGEMENT OPTIONS:

➡ *AVOID COMBINATION.* Avoid combined use of clomipramine or imipramine with non-selective MAOIs.

REFERENCES:

Kline NS. Experimental use of monoamine oxidase inhibitors with tricyclic antidepressants (Questions and Answers). *JAMA.* 1974;227:807.

De La Fuente RJ, et al. Mania induced by tricyclic-MAOI combination therapy in bipolar treatment-resistant disorder: case reports. *J Clin Psychiatry.* 1986;47:40.

Beaumont G. Drug interactions with clomipramine (*Anafranil*). *J Int Med Res.* 1973;1:480.

White K, et al. The combined use of MAOIs and tricyclics. *J Clin Psychiatry.* 1984;45:67.

Winston F. Combined antidepressant therapy. *Br J Psychiatry.* 1971;118:301.

Schuckit U, et al. Tricyclic antidepressants and monoamine oxidase inhibitors. Combination therapy in the treatment of depression. *Arch Gen Psychiatry.* 1971;24:509.

Spiker DG, et al. Combining tricyclic and monoamine oxidase inhibitor antidepressants. *Arch Gen Psychiatry.* 1976;33:828.

Ananth J, et al. A review of combined tricyclic and MAOI therapy. *Compr Psychiatry.* 1977;18:221.

White K. Tricyclic overdose in a patient given combined tricyclic-MAOI treatment. *Am J Psychiatry.* 1978;135:1411.

Young JPR, et al. Controlled trial of trimipramine, monoamine oxidase inhibitors, and combined treatment in depressed outpatients. *BMJ.* 1979;2:1315.

White K. Combined tricyclic and monoamine-oxidase inhibitor antidepressant treatment. *West J Med.* 1983;138:406.

Clonazepam (eg, *Klonopin*)

Valproic Acid (eg, *Depakene*)

SUMMARY: Absence seizures have been reported in patients receiving valproic acid and clonazepam, but a causal relationship has not been established.

RISK FACTORS: No specific risk factors are known.

RELATED DRUGS: No information is available.

MANAGEMENT OPTIONS:

➡ *Monitor.* If absence seizures increase with combined clonazepam and valproic acid, consider an alternative anticonvulsant regimen.

REFERENCES:

Jeavons PM, et al. Treatment of generalized epilepsies of childhood and adolescence with sodium valproate ("epilim"). *Dev Med Child Neurol.* 1977;19:9.

Browne TR. Interaction between clonazepam and sodium valproate. *N Engl J Med.* 1979;300:678.

Clonidine (eg, *Catapres*)

Cyclosporine (eg, *Neoral*)

SUMMARY: Limited clinical evidence suggests that clonidine increases cyclosporine blood concentrations; more study is needed to establish the incidence and magnitude of this interaction.

RISK FACTORS: No specific risk factors are known.

RELATED DRUGS: The effect of clonidine on tacrolimus (*Prograf*) is not established, but the drug interactions of cyclosporine and tacrolimus tend to be similar.

MANAGEMENT OPTIONS:

➡ *Monitor.* Monitor for altered cyclosporine blood concentrations if clonidine is initiated, discontinued, or changed in dosage; adjust cyclosporine dose as needed.

REFERENCES:

Gilbert RD, et al. Interaction between clonidine and cyclosporine A. *Nephron.* 1995;71:105.

Luke J, et al. Prevention of cyclosporine-induced nephrotoxicity with transdermal clonidine. *Clin Pharmacol.* 1990;9:49.

Clonidine (eg, *Catapres*)

Desipramine (eg, *Norpramin*)

SUMMARY: Tricyclic antidepressants (TCAs) such as desipramine can inhibit the antihypertensive response to clonidine; preliminary evidence indicates that TCAs also may enhance the hypertensive response to abrupt clonidine withdrawal.

RISK FACTORS:

➡ *Dosage Regimen.* Abrupt withdrawal of clonidine in the presence of a TCA may lead to an exaggerated hypertensive response.

RELATED DRUGS: Little is known regarding the effect of other TCAs on clonidine response; assume that they interact until proven otherwise. Trazodone (eg, *Desyrel*) reportedly inhibits the hypotensive response to clonidine, but more evidence is needed. Theoretically, maprotiline (eg, *Ludiomil*) would be less likely to interact with clonidine than other TCAs, but clinical studies are lacking. The tetracyclic drug mianserin has minimal effects on clonidine response in both healthy subjects and patients with essential hypertension. Clonidine-like drugs such as guanabenz (eg, *Wytensin*) and guanfacine (*Tenex*) theoretically also would interact with TCAs.

MANAGEMENT OPTIONS:

➡ *Avoid Unless Benefit Outweighs Risk.* If possible, avoid concomitant use of clonidine and tricyclic antidepressants. Since TCAs also appear to interact with guanethidine (*Ismelin*), bethanidine, and debrisoquin, these drugs would not be suitable alternatives. Methyldopa (eg, *Aldomet*) apparently can be used safely with TCAs, but methyldopa has other disadvantages. In any case, blood monitor pressure if TCAs are initiated, discontinued, or changed in dosage in a patient on antihypertensive drugs.

➡ *Monitor.* If TCAs and clonidine are used concurrently, monitor blood pressure carefully when the TCA is started and also if the clonidine is withdrawn. Gradual tapering of the clonidine dosage may be helpful in reducing the likelihood of severe rebound hypertension.

REFERENCES:

Gutkind JS, et al. Differential pharmacological interaction of clonidine and guanabenz with antidepressive drugs. *Clin Exp Hypertens.* 1987;A9:1531.

Briant RH, et al. Interaction between clonidine and desipramine in man. *BMJ.* 1973;1:522.

Hui KK. Hypertensive crisis induced by interaction of clonidine with imipramine. *J Am Geriatr Soc.* 1983;31:164.

Stiff JL, et al. Clonidine withdrawal complicated by amitriptyline therapy. *Anesthesiology.* 1983;59:73.

Barnes JS, et al. Lack of interaction between tricyclic antidepressants and clonidine at the alpha-2-adrenoceptor on human platelets. *Clin Pharmacol Ther.* 1982;32:744.

Elliott HL, et al. Pharmacodynamics studies on mianserin and its interaction with clonidine. *Eur J Clin Pharmacol.* 1981;21:97.

Elliot HL, et al. Absence of an effect of mianserin on the actions of clonidine or methyldopa in hypertensive patients. *Eur J Clin Pharmacol.* 1983;24:15.

Elliot HL, et al. Assessment of the interaction between mianserin and centrally-acting antihypertensive drugs. *Br J Clin Pharmacol.* 1983;15:323S.

Clonidine (eg, *Catapres*)

Insulin

SUMMARY: Clonidine may diminish the symptoms of hypoglycemia.

RISK FACTORS: No specific risk factors are known.

RELATED DRUGS: Guanfacine (*Tenex*) and guanabenz (eg, *Wytensin*) theoretically would produce a similar effect during hypoglycemic episodes.

MANAGEMENT OPTIONS:

➡ *Monitor.* Patients receiving antidiabetic drugs and clonidine should be aware that clonidine may suppress the signs and symptoms of hypoglycemia.

REFERENCES:

Hedeland H, et al. The effect of insulin-induced hypoglycaemia on plasma renin activity and urinary catecholamines before and following clonidine (*Catapres*) in man. *Acta Endocrinol.* 1972;71:321.

Guthrie GP, et al. Effect of transdermal clonidine on the endocrine responses to insulin-induced hypoglycemia in essential hypertension. *Clin Pharmacol Ther.* 1989;45:417.

Clonidine (eg, *Duraclon*)

Mirtazapine (*Remeron*)

SUMMARY: A man with well-controlled hypertension developed a severe hypertensive reaction after mirtazapine was added to his therapy.

RISK FACTORS: No specific risk factors are known.

RELATED DRUGS: Tricyclic antidepressants (TCAs) also antagonize the antihypertensive response to clonidine, and they would not be appropriate substitutes for mirtazapine in a patient on clonidine. Trazodone (eg, *Desyrel*) reportedly inhibits the hypotensive response to clonidine but more evidence is needed. Mianserin has minimal effects on clonidine response in healthy subjects and hypertensive patients. Antihypertensive drugs such as guanabenz (eg, *Wytensin*) and guanfacine (*Tenex*) stimulate central α2-receptors, and theoretically would interact with mirtazapine or TCAs in the same manner as clonidine.

MANAGEMENT OPTIONS:

➡ *Use Alternative.* In patients on clonidine, use antidepressants other than mirtazapine or TCAs (see Related Drugs).

REFERENCES:

Abo-Zena RA, et al. Hypertensive urgency induced by an interaction of mirtazapine and clonidine. *Pharmacotherapy.* 2000;20:476-78.

Barnes JS, et al. Lack of interaction between tricyclic antidepressants and clonidine at the alpha 2-adrenoceptor on human platelets. *Clin Pharmacol Ther.* 1982;32:744-48.

Elliott HL, et al. Pharmacodynamic studies on mianserin and its interaction with clonidine. *Eur J Clin Pharmacol.* 1981;21:97-102.

Elliott HL, et al. Absence of an effect of mianserin on the actions of clonidine or methyldopa in hypertensive patients. *Eur J Clin Pharmacol.* 1983;24:15-19.

Clonidine (eg, *Catapres*)

Nitroprusside

SUMMARY: Cases of severe hypotensive reactions with the combined use of clonidine and nitroprusside have been reported.

RISK FACTORS: No specific risk factors are known.

RELATED DRUGS: Although little is known regarding the effect of centrally acting alpha-agonists other than clonidine, such as guanabenz (eg, *Wytensin*) and guanfacine (*Tenex*), consider the possibility that they interact with nitroprusside until clinical information is available.

MANAGEMENT OPTIONS:

➡ ***Monitor.*** Monitor for excessive hypotensive effects when clonidine is used in patients who are receiving nitroprusside or who have recently received it.

REFERENCES:

Cohen IM, et al. Danger in nitroprusside therapy. *Ann Intern Med.* 1976;85:205.

Clonidine (eg, *Catapres*)

Propranolol (eg, *Inderal*)

SUMMARY: Hypertension occurring upon withdrawal of clonidine may be exacerbated by noncardioselective (eg, propranolol, nadolol [eg, *Corgard*]) beta blocker therapy.

RISK FACTORS:

➡ ***Order of Drug Administration.*** Withdrawal of clonidine during noncardioselective beta blocker therapy.

RELATED DRUGS: Centrally acting alpha-agonists other than clonidine, such as guanabenz (eg, *Wystensin*) and guanfacine (*Tenex*), can produce rebound hypertension when discontinued; thus, assume that beta-adrenergic blockers can enhance this hypertensive reaction until proven otherwise.

MANAGEMENT OPTIONS:

➡ ***Consider Alternative.*** The use of labetalol (*Normodyne*) (which has both alpha- and beta-blocking activity) may prove useful in preventing rebound hypertension following clonidine withdrawal. Cardioselective beta blockers (eg, atenolol [eg, *Tenormin*], metoprolol [eg, *Lopressor*]) would be less likely to produce rebound hypertension.

➡ ***Circumvent/Minimize.*** In patients receiving both nonselective beta-adrenergic blockers and clonidine, the beta blocker could be withdrawn before the clonidine to reduce the danger of rebound hypertension.

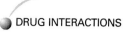
➡ **Monitor.** If clonidine is withdrawn while the patient remains on a beta-adrenergic blocker, monitor the patient very carefully for a hypertensive response.

REFERENCES:

Harris AL. Clonidine withdrawal and blockade. *Lancet.* 1976;1:596.

Cairns SA, et al. Clonidine withdrawal. *Lancet.* 1976;1:368.

Bailey RR, et al. Rapid clonidine withdrawal with blood pressure overshoot exaggerated by beta blockade. *BMJ.* 1976;2:942.

Strauss FG, et al. Withdrawal of antihypertensive therapy. *JAMA.* 1977;238:1734.

Vernon C, et al. Fatal rebound hypertension after abrupt withdrawal of clonidine and propranolol. *Br J Clin Pract.* 1979;33:112.

Warren SE, et al. Clonidine and propranolol paradoxical hypertension. *Arch Intern Med.* 1979;139:253.

Lilja M, et al. Interaction of clonidine and beta blockers. *Acta Med Scand.* 1980;207:173.

Rosenthal T, et al. Use of labetalol in hypertensive patients during discontinuation of clonidine therapy. *Eur J Clin Pharmacol.* 1981;20:237.

Saarimaa H. Combination of clonidine and sotalol in hypertension. *BMJ.* 1976;1:810.

Clopidogrel (*Plavix*)

Rifampin (eg, *Rifadin*)

SUMMARY: Rifampin appears to enhance the antiplatelet effects of clopidogrel, but the clinical importance of this effect is not established.

RISK FACTORS: No specific risk factors are known.

RELATED DRUGS: Although clinical information is not available, other CYP3A4 inducers would also be expected to increase clopidogrel effect.

MANAGEMENT OPTIONS:

➡ **Monitor.** Consider monitoring platelet function if rifampin is initiated, discontinued, or changed in dosage. Adjustments in clopidogrel dose may be needed.

REFERENCES:

Clarke TA, et al. The metabolism of clopidogrel is catalyzed by human cytochrome P450 3A and is inhibited by atorvastatin. *Drug Metab Dispos.* 2003;31:53-59.

Lau WC, et al. Atorvastatin reduces the ability of clopidogrel to inhibit platelet aggregation: a new drug-drug interaction. *Circulation.* 2003;107:32-37.

Clotrimazole (eg, *Mycelex*)

Tacrolimus (*Prograf*)

SUMMARY: Clotrimazole troche administration appears to result in increased tacrolimus concentrations and possibly enhanced nephrotoxicity; more study is needed to clarify this interaction.

RISK FACTORS: No specific risk factors are known.

RELATED DRUGS: Fluconazole (*Diflucan*) (and perhaps other antifungal agents) administration increases tacrolimus concentration. Cyclosporine (eg, *Neoral*) may be similarly affected by clotrimazole.

MANAGEMENT OPTIONS:

➡ *Monitor.* Until more information is available, monitor patients taking tacrolimus carefully for increased serum concentrations of tacrolimus and creatinine during coadministration of clotrimazole.

REFERENCES:

Mieles L, et al. Interaction between FK506 and clotrimazole in a liver transplant recipient. *Transplantation.* 1991;52:1086-87.

Clozapine (eg, *Clozaril*)

Diazepam (eg, *Valium*)

SUMMARY: Isolated cases of cardiorespiratory collapse have been reported in patients receiving diazepam and clozapine, but a causal relationship has not been established.

RISK FACTORS: No specific risk factors are known.

RELATED DRUGS: Lorazepam (eg, *Ativan*) also has been associated with similar reactions when combined with clozapine, but a causal relationship has not been established.

MANAGEMENT OPTIONS:

➡ *Monitor.* Although a causal relationship has not been established for this interaction, the severity of the reaction dictates that patients receiving clozapine and diazepam be monitored closely for evidence of respiratory depression and hypotension, especially during the first few weeks of therapy and after an increase in the dose of either drug. Until more information is available, the same precautions also should pertain to the use of clozapine concurrently with benzodiazepines other than diazepam.

REFERENCES:

Sassim N, et al. Adverse drug reactions with clozapine and simultaneous application of benzodiazepines. *Pharmacopsychiatry.* 1988;21:306-07.

Finkel M, et al. Clozapine—a novel antipsychotic agent. *N Engl J Med.* 1991;325:518.

Frankenburg F, et al. Clozapine—a novel antipsychotic agent. *N Engl J Med.* 1991;325:518.

Clozapine (eg, *Clozaril*)

Erythromycin (eg, *E-Mycin*)

SUMMARY: A patient receiving clozapine developed elevated plasma concentrations and a seizure following the addition of erythromycin therapy.

RISK FACTORS: No specific risk factors are known.

RELATED DRUGS: Troleandomycin (*TAO*) or clarithromycin (*Biaxin*) may inhibit the metabolism of clozapine. Azithromycin (*Zithromax*) and dirithromycin (*Dynabac*) would be unlikely to inhibit the metabolism of clozapine.

MANAGEMENT OPTIONS:

➡ **Use Alternative.** Noninteracting antibiotics (eg, azithromycin, dirithromycin) are preferable in patients receiving clozapine.

REFERENCES:

Funderburg LG, et al. Seizure following the addition of erythromycin to clozapine treatment. *Am J Psychiatry.* 1994;151:1840.

 Clozapine (eg, *Clozaril*)

Fluvoxamine (*Luvox*)

SUMMARY: Fluvoxamine can markedly increase clozapine plasma concentrations; dosage adjustments are likely to be needed.

RISK FACTORS: No specific risk factors are known.

RELATED DRUGS: The effect of selective serotonin reuptake inhibitors (SSRIs) other than fluvoxamine on clozapine is not established, but fluoxetine (*Prozac*), paroxetine (*Paxil*), and sertraline (*Zoloft*) appear to have little effect on cytochrome P4501A2.

MANAGEMENT OPTIONS:

➡ **Use Alternative.** Given the large magnitude of the increases in clozapine plasma concentrations because of fluvoxamine, an SSRI other than fluvoxamine generally would be preferable. If fluvoxamine is used, adjustments in clozapine dosage are likely to be needed. Monitor for altered clozapine response if fluvoxamine therapy is initiated, discontinued, or changed in dosage.

REFERENCES:

Hiemke C, et al. Elevated levels of clozapine in serum after addition of fluvoxamine. *J Clin Psychopharmacol.* 1994;14:279.

Jerling M, et al. Fluvoxamine inhibition and carbamazepine induction of the metabolism of clozapine: evidence from a therapeutic drug monitoring service. *Ther Drug Monit.* 1994;16:368.

 Clozapine (eg, *Clozaril*)

Lorazepam (eg, *Ativan*)

SUMMARY: Isolated cases of cardiovascular or respiratory collapse have been reported in patients receiving lorazepam and clozapine, but a causal relationship has not been established.

RISK FACTORS: No specific risk factors are known.

RELATED DRUGS: Diazepam (eg, *Valium*) also has been associated with similar reactions when combined with clozapine, but a causal relationship has not been established.

MANAGEMENT OPTIONS:

➡ **Monitor.** Although a causal relationship has not been established for this interaction, the severity of the reaction dictates that patients receiving clozapine and lorazepam be monitored closely for evidence of respiratory depression and hypotension, especially during the first few weeks of therapy and after an increase in the dose of either drug. Until more information is available, the same precautions also should pertain to the use of clozapine concurrently with benzodiazepines other than lorazepam.

REFERENCES:

Friedman LJ, et al. Clozapine—a novel antipsychotic agent. *N Engl J Med.* 1991;325:518-519.

Sassim N, et al. Adverse drug reactions with clozapine and simultaneous application of benzodiazepines. *Pharmacopsychiatry.* 1988;21:306-307.

Klimke A, et al. Sudden death after intravenous application of lorazepam in a patient treated with clozapine. *Am J Psychiatry.* 1994;151:780.

Finkel M, et al. Clozapine—a novel antipsychotic agent. *N Engl J Med.* 1991;325:518.

Clozapine (*Clozaril*)

Valproic Acid (eg, *Depakene*)

SUMMARY: Several patients stabilized on clozapine developed substantial reductions in clozapine total serum concentrations after valproic acid was started, but clozapine therapeutic response was not affected.

RISK FACTORS: No specific risk factors are known.

RELATED DRUGS: No information is available.

MANAGEMENT OPTIONS:

➡ ***Monitor.*** Until more data are available, monitor for altered clozapine response if valproic acid therapy is initiated, discontinued, or changed in dosage. When interpreting clozapine serum concentrations, keep in mind that if displacement of clozapine from plasma protein binding is involved, subtherapeutic total clozapine levels may not indicate subtherapeutic unbound levels.

REFERENCES:

Finley P, et al. Potential impact of valproic acid therapy on clozapine disposition. *Biol Psychiatry.* 1994;36:487.

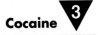

Cocaine

Disulfiram (*Antabuse*)

SUMMARY: Disulfiram may substantially increase cocaine plasma concentrations and cardiovascular effects, but the clinical importance of this effect is not established.

RISK FACTORS: No specific risk factors are known.

RELATED DRUGS: No information is available.

MANAGEMENT OPTIONS:

➡ ***Circumvent/Minimize.*** Inform patients receiving disulfiram that cocaine may have greater toxicity.

REFERENCES:

McCance-Katz EF, et al. Disulfiram effects on acute cocaine administration. *Drug Alcohol Depend.* 1998;52:27.

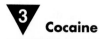

▼③ Cocaine

Propranolol (eg, *Inderal*)

SUMMARY: Propranolol increases the angina-inducing potential of cocaine; other beta-adrenergic blockers would be expected to have similar effects.

RISK FACTORS: No specific risk factors are known.

RELATED DRUGS: Other beta blockers are likely to produce a similar reaction.

MANAGEMENT OPTIONS:

➥ *Consider Alternative.* The use of cocaine for local anesthesia might pose an increased risk to patients taking beta blockers. Consider other local anesthetics for use.

➥ *Monitor.* Caution patients, particularly those with coronary artery disease, taking beta-adrenergic blockers regarding the potential for angina during cocaine use.

REFERENCES:

Lange RA, et al. Potentiation of cocaine-induced coronary vasoconstriction by beta-adrenergic blockade. *Ann Intern Med.* 1990;112:897.

Codeine

Quinidine (eg, *Quinora*)

SUMMARY: Quinidine inhibits the bioactivation of codeine to morphine, thus reducing the analgesic effect of codeine.

RISK FACTORS:

➥ *Pharmacogenetics.* Only patients with the extensive metabolizer CYP2D6 phenotype (EMs) would be expected to experience this interaction. Poor metabolizers (PMs) do not have the gene for production of CYP2D6, so there would be no CYP2D6 for the quinidine to inhibit. Approximately 8% of whites are deficient in CYP2D6, but the deficiency is rare in Asians, usually no more than 2%.

RELATED DRUGS: The analgesic effect of dihydrocodeine (eg, *Synalgos-DC*) and hydro-codone (eg, *Vicodin*) also may be dependent on conversion to morphine-like active metabolites, and early evidence suggests that quinidine can reduce their analgesic efficacy. Tramadol (*Ultram*) appears to be partially dependent upon CYP2D6 for analgesic activity, but theoretically would be less affected than codeine by quinidine therapy. Early pharmacodynamic evidence suggest that oxycodone (eg, *Percodan*) does not require conversion by CYP2D6 to an active metabolite. Theoretically, oxycodone would not be affected by quinidine, but more study is needed.

MANAGEMENT OPTIONS:

➥ *Consider Alternative.* Consider use of an analgesic other than codeine, dihydrocodeine, hydrocodone, or tramadol. (See Related Drugs.)

➥ *Monitor.* If codeine and quinidine are used together, monitor for reduced analgesic effect.

REFERENCES:

Tseng C-Y, et al. Formation of morphine from codeine in Chinese subjects of different CYP2D6 genotypes. *Clin Pharmacol Ther.* 1996;60:177.

Straka RJ, et al. Comparison of the prevalence of the poor metabolizer phenotype for CYP2D6 between 203 Hmong subjects and 280 white subjects residing in Minnesota. *Clin Pharmacol Ther*. 1995;58:29.

Sindrup SH, et al. Codeine increases pain thresholds to copper vapor laser stimuli in extensive but not poor metabolizers of sparteine. *Clin Pharmacol Ther*. 1990;48:686.

Poulsen L, et al. Codeine and morphine in extensive and poor metabolizers of sparteine: pharmacokinetics, analgesic effect and side effects. *Eur J Clin Pharmacol*. 1996;51:289.

Desmeules J, et al. Impact of genetic and environmental factors on codeine analgesia. *Clin Pharmacol Ther*. 1989;45:122.

Sindrup SH, et al. The effect of quinidine on the analgesic effect of codeine. *Eur J Clin Pharmacol*. 1992;42:587.

Sindrup SH, et al. Impact of quinidine on plasma and cerebrospinal fluid concentrations of codeine and morphine after codeine intake. *Eur J Clin Pharmacol*. 1996;49:503.

Caraco Y, et al. Pharmacogenetic determination of the effects of codeine and prediction of drug interactions. *J Pharmacol Exp Ther*. 1996;278:1165.

Mikus G, et al. Effect of codeine on gastrointestinal motility in relation to CYP2D6 phenotype. *Clin Pharmacol Ther*. 1997;61:459.

Fromm MF, et al. Dihydrocodeine: a new opioid substrate for the polymorphic CYP2D6 in humans. *Clin Pharmacol Ther*. 1995;58:374.

Hufschmid E, et al. Exploration of the metabolism of dihydrocodeine via determination of its metabolites in human urine using micellar electrokinetic capillary chromatography. *J Chromatogr B Biome Appl*. 1995;668:159.

Otton SV, et al. CYP2D6 phenotype determines the metabolic conversion of hydrocodone to hydromorphone. *Clin Pharmacol Ther*. 1993;54:463.

Poulsen L, et al. The hypoalgesic effect of tramadol in relation to CYP2D6. *Clin Pharmacol Ther*. 1996;60:636.

Poyhia R, et al. A review of oxycodone's clinical pharmacokinetics and pharmacodynamics. *J Pain Symptom Manage*. 1993;8:63.

Kaiko RF, et al. Phamacokinetic-phamacodynamic relationships of controlled-release oxycodone. *Clin Pharmacol Ther*. 1996;59:52.

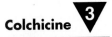

Colchicine

Cyclosporine (eg, *Neoral*)

SUMMARY: Cyclosporine blood concentrations increased and nephrotoxicity developed after administration of colchicine in renal transplant patients.

RISK FACTORS: No specific risk factors are known.

RELATED DRUGS: Tacrolimus (*Prograf*) and cyclosporine tend to have similar interactions, but it is not known if tacrolimus interacts with colchicine.

MANAGEMENT OPTIONS:

➡ *Monitor.* Monitor for altered cyclosporine blood concentrations and renal function if colchicine is initiated, discontinued or changed in dosage. *Note:* Cyclosporine commonly induces hyperuricemia by decreasing urate clearance. Colchicine must be used with caution in patients with decreased renal function because they are at increased risk for neuromuscular toxicity and bone marrow dysplasia.

REFERENCES:

Menta R, et al. Reversible acute cyclosporine nephrotoxicity induced by colchicine administration. *Nephrol Dial Transplant*. 1987;2:380.

Lin HY, et al. Cyclosporine-induced hyperuricemia and gout. *N Engl J Med*. 1989;321:287.

Kuncl RE, et al. Colchicine myopathy and neuropathy. *N Engl J Med*. 1987;316:1562.

Yussim A, et al. Gastrointestinal, hepatorenal, and neuromuscular toxicity caused by cyclosporine-colchicine interaction in renal transplantation. *Transplant Proc*. 1994;26:2825.

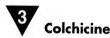

 Colchicine

Erythromycin (eg, *E-Mycin*)

SUMMARY: A patient developed severe colchicine toxicity following 2 weeks of erythromycin coadministration.

RISK FACTORS: No specific risk factors are known.

RELATED DRUGS: Troleandomycin (*TAO*) or clarithromycin (*Biaxin*) also may inhibit the metabolism of colchicine, provided this interaction is confirmed.

MANAGEMENT OPTIONS:

➡ *Monitor.* Pending further reports of the concomitant usage of erythromycin and colchicine, monitor patients receiving both drugs for evidence of colchicine toxicity (eg, fever, GI symptoms, leukopenia).

REFERENCES:

Caraco Y, et al. Acute colchicine intoxication—possible role of erythromycin administration. *J Rheumatol.* 1992;19:494.

 Colestipol (*Colestid*)

Diclofenac (eg, *Voltaren*)

SUMMARY: Single dose studies suggest that colestipol moderately reduces the bioavailability of diclofenac; the clinical importance of this effect is not established, but reduced diclofenac effect may occur.

RISK FACTORS: No specific risk factors are known.

RELATED DRUGS: Cholestyramine (eg, *Questran*) also appears to inhibit the absorption of diclofenac, and to a greater extent than colestipol.

MANAGEMENT OPTIONS:

➡ *Circumvent/Minimize.* Give the diclofenac 2 hours before or 6 hours after the colestipol to optimize the absorption of the diclofenac. However, because diclofenac undergoes enterohepatic circulation, reduced diclofenac plasma concentrations may occur even if the doses are separated.

➡ *Monitor.* Monitor for reduced diclofenac effect, regardless of how far apart the doses are separated.

REFERENCES:

Al-balla SR, et al. The effects of cholestyramine and colestipol on the absorption of diclofenac in man. *Int J Clin Pharmacol Ther.* 1994;32:441.

Colestipol (*Colestid*)

Furosemide (eg, *Lasix*)

SUMMARY: Study in healthy subjects suggests that colestipol considerably reduces the bioavailability and diuretic response of furosemide.

RISK FACTORS: No specific risk factors are known.

RELATED DRUGS: Cholestyramine (eg, *Questran*) also substantially reduces the bioavailability of furosemide.

MANAGEMENT OPTIONS:

➡ *Circumvent/Minimize.* Although the ability to circumvent the interaction by separating doses of furosemide from colestipol has not been studied systematically, giving furosemide 2 hours before or 6 hours after the colestipol would be expected to minimize the interaction.

➡ *Monitor.* Monitor for altered furosemide response if colestipol therapy is initiated, discontinued, changed in dosage, or if the interval between doses of the 2 drugs is changed.

REFERENCES:

Neuvonen PJ, et al. Effects of resins and activated charcoal on the absorption of digoxin, carbamazepine and furosemide. *Br J Clin Pharmacol.* 1988;25:229.

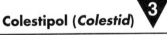

Colestipol (*Colestid*)

Gemfibrozil (eg, *Lopid*)

SUMMARY: Colestipol appears to reduce the bioavailability of gemfibrozil if the drugs are given concurrently, but not if the doses are separated by at least 2 hours.

RISK FACTORS: No specific risk factors are known.

RELATED DRUGS: Cholestyramine (eg, *Questran*) probably also inhibits the absorption of gemfibrozil.

MANAGEMENT OPTIONS:

➡ *Circumvent/Minimize.* Until more is known about this interaction, it would be prudent to separate doses of gemfibrozil and colestipol (or cholestyramine) by at least 2 hours.

➡ *Monitor.* Monitor for reduced gemfibrozil response if colestipol orcholestyramine is also given.

REFERENCES:

Forland SC, et al. Apparent reduced absorption of gemfibrozil when given with colestipol. *J Clin Pharmacol.* 1990;30:29.

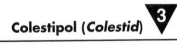

Colestipol (*Colestid*)

Tetracycline

SUMMARY: Colestipol reduces the bioavailability of tetracycline; however, the clinical importance of this interaction is not established.

RISK FACTORS: No specific risk factors are known.

RELATED DRUGS: Cholestyramine (eg, *Questran*) might reduce absorption of tetracycline as well.

MANAGEMENT OPTIONS:

➡ *Circumvent/Minimize.* Until further information is available, patients receiving colestipol and tetracycline should separate the doses in an attempt to minimize the effect of colestipol on tetracycline absorption. Administer tetracycline 2 hours before or at least 3 hours after colestipol.

➡ **Monitor.** If doses of tetracycline and bile acid binding resin must be administered together, monitor patient for reduced antibiotic effect.

REFERENCES:

Friedman H, et al. Impaired absorption of tetracycline by colestipol is not reversed by orange juice. *J Clin Pharmacol.* 1989;29:748.

Colestipol (*Colestid*)

Thiazides

SUMMARY: Colestipol has been reported to reduce the serum concentrations of thiazides and may lessen their diuretic effect.

RISK FACTORS: No specific risk factors are known.

RELATED DRUGS: Assume that all thiazides interact with colestipol until proved otherwise. Cholestyramine (eg, *Questran*) also inhibits thiazide diuretic absorption.

MANAGEMENT OPTIONS:

➡ **Circumvent/Minimize.** Take thiazides at least 2 hours before or 6 hours after the colestipol, and try to maintain a relatively constant interval and sequence of administration of the 2 drugs.

➡ **Monitor.** Monitor for altered thiazide response if colestipol therapy is initiated, discontinued, changed in dosage, or if the interval between doses of the 2 drugs is changed.

REFERENCES:

Kauffman RE, et al. Effect of colestipol on gastrointestinal absorption of chlorothiazide in man. *Clin Pharmacol Ther.* 1973;14:886.

Hunninghake DB, et al. The effect of cholestyramine and colestipol on the absorption of hydrochlorothiazide. *Int J Clin Pharmacol Ther Toxicol.* 1982;20:151.

Contraceptives, Oral (eg, *Ortho-Novum*)

Felbamate (*Felbatol*)

SUMMARY: Felbamate substantially reduced plasma gestodene concentrations and slightly reduced plasma ethinyl estradiol concentrations in women on an oral contraceptive containing ethinyl estradiol and gestodene, but the extent to which felbamate reduces oral contraceptive efficacy is not established.

RISK FACTORS: No specific risk factors are known.

RELATED DRUGS: The effect of felbamate on progestins other than gestodene or estrogens other than ethinyl estradiol is not established, but an interaction could occur.

MANAGEMENT OPTIONS:

➡ **Consider Alternative.** Consider adding other means of contraception to the oral contraceptive, especially during the first 2 to 3 months of combined therapy with felbamate. Alternatively, some studies have recommended using a higher-dose oral contraceptive to maintain adequate hormonal concentrations. This appears to be a reasonable recommendation, but the magnitude of the required dosage increase is likely to vary considerably from one patient to another.

➡ *Monitor.* Spotting or breakthrough bleeding in patients taking oral contraceptives and felbamate could indicate that the drugs are interacting, although lack of breakthrough bleeding does not ensure contraceptive protection.

REFERENCES:

Saano V, et al. Effects of felbamate on the pharmacokinetics of a low-dose combination oral contraceptive. *Clin Pharmacol Ther.* 1995;58(5):523-31.

Wilbur K, et al. Pharmacokinetic drug interactions between oral contraceptives and second-generation anticonvulsants. *Clin Pharmacokinet.* 2000;38(4):355-65.

Contraceptives, Oral (eg, *Ortho-Novum*)
Oxcarbazepine (*Trileptal*)

SUMMARY: Two studies suggest that oxcarbazepine reduces the plasma concentrations of ethinyl estradiol and levonorgestrel, and may reduce the efficacy of oral contraceptives.

RISK FACTORS: No specific risk factors are known.

RELATED DRUGS: The effect of oxcarbazepine on progestins other than levonorgestrel or estrogens other than ethinyl estradiol is not established, but an interaction could occur.

MANAGEMENT OPTIONS:

➡ *Consider Alternative.* Consider adding other means of contraception to the oral contraceptives, especially during the first 2 to 3 months of combined therapy with oxcarbazepine. Alternatively, some studies have recommended using a higher-dose oral contraceptive to maintain adequate hormonal concentrations. This appears to be a reasonable recommendation, but the magnitude of the required dosage increase is likely to vary considerably from one patient to another.

➡ *Monitor.* Spotting or breakthrough bleeding in patients taking oral contraceptives and oxcarbazepine could indicate that the drugs are interacting, although lack of breakthrough bleeding does not ensure contraceptive protection.

REFERENCES:

Fattore C, et al. Induction of ethinylestradiol and levonorgestrel metabolism by oxycarbazepine in healthy women. *Epilepsia.* 1999;40:783-787.

Klosterskov Jensen P, et al. Possible interaction between oxcarbazepine and an oral contraceptive. *Epilepsia.* 1992;33:1149-1152.

Contraceptives, Oral (eg, *Ortho-Novum*)
Phenobarbital (eg, *Bellatal*)

SUMMARY: Phenobarbital may reduce the efficacy of oral contraceptives; menstrual irregularities and unintended pregnancies may occur.

RISK FACTORS:

➡ *Dosage Regimen.* It is likely that patients taking low-dose oral contraceptives that contain the lowest doses of steroids are most susceptible to this interaction.

RELATED DRUGS: All barbiturates are likely to enhance estrogen metabolism.

MANAGEMENT OPTIONS:

➡ *Circumvent/Minimize.* Patients receiving chronic barbiturate therapy may require oral contraceptives with a higher estrogen content. If barbiturate use is short-term, use alternative methods of contraception (in addition to the oral contraceptives) during, and for at least several weeks after, barbiturate therapy has been discontinued.

➡ *Monitor.* Spotting or breakthrough bleeding may be an indication that significant enzyme induction is occurring, but a lack of menstrual irregularities does not ensure that the interaction has not occurred.

REFERENCES:

Janz D, et al. Letter: Anti-epileptic drugs and failure of oral contraceptives. *Lancet.* 1974;1:1113.

Conney AH. Pharmacological implications of microsomal enzyme induction. *Pharmacol Rev.* 1967;19:317-366.

Robertson YR, et al. Interactions between oral contraceptives and other drugs: a review. *Curr Med Res Opin.* 1976;3:647.

Hempel E, et al. Drug stimulated biotransformation of hormonal steroid contraceptives: clinical implications. *Drugs.* 1976;12:442-448.

Contraceptives, Oral (eg, *Ortho-Novum*)

Phenytoin (eg, *Dilantin*)

SUMMARY: Phenytoin and other enzyme-inducing anticonvulsants, such as barbiturates, carbamazepine, and primidone, may inhibit the effect of oral contraceptives resulting in menstrual irregularities and unplanned pregnancies.

RISK FACTORS: No specific risk factors are known.

RELATED DRUGS: Valproic acid (eg, *Depakene*) does not appear to affect the pharmacokinetics of oral contraceptives; clinical evidence and theoretical considerations suggest that benzodiazepine anticonvulsants are unlikely to affect oral contraceptive efficacy. Carbamazepine (eg, *Tegretol*) and primidone (eg, *Mysoline*) may inhibit the effect of oral contraceptives resulting in menstrual irregularities and unplanned pregnancies.

MANAGEMENT OPTIONS:

➡ *Consider Alternative.* When pregnancy is to be avoided in women receiving enzyme-inducing anticonvulsants such as carbamazepine, phenobarbital, phenytoin, and primidone, use a means of contraception other than oral contraceptives. Alternatively, some studies have recommended using a higher estrogen content oral contraceptive for women being treated with an enzyme reducing drug. This method would work best for women on a relatively stable anticonvulsant regimen.

➡ *Monitor.* Individualize this method based on patient response (eg, lack of breakthrough bleeding). Spotting or breakthrough bleeding in patients who are taking oral contraceptives and enzyme-inducing anticonvulsants could indicate that the drugs are interacting, although lack of breakthrough bleeding does not ensure contraceptive protection. Also be alert for evidence of increased phenytoin effect in patients taking oral contraceptives.

REFERENCES:

Hooper WD, et al. Plasma protein binding of diphenylhydantoin. Effects of sex hormones, renal and hepatic disease. *Clin Pharmacol Ther.* 1974; 15:276.

Kutt H, et al. Management of epilepsy with diphenylhydantoin sodium. *JAMA.* 1968;203:969.

Kutt H, et al. Metabolism of diphenylhydantoin by rat liver microsomes. I. Characteristics of the reaction. *Biochem Pharmacol.* 1970;19:675.

Espir M, et al. Epilepsy and oral contraception. *BMJ.* 1969;1:294.

McArthur J. Oral contraceptives and epilepsy (Notes and Comments). *BMJ.* 1967;3:162.

Kenyon IE. Unplanned pregnancy in an epileptic. *BMJ.* 1972;1:686.

Janz D, et al. Anti-epileptic drugs and failure of oral contraceptives. *Lancet.* 1974;1:113.

Laengner H, et al. Antiepileptic drugs and failure of oral contraceptives. *Lancet.* 1974;2:600.

Robertson YR, et al. Interactions between oral contraceptives and other drugs:a review. *Curr Med Res Opin.* 1976;3:647.

Coulam CB, et al. Do anticonvulsants reduce the efficacy of oral contraceptives? *Epilepsia.* 1979;20:519.

Crawford P, et al. The lack of effect of sodium valproate on the pharmacokinetics or oral contraceptive steroids. *Contraception.* 1986;33:23.

Haukkamaa M. Contraception by Norplant subdermal capsules is not reliable in epileptic patients on anticonvulsant treatment. *Contraception.* 1986;33:559.

Mattson RH, et al. Use of oral contraceptives by women with epilepsy. *JAMA.* 1986;256:238.

Contraceptives, Oral (eg, *Ortho-Novum*)

Prednisolone (eg, *Prelone*)

SUMMARY: Oral contraceptives and estrogens may enhance the effect of hydrocortisone, prednisolone, and possibly other corticosteroids; adjustments in corticosteroid dosage may be required.

RISK FACTORS: No specific risk factors are known.

RELATED DRUGS: Most combinations of oral contraceptives and corticosteroids probably interact.

MANAGEMENT OPTIONS:

➡ *Monitor.* In patients receiving both corticosteroids and oral contraceptives estrogen, watch for evidence of excessive corticosteroid effects. It may be necessary to reduce the dose of the corticosteroid.

REFERENCES:

Nelson DH, et al. Potentiation of the biologic effect of administered cortisol by estrogen treatment. *J Clin Endocrinol Metab.* 1963;23:261.

Spangler AS, et al. Enhancement of the anti-inflammatory action of hydrocortisone by estrogen. *J Clin Endocrinol.* 1969;29:650.

Kozower M, et al. Decreased clearance of prednisolone, a factor in the development of corticosteroid side effects. *J Clin Endocrinol Metab.* 1974;38:407.

Boekenoogen SJ, et al. Prednisolone disposition and protein binding in oral contraceptive users. *J Clin Endocrinol Metab.* 1983;56:702.

Contraceptives, Oral (eg, *Ortho-Novum*)
Rifabutin (*Mycobutin*)

SUMMARY: Rifabutin can reduce the plasma concentrations of ethinyl estradiol and norethindrone and may reduce oral contraceptive effectiveness; unintended pregnancy may result.

RISK FACTORS: No specific risk factors are known.

RELATED DRUGS: All oral contraceptives would be expected to interact in a similar manner with rifabutin. Rifampin is also known to reduce the plasma concentrations of estrogens.

MANAGEMENT OPTIONS:

➡ *Consider Alternative.* Patients receiving rifabutin should use contraceptive methods other than oral contraceptives or use additional contraceptive methods during and for at least 1 cycle after rifabutin is discontinued.

➡ *Monitor.* Watch for evidence of reduced estrogen effect, including menstrual irregularities, as evidence of reduced estrogen concentrations. Counsel patients taking oral contraceptives on the risk of pregnancy during rifabutin administration.

REFERENCES:

LeBel M, et al. Effects of rifabutin and rifampicin on the pharmacokinetics of ethinylestradiol and norethindrone. *J Clin Pharmacol*. 1998;38:1042-1050.

Barditch-Crovo P, et al. The effects of rifampin and rifabutin on the pharmacokinetics and pharmacodynamics of a combination oral contraceptive. *Clin Pharmacol Ther*. 1999;65:428-438.

Contraceptives, Oral (eg, *Ortho-Novum*)
Rifampin (eg, *Rifadin*)

SUMMARY: Rifampin can reduce the plasma concentrations of ethinyl estradiol and norethindrone and may reduce oral contraceptive effectiveness; unintended pregnancy may result.

RISK FACTORS: No specific risk factors are known.

RELATED DRUGS: All oral contraceptives would be expected to interact in a similar manner with rifampin. Rifabutin is also known to reduce the plasma concentrations of estrogens.

MANAGEMENT OPTIONS:

➡ *Consider Alternative.* Patients receiving rifampin should use contraceptive methods other than oral contraceptives or use additional contraceptive methods during and for at least 1 cycle after rifampin is discontinued.

➡ *Monitor.* Watch for evidence of reduced estrogen effect, including menstrual irregularities, as evidence of reduced estrogen concentrations. Counsel patients taking oral contraceptives on the risk of pregnancy during rifampin administration.

REFERENCES:

LeBel M, et al. Effects of rifabutin and rifampicin on the pharmacokinetics of ethinylestradiol and norethindrone. *J Clin Pharmacol*. 1998;38:1042-1050.

Barditch-Crovo P, et al. The effects of rifampin and rifabutin on the pharmacokinetics and pharmacodynamics of a combination oral contraceptive. *Clin Pharmacol Ther*. 1999;65:428-438.

Back DJ, et al. The effect of rifampicin on the pharmacokinetics of ethynylestradiol in women. *Contraception*. 1980;21:135-143.

Skolnick JL, et al. Rifampin, oral contraceptives, and pregnancy. *JAMA*. 1976;236:1382.

Meyer B, et al. A model to detect interactions between roxithromycin and oral contraceptives. *Clin Pharmacol Ther*. 1990;47:671-674.

Contraceptives, Oral (eg, *Ortho-Novum*)

Ritonavir (*Norvir*)

SUMMARY: Ritonavir is reported to reduce ethinyl estradiol concentrations. Loss of contraceptive activity could occur.

RISK FACTORS: No specific risk factors are known.

RELATED DRUGS: Indinavir (*Crixivan*) has been noted to increase ethinyl estradiol concentrations 24%. The effect of ritonavir on other estrogens is unknown. While no data are available, saquinavir (*Fortovase*) and nelfinavir (*Viracept*) would be less likely to interact with ethinyl estradiol.

MANAGEMENT OPTIONS:

➡ ***Consider Alternative.*** Patients receiving ritonavir and oral contraceptives should utilize an alternative method of birth control during ritonavir administration and for at least 1 cycle following its discontinuation. Indinavir does not appear to reduce oral contraceptive concentrations and could be considered as an alternative antiviral agent.

➡ ***Monitor.*** Monitor patients for signs that may indicate insufficient estrogen concentrations such as breakthrough bleeding.

REFERENCES:

Shenfield GM. Oral contraceptives. Are drug interactions of clinical significance? *Drug Saf*. 1993;9:21-37.

Product information. Ritonavir (*Norvir*). Abbott Laboratories. 1996.

Product information. Indinavir (*Crixivan*). Merck and Company, Inc. 1996.

Contraceptives, Oral (eg, *Ortho-Novum*)

Selegiline (eg, *Eldepryl*)

SUMMARY: Women on oral contraceptives appear to have considerably higher serum concentrations of selegiline, but the extent to which this increases the risk of selegiline drug interactions or adverse effects is not established.

RISK FACTORS: No specific risk factors are known.

RELATED DRUGS: No information is available.

MANAGEMENT OPTIONS:

➡ ***Consider Alternative.*** In patients receiving selegiline, consider advising use of contraceptive methods other than oral contraceptives. When selegiline is being used for parkinsonism, most patients would not be of an age to need contraception, but selegiline is occasionally used for disorders other than parkinsonism.

➡ ***Monitor.*** When selegiline is used in women taking oral contraceptives, watch for evidence of nonselective MAO inhibition (eg, hypertensive reactions to tyramine or sympathomimetics, serotonin syndrome when combined with other serotonergic drugs).

REFERENCES:

Laine K, et al. Dose linearity study of selegiline pharmacokinetics after oral administration: evidence for strong drug interaction with female sex steroids. *Br J Clin Pharmacol.* 1999;47:249-254.

Contraceptives, Oral (eg, *Ortho-Novum*)

St. John's Wort

SUMMARY: Several cases of menstrual breakthrough bleeding and at least 1 unintended pregnancy have been reported in association with use of St. John's wort in patients taking oral contraceptives. Although a causal relationship has not been established, patients on oral contraceptives should avoid St. John's wort or consider using additional contraceptive methods.

RISK FACTORS: No specific risk factors are known.

RELATED DRUGS: No information is available.

MANAGEMENT OPTIONS:

➡ *Consider Alternative.* In patients receiving oral contraceptives, consider using alternative antidepressants. Selective serotonin reuptake inhibitors (SSRIs) are not known to induce CYP3A4. SSRIs include fluoxetine (*Prozac*), paroxetine (*Paxil*), sertraline (*Zoloft*), and citalopram (*Celexa*).

➡ *Circumvent/Minimize.* Consider the use of additional forms of contraception if St. John's wort is used with oral contraceptives.

➡ *Monitor.* Menstrual irregularities, such as breakthrough bleeding, may be signs of reduced oral contraceptive efficacy, but the absence of menstrual irregularities does not ensure adequate contraception.

REFERENCES:

Yue QY, et al. Safety of St. John's wort. *Lancet.* 2000;355:576-577.

Ruschitzka F, et al. Acute heart transplant rejection due to Saint John's wort. *Lancet.* 2000;355:548-549.

Piscitelli SC, et al. Indinavir concentrations and St. John's wort. *Lancet.* 2000;355:547-548.

Johne A, et al. Pharmacokinetic interaction of digoxin with an herbal extract from St. John's wort (*hypericum perforatum*). *Clin Pharmacol Ther.* 1999;66:338-345.

Schwarz UI, et al. Unwanted pregnancy on self-medication with St. John's wort despite hormonal contraception. *Br J Clin Pharmacol.* 2003;55:112-113.

Contraceptives, Oral (eg, *Ortho-Novum*)

Tetracycline (eg, *Sumycin*)

SUMMARY: Case reports suggest that tetracycline can reduce the effectiveness of oral contraceptives; a prospective study failed to demonstrate an effect in a small number of women.

RISK FACTORS: No specific risk factors are known.

RELATED DRUGS: Other oral antibiotics have been associated with oral contraceptive failure.

MANAGEMENT OPTIONS:

➡ *Monitor.* Although evidence of interaction between tetracyclines and oral contraceptives is limited, counsel women taking oral contraceptives to use additional forms of contraception during tetracycline therapy.

REFERENCES:

Orme ML. The clinical pharmacology of oral contraceptive steroids. *Br J Clin Pharmacol.* 1982;14:31-42.

Bacon JF, et al. Pregnancy attributable to interaction between tetracycline and oral contraceptives. *Br Med J.* 1980;280:293.

DeSano EA, et al. Possible interactions of antihistamines and antibiotics with oral contraceptive effectiveness. *Fertil Steril.* 1982;37:853-854.

Back DJ, et al. Evaluation of Committee on Safety of Medicines yellow card reports on oral contraceptive-drug interactions with anticonvulsants and antibiotics. *Br J Clin Pharmacol.* 1988;25:527-532.

Murphy AA, et al. The effect of tetracycline on levels of oral contraceptives. *Am J Obstet Gynecol.* 1991;164:28-33.

Neely JL, et al. The effect of doxycycline on serum levels of ethinyl estradiol, norethindrone, and endogenous progesterone. *Obstet Gynecol.* 1991;77:416-420.

Contraceptives, Oral (eg, *Ortho-Novum*)

Topiramate (*Topamax*)

SUMMARY: Topiramate can moderately reduce serum concentrations of ethinyl estradiol, but the degree to which this would increase the risk of contraceptive failure is not established.

RISK FACTORS: No specific risk factors are known.

RELATED DRUGS: The effect of topiramate on estrogens other than ethinyl estradiol is not established, but an interaction could occur.

MANAGEMENT OPTIONS:

➡ *Consider Alternative.* Consider adding other means of contraception to the oral contraceptive, especially during the first 2 to 3 months of combined therapy with topiramate. Alternatively, some have recommended using a higher-dose oral contraceptive to maintain adequate hormonal concentrations. This appears to be a reasonable recommendation, but the magnitude of the required dosage increase is likely to vary considerably from one patient to another.

➡ *Monitor.* Spotting or breakthrough bleeding in patients taking oral contraceptives and topiramate could indicate that the drugs are interacting, although lack of breakthrough bleeding does not ensure contraceptive protection.

REFERENCES:

Rosenfeld WE, et al. Effect of topiramate on the pharmacokinetics of an oral contraceptive containing norethindrone and ethinyl estradiol in patients with epilepsy. *Epilepsia.* 1997;38(3):317-23.

Contraceptives, Oral (eg, *Ortho-Novum*)

Warfarin (eg, *Coumadin*)

SUMMARY: Oral contraceptives have been reported to increase and decrease the anticoagulant response, depending upon the oral anticoagulant. Most patients requiring oral anticoagulants should avoid oral contraceptives because they may increase the risk of thromboembolic disorders.

RISK FACTORS: No specific risk factors are known.

RELATED DRUGS: No information is available.

MANAGEMENT OPTIONS:

➡ *Avoid Unless Benefit Outweighs Risk.* Patients on oral anticoagulants generally should avoid oral contraceptives because the contraceptives may increase the risk of thromboembolic disorders.

➡ *Monitor.* If an oral contraceptive must be used in a patient receiving an oral anticoagulant, monitor for altered hypoprothrombinemic response when the oral contraceptive is initiated, discontinued, or if the hormone content of the oral contraceptive is changed.

REFERENCES:

Schrogie JJ, et al. Effect of oral contraceptives on vitamin K-dependent clotting activity. *Clin Pharmacol Ther.* 1967;8:670.

de Teresa E, et al. Interaction between anticoagulants and contraceptives: an unexpected finding. *BMJ.* 1979;2:1260.

Monig H, et al. Effect of oral contraceptive steroids on the pharmacokinetics of phenprocoumon. *Br J Clin Pharmacol.* 1990;30:115.

 Contrast Media

Propranolol (eg, *Inderal*)

SUMMARY: Patients taking beta blockers like propranolol are at increased risk for anaphylaxis following the administration of IV contrast media.

RISK FACTORS:

➡ *Concurrent Diseases.* Patients with a prior history of anaphylactoid reactions may be at particular risk.

RELATED DRUGS: Consider all beta blockers to increase the risk of anaphylaxis following contrast media.

MANAGEMENT OPTIONS:

➡ *Circumvent/Minimize.* While the overall incidence of anaphylaxis is low following contrast media, the use of lower osmolality contrast agents or pretreatment with antihistamines and corticosteroids might be considered for patients taking beta blockers.

➡ *Monitor.* Watch for an increased incidence of anaphylaxis in patients taking beta blockers who receive contrast media.

REFERENCES:

Lang DM, et al. Increased risk for anaphylactoid reaction from contrast media in patients on beta-adrenergic blockers or with asthma. *Ann Intern Med.* 1991;115:270.

Jacobs RL, et al. Potentiated anaphylaxis in patients with drug-induced beta-adrenergic blockade. *J Allergy Clin Immunol.* 1981;68:125.

Hannaway PJ, et al. Severe anaphylaxis and drug-induced beta-blockade. *N Engl J Med.* 1983;302:1536.

Cyclobenzaprine (eg, *Flexeril*)

Droperidol (eg, *Inapsine*)

SUMMARY: A patient receiving cyclobenzaprine and fluoxetine (*Prozac*) developed ventricular tachycardia and fibrillation after droperidol was added, but the relative contribution of each drug to the adverse effect is not clear.

RISK FACTORS: No specific risk factors are known.

RELATED DRUGS: Theoretically, antipsychotic drugs other than droperidol that also prolong the QT interval could produce similar effects.

MANAGEMENT OPTIONS:

➡ *Monitor.* Monitor for evidence of polymorphic ventricular tachycardia (eg, lightheadedness, fainting). Monitor the ECG for excessive prolongation of the QTc interval.

REFERENCES:
Michalets EL, et al. Torsade de pointes resulting from the addition of droperidol to an existing cytochrome P450 drug interaction. *Ann Pharmacother.* 1998;32:761.

Cyclobenzaprine (eg, *Flexeril*)

Fluoxetine (*Prozac*)

SUMMARY: A patient receiving cyclobenzaprine and fluoxetine developed ventricular tachycardia and fibrillation after droperidol was added, but the relative contribution of each drug to the adverse effect is not clear.

RISK FACTORS: No specific risk factors are known.

RELATED DRUGS: No information is available.

MANAGEMENT OPTIONS:

➡ *Monitor.* Monitor for evidence of polymorphic ventricular tachycardia (eg, lightheadedness, fainting). Monitor the ECG for excessive prolongation of the QTc interval.

REFERENCES:
Michalets EL, et al. Torsade de pointes resulting from the addition of droperidol to an existing cytochrome P450 drug interaction. *Ann Pharmacother.* 1998;32:761.

Cyclophosphamide (eg, *Cytoxan*)

Digoxin (eg, *Lanoxin*)

SUMMARY: Patients receiving cancer chemotherapy may have impaired absorption of Lanoxin tablets; the magnitude of the reduction appears sufficient to reduce the therapeutic effect of digoxin in some patients. The absorption of digoxin capsules and digitoxin (*Crystodigin*) does not appear to be affected by cytotoxic drugs.

RISK FACTORS: No specific risk factors are known.

RELATED DRUGS: Other cytotoxic drugs also may inhibit the absorption of digoxin. Unlike digoxin, digitoxin absorption does not appear to be reduced by cytotoxic drugs.

MANAGEMENT OPTIONS:

➡ *Consider Alternative.* Digoxin capsules appear less likely to interact with cytotoxic drugs.

➡ *Monitor.* Be alert for evidence of reduced digoxin response during cytotoxic drug therapy. If oral doses of digoxin are increased to compensate for this effect, it is likely that reductions in digoxin dosage would be required if the cytotoxic drugs are stopped for more than a few days.

REFERENCES:

Kuhlmann J, et al. Effects of cytotoxic drugs on plasma level and renal excretion of beta-acetyldigoxin. *Clin Pharmacol Ther.* 1981;30:518.

Bjornsson TD, et al. Effects of high-dose cancer chemotherapy on the absorption of digoxin in two different formulations. *Clin Pharmacol Ther.* 1986;39:25.

Kuhlmann J, et al. Cytostatic drugs are without significant effect on digitoxin plasma level and renal excretion. *Clin Pharmacol Ther.* 1982;32:646

Cyclophosphamide (eg, *Cytoxan*)

Succinylcholine (eg, *Anectine*)

SUMMARY: Cyclophosphamide may prolong the neuromuscular blocking effect of succinylcholine.

RISK FACTORS: No specific risk factors are known.

RELATED DRUGS: No information is available.

MANAGEMENT OPTIONS:

➡ *Monitor.* Monitor patients for prolonged succinylcholine effect in patients also receiving cyclophosphamide (and probably other antineoplastics). Plasma pseudo-cholinesterase determinations may be desirable prior to succinylcholine administration. Avoidance of succinylcholine or cyclophosphamide has been recommended if the patient has significantly depressed pseudocholinesterase levels.

REFERENCES:

Walker IR, et al. Cyclophosphamide, cholinesterase and anaesthesia. *Aust NZ J Med.* 1972;2:247.

Mone JG, et al. Qualitative and quantitative defects of pseudocholinesterase activity. *Anaesthesia.* 1967;22:55.

Smith RM Jr, et al. Succinylcholine-pantothenyl alcohol: a reappraisal. *Anesth Analg Curr Res.* 1969;48:205.

Zsigmond EK, et al. The effect of a series of anticancer drugs on plasma cholinesterase activity. *Can Anaesth Soc J.* 1972;19:75.

Wolff H. Die Hemmung der Serumcholinesterase durch Cyclophosphamid (*Endoxan*). *Klin Wochenschr.* 1965;43:819.

Cyclophosphamide (eg, *Cytoxan*)

Warfarin (eg, *Coumadin*)

SUMMARY: Cyclophosphamide appeared to inhibit the hypoprothrombinemic response to warfarin in one patient; more study is needed.

RISK FACTORS: No specific risk factors are known.

RELATED DRUGS: The effect of cyclophosphamide on oral anticoagulants other than warfarin is not established, but be alert for the possibility. Several other cytotoxic drugs have been reported to affect warfarin response.

MANAGEMENT OPTIONS:

➡ **Monitor.** Watch for an alteration in the hypoprothrombinemic response to oral anticoagulants if cyclophosphamide is initiated, discontinued, or changed in dosage; adjust oral anticoagulant dosage as needed.

REFERENCES:

Tashima CK. Cyclophosphamide effect on coumarin anticoagulation. *South Med J.* 1979;72:633.

Cycloserine (*Seromycin*)
Isoniazid (INH)

SUMMARY: The combined use of cycloserine and INH may result in increased central nervous system (CNS) toxicity.

RISK FACTORS: No specific risk factors are known.

RELATED DRUGS: No information is available.

MANAGEMENT OPTIONS:

➡ **Monitor.** Monitor patients receiving cycloserine and INH more closely for signs of CNS toxicity including dizziness or drowsiness.

REFERENCES:

Mattila MJ, et al. Serum levels, urinary excretion, and side-effects of cycloserine in the presence of isoniazid and p-aminosalicyclic acid. *Scand J Respir Dis.* 1969;50:291.

Cyclosporine (eg, *Neoral*)
Contraceptives, Oral (eg, *Ortho-Novum*)

SUMMARY: Isolated cases of elevated plasma cyclosporine concentrations have been observed following oral contraceptive use.

RISK FACTORS: No specific risk factors are known.

RELATED DRUGS: The effect of replacement estrogen therapy on cyclosporine is not established; given the lower doses of estrogen used in replacement therapy, an interaction seems less likely.

MANAGEMENT OPTIONS:

➡ **Consider Alternative.** Although this interaction is not well documented, consider using contraception other than oral contraceptives in patients receiving cyclosporine, because the consequences are potentially severe.

➡ **Monitor.** If oral contraceptives are used, monitor the patient's clinical response and cyclosporine serum concentrations. When cyclosporine therapy is started in a patient who is already taking oral contraceptives, anticipate the possibility that cyclosporine dosage requirements may be lower than expected. In a patient stabilized on both cyclosporine and an oral contraceptive, discontinuation of the contraceptive may cause a fall in cyclosporine blood concentrations. In both situations, carefully monitor the clinical response of the patient and adjust the cyclosporine dose as necessary. Based on the case reported and theoretical considerations, the changes in cyclosporine concentrations caused by hormone therapy probably occur gradually over several weeks. Keep this in mind when monitoring patients for this interaction.

REFERENCES:

Chambers DM, et al. Antipyrine elimination in saliva after low-dose combined or progestogen only oral contraceptive steroids. *Br J Clin Phamacol.* 1982;13:229.

Abernethy DR, et al. Impairment of antipyrine metabolism by low-dose oral contraceptive steroids. *Clin Pharmacol Ther.* 1981;29:106.

O'Malley K, et al. Increased antipyrine half-life in women taking oral contraceptives. *Scot Med J.* 1970;15:454.

Deray G. Oral contraceptive interaction with cyclosporine. *Lancet.* 1987;1:158.

Maurer G. Metabolism of cyclosporine. *Transplant Proc.* 1985;17(Suppl. 1):19.

 ## Cyclosporine (eg, *Neoral*)

Danazol (eg, *Danocrine*)

SUMMARY: Preliminary case reports suggest that danazol and other androgens can increase serum cyclosporine concentrations and may result in cyclosporine toxicity.

RISK FACTORS: No specific risk factors are known.

RELATED DRUGS: Tacrolimus (*Prograf*), like cyclosporine, is metabolized by CYP3A4, and its effect also appears to be increased by danazol. Other androgens appear to interact similarly.

MANAGEMENT OPTIONS:

➡ *Avoid Unless Benefit Outweighs Risk.* Although this interaction is based upon isolated cases, the potentially severe consequences warrant avoiding the use of anabolic steroids in patients receiving cyclosporine.

➡ *Monitor.* If anabolic steroids are started in a patient receiving cyclosporine, monitor the patient's cyclosporine response and serum concentrations carefully. When cyclosporine therapy is started in a patient who is already taking anabolic steroids, the cyclosporine dose requirements may be lower than expected. In a patient stabilized on both cyclosporine and anabolic steroids, stopping the hormone may cause a fall in cyclosporine blood concentrations; monitor the clinical response of the patient carefully and increase the cyclosporine dose as necessary. Based upon the cases reported as well as theoretical considerations, the changes in cyclosporine concentrations caused by such hormones probably occur gradually over several weeks; keep this in mind when monitoring for this interaction.

REFERENCES:

Kramer G, et al. Carbamazepine-danazol drug interaction: its mechanism examined by a stable isotope technique. *Ther Drug Monit.* 1986;8:387.

Hvidberg EF, et al. Studies of the interaction of phenylbutazone, oxyphenbutazone and methandrostenolone in man. *Proc Soc Exp Biol Med.* 1968;129:438.

Moller BB, et al. Toxicity of cyclosporine during treatment with androgens. *N Engl J Med.* 1985;313:1416.

Ross WB, et al. Cyclosporine interaction with danazol and noresthisterone. *Lancet.* 1986;1:330.

Shapiro R, et al. FK 506 interaction with danazol. *Lancet.* 1993;341:1344.

Cyclosporine (eg, *Neoral*)

Diclofenac (eg, *Voltaren*)

SUMMARY: Diclofenac has been associated with increased serum concentrations of creatinine and potassium as well as increased blood pressure in a number of patients receiving cyclosporine.

RISK FACTORS: No specific risk factors are known.

RELATED DRUGS: Sulindac (eg, *Clinoril*) was associated with increased serum cyclosporine and serum creatinine concentrations in 1 patient. On the other hand, indomethacin (*Indocin*) and ketoprofen (eg, *Orudis*) appeared *less* likely than diclofenac to interact with cyclosporine in another patient. Given the paucity of data, the relative likelihood of various NSAIDs to increase cyclosporine-induced nephrotoxicity cannot be determined. Assume that all NSAIDs are capable of interacting with cyclosporine until evidence to the contrary is available.

MANAGEMENT OPTIONS:

➡ *Consider Alternative.* Until the clinical importance of this potential interaction is better defined, patients taking cyclosporine should use diclofenac or other NSAIDs only when the expected benefit clearly outweighs the risk of nephrotoxicity.

➡ *Monitor.* If the combination is used, monitor the patient's renal function carefully and be prepared to discontinue one or both drugs.

REFERENCES:
Branthwaite JP, et al. Cyclosporin and diclofenac interaction in rheumatoid arthritis. *Lancet.* 1991;337:252.

Deray G, et al. Enhancement of cyclosporine A nephrotoxicity of diclofenac. *Clin Nephrol.* 1987;27:213.

Sesin GP, et al. Sulindac-induced elevation of serum cyclosporine concentration. *Clin Pharm.* 1989;8:445.

Cyclosporine (eg, *Neoral*)

Digoxin (eg, *Lanoxin*)

SUMMARY: The administration of cyclosporine to patients stabilized on digoxin may result in increased digoxin serum concentrations and digoxin toxicity.

RISK FACTORS: No specific risk factors are known.

RELATED DRUGS: Tacrolimus (*Prograf*) may produce a similar interaction with digoxin, but data are not available.

MANAGEMENT OPTIONS:

➡ *Circumvent/Minimize.* A reduction in the digoxin dosage may be required. With the discontinuation of cyclosporine, patients may require increased digoxin dosages.

➡ *Monitor.* Until more data regarding this interaction are available, monitor patients maintained on digoxin carefully for digitalis toxicity if cyclosporine is added to their regimen.

REFERENCES:
Dorian P, et al. Digoxin-cyclosporine interaction: severe digitalis toxicity after cyclosporine treatment. *Clin Invest Med.* 1988;11:108.

Robieux LC, et al. The effect of cardiac transplantation and cyclosporin therapy on digoxin pharmacokinetics. *J Clin Pharmacol*. 1992;32:338.

Okamura N, et al. Digoxin-cyclosporin A interaction: modulation of the multidrug transporter P-glycoprotein in the kidney. *J Pharmacol Exp Ther*. 1993;266:1614.

Cyclosporine (eg, *Neoral*)

Diltiazem (eg, *Cardizem*)

SUMMARY: Cyclosporine blood concentrations are increased by diltiazem; renal toxicity has been reported with the elevated cyclosporine concentrations.

RISK FACTORS: No specific risk factors are known.

RELATED DRUGS: Nicardipine (eg, *Cardene*) and verapamil (eg, *Calan*) inhibit cyclosporine metabolism while isradipine (*DynaCirc*), nifedipine (eg, *Procardia*), amlodipine (*Norvasc*), and nitrendipine have minimal effect. Diltiazem may affect tacrolimus (*Prograf*) in a similar manner.

MANAGEMENT OPTIONS:

➡ **Consider Alternative.** Calcium channel blockers that do not appear to alter cyclosporine pharmacokinetics include isradipine, nitrendipine, and amlodipine.

➡ **Circumvent/Minimize.** Reduce cyclosporine dosage and monitor blood concentrations when diltiazem is coadministered.

➡ **Monitor.** Observe patients receiving both drugs for increased cyclosporine concentrations and decreasing renal function.

REFERENCES:

Pochet JM, et al. Cyclosporine-diltiazem interactions. *Lancet*. 1986;1:979.

Smith CL, et al. Clinical and medicoeconomic impact of the cyclosporine-diltiazem interaction in renal transplant recipients. *Pharmacotherapy*. 1994;14:471.

Chrysostomou A, et al. Diltiazem in renal allograft recipients receiving cyclosporine. *Transplantation*. 1993;55:300.

Wagner K, et al. Interaction of cyclosporin and calcium antagonists. *Transplant Proc*. 1989;21:1453.

Sabate I, et al. Cyclosporin-diltiazem interaction: comparison of cyclosporin levels measured with two monoclonal antibodies. *Transplant Proc*. 1989;21:1460.

Roy LF, et al. Short-term effects of calcium antagonists on hemodynamics and cyclosporine pharmacokinetics in heart-transplant and kidney-transplant patients. *Clin Pharmacol Ther*. 1989;46:657.

Campistol JM, et al. Interactions between cyclosporine and diltiazem in renal transplant patients. *Nephron*. 1991;57:241.

Bourge RC, et al. Diltiazem-cyclosporine interaction in cardiac transplant recipients: impact on cyclosporine dose and medication costs. *Am J Med*. 1991;90:402.

Martinez F, et al. No clinically significant interaction between cyclosporin and isradipine. *Nephron*. 1991;59:658.

Copur MS, et al. Effects of nitrendipine on blood pressure and blood cyclosporine A level in patients with posttransplant hypertension. *Nephron*. 1989;52:227.

Toupance O, et al. Antihypertensive effect of amlodipine and lack of interference with cyclosporine metabolism in renal transplant recipients. *Hypertension*. 1994;24:297.

Cyclosporine (eg, *Neoral*)

Doxorubicin (eg, *Adriamycin*)

SUMMARY: A patient receiving cyclosporine and doxorubicin developed CNS toxicity including coma and seizures; causation has not been established.

RISK FACTORS: No specific risk factors are known.

RELATED DRUGS: The effect of tacrolimus (*Prograf*) on doxorubicin is not established.

MANAGEMENT OPTIONS:

➡ *Monitor.* Until further information is available, carefully observe patients taking cyclosporine for changing mental status and CNS toxicity if they receive doxorubicin.

REFERENCES:

Barbui T, et al. Neurological symptoms and coma associated with doxorubicin administration during chronic cyclosporine therapy. *Lancet*. 1992;339:1421.

Cyclosporine (eg, *Neoral*)

Enalapril (*Vasotec*)

SUMMARY: Initiation of enalapril therapy in 2 renal transplant patients receiving cyclosporine was associated with acute renal failure; more study is needed to assess the clinical importance of this purported interaction.

RISK FACTORS:

➡ *Other Drugs.* Diuretic-induced hypovolemia is a possible risk factor.

RELATED DRUGS: Based on the proposed mechanism, expect other ACE inhibitors to interact with cyclosporine in a similar manner.

MANAGEMENT OPTIONS:

➡ *Monitor.* Until further information is available, initiate ACE inhibitors cautiously in patients receiving cyclosporine; monitor renal function carefully.

REFERENCES:

Murray BM, et al. Enalapril-associated acute renal failure in renal transplants: possible role of cyclosporine. *Am J Kidney Dis*. 1990;16:66.

Funck-Brentano C, et al. Reversible renal failure after combined treatment with enalapril and furosemide in a patient with congestive heart failure. *Br Heart J*. 1986;55:596.

Cyclosporine (eg, *Neoral*)

Erythromycin (eg, *E-Mycin*)

SUMMARY: The combination of cyclosporine and erythromycin should be used with caution because of the potential for elevated cyclosporine concentrations and nephrotoxicity.

RISK FACTORS: No specific risk factors are known.

RELATED DRUGS: Troleandomycin (*TAO*) or clarithromycin (*Biaxin*) also may inhibit the metabolism of cyclosporine. Tacrolimus (*Prograf*) is affected similarly by erythromycin administration. Azithromycin (*Zithromax*) does not appear to affect cyclosporine.

MANAGEMENT OPTIONS:

➡ *Circumvent/Minimize.* Cyclosporine doses may require reduction during erythromycin administration.

➡ *Monitor.* Monitor renal function and cyclosporine concentrations when erythromycin is added to or deleted from the regimen of patients receiving cyclosporine.

REFERENCES:

Ptachcinski RJ, et al. Effect of erythromycin on cyclosporine levels. *N Engl J Med.* 1985;313:1416.

Kohan DE. Possible interaction between cyclosporine and erythromycin. *N Engl J Med.* 1986;314:448.

Freeman DJ, et al. Cyclosporin-erythromycin interaction in normal subjects. *Br J Clin Pharmacol.* 1987;23:776.

Godin JRP, et al. Erythromycin-cyclosporin interaction. *Drug Intell Clin Pharm.* 1986;20:504.

Hourmant M, et al. Co-administration of erythromycin results in an increase of blood cyclosporine to toxic levels. *Transplant Proc.* 1985;17:2723.

Kessler M, et al. Interaction between cyclosporine and erythromycin in a kidney transplant patient. *Eur J Clin Pharmacol.* 1986;30:633.

Grino JM, et al. Erythromycin and cyclosporine. *Ann Intern Med.* 1986;105:467.

Jensen CWB, et al. Exacerbation of cyclosporine toxicity of concomitant administration of erythromycin. *Transplantation.* 1987;43:263.

Wadhwa NK, et al. Interaction between erythromycin and cyclosporine in a kidney and pancreas allograft recipient. *Ther Drug Monit.* 1987;9:123.

Gupta SK, et al. Cyclosporin-erythromycin interaction in renal transplant patients. *Br J Clin Pharmacol.* 1989;27:475.

Koselj M, et al. Drug interaction between cyclosporine and rifampicin, erythromycin, and azoles in kidney recipients with opportunistic infections. *Transplant Proc.* 1994;26:2823.

Cyclosporine (eg, *Neoral*)

Etoposide (eg, *VePesid*)

SUMMARY: High-dose cyclosporine may improve tumor response to etoposide, but also increases toxicity; adjustments to etoposide dose may be necessary.

RISK FACTORS: No specific risk factors are known.

RELATED DRUGS: No information is available.

MANAGEMENT OPTIONS:

➡ *Circumvent/Minimize.* The authors recommend halving the etoposide dose if high-dose cyclosporine is used concurrently.

➡ *Monitor.* Closely monitor patients on this combination, especially for hypersensitivity reactions such as rash, fever, and bronchospasm.

REFERENCES:

Bisogno G, et al. High-dose cyclosporin with etoposide—toxicity and pharmacokinetic interaction in children with solid tumors. *Br J Cancer.* 1998;77:2304.

Cyclosporine (eg, *Neoral*)

Felodipine (*Plendil*)

SUMMARY: When cyclosporine and felodipine are coadministered, cyclosporine markedly increases felodipine concentrations while the concentrations of cyclosporine are minimally increased.

RISK FACTORS:

➡ *Route of Administration.* The administration of oral cyclosporine would be expected to produce a greater effect on felodipine concentrations than IV cyclosporine.

RELATED DRUGS: It is possible that other dihydropyridines that have a large first-pass clearance (eg, nitrendipine) may be similarly affected by cyclosporine coadministration. Dihydropyridines that have less first-pass metabolism include amlodipine (*Norvasc*).

MANAGEMENT OPTIONS:

➡ *Consider Alternative.* Patients receiving cyclosporine could be treated with a dihydropyridine that has less first-pass metabolism than felodipine (see Related Drugs) or a different class of antihypertensive could be selected.

➡ *Circumvent/Minimize.* Avoid taking felodipine with cyclosporine. Separate the doses by at least 2 hours.

➡ *Monitor.* If felodipine and cyclosporine are administered together, watch for excessive hypotensive effects.

REFERENCES:

Madsen JK, et al. Pharmacokinetic interaction between cyclosporine and the dihydropyridine calcium antagonist felodipine. *Eur J Clin Pharmacol.* 1996;50:203.

Cyclosporine (eg, *Neoral*)

Fluconazole (*Diflucan*)

SUMMARY: Fluconazole appears to increase cyclosporine plasma concentrations, particularly at higher fluconazole doses; cyclosporine toxicity could result in some patients.

RISK FACTORS:

➡ *Dosage Regimen.* Fluconazole doses higher than 100 mg/day might increase the likelihood of the interaction.

RELATED DRUGS: Fluconazole inhibits tacrolimus (*Prograf*) metabolism. Ketoconazole (eg, *Nizoral*), miconazole, and itraconazole (*Sporanox*) are also inhibitors of cyclosporine metabolism.

MANAGEMENT OPTIONS:

➡ *Monitor.* Until more studies have been done, monitor cyclosporine plasma concentrations and renal function when fluconazole is administered. Cyclosporine dosage adjustments may be required in some patients.

REFERENCES:

Lopez-Gill JA. Fluconazole-cyclosporine interaction: a dose-dependent effect? *Ann Pharmacother.* 1993;27:427.

Collingnon P, et al. Interaction of fluconazole with cyclosporin. *Lancet.* 1989;1:1262.

Kruger HU, et al. No severe interactions between fluconazole, a triazole antifungal agent, with cyclosporin. *Bone Marrow Trans.* 1988;3:271.

Ehninger G, et al. Interaction of fluconazole with cyclosporin. *Lancet.* 1989;2:104.

Graves NM, et al. Increased cyclosporine levels as a result of simultaneous fluconazole and cyclosporine therapy in renal transplant recipients: a double-blind, randomized pharmacokinetic and safety study. *Transplant Proc.* 1991;23:1041.

Lazar J, et al. Drug interactions with fluconazole. *Rev Infect Dis.* 1990;12(Suppl. 3):S327.

Kruger HU, et al. Absence of significant interaction of fluconazole with cyclosporin. *J Antimicrob Chemother.* 1989;24:781.

Torregrosa V, et al. Interaction of fluconazole with cyclosporin A. *Nephron.* 1992;60:125.

Back DJ, et al. Comparative effects of the antimycotic drugs ketoconazole, fluconazole, itraconazole and terbinafine on the metabolism of cyclosporin by human liver microsomes. *Br J Clin Pharmacol.* 1991;32:624.

Cyclosporine (eg, *Neoral*)

Gentamicin (eg, *Garamycin*)

SUMMARY: Cyclosporine and gentamicin are both nephrotoxic and produce additive renal damage when administered together.

RISK FACTORS: No specific risk factors are known.

RELATED DRUGS: Other aminoglycosides may produce additive nephrotoxicity with cyclosporine. The effect of aminoglycosides on tacrolimus (*Prograf*) nephrotoxicity is unknown.

MANAGEMENT OPTIONS:

➡ *Consider Alternative.* If possible, avoid the administration of aminoglycosides in patients receiving cyclosporine for immunosuppression after renal transplantation.

➡ *Monitor.* Monitor patients receiving the combination for reduced renal function.

REFERENCES:

Tremeer A, et al. Severe nephrotoxicity caused by the combined use of gentamicin and cyclosporine in renal allograft recipients. *Transplantation.* 1986;42:220.

Whiting PH, et al. The enhancement of cyclosporine A-induced nephrotoxicity by gentamicin. *Biochem Pharmacol.* 1983;32:2025.

Cyclosporine (eg, *Neoral*)

Glipizide (eg, *Glucotrol*)

SUMMARY: Glipizide administration appears to increase cyclosporine concentrations; nephrotoxicity could occur.

RISK FACTORS: No specific risk factors are known.

RELATED DRUGS: Other sulfonylureas may affect cyclosporine in a similar manner. It is possible that tacrolimus (*Prograf*) interacts with glipizide.

MANAGEMENT OPTIONS:

➡ *Circumvent/Minimize.* Cyclosporine doses may require adjustment to avoid cyclosporine-induced renal toxicity.

➡ **Monitor.** Until further information is available, monitor patients stabilized on cyclosporine for increased cyclosporine concentrations following the addition of glipizide.

REFERENCES:
Chidester PD, et al. Interaction between glipizide and cyclosporine: report of two cases. *Transplant Proc.* 1993;25:2136.

Cyclosporine (eg, *Neoral*)

Grapefruit Juice

SUMMARY: Grapefruit juice can increase cyclosporine blood concentrations; adjustments in cyclosporine dosage may be necessary.

RISK FACTORS: No specific risk factors are known.

RELATED DRUGS: Like cyclosporine, tacrolimus (*Prograf*) also undergoes first-pass metabolism by CYP3A4. Thus, grapefruit juice probably also increases tacrolimus blood concentrations.

MANAGEMENT OPTIONS:

➡ **Consider Alternative.** Orange juice does not appear to interact with cyclosporine.

➡ **Circumvent/Minimize.** Advise patients on cyclosporine to avoid grapefruit juice (unless the combination is being used intentionally to elevate cyclosporine blood levels). Separating doses of grapefruit juice from cyclosporine may not eliminate the interaction completely, since the inhibitory effect of grapefruit juice on CYP3A4 can last for several hours.

➡ **Monitor.** If grapefruit juice is taken concurrently with cyclosporine, carefully monitor the patient's response to cyclosporine, especially if grapefruit juice is initiated, discontinued, or if the interval between the cyclosporine and grapefruit juice is changed.

REFERENCES:
Yee G, et al. Effect of grapefruit juice on blood cyclosporin concentration. *Lancet.* 1995;345:955.

Ducharme MP, et al. Trough concentrations of cyclosporine in blood following administration with grapefruit juice. *Br J Clin Pharmacol.* 1993;36:457.

Proppe DG, et al. Influence of chronic ingestion of grapefruit juice on steady-state blood concentrations of cyclosporine A in renal transplant patients with stable graft function. *Br J Clin Pharmacol.* 1995;39:337.

Herlitz H, et al. Grapefruit juice: a possible source of variability in blood concentration of cyclosporin A. *Nephrol Dial Transplant.* 1993;8:375.

Hollander AAMJ, et al. The effect of grapefruit juice on cyclosporine and prednisone metabolism in transplant patients. *Clin Pharmacol Ther.* 1995;57:318.

Cyclosporine (eg, *Neoral*)

Griseofulvin (eg, *Grisactin*)

SUMMARY: Griseofulvin administration decreased the blood concentrations of cyclosporine in 1 patient; cyclosporine efficacy could be reduced during griseofulvin administration.

RISK FACTORS: No specific risk factors are known.

RELATED DRUGS: Griseofulvin may affect tacrolimus (*Prograf*) similarly. Other antifungal agents (eg, ketoconazole [eg, *Nizoral*]) may reduce cyclosporine metabolism.

MANAGEMENT OPTIONS:

➡ ***Circumvent/Minimize.*** Cyclosporine doses may have to be increased during griseofulvin therapy and decreased when griseofulvin is discontinued.

➡ ***Monitor.*** Monitor cyclosporine concentrations and signs of transplant rejection when griseofulvin is added to or removed from the therapy of a patient receiving cyclosporine.

REFERENCES:

Abu-Romeh SH, et al. Cyclosporin A and griseofulvin: another drug interaction. *Nephron.* 1991;58:237.

Klintmalm G, et al. High dose methylprednisolone increases plasma cyclosporin levels in renal transplant recipients. *Lancet.* 1984;1:731.

Cyclosporine (eg, *Neoral*)

Imipenem (*Primaxin*)

SUMMARY: Taking imipenem with cyclosporine resulted in acute CNS toxicity in 1 patient.

RISK FACTORS: No specific risk factors are known.

RELATED DRUGS: A similar interaction with tacrolimus (*Prograf*) and imipenem may occur, but data are not available.

MANAGEMENT OPTIONS:

➡ ***Monitor.*** Until more information about this is available, carefully observe patients receiving both drugs for CNS toxic symptoms and altered cyclosporine serum concentrations.

REFERENCES:

Zazgornik J, et al. Potentiation of neurotoxic side effects by co-administration of imipenem to cyclosporine therapy in a kidney transplant recipient—synergism of side effects or drug interaction? *Clin Nephrol.* 1986;26:265.

Cyclosporine (eg, *Neoral*)

Indomethacin (eg, *Indocin*)

SUMMARY: Some nonsteroidal anti-inflammatory drugs (NSAIDs) may increase the risk of cyclosporine nephrotoxicity, but little clinical information is available for indomethacin.

RISK FACTORS: No specific risk factors are known.

RELATED DRUGS: Another NSAID, diclofenac (eg, *Voltaren*), has been associated with impaired renal function in a number of patients receiving cyclosporine; and sulindac (eg, *Clinoril*) was associated with increased serum cyclosporine and serum creatinine concentrations in 1 patient. However, because little is known regarding the effect of other NSAIDs on cyclosporine response, assume that all NSAIDs are capable of interacting with cyclosporine until evidence to the contrary is available.

MANAGEMENT OPTIONS:

➡ *Consider Alternative.* Even though there is little clinical information available regarding the effect of indomethacin on the response to cyclosporine, use all NSAIDs cautiously in patients taking cyclosporine.

➡ *Monitor.* If the combination is used, monitor the patient's renal function carefully and be prepared to discontinue one or both drugs.

REFERENCES:
Whiting PM, et al. Drug interactions with cyclosporine; implications from animal studies. *Transplant Proc.* 1986;18(Suppl. 5):56.

Branthwaite JP, et al. Cyclosporin and diclofenac interaction in rheumatoid arthritis. *Lancet.* 1991;337:252.

Deray G, et al. Enhancement of cyclosporine A nephrotoxicity of diclofenac. *Clin Nephrol.* 1987;27:213.

Sesin GP, et al. Sulindac-induced elevation of serum cyclosporine concentration. *Clin Pharm.* 1989;8:445.

Cyclosporine (eg, *Neoral*)

Itraconazole (*Sporanox*)

SUMMARY: Itraconazole may increase cyclosporine serum concentrations; nephrotoxicity may result.

RISK FACTORS: No specific risk factors are known.

RELATED DRUGS: Ketoconazole (eg, *Nizoral*), miconazole, and fluconazole (*Diflucan*) are also inhibitors of cyclosporine metabolism. Itraconazole may affect tacrolimus (*Prograf*) similarly.

MANAGEMENT OPTIONS:

➡ *Monitor.* Monitor cyclosporine concentrations and renal function when itraconazole is added to or removed from the therapy of patients taking cyclosporine.

REFERENCES:
Kwan JTC, et al. Interaction of cyclosporine and itraconazole. *Lancet.* 1987;2:282.

Trenk D, et al. Time course of cyclosporin/itraconazole interaction. *Lancet.* 1987;2:1335.

Novakova I, et al. Itraconazole and cyclosporin nephrotoxicity. *Lancet.* 1987;2:920.

Kramer MR, et al. Cyclosporin and itraconazole interaction in heart and lung transplant recipients. *Ann Intern Med.* 1990;113:327.

Back DJ, et al. Comparative effects of the antimycotic drugs ketoconazole, fluconazole, itraconazole, and terbinafine on the metabolism of cyclosporin by human liver microsomes. *Br J Clin Pharmacol.* 1991;32:624.

Berenguer J, et al. Itraconazole for experimental pulmonary aspergillosis: comparison with amphotericin B, interaction with cyclosporine A, and correlation between therapeutic response and itraconazole concentrations in plasma. *Antimicrob Agents Chemother.* 1994;38:1303.

Cyclosporine (eg, *Neoral*)

Josamycin

SUMMARY: Josamycin, a macrolide antibiotic, appears to increase cyclosporine plasma concentrations, but additional study is needed to assess the incidence and magnitude of this effect.

RISK FACTORS: No specific risk factors are known.

RELATED DRUGS: Tacrolimus (*Prograf*) is likely to be affected similarly by josamycin administration. Other macrolides (eg, erythromycin, troleandomycin [*TAO*], clarithromycin [*Biaxin*]) are known to inhibit cyclosporine metabolism. Azithromycin (*Zithromax*) and dirithromycin (*Dynabac*) would be unlikely to inhibit cyclosporine metabolism.

MANAGEMENT OPTIONS:

➡ *Monitor.* Monitor patients receiving cyclosporine for elevated cyclosporine concentrations and nephrotoxicity if josamycin is administered. Cyclosporine concentrations may decline following discontinuation of josamycin dosing.

REFERENCES:

Kreft-Jais C, et al. Effect of josamycin on plasma cyclosporine levels. *Eur J Clin Pharmacol.* 1987;32:327.

Azana J, et al. Possible interaction between cyclosporine and josamycin: a description of three cases. *Clin Pharmacol Ther.* 1992;51:572.

Torregrosa JV, et al. Interaction of josamycin with cyclosporin A. *Nephron.* 1993;65:476.

Cyclosporine (eg, *Neoral*)

Ketoconazole (eg, *Nizoral*)

SUMMARY: Ketoconazole appears to increase the serum concentration of cyclosporine, thereby increasing the risk of cyclosporine-induced renal toxicity.

RISK FACTORS: No specific risk factors are known.

RELATED DRUGS: Other antifungal agents (eg, miconazole, itraconazole [*Sporanox*], fluconazole [*Diflucan*]) are likely to increase cyclosporine concentrations. It is likely that tacrolimus (*Prograf*) concentrations will be increased by ketoconazole and other antifungal agents.

MANAGEMENT OPTIONS:

➡ *Circumvent/Minimize.* Cyclosporine dose reduction is usually necessary when administered with ketoconazole.

➡ *Monitor.* Monitor cyclosporine concentrations and renal function when ketoconazole is prescribed during cyclosporine therapy. In patients stabilized on both drugs, large reductions in cyclosporine concentrations may occur when ketoconazole is discontinued.

REFERENCES:

First MR, et al. Cyclosporine-ketoconazole interaction. *Transplantation.* 1993;55:1000.

Sorenson AL, et al. Effects of ketoconazole on cyclosporine metabolism in renal allograft recipients. *Transplant Proc.* 1994;26:2822.

Shepard JH, et al. Cyclosporine-ketoconazole: a potentially dangerous drug-drug interaction. *Clin Pharm.* 1986;5:648.

Nolan PE, et al. Potentially favorable pharmacokinetic interaction between cyclosporine and ketoconazole in cardiac transplant recipients. *Pharmacotherapy.* 1989;9:192.

First MR, et al. Concomitant administration of cyclosporin and ketoconazole in renal transplant recipients. *Lancet.* 1989;2:1198.

Charles BG, et al. The ketoconazole-cyclosporin interaction in an elderly renal transplant patient. *Aust N Z J Med.* 1989;19:292.

Back DJ, et al. Comparative effects of the antimycotic drugs ketoconazole, fluconazole, itraconazole, and terbinafine on the metabolism of cyclosporin by human liver microsomes. *Br J Clin Pharmacol.* 1991;32:624.

Gomez DY, et al. The effects of ketoconazole on the intestinal metabolism and bioavailability of cyclosporine. *Clin Pharmacol Ther.* 1995;58:15.

Cyclosporine (eg, *Neoral*)

Ketoprofen (eg, *Orudis*)

SUMMARY: Although some nonsteroidal anti-inflammatory drugs (NSAIDs) may increase the risk of cyclosporine nephrotoxicity, little clinical information is available for ketoprofen.

RISK FACTORS: No specific risk factors are known.

RELATED DRUGS: Another NSAID, diclofenac (eg, *Voltaren*), has been associated with impaired renal function in a number of patients receiving cyclosporine; and sulindac (eg, *Clinoril*) was associated with increased serum cyclosporine and serum creatinine concentrations in 1 patient. However, since little is known regarding the effect of other NSAIDs on cyclosporine response, assume that all NSAIDs are capable of interacting with cyclosporine until evidence to the contrary is available.

MANAGEMENT OPTIONS:

➡ ***Consider Alternative.*** Although little clinical information is available regarding the effect of ketoprofen on the response to cyclosporine, use all NSAIDs cautiously in patients receiving cyclosporine.

➡ ***Monitor.*** If the combination is used, monitor the patient's renal function carefully and be prepared to discontinue one or both drugs.

REFERENCES:

Branthwaite JP, et al. Cyclosporin and diclofenac interaction in rheumatoid arthritis. *Lancet*. 1991;337:252.

Deray G, et al. Enhancement of cyclosporine A nephrotoxicity of diclofenac. *Clin Nephrol*. 1987;27:213.

Sesin GP, et al. Sulindac-induced elevation of serum cyclosporine concentration. *Clin Pharm*. 1989;8:445.

Cyclosporine (eg, *Neoral*)

Mefenamic Acid (*Ponstel*)

SUMMARY: A renal transplant patient rapidly developed nephrotoxicity and an increase in plasma cyclosporine concentration following the use of mefenamic acid, but the clinical importance is not established.

RISK FACTORS: No specific risk factors are known.

RELATED DRUGS: Several NSAIDs (eg, diclofenac [eg, *Voltaren*], sulindac [eg, *Clinoril*]) have been associated with impaired renal function or increased cyclosporine blood concentrations. The relative likelihood of various NSAIDs to increase cyclosporine-induced nephrotoxicity is not established, but assume that all NSAIDs are capable of interacting with cyclosporine until evidence to the contrary is available.

MANAGEMENT OPTIONS:

➡ ***Consider Alternative.*** Until the clinical importance of this potential interaction is better defined, use mefenamic acid (or other NSAIDs) in patients receiving cyclosporine only when the expected benefit clearly outweighs the risk of excessive cyclosporine response and nephrotoxicity.

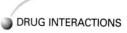

➧ **Monitor.** If the combination is used, monitor the patient's renal function and cyclosporine concentrations carefully, and be prepared to discontinue one or both drugs.

REFERENCES:

Agar JWM. Cyclosporin A and mefenamic acid in a renal transplant patient. *Aust N Z J Med.* 1991;21:784.

 Cyclosporine (eg, *Neoral*)

Melphalan (*Alkeran*)

SUMMARY: Preliminary evidence indicates that melphalan may increase the likelihood of nephrotoxicity in patients receiving cyclosporine.

RISK FACTORS: No specific risk factors are known.

RELATED DRUGS: No information is available.

MANAGEMENT OPTIONS:

➧ **Monitor.** Monitor renal function carefully in patients receiving concurrent therapy with cyclosporine and melphalan.

REFERENCES:

Morgenstern GR, et al. Cyclosporin interaction with ketoconazole and melphalan. *Lancet.* 1982;2:1342.

 Cyclosporine (eg, *Neoral*)

Methotrexate

SUMMARY: The combination of methotrexate and cyclosporine in the treatment of psoriasis appears to increase toxicity.

RISK FACTORS: No specific risk factors are known.

RELATED DRUGS: No information is available.

MANAGEMENT OPTIONS:

➧ **Monitor.** Carefully monitor patients receiving methotrexate and cyclosporine for toxicity from both agents. Monitor cyclosporine and methotrexate concentrations; the dosage of either drug may require adjustment.

REFERENCES:

Powles AV, et al. Cyclosporin toxicity. *Lancet.* 1990;335:610.

Korstanje MJ, et al. Cyclosporine and methotrexate: a dangerous combination. *J Am Acad Derm.* 1990;23:320.

 Cyclosporine (eg, *Neoral*)

Metoclopramide (eg, *Reglan*)

SUMMARY: Metoclopramide increases the bioavailability and serum concentrations of single-dose cyclosporine, probably by increasing gastric emptying; nevertheless, it is not known how often this effect would cause clinical difficulties.

RISK FACTORS: No specific risk factors are known.

RELATED DRUGS: The effect of cisapride on cyclosporine is not established, but caution is in order as both are metabolized by CYP3A4. Competition for metabolism is theoretically possible.

MANAGEMENT OPTIONS:

➡ **Monitor.** Until multiple-dose studies are performed, monitor cyclosporine serum concentrations and responses carefully when metoclopramide is given concurrently. It may be necessary to reduce the cyclosporine dose in some patients.

REFERENCES:

Yee GC, et al. Cyclosporine. In: Evans WE, et al, eds. *Applied Pharmacokinetics: Principles of Therapeutic Drug Monitoring.* 3rd ed. Vancouver: Applied Therapeutics, Inc.; 1992:28–1–28–40.

Wadhwa NK, et al. The effect of oral metoclopramide on the absorption of cyclosporine. *Transplantation.* 1987;43:211-213.

Cyclosporine (eg, *Neoral*)

Miconazole (eg, *Monistat*)

SUMMARY: Miconazole administration to a patient receiving cyclosporine appears to increase cyclosporine concentrations; the clinical significance of this increase is unknown.

RISK FACTORS: No specific risk factors are known.

RELATED DRUGS: Other antifungal agents (ketoconazole, itraconazole [eg, *Sporanox*], fluconazole) are likely to increase cyclosporine concentrations. Miconazole may produce a similar reaction with tacrolimus (eg, *Prograf*).

MANAGEMENT OPTIONS:

➡ **Monitor.** Until further studies of this interaction are available, closely monitor patients stabilized on cyclosporine for increased concentrations of cyclosporine when miconazole is administered.

REFERENCES:

Horton CM, et al. Cyclosporine interactions with miconazole and other azole-antimycotics: a case report and review of the literature. *J Heart Lung Transplant.* 1992;11:1127-1132.

Canafax DM, et al. Increased cyclosporine levels as a result of simultaneous fluconazole and cyclosporine therapy in renal transplant recipients: a double-blind, randomized pharmacokinetic and safety study. *Transplant Proc.* 1991;23:1041-1042.

Cyclosporine (eg, *Sandimmune*)

Modafinil (*Provigil*)

SUMMARY: Limited clinical evidence and theoretical considerations suggest that modafinil can reduce cyclosporine blood concentrations; monitor patients carefully.

RISK FACTORS: No specific risk factors are known.

RELATED DRUGS: No information is available.

MANAGEMENT OPTIONS:

➡ **Circumvent/Minimize.** Given the importance of maintaining adequate cyclosporine blood concentrations in transplant patients, avoid concurrent use of modafinil and cyclosporine if possible.

➡ **Monitor.** If modafinil is used concurrently with cyclosporine, monitor cyclosporine blood concentrations carefully when modafinil is initiated, discontinued, or changed in dosage. Note that the onset and offset of enzyme induction can be gradual, so continue cyclosporine monitoring until it is clear that blood concentrations are stable.

REFERENCES:

Product information. Modafinil (*Provigil*). Cephalon, Inc. 2002.

Robertson P, et al. Effect of modafinil on the pharmacokinetics of ethinyl estradiol and triazolam in healthy volunteers. *Clin Pharmacol Ther.* 2002;71:46-56.

Cyclosporine (eg, *Neoral*)

Nafcillin

SUMMARY: Nafcillin therapy reduced cyclosporine blood concentrations during coadministration; the clinical significance of this interaction is unknown, but a reduction in cyclosporine activity may be anticipated.

RISK FACTORS: No specific risk factors are known.

RELATED DRUGS: If this interaction is substantiated, tacrolimus (*Prograf*) is likely to be affected similarly.

MANAGEMENT OPTIONS:

➡ **Monitor.** Monitor patients receiving cyclosporine for reduced blood concentrations of cyclosporine and evidence of organ rejection during nafcillin administration.

REFERENCES:

Veremis SA, et al. Subtherapeutic cyclosporine concentrations during nafcillin therapy. *Transplantation.* 1987;43:913.

Cyclosporine (eg, *Neoral*)

Naproxen (eg, *Naprosyn*)

SUMMARY: Impaired renal function appears to be greater with naproxen plus cyclosporine than with either drug alone.

RISK FACTORS: No specific risk factors are known.

RELATED DRUGS: In patients receiving cyclosporine, several NSAIDs have been associated with impaired renal function or increased cyclosporine blood concentrations. The relative likelihood of various NSAIDs to increase cyclosporine-induced nephrotoxicity is not established, but assume that all NSAIDs are capable of interacting with cyclosporine until evidence to the contrary is available.

MANAGEMENT OPTIONS:

➡ **Consider Alternative.** Until the clinical importance of this potential interaction is better defined, use naproxen (or other NSAIDs) in patients receiving cyclosporine only when the expected benefit clearly outweighs the risk of excessive cyclosporine response and nephrotoxicity.

➡ **Monitor.** If the combination is used, monitor the patient's renal function carefully and be prepared to discontinue one or both drugs.

REFERENCES:

Sesin GP, et al. Sulindac-induced elevation of serum cyclosporine concentrations. *Clin Pharm.* 1989;8:445.

Branthwaite JP, et al. Cyclosporin and diclofenac interaction in rheumatoid arthritis. *Lancet*. 1991;337:252.

Deray G, et al. Enhancement of cyclosporine A nephrotoxicity by diclofenac. *Clin Nephrol*. 1987;27:213.

Altman RD, et al. Interaction of cyclosporine A and nonsteroidal antiinflammatory drugs on renal function in patients with rheumatoid arthritis. *Am J Med*. 1992;93:396.

Cyclosporine (*Neoral*)

Nicardipine (eg, *Cardene*)

SUMMARY: Cyclosporine blood concentrations are increased by nicardipine; cyclosporine toxicity could result.

RISK FACTORS: No specific risk factors are known.

RELATED DRUGS: Diltiazem (eg, *Cardizem*) and verapamil (eg, *Calan*) inhibit cyclosporine metabolism while isradipine (*DynaCirc*), nifedipine (eg, *Procardia*), amlodipine (*Norvasc*) and nitrendipine have minimal effect. Nicardipine may affect tacrolimus (*Prograf*) in a similar manner.

MANAGEMENT OPTIONS:

➡ *Consider Alternative.* Calcium channel blockers that do not appear to alter cyclosporine pharmacokinetics include isradipine, nitrendipine, and amlodipine.

➡ *Circumvent/Minimize.* Reduce cyclosporine dosage and monitor blood concentrations when nicardipine is coadministered.

➡ *Monitor.* Observe patients receiving both drugs for increased cyclosporine concentrations and decreasing renal function.

REFERENCES:

Bourbigot B, et al. Nicardipine increases cyclosporine blood levels. *Lancet*. 1986;1:1447.

Cantarovich M, et al. Confirmation of the interaction between cyclosporine and the calcium channel blocker nicardipine in renal transplant patients. *Clin Nephrol*. 1987;29:190.

Todd P, et al. Nicardipine interacts with cyclosporin. *Br J Dermatol*. 1989;121:820.

Martinez F, et al. No clinically significant interaction between cyclosporin and isradipine. *Nephron*. 1991;59:658.

Coupur MS, et al. Effects of nitrendipine on blood pressure and blood cyclosporine A level in patients with posttransplant hypertension. *Nephron*. 1989;52:227.

Toupance O, et al. Antihypertensive effect of amlodipine and lack of interference with cyclosporine metabolism in renal transplant recipients. *Hypertension*. 1994;24:297.

Cyclosporine (eg, *Neoral*)

Phenobarbital

SUMMARY: Phenobarbital (and probably other barbiturates) can reduce the effect of cyclosporine; adjustments in cyclosporine dose may be needed.

RISK FACTORS: No specific risk factors are known.

RELATED DRUGS: Expect other barbiturates to reduce cyclosporine response until evidence to the contrary appears.

MANAGEMENT OPTIONS:

➡ *Consider Alternative.* If the barbiturate is being used as a sedative-hypnotic, consider using a benzodiazepine in place of the barbiturate.

➡ *Monitor.* In a patient stabilized on cyclosporine, monitor for altered cyclosporine response if barbiturate therapy is started or stopped or if the barbiturate dose is changed. Note that the enzyme inducing effects of barbiturates tend to have a gradual onset and offset (at least 1 to 2 weeks, depending on the barbiturate). When initiating cyclosporine therapy in a patient receiving a barbiturate, be aware that the cyclosporine dosage requirements may be higher than anticipated.

REFERENCES:

Burckart GJ, et al. Usefulness of cyclosporine monitoring questioned. *Clin Pharm.* 1984;3:243.

Kerr KE. Drug interactions with cyclosporine. *Clin Pharm.* 1984;3:346.

Carstensen H, et al. Interaction between cyclosporine A and phenobarbitone. *Br J Clin Pharmacol.* 1986;21:550.

Offermann G, et al. Low cyclosporin A blood levels and acute graft rejection in a renal transplant recipient during rifampin treatment. *Am J Nephrol.* 1985;5:385.

Cockburn ITR, et al. An appraisal of drug interactions with Sandummun.® *Transplant Proc.* 1989;21:3845.

Cyclosporine (eg, *Neoral*)

Phenytoin (eg, *Dilantin*)

SUMMARY: Phenytoin markedly reduces serum cyclosporine concentrations and is likely to increase cyclosporine dosage requirements.

RISK FACTORS: No specific risk factors are known.

RELATED DRUGS: Other enzyme-inducing anticonvulsants also appear to reduce blood cyclosporine concentrations. Tacrolimus (*Prograf*) is probably affected similarly by enzyme inducers.

MANAGEMENT OPTIONS:

➡ *Circumvent/Minimize.* When initiating cyclosporine therapy in a patient receiving phenytoin, be aware that the cyclosporine dosage requirements may be higher than anticipated.

➡ *Monitor.* In a patient stabilized on cyclosporine, monitor for altered cyclosporine response if phenytoin therapy is started, stopped or if the dose is changed. Starting phenytoin therapy may increase the risk of rejection in patients on cyclosporine.

REFERENCES:

Keown PA, et al. The effects and side effects of cyclosporine; relationship to drug pharmacokinetics. *Transplant Proc.* 1982;14:659.

Freeman DJ, et al. Evaluation of cyclosporin-phenytoin interaction with observations of cyclosporin metabolites. *Br J Clin Pharmacol.* 1984;18:887.

Keown PA, et al. Interaction between phenytoin and cyclosporine following organ transplantation. *Transplantation.* 1984;38:304.

Rowland M, et al. Cyclosporin-phenytoin interaction: re-evaluation using metabolite data. *Br J Clin Pharmacol.* 1987;24:329.

Cyclosporine (eg, *Neoral*)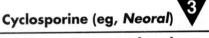

Prednisolone (eg, *Prelone*)

SUMMARY: The concurrent use of cyclosporine and methylprednisolone may increase the plasma concentrations of both drugs; isolated case reports indicate that the combination may result in seizures. The clinical importance of these findings is unclear.

RISK FACTORS: No specific risk factors are known.

RELATED DRUGS: There is little evidence of drug interactions when combining cyclosporine with other corticosteroids, but it is possible that they interact as well. Tacrolimus (*Prograf*) may interact with corticosteroids, but little information is available.

MANAGEMENT OPTIONS:

➡ ***Monitor.*** Although cyclosporine and corticosteroids commonly are used concurrently, be alert for evidence of increased response to both drugs.

REFERENCES:

Durrant S, et al. Cyclosporin A, methylprednisolone, and convulsions. *Lancet*. 1982;2:829.

Boogaerts MA, et al. Cyclosporin, methylprednisolone, and convulsions. *Lancet*. 1982;2:1216.

Ost L. Effects of cyclosporin on prednisolone metabolism. *Lancet*. 1984;1:451.

Klintmalm G, et al. High dose methylprednisolone increases plasma cyclosporin levels in renal transplant recipients. *Lancet*. 1984;1:731.

Cyclosporine (eg, *Neoral*)

Probucol

SUMMARY: A preliminary report suggests that probucol slightly reduces blood cyclosporine concentrations, but the clinical importance of this effect is unknown.

RISK FACTORS: No specific risk factors are known.

RELATED DRUGS: No information is available.

MANAGEMENT OPTIONS:

➡ ***Monitor.*** Although the interaction is not well documented, it would be prudent to monitor patients for altered cyclosporine blood levels and response if probucol is initiated or discontinued.

REFERENCES:

Chen P, et al. Clinical pharmacokinetic interaction of cyclosporine and probucol studied using a HPLC assay procedure. *Pharm Res*. 1990;7:S-254.

Corder CN, et al. Interference with steady state cyclosporine levels by probucol. *Clin Pharmacol Ther*. 1990;47:204.

Gallego C, et al. Interaction between probucol and cyclosporine in renal transplant patients. *Ann Pharmacother*. 1994;28:940.

Sundararajan V, et al. Interaction of cyclosporine and probucol in heart transplant patients. *Transplant Proc*. 1991;23:2028.

Cyclosporine (eg, *Neoral*)

Pyrazinamide

SUMMARY: The administration of pyrazinamide to a patient receiving cyclosporine resulted in a need to increase cyclosporine doses to maintain therapeutic plasma concentrations of cyclosporine.

RISK FACTORS: No specific risk factors are known.

RELATED DRUGS: If this interaction is substantiated, tacrolimus (*Prograf*) is likely to be affected similarly.

MANAGEMENT OPTIONS:

➡ *Circumvent/Minimize.* Cyclosporine dosages may need to be increased during the coadministration of pyrazinamide to maintain therapeutic concentrations.

➡ *Monitor.* Until further information regarding this interaction is available, monitor patients stabilized on cyclosporine for reduced concentrations if pyrazinamide therapy is initiated.

REFERENCES:

del Cerro LAJ, et al. Effect of pyrazinamide on cyclosporine levels. *Nephron.* 1992;62:113.

Cyclosporine (eg, *Neoral*)

Quinupristin/Dalfopristin (*Synercid*)

SUMMARY: The blood concentration of cyclosporine was increased by coadministration of quinupristin/dalfopristin; reduced doses of cyclosporine may be necessary.

RISK FACTORS: No specific risk factors are known.

RELATED DRUGS: Tacrolimus (*Prograf*) would probably be affected by quinupristin/dalfopristin in a similar manner.

MANAGEMENT OPTIONS:

➡ *Monitor.* Carefully monitor patients stabilized on cyclosporine for increasing cyclosporine concentrations when quinupristin/dalfopristin is added. Cyclosporine dosages may need to be reduced during coadministration with quinupristin/dalfopristin.

REFERENCES:

Product information. Quinupristin/dalfopristin (*Synercid*). Rhône-Poulenc Rorer. 1999.

Cyclosporine (eg, *Neoral*)

Rifampin (eg, *Rifadin*)

SUMMARY: Rifampin may reduce cyclosporine concentrations and cause therapeutic failure.

RISK FACTORS: No specific risk factors are known.

RELATED DRUGS: Tacrolimus (*Prograf*) is likely to be affected similarly by rifampin administration.

MANAGEMENT OPTIONS:

➡ ***Avoid Unless Benefit Outweighs Risk.*** Coadminister rifampin and cyclosporine only with careful monitoring of cyclosporine concentrations.

➡ ***Monitor.*** Monitor cyclosporine blood concentrations when cyclosporine and rifampin are used simultaneously. The addition of rifampin to cyclosporine regimens may require a 2- to 4-fold increase in cyclosporine dosages to maintain therapeutic blood concentrations. The discontinuation of rifampin may cause cyclosporine concentrations to increase over 5 to 10 days, possibly resulting in toxicity. Dosage reduction will probably be required, particularly in patients who have had their dosage increased as a result of rifampin administration.

REFERENCES:

Hebert MF, et al. Bioavailability of cyclosporine with concomitant rifampin administration is markedly less than predicted by hepatic enzyme induction. *Clin Pharmacol Ther.* 1992;52:453-457.

Combalbert J, et al. Metabolism of cyclosporin A. IV. Purification and identification of the rifampicin-inducible human liver cytochrome P450 (cyclosporin A oxidase) as a product of P450IIIA gene subfamily. *Drug Metab Disp.* 1989;17:197-207.

Hebert MF, et al. Clinical evidence of metabolic differences between intestinal and hepatic cytochrome P450. *Clin Pharmacol Ther.* 1993;53:190.

Modry DL, et al. Acute rejection and massive cyclosporine requirements in heart transplant recipients treated with rifampin. *Transplantation.* 1985;39:313-.314

Howard PL, et al. Cyclosporine-rifampin drug interaction. *Drug Intell Clin Pharm.* 1985;19:763-764.

Cassidy MJ, et al. Effect of rifampicin on cyclosporin A blood levels in a renal transplant recipient. *Nephron.* 1985;41:207-208.

Van Buren D, et al. The antagonistic effect of rifampin upon cyclosporine bioavailability. *Transplant Proc.* 1984;16:1642-1645.

Offermann G, et al. Low cyclosporin A blood levels and acute graft rejection in a renal transplant recipient during rifampin treatment. *Am J Nephrol.* 1985;5:385-387.

Koselj M, et al. Drug interaction between cyclosporine and rifampicin, erythromycin, and azoles in kidney recipients with opportunistic infections. *Transplant Proc.* 1994;26:2823-2824.

Cyclosporine (eg, *Neoral*)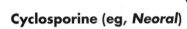

Roxithromycin

SUMMARY: Roxithromycin administration appears to increase cyclosporine concentrations; and cyclosporine appears to increase the concentration of roxithromycin. The clinical significance of these effects is not established.

RISK FACTORS: No specific risk factors are known.

RELATED DRUGS: Other macrolide antibiotics including erythromycin (eg, *E-Mycin*), troleandomycin (*TAO*), and clarithromycin (*Biaxin*) may inhibit the metabolism of cyclosporine. Azithromycin (*Zithromax*) would not interact with cyclosporine. Roxithromycin may have a similar effect on tacrolimus (*Prograf*) elimination.

MANAGEMENT OPTIONS:

➡ ***Monitor.*** Until more studies of these interactions are available, monitor patients stabilized on cyclosporine for changing cyclosporine concentrations when roxithromycin is added to or deleted from their dosage regimens.

REFERENCES:

Billaud EM, et al. Interaction between roxithromycin and cyclosporin in heart transplant patients. *Clin Pharmacokinet.* 1990;19:499-502.

Moravek J, et al. Pharmacokinetics of roxithromycin in kidney grafted patients under cyclosporin A or azathioprine immunosuppression and in healthy volunteers. *Int J Clin Pharmacol Ther Toxicol.* 1990;28:262-267.

Cyclosporine (eg, *Neoral*)

St. John's Wort

SUMMARY: Two heart transplant patients receiving cyclosporine developed acute rejection reactions after starting therapy with St. John's wort; monitor patients for altered cyclosporine effect if St. John's wort is used concurrently.

RISK FACTORS: No specific risk factors are known.

RELATED DRUGS: Theoretically, St. John's wort would also reduce the serum plasma concentrations of related immunosuppressants that are metabolized by CYP3A4 and may be transported by p-glycoprotein. Examples include tacrolimus (*Prograf*) and sirolimus (*Rapamune*).

MANAGEMENT OPTIONS:

➡ *Use Alternative.* The use of antidepressants other than St. John's wort in patients receiving cyclosporine (and perhaps also tacrolimus or sirolimus) is preferable. Selective serotonin reuptake inhibitors and related antidepressants (eg, paroxetine [*Paxil*], sertraline [*Zoloft*], citalopram [*Celexa*], venlafaxine [*Effexor*]) are not known to induce or inhibit CYP3A4 to a clinically important extent. Fluoxetine (eg, *Prozac*) appears to be a weak inhibitor of CYP3A4, fluvoxamine (*Luvox*) is a moderate CYP3A4 inhibitor, and nefazodone (*Serzone*) is a potent inhibitor of CYP3A4.

➡ *Monitor.* If St. John's wort is used with cyclosporine, tacrolimus, or sirolimus, monitor the patient for reduced immunosuppressant effect.

REFERENCES:

Ruschitzka F, et al. Acute heart transplant rejection due to Saint John's wort (*Hypericum perforatum*). *Lancet*. 2000;355:548-549.

Yue QY, et al. Safety of St. John's wort. *Lancet*. 2000;355:576-577.

Piscitelli SC, et al. Indinavir concentrations and St. John's wort. *Lancet*. 2000;355:547-548.

Johne A, et al. Pharmacokinetic interaction of digoxin with an herbal extract from St. John's wort (*Hypericum perforatum*). *Clin Pharmacol Ther*. 1999;66:338-345.

Cyclosporine (eg, *Neoral*)

Sulindac (eg, *Clinoril*)

SUMMARY: Impaired renal function appears to be greater with sulindac plus cyclosporine than with either drug alone; sulindac has also been reported to increase serum cyclosporine concentrations.

RISK FACTORS: No specific risk factors are known.

RELATED DRUGS: In patients receiving cyclosporine, several NSAIDs have been associated with impaired renal function or increased cyclosporine blood concentrations. The relative likelihood of various NSAIDs to increase cyclosporine-induced nephrotoxicity is not established, but assume that all NSAIDs are capable of interacting with cyclosporine until evidence to the contrary is available.

MANAGEMENT OPTIONS:

➡ *Consider Alternative.* Until the clinical importance of this potential interaction is better defined, use sulindac (or other NSAIDs) in patients receiving cyclosporine only when the expected benefit clearly outweighs the risk of excessive cyclosporine response and nephrotoxicity.

➡ *Monitor.* If the combination is used, monitor the patient's renal function carefully and be prepared to discontinue one or both drugs.

REFERENCES:

Sesin GP, et al. Sulindac-induced elevation of serum cyclosporine concentrations. *Clin Pharm.* 1989;8:445.

Branthwaite JP, et al. Cyclosporin and diclofenac interaction in rheumatoid arthritis. *Lancet.* 1991;337:252.

Deray G, et al. Enhancement of cyclosporine A nephrotoxicity by diclofenac. *Clin Nephrol.* 1987;27:213.

Altman RD, et al. Interaction of cyclosporine A and nonsteroidal antiinflammatory drugs on renal function in patients with rheumatoid arthritis. *Am J Med.* 1992;93:396.

Cyclosporine (eg, *Neoral*)

Sulphadimidine

SUMMARY: Some sulfonamides can reduce the plasma concentration of cyclosporine, potentially reducing its efficacy.

RISK FACTORS:

➡ *Dosage Regimen.* IV administration of sulphadimidine is a probable risk factor.

RELATED DRUGS: Tacrolimus (*Prograf*) concentrations may be reduced in a similar manner.

MANAGEMENT OPTIONS:

➡ *Circumvent/Minimize.* Oral TMP-SMZ did not affect cyclosporine plasma concentrations.

➡ *Monitor.* During the administration of sulfadimidine to patients receiving cyclosporine, monitor plasma cyclosporine concentrations.

REFERENCES:

Jones DK, et al. Serious interaction between cyclosporine A and sulphadimidine. *BMJ.* 1986;292:728.

Wallwork H, et al. Cyclosporine and intravenous sulphadimidine and trimethoprim therapy. *Lancet.* 1983;1:366.

Spes CH, et al. Sulfadiazine therapy for toxoplasmosis in heart transplant recipients decreases cyclosporine concentration. *Clin Investig.* 1992;70:752.

Cyclosporine (eg, *Neoral*)

Ticlopidine (eg, *Ticlid*)

SUMMARY: A patient with nephrotic syndrome developed a marked reduction in blood cyclosporine concentrations during ticlopidine therapy; a causal relationship was likely in this patient, but more study is needed to assess the clinical importance.

RISK FACTORS: No specific risk factors are known.

RELATED DRUGS: No information is available.

MANAGEMENT OPTIONS:

➡ *Monitor.* Until more information is available, monitor cyclosporine blood concentrations and therapeutic response carefully if ticlopidine is initiated or discontinued in patients taking cyclosporine.

REFERENCES:

Birmele B, et al. Interaction of cyclosporin and ticlopidine. *Nephrol Dial Transplant.* 1991;6:150.

 Cyclosporine (eg, *Neoral*)

Verapamil (eg, *Calan*)

SUMMARY: Cyclosporine blood concentrations are increased by verapamil; cyclosporine toxicity could result.

RISK FACTORS: No specific risk factors are known.

RELATED DRUGS: Diltiazem (eg, *Cardizem*) and nicardipine (eg, *Cardene*) inhibit cyclosporine metabolism while isradipine (*DynaCirc*), nifedipine (eg, *Procardia*), amlodipine (*Norvasc*), and nitrendipine have minimal effect. Verapamil may affect tacrolimus (*Prograf*) in a similar manner.

MANAGEMENT OPTIONS:

➡ *Consider Alternative.* Calcium channel blockers that do not appear to alter cyclosporine pharmacokinetics include isradipine, nitrendipine, and amlodipine.

➡ *Circumvent/Minimize.* Reduce cyclosporine dosage and monitor blood concentrations when verapamil is coadministered.

➡ *Monitor.* Observe patients receiving both drugs for increased cyclosporine concentrations and decreasing renal function.

REFERENCES:

Lindholm A, et al. Verapamil inhibits cyclosporin metabolism. *Lancet.* 1987;1:1262.

Maggio TG, et al. Increased cyclosporine blood concentrations due to verapamil administration. *Drug Intell Clin Pharm.* 1988;22:705.

Robson RA, et al. Cyclosporin-verapamil interactions. *Br J Clin Pharmacol.* 1988;25:402.

Sabate I, et al. Evaluation of cyclosporin-verapamil interactions, with observations on patient cyclosporin and metabolites. *Clin Chem.* 1988;34:2151.

Howard RL, et al. The effect of calcium channel blockers on the cyclosporine dose requirement in renal transplant patients. *Ren Fail.* 1990;12;89.

Martinez F, et al. No clinically significant interaction between cyclosporin and isradipine. *Nephron.* 1991;59:658.

Coupur MS, et al. Effects of nitrendipine on blood pressure and blood cyclosporine A level in patients with posttransplant hypertension. *Nephron.* 1989;52:227.

Toupance O, et al. Antihypertensive effect of amlodipine and lack of interference with cyclosporine metabolism in renal transplant recipients. *Hypertension.* 1994;24:297.

Cyclosporine (eg, *Neoral*)

Voriconazole (*Vfend*)

SUMMARY: Cyclosporine blood concentrations are increased by concurrent voriconazole administration.

RISK FACTORS:

➡ ***Pharmacogenetics.*** Patients who are poor metabolizers for CYP2C19 will have higher voriconazole concentrations and thus are likely to have an interaction of larger magnitude.

RELATED DRUGS: Tacrolimus (eg, *Prograf*) is similarly affected by voriconazole administration. Sirolimus (*Rapamune*) concentrations are increased to a greater extent than cyclosporine by voriconazole. The metabolism of other immunosuppressants such as everolimus (*Certican*) is likely to be decreased by voriconazole. Other azole antifungal agents including ketoconazole (eg, *Nizoral*), fluconazole (*Diflucan*), and itraconazole (eg, *Sporanox*) are known to reduce the metabolism of cyclosporine.

MANAGEMENT OPTIONS:

➡ ***Circumvent/Minimize.*** A reduction in cyclosporine dose may be required during treatment with voriconazole.

➡ ***Monitor.*** Carefully monitor patients for elevated cyclosporine concentrations or evidence of cyclosporine toxicity (eg, increased serum creatinine) during voriconazole coadministration. When voriconazole is discontinued, monitor for decreasing cyclosporine concentrations

REFERENCES:

Romero AJ et al. Effect of voriconazole on the pharmacokinetics of cyclosporine in renal transplant patients. *Clin Pharmacol Ther.* 2002;71:226-234.

Cyclosporine (eg, *Sandimmune*)

Wine, Red

SUMMARY: Red wine moderately reduced cyclosporine blood concentrations following use of *Sandimmune*; the effect of red wine on *Neoral* is not established.

RISK FACTORS:

➡ ***Pharmacogenetics.*** Although data are limited (9 Caucasians and 3 Asians), the Asians experienced a smaller decrease (14%) than the Caucasians (35%). More study is needed to determine whether this difference is real.

RELATED DRUGS: The microemulsion form of cyclosporine (*Neoral*) is better absorbed than the standard formulation used in this study (*Sandimmune*). Thus, these results do not necessarily apply to patients taking *Neoral*. Theoretically, *Neoral* would be less likely to be affected than *Sandimmune*. The effect of other red wines on cyclosporine is not known, but it is likely that some would have a greater effect on cyclosporine, and some would have less. Preliminary results from the same authors suggest that white wine may not affect cyclosporine bioavailability.

MANAGEMENT OPTIONS:

➡ *Consider Alternative.* Preliminary evidence suggests that white wine may be less likely to interact. Theoretically, the microemulsion form of cyclosporine would be less likely to interact.

➡ *Circumvent/Minimize.* In patients receiving the standard cyclosporine formulation (eg, *Sandimmune*) it may be prudent for them to avoid red wine. The effect of separating doses of *Sandimmune* from red wine is not known.

➡ *Monitor.* Be alert for altered cyclosporine blood concentrations if patients ingest red wine.

REFERENCES:

Tsunoda SM, et al. Red wine decreases cyclosporine bioavailability. *Clin Pharmacol Ther.* 2001;70:462-467.

Cyproheptadine (*Periactin*)

Fluoxetine (eg, *Prozac*)

SUMMARY: Some patients on fluoxetine have developed a worsening of depression when cyproheptadine was added, but this has not been a consistent finding; more study is needed.

RISK FACTORS: No specific risk factors are known.

RELATED DRUGS: Theoretically, other selective serotonin reuptake inhibitors would interact similarly with cyproheptadine.

MANAGEMENT OPTIONS:

➡ *Monitor.* Until more information is available, monitor for reduced antidepressant response to fluoxetine if cyproheptadine is started.

REFERENCES:

Feder R. Reversal of antidepressant activity of fluoxetine by cyproheptadine in three patients. *J Clin Psychiatry.* 1991;52:163.

McCormick S, et al. Reversal of fluoxetine-induced anorgasmia by cyproheptadine in two patients. *J Clin Psychiatry.* 1990;51:383.

Danazol (eg, *Danocrine*)

Lovastatin (*Mevacor*)

SUMMARY: A patient developed myositis with rhabdomyolysis after danazol was added to his lovastatin therapy; although a causal relationship was not proved, the reaction is consistent with the known interactive properties of the drugs.

RISK FACTORS: No specific risk factors are known.

RELATED DRUGS: It is not known whether androgens other than danazol interact with lovastatin, but consider the possibility. The effect of danazol on other hepatic hydroxymethylglutaryl coenzyme A reductase inhibitors is not established. Because pravastatin (*Pravachol*) and fluvastatin (*Lescol*) appear less likely to interact with cyclosporine than lovastatin, they also may be less likely to interact with danazol.

MANAGEMENT OPTIONS:

➡ *Consider Alternative.* See Related Drugs.

➡ *Monitor.* If the combination is used, monitor the patient for evidence of myositis. Advise patients to contact health care provider if developing unexpected muscle pain or weakness.

REFERENCES:

Dallaire M, et al. Severe rhabdomyolysis in a patient receiving lovastatin, danazol, and doxycycline [in French]. *CMAJ*. 1994;150:1991.

Danazol (eg, *Danocrine*)

Warfarin (eg, *Coumadin*)

SUMMARY: Several cases of enhanced hypoprothrombinemic response to warfarin following danazol therapy have been reported.

RISK FACTORS: No specific risk factors are known.

RELATED DRUGS: Anabolic steroids other than danazol are known to increase the hypoprothrombinemic response to oral anticoagulants. Oral anticoagulants other than warfarin also are likely to interact with danazol.

MANAGEMENT OPTIONS:

➡ *Avoid Unless Benefit Outweighs Risk.* Avoid concomitant therapy with oral anticoagulants and danazol if possible.

➡ *Monitor.* If the combination is used, watch for an alteration in the hypoprothrombinemic response to oral anticoagulants if danazol is initiated, discontinued, or changed in dosage; adjust oral anticoagulant dosage as needed. It is possible that danazol, by increasing fibrinolytic activity, increases the bleeding risk in anticoagulated patients even when the warfarin dose has been adjusted to achieve the desired hypoprothrombinemic response. Thus, give careful attention to early detection of bleeding.

REFERENCES:

Goulbourne IA, et al. An interaction between danazol and warfarin: case report. *Br J Obstet Gynaecol*. 1981;88:950.

Small M, et al. Danazol and oral anticoagulants. *Scott Med J.* 1982;27:331.

Meeks ML, et al. Danazol increases the anticoagulant effect of warfarin. *Ann Pharmacother.* 1992;26:641.

Danshen

Warfarin (eg, *Coumadin*)

SUMMARY: Danshen has been reported to increase the bleeding risk in patients on warfarin, but more study is needed to establish the clinical importance of this interaction.

RISK FACTORS: No specific risk factors are known.

RELATED DRUGS: Theoretically, danshen could increase the bleeding risk in patients on other oral anticoagulants such as acenocoumarol and phenprocoumon.

MANAGEMENT OPTIONS:

➡ *Consider Alternative.* In patients receiving warfarin or other oral anticoagulants, consider using an alternative to danshen.

➡ *Monitor.* In patients receiving warfarin or other oral anticoagulants, monitor the INR when danshen is started, stopped, or changed in dosage. Note that some of the purported mechanisms (eg, platelet inhibition) would not be reflected in an increased INR, so an INR in the desired range does not ensure that there is not an increased risk of bleeding.

REFERENCES:

Chan TK. Interaction between warfarin and danshen (*Salvia miltiorrhiza*). *Ann Pharmacother.* 2001;35:501.

Dapsone

Didanosine (*Videx*)

SUMMARY: Dapsone failed to prevent pneumocystis infections in patients being treated with didanosine for human immunodeficiency virus (HIV).

RISK FACTORS: No specific risk factors are known.

RELATED DRUGS: No information is available.

MANAGEMENT OPTIONS:

➡ *Circumvent/Minimize.* Administer dapsone 2 to 3 hours before didanosine to avoid a reduction in dapsone absorption.

➡ *Monitor.* Watch patients receiving the combination for reduced dapsone efficacy.

REFERENCES:

Metroka CE, et al. Failure of prophylaxis with dapsone in patients taking dideoxyinosine. *N Engl J Med.* 1991;325:737.

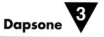

Dapsone

Probenecid

SUMMARY: Probenecid may increase serum dapsone concentrations, but the clinical importance of this effect is not established.

RISK FACTORS: No specific risk factors are known.

RELATED DRUGS: No information is available.

MANAGEMENT OPTIONS:

➡ *Circumvent/Minimize.* The dapsone dose may need to be reduced in some patients taking concomitant probenecid.

➡ *Monitor.* Monitor patients taking dapsone and probenecid for evidence of increased dapsone serum concentrations including hemolytic anemia, methemoglobinemia, and peripheral neuropathy with muscle weakness.

REFERENCES:

Goodwin CS, et al. Inhibition of dapsone excretion by probenecid. *Lancet.* 1969;2:884.

Dapsone

Rifampin (eg, *Rifadin*)

SUMMARY: Rifampin reduces dapsone serum concentrations; methemoglobin concentrations were increased.

RISK FACTORS: No specific risk factors are known.

RELATED DRUGS: No information is available.

MANAGEMENT OPTIONS:

➡ *Circumvent/Minimize.* Dapsone doses may need to be increased during rifampin administration.

➡ *Monitor.* Monitor patients for methemoglobin accumulation during rifampin coadministration. Observe patients being treated for pneumocystis for reduced efficacy.

REFERENCES:

Pieters FAJM, et al. Influence of once-monthly rifampicin and daily clofazimine on the pharmacokinetics of dapsone in leprosy patients in Nigeria. *Eur J Clin Pharmacol.* 1988;34:73.

George J, et al. Drug interaction during multidrug regimens for treatment of leprosy. *Indian J Med Res.* 1988;87:151.

Balakrishnan S, et al. Drug interactions. The influence of rifampicin and clofazimine on the urinary excretion of DDS. *Lepr India.* 1981;53:17.

Balakrishnan S, et al. Influence of rifampicin on DDS excretion in urine. *Lepr India.* 1979;51:54.

Horowitz HW, et al. Drug interactions in use of dapsone for Pneumocystis carinii prophylaxis. *Lancet.* 1992;339:747.

Occhipinti DJ, et al. Influence of rifampin and clarithromycin on dapsone disposition and methemoglobin concentrations. *Clin Pharmacol Ther.* 1995;57:163.

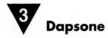

 Dapsone

Trimethoprim (eg, *Proloprim*)

SUMMARY: Trimethoprim appears to increase dapsone serum concentrations and effects; dapsone increases trimethoprim concentrations.

RISK FACTORS: No specific risk factors are known.

RELATED DRUGS: Trimethoprim-sulfamethoxazole (eg, *Bactrim*) also may produce similar effects.

MANAGEMENT OPTIONS:

➡ *Monitor.* Monitor methemoglobin levels of patients receiving dapsone plus trimethoprim for increased dapsone toxicity.

REFERENCES:

Lee BL, et al. Dapsone, trimethoprim, and sulfamethoxazole plasma levels during treatment of pneumocystis pneumonia in patients with the acquired immunodeficiency syndrome (AIDS). *Ann Intern Med.* 1989;110:606.

Debrisoquin[†]

Desipramine (eg, *Norpramin*)

SUMMARY: Desipramine and other tricyclic antidepressants appear to inhibit the antihypertensive response to debrisoquin.

RISK FACTORS: No specific risk factors are known.

RELATED DRUGS: Amitriptyline reduced antihypertensive response to debrisoquin. The effect of other tricyclic antidepressants on the response to debrisoquin is not known, but assume that they interact until proven otherwise.

MANAGEMENT OPTIONS:

➡ *Consider Alternative.* Although limited clinical evidence is available, it would be prudent to avoid the use of tricyclic antidepressants in patients receiving debrisoquin.

➡ *Monitor.* If the combination is used, monitor for altered debrisoquin effect if TCAs are initiated, discontinued, or changed in dosage; adjust debrisoquin dose as needed.

REFERENCES:

Mitchell JR, et al. Guanethidine and related agents. III. Antagonism by drugs which inhibit the norepinephrine pump in man. *J Clin Invest.* 1970;49:1596.

Skinner C, et al. Antagonism of the hypotensive action of bethanidine and debrisoquine by tricyclic antidepressants. *Lancet.* 1969;2:564.

† Not available in the US.

Delavirdine (*Rescriptor*)

Omeprazole (*Prilosec*)

SUMMARY: The absorption of delavirdine is reduced when gastric pH is increased; a reduction in antiviral efficacy may result.

RISK FACTORS: No specific risk factors are known.

RELATED DRUGS: Other proton pump inhibitors (eg, lansoprazole [*Prevacid*], rabeprazole [*Aciphex*], pantoprazole [*Protonix*]) or H$_2$-receptor antagonists (eg, cimetidine [eg, *Tagamet*], ranitidine [eg, *Zantac*], famotidine [eg, *Pepcid*], nizatidine [*Axid*]) may also reduce the absorption of delavirdine.

MANAGEMENT OPTIONS:

➡ *Circumvent/Minimize.* Pending further study of this potential interaction, patients receiving delavirdine should avoid drugs that produce reduced gastric acidity at the time of delavirdine administration. The use of antacids separated by 3 to 4 hours from the administration of delavirdine may reduce their affect on delavirdine absorption.

➡ *Monitor.* Monitor patients taking delavirdine and acid suppressing drugs for a reduced antiviral effect.

REFERENCES:

Morse GD, et al. Gastric acidification increases delavirdine (DLV) mesylate exposure in HIV + subjects with gastric hypoacidity. *Clin Pharmacol Ther.* 1996;59:141.

Product information. Delavirdine (*Rescriptor*). Pharmacia and Upjohn. 1999.

Delavirdine (*Rescriptor*)

Paclitaxel (*Taxol*)

SUMMARY: Two patients on combined therapy with delavirdine and saquinavir (*Fortovase*) developed unexpectedly severe paclitaxel toxicity, but a causal relationship was not established.

RISK FACTORS: No specific risk factors are known.

RELATED DRUGS: Little is known about the effect of other antiretroviral agents on paclitaxel toxicity. Theoretically, any antiretroviral agent that inhibits CYP3A4 may be expected to increase paclitaxel serum concentrations, including ritonavir (*Norvir*), indinavir, nelfinavir (*Viracept*), and amprenavir (*Agenerase*).

MANAGEMENT OPTIONS:

➡ *Monitor.* Monitor patients on delavirdine or other antiretroviral agents that inhibit CYP3A4 for excessive paclitaxel toxicity and reduce paclitaxel doses if necessary.

REFERENCES:

Schwartz JD, et al. Potential interaction of antiretroviral therapy with paclitaxel in patients with AIDS-related Kaposi's sarcoma. *AIDS.* 1999; 13:283-84.

Delavirdine (*Rescriptor*)

Rifabutin (*Mycobutin*)

SUMMARY: Rifabutin significantly reduces the plasma concentration of delavirdine; if coadministration cannot be avoided, delavirdine doses may need to be increased.

RISK FACTORS: No specific risk factors are known.

RELATED DRUGS: Rifampin (eg, *Rifadin*) is known to be an inducer of CYP3A4 and is likely to reduce the plasma concentration of delavirdine.

MANAGEMENT OPTIONS:

➡ ***Circumvent/Minimize.*** The dose of delavirdine may need to be increased during coadministration with rifabutin.

➡ ***Monitor.*** Monitor patients receiving rifabutin and delavirdine for reduced antiviral effect.

REFERENCES:

Borin MT, et al. Pharmacokinetic study of the interaction between rifabutin and delavirdine mesylate in HIV-1 infected patients. *Antiviral Res.* 1997;35:53.

Delavirdine (*Rescriptor*)

Rifampin (eg, *Rifadin*)

SUMMARY: Rifampin administration reduces the plasma concentrations of delavirdine; a loss of antiviral efficacy is likely to result.

RISK FACTORS: No specific risk factors are known.

RELATED DRUGS: Rifabutin (*Mycobutin*) also increases the clearance of delavirdine but to a somewhat lesser (5-fold increase) extent.

MANAGEMENT OPTIONS:

➡ ***Consider Alternative.*** In view of the magnitude of this interaction, avoiding the use of rifampin in patients taking delavirdine seems prudent.

➡ ***Monitor.*** Monitor patients receiving delavirdine for loss of efficacy if rifampin or rifabutin are administered.

REFERENCES:

Borin MT, et al. Pharmacokinetic study of the interaction between rifampin and delavirdine mesylate. *Clin Pharmacol Ther.* 1997;61:544–53.

Borin MT, et al. Effect of rifabutin on delavirdine pharmacokinetics in HIV positive patients. Presented at the 34th Interscience Conference on Antimicrobial Agents and Chemotherapy, Orlando, Florida, 1994.

Desipramine (eg, *Norpramin*)

Fluoxetine (*Prozac*)

SUMMARY: Patients receiving desipramine or other tricyclic antidepressants (TCAs) may manifest marked increases in their antidepressant plasma concentration when fluoxetine is added; some may develop symptoms of antidepressant toxicity.

RISK FACTORS: No specific risk factors are known.

RELATED DRUGS: Five patients receiving antidepressants including desipramine, imipramine, nortriptyline, and trazodone (eg, *Desyrel*) developed marked increases in their plasma antidepressant concentrations after the addition of fluoxetine. Within 1 or 2 weeks of starting fluoxetine, 3 of the patients developed adverse effects characteristic of the antidepressant they were receiving (eg, anticholinergic symptoms, sedation). Three other patients developed elevated plasma cyclic concentrations and cyclic toxicity such as seizures and delirium after fluoxetine was added to TCA (desipramine, imipramine, or doxepin [eg, *Sinequan*]) therapy. In 8 depressed patients given fluoxetine plus trazodone, 3 had a good response but 5 experienced intolerable side effects (eg, headaches, dizziness, sedation, fatigue) or did not respond. Paroxetine (*Paxil*) is also a potent inhibitor of CYP2D6 and can increase serum desipramine concentrations substantially.

MANAGEMENT OPTIONS:

➡ ***Monitor.*** Monitor patients for increased antidepressant plasma levels and toxicity when fluoxetine is used concurrently; adjustment of the antidepressant dosage is likely to be required. Because of the slow elimination of fluoxetine and its active metabolite, its effect on the metabolism of other antidepressants is likely to dissipate gradually over 2 to 4 weeks.

REFERENCES:

Bell IR, et al. Fluoxetine induces elevation of desipramine level and exacerbation of geriatric nonpsychotic depression. *J Clin Psychopharmacol.* 1988;8:447.

Aranow RB, et al. Elevated antidepressant plasma levels after addition of fluoxetine. *Am J Psychiatry.* 1989;146:911.

Preskorn SH, et al. Serious adverse effects of combining fluoxetine and tricyclic antidepressants. *Am J Psychiatry.* 1990;147:532.

Kahn DG, et al. Increased plasma nortriptyline concentration in a patient cotreated with fluoxetine. *J Clin Psychiatry.* 1990;51:36.

Brosen K, et al. Fluoxetine and norfluoxetine are potent inhibitors of P450IID6: the source of sparteine/debrisoquine oxidation polymorphism. *Br J Clin Pharmacol.* 1991;32:136.

Muller N, et al. Extremely long plasma half-life of amitriptyline in a woman with the cytochrome P450IID6 29/ 29-Kilobase Wild-Type Allele: a slowly reversible interaction with fluoxetine. *Ther Drug Monit.* 1991;13:533.

Bergstrom RF, et al. Quantification and mechanism of the fluoxetine and tricyclic antidepressant interaction. *Clin Pharmacol Ther.* 1992;51:239.

Nierenberg AA, et al. Possible trazodone potentiation of fluoxetine:a case series. *J Clin Psychiatry.* 1992;53:83.

Desipramine (eg, *Norpramin*)

Guanethidine (*Ismelin*)

SUMMARY: Tricyclic antidepressants (TCAs) consistently inhibit the antihypertensive response to guanethidine.

RISK FACTORS: No specific risk factors are known.

RELATED DRUGS: In one case report, an interaction between guanethidine and imipramine (eg, *Tofranil*) was implicated in producing cardiac standstill and death. However, a causal relationship was not established. Limited clinical evidence indicates that guanethidine's antihypertensive response is unaffected by mianserin, and is only occasionally affected by maprotiline (eg, *Ludiomil*)., Guanadrel (*Hylorel*) is pharmacologically similar to guanethidine and also may be inhibited by TCAs. Methyldopa (eg, *Aldomet*) may be less likely to interact with tricyclic antidepressants than guanethidine, but more information is needed.

MANAGEMENT OPTIONS:

➤ *Consider Alternative.* Although satisfactory control of hypertension can sometimes be achieved by alteration in guanethidine dosage, it is preferable to avoid the combination when possible. Maprotiline may be less likely to interact with guanethidine than tricyclic antidepressants.

➤ *Monitor.* If the combination is used, monitor patients for rising blood pressures when TCAs are started and for hypotension when cyclics are stopped.

REFERENCES:

Oates JA, et al. Effect of doxepin on the norepinephrine pump. A preliminary report. *Psychosomatics.* 1969;10:12.

Mitchell JR, et al. Antagonism of the antihypertensive action of guanethidine sulfate by desipramine hydrochloride. *JAMA.* 1967;202:973.

Feagin OT, et al. Uptake and release of guanethidine and bethanidine by the adrenergic neuron. *J Clin Invest.* 1969;48:23a.

Mitchell JR, et al. Guanethidine and related agents. III. Antagonism by drugs which inhibit the norepinephrine pump in man. *J Clin Invest.* 1970;49:1596.

Ober KF, et al. Drug interactions with guanethidine. *Clin Pharmacol Ther.* 1973;14:190.

Gulati OD, et al. Antagonism of adrenergic neuron blockade in hypertensive subjects. *Clin Pharmacol Ther.* 1966;7:510.

Stone CA, et al. Antagonism of certain effects of catecholamine depleting agents by antidepressant and related drugs. *J Pharmacol Exp Ther.* 1964;144:196.

Leishman AWD, et al. Antagonism of guanethidine by imipramine. *Lancet.* 1963;1:112.

Pitts NE. The clinical evaluation of doxepin. A new psychotherapeutic agent. *Psychosomatics.* 1969;10:164.

Meyer JF, et al. Insidious and prolonged antagonism of guanethidine by amitriptyline. *JAMA.* 1970;213:1487.

Lahti RA, et al. The tricyclic antidepressants: inhibition of norepinephrine uptake as related to potentiation of norepinephrine and clinical efficacy. *Biochem Pharmacol.* 1971;20:482.

Williams RB Jr, et al. Cardiac complications of tricyclic antidepressant therapy. *Ann Intern Med.* 1971;74:395.

Boston Collaborative Drug Surveillance Program. Adverse reactions to the tricyclic antidepressant drugs. *Lancet.* 1972;1:529.

Mitchell JR, et al. Guanethidine and related agents. I. Mechanism of the selective blockade of adrenergic neurons and its antagonism by drugs. *J Pharmacol Exp Ther.* 1970;172:100.

Ghose K, et al. Autonomic actions and interactions of mianserin hydrochloride (org. GB 94) and amitriptyline in patients with depressive illness. *Psychopharmacology.* 1976;49:201.

Smith AJ, et al. Interaction between postganglionic sympathetic blocking drugs and antidepressants. *J Int Med Res*. 1975;3(Suppl. 2):55.

Briant RH, et al. The assessment of potential drug interaction with a new tricyclic antidepressant drug. *Br J Clin Pharmacol*. 1974;1:113.

Burgess CD, et al. Cardiovascular responses to mianserin hydrochloride: A comparison with tricyclic antidepressant drugs. *Br J Clin Pharmacol*. 1978;5:215.

Desipramine (eg, *Norpramin*)
Ritonavir (*Norvir*)

SUMMARY: Desipramine concentrations are markedly increased by ritonavir administration; toxicity could result.

RISK FACTORS: No specific risk factors are known.

RELATED DRUGS: Other tricyclic antidepressants may be similarly affected by ritonavir. Indinavir (*Crixivan*) may inhibit the metabolism of tricyclic antidepressants; the magnitude of any inhibition is unknown.

MANAGEMENT OPTIONS:

➡ *Circumvent/Minimize.* Dosage of desipramine may require reduction.

➡ *Monitor.* Monitor patients stabilized on desipramine and other tricyclic antidepressants for cardiac, central nervous system, and anticholinergic side effects.

REFERENCES:
Product information. Ritonavir (*Norvir*). Abbott Laboratories. 1996.

Desipramine (eg, *Norpramin*)
Venlafaxine (eg, *Effexor*)

SUMMARY: Study in healthy subjects suggests that venlafaxine increases desipramine serum concentrations, but the extent to which this increases the risk of desipramine toxicity is not established.

RISK FACTORS:

➡ *Pharmacogenetics.* Only patients who have CYP2D6 would be expected to experience this interaction.

RELATED DRUGS: Theoretically, other tricyclic antidepressants that are metabolized by CYP2D6 such as amitriptyline (eg, *Elavil*) would be similarly affected.

MANAGEMENT OPTIONS:

➡ *Monitor.* Monitor for altered desipramine effect if venlafaxine is initiated, discontinued, or changed in dosage.

REFERENCES:
Albers LJ, et al. Effect of venlafaxine on imipramine metabolism. *Psychiatry Res*. 2000;96:235-243.

Dexfenfluramine

Fluoxetine (*Prozac*)

SUMMARY: Cotherapy with dexfenfluramine and selective serotonin reuptake inhibitors (SSRIs) such as fluoxetine theoretically could result in serotonin syndrome.

RISK FACTORS: No specific risk factors are known.

RELATED DRUGS: Avoid dexfenfluramine in combinations with other SSRIs such as paroxetine, sertraline, and fluvoxamine. Dexfenfluramine is the S-enantiomer of the racemate fenfluramine, so the 2 drugs probably interact in a similar way with SSRIs.

MANAGEMENT OPTIONS:

➡ *Avoid Unless Benefit Outweighs Risk.* Patients should avoid the use of SSRIs with either dexfenfluramine or fenfluramine, unless the combinations are found to be safe in well controlled clinical trials. There is also a medicolegal risk in using the combinations, since the manufacturer's information states that cotherapy should be avoided.

➡ *Monitor.* If the combination is used, be alert for evidence of serotonin syndrome which can result in neurotoxicity (eg, myoclonus, tremors, rigidity, incoordination, restlessness, hyperreflexia, seizures, coma); psychiatric symptoms (eg, agitation, confusion, hypomania); and temperature regulation abnormalities (eg, fever, sweating).

REFERENCES:

Gross AS, et al. The influence of the sparteine/debrisoquine genetic polymorphism on the disposition of dexfenfluramine. *Br J Clin Pharmacol*. 1996;41:311.

Product Information. Dexfenfluramine (*Redux*). Wyeth-Ayerst Laboratories. 1996.

 Dexfenfluramine

AVOID Phenelzine (*Nardil*)

SUMMARY: Cotherapy with dexfenfluramine and nonselective monoamine oxidase inhibitors (MAOIs) such as phenelzine theoretically could result in serotonin syndrome.

RISK FACTORS: No specific risk factors are known.

RELATED DRUGS: Dexfenfluramine also is contraindicated with other nonselective MAOIs such as tranylcypromine and isocarboxazid (*Marplan*). Given that selegiline (eg, *Eldepryl*) can sometimes act as a nonselective MAOI (especially if given in large doses), it also might interact adversely with dexfenfluramine. Dexfenfluramine is the S-enantiomer of the racemate fenfluramine, so the 2 drugs probably interact in a similar way with nonselective MAOIs.

MANAGEMENT OPTIONS:

➡ *AVOID COMBINATION.* Patients should avoid any combination of a nonselective MAOI with either dexfenfluramine or fenfluramine.

REFERENCES:

Gross AS, et al. The influence of the sparteine/debrisoquine genetic polymorphism on the disposition of dexfenfluramine. *Br J Clin Pharmacol*. 1996;41:311.

Product information. Dexfenfluramine (*Redux*). Wyeth-Ayerst Laboratories. 1996.

Dextroamphetamine (eg, *Dexedrine*)

Furazolidone (*Furoxone*)

SUMMARY: Amphetamines may induce a hypertensive response in patients taking furazolidone.

RISK FACTORS: No specific risk factors are known.

RELATED DRUGS: One would expect an enhanced response to other sympathomimetics with indirect activity (eg, ephedrine), but this apparently has not been studied.

MANAGEMENT OPTIONS:

➡ *Consider Alternative.* Patients receiving furazolidone probably should avoid taking amphetamines.

➡ *Monitor.* Watch for increased blood pressure if amphetamine and furazolidone are coadministered.

REFERENCES:

Pettinger WA, et al. Inhibition of monoamine oxidase in man by furazolidone. *Clin Pharmacol Ther.* 1968;9:442-447.

Dextroamphetamine (eg, *Dexedrine*)

Guanethidine (*Ismelin*)

SUMMARY: Amphetamines, and probably related sympathomimetics, inhibit the antihypertensive response to guanethidine.

RISK FACTORS: No specific risk factors are known.

RELATED DRUGS: Although little is known regarding other sympathomimetics, their pharmacologic similarity to amphetamines suggests that they are likely to inhibit guanethidine's effect as well. Guanadrel (*Hylorel*) is similar to guanethidine and also may be inhibited by amphetamines.

MANAGEMENT OPTIONS:

➡ *Consider Alternative.* Consider using an alternative to amphetamine or guanethidine.

➡ *Monitor.* If the combination is used, monitor for inhibition of antihypertensive response to guanethidine or guanadrel.

REFERENCES:

Ober KF, et al. Drug interactions with guanethidine. *Clin Pharmacol Ther.* 1973;14:190-195.

Feagin OT, et al. Uptake and release of guanethidine and bethanidine by the adrenergic neuron. *J Clin Invest.* 1969;48:23a.

Day MD, et al. Antagonism of guanethidine and bretylium by various agents. *Lancet.* 1962;2:1282.

Gulati OD, et al. Antagonism of adrenergic neuron blockade in hypertensive subjects. *Clin Pharmacol Ther.* 1966;7:510-514.

Starke K. Interactions of guanethidine and indirect-acting sympathomimetic amines. *Arch Int Pharmacodyn Ther.* 1972;195:309-314.

Dextroamphetamine (eg, *Dexedrine*)

Imipramine (eg, *Tofranil*)

SUMMARY: Theoretically, tricyclic antidepressants (TCAs) such as imipramine would increase the effect of amphetamines, but clinical evidence is lacking.

RISK FACTORS: No specific risk factors are known.

RELATED DRUGS: Other amphetamines may be similarly affected.

MANAGEMENT OPTIONS:

→ *Circumvent/Minimize.* Patients receiving tricyclic antidepressants should avoid recreational use of amphetamines. The risk of therapeutic use of amphetamines with tricyclic antidepressants is not established.

→ *Monitor.* Monitor for adverse cardiovascular effects in patients on the combination.

REFERENCES:

Raisfeld IH. Cardiovascular complications of antidepressant therapy. *Am Heart J*. 1972;83:129-133.

Beaumont G. Drug interactions with clomipramine (*Anafranil*). *J Int Med Res*. 1973;1:480.

Dextroamphetamine (eg, *Dexedrine*)

AVOID Tranylcypromine (*Parnate*)

SUMMARY: Severe hypertensive reactions have occurred when amphetamines were ingested by patients taking monoamine oxidase inhibitors (MAOIs).

RISK FACTORS: No specific risk factors are known.

RELATED DRUGS: Although methylphenidate (eg, *Ritalin*) has amphetamine-like pharmacologic activity, some evidence indicates that the reactions it causes when used with MAOIs are less severe than those caused by amphetamines. Nevertheless, use methylphenidate cautiously in combination with MAOIs., All nonselective MAOIs probably interact similarly with amphetamines: isocarboxazid (*Marplan*), phenelzine, tranylcypromine. Furazolidone (*Furoxone*), another MAOI, has been shown to increase pressor sensitivity to amphetamines., Selegiline (eg, *Eldepryl*) has been reported to enhance the pressor effect of tyramine, particularly following doses greater than 10 mg/day; it could theoretically interact with amphetamines as well. Type B MAOIs (eg, selegiline) should be less likely than the type A MAOIs (eg, moclobemide[†]) to interact with drugs that release catecholamines (eg, amphetamines). Nevertheless, little is known regarding drug interactions with type B MAOIs. Use cautiously until more data are available.

MANAGEMENT OPTIONS:

→ *AVOID COMBINATION.* Amphetamines should not be given to patients receiving a nonselective MAOI. Phentolamine (*Regitine*) appears to be the logical therapy for severe hypertension resulting from this interaction, since it blocks the alpha effects of the released norepinephrine. Remember that the effects of nonselective MAOIs should be assumed to persist for 2 weeks after they are discontinued.

REFERENCES:

Zeck P. The dangers of some antidepressant drugs. *Med J Aust*. 1961;2:607.

Krisko I, et al. Severe hyperpyrexia due to tranylcypromineamphetamine toxicity. *Ann Intern Med.* 1969;70:559.

Brownlee G, et al. Potentiation of amphetamine and pethidine by monoamine oxidase inhibitors. *Lancet.* 1963;1:669.

Goldberg LI. Monoamine oxidase inhibitors. Adverse reactions and possible mechanisms. *JAMA.* 1964;190:456.

Sjoqvist F. Psychotropic drugs (2). Interaction between monoamine oxidase (MAO) inhibitors and other substances. *Proc R Soc Med.* 1965;58:967.

Pettinger WA, et al. Inhibition of monoamine oxidase in man by furazolidone. *Clin Pharmacol Ther.* 1968;9:442.

Pettinger WA, et al. Supersensitivity to tyramine during monoamine oxidase inhibition in man. Mechanism at the level of the adrenergic neuron. *Clin Pharmacol Ther.* 1968;9:341.

Lloyd JTA, et al. Death after combined dexamphetamine and phenelzine. *BMJ.* 1965;2:168.

Product information. Dextroamphetamine (*Dexedrine*). 1990.

Schulz R, et al. Tyramine kinetics and pressor sensitivity during monoamine oxidase inhibition by selegiline. *Clin Pharmacol Ther.* 1989;46:528.

† Not available in the US.

Dextromethorphan (eg, *Robitussin-DM*)

Fluoxetine (*Prozac*)

SUMMARY: A patient receiving fluoxetine developed visual hallucinations when she began to take dextromethorphan for her cough. A causal relationship was not established, but theoretical considerations suggest that an interaction may have occurred.

RISK FACTORS: No specific risk factors are known.

RELATED DRUGS: A patient on paroxetine (*Paxil*) developed symptoms of serotonin syndrome after taking dextromethorphan, but a causal relationship was not established. Sertraline (*Zoloft*) and fluvoxamine (*Luvox*) appear to have less effect on CYP2D6 than fluoxetine and paroxetine, but little is known regarding their use with dextromethorphan. When considering codeine as an alternative to dextromethorphan, keep in mind that inhibitors of CYP2D6 may reduce the analgesic effect of codeine by inhibiting its conversion to morphine. The extent to which the antitussive effect of codeine is affected by inhibitors of CYP2D6 is not established.

MANAGEMENT OPTIONS:

➡ *Consider Alternative.* Although clinical data are very limited, there are theoretical reasons for limiting the use of dextromethorphan in patients taking fluoxetine (or other selective serotonin reuptake inhibitors). Moreover, the limited therapeutic usefulness of dextromethorphan in many patients is another reason for avoiding it in patients receiving fluoxetine, even though the risk of the combination is not established.

➡ *Monitor.* If the combination is used, monitor for evidence of serotonin syndrome which can result in neurologic findings (eg, dizziness, tremor, myoclonus, rigidity, seizures, incoordination, and coma), psychiatric symptoms (eg, agitation, confusion, hypomania), and disorders of temperature regulation (eg, fever, sweating, shivering); severe cases can be fatal.

REFERENCES:

Achamallah NS. Visual hallucinations after combining fluoxetine and dextromethorphan. *Am J Med.* 1992;149:1406.

Crewe HK, et al. The effect of selective serotonin re-uptake inhibitors on cytochrome P4052D6 (CYP2D6) activity in human liver microsomes. *Br J Clin Pharmacol.* 1992; 34:262.

Dextromethorphan (eg, *Robitussin-DM*)

AVOID **Moclobemide†**

SUMMARY: Since dextromethorphan can cause serotonin syndrome when administered with nonselective monoamine oxidase inhibitors (MAOIs), cotherapy of dextromethorphan with moclobemide or other MAO-A inhibitors would theoretically produce the same effect.

RISK FACTORS: No specific risk factors are known.

RELATED DRUGS: Since serotonin is metabolized by MAO-A, one would expect all type A monoamine oxidase inhibitors to interact with dextromethorphan.

MANAGEMENT OPTIONS:

➡ *AVOID COMBINATION.* Dextromethorphan is contraindicated in patients receiving nonselective or type A MAO inhibitors.

REFERENCES:

Rivers N, et al. Possible lethal reaction between Nardil and dextromethorphan. *Can Med Assoc J.* 1970;103:85.

Sovner R, et al. Interaction between dextromethorphan and monoamine oxidase inhibitor therapy with isocarboxazid. *N Engl J Med.* 1988;319:1671.

Nierenberg DW, et al. The central nervous system serotonin syndrome. *Clin Pharmacol Ther.* 1993;53:84.

Amrein R, et al. Interactions of moclobemide with concomitantly administered medication: evidence from pharmacological and clinical studies. *Psychopharmacology.* 1992;106:S24.

† Not available in the US.

 Dextromethorphan (eg, *Robitussin-DM*)

AVOID **Phenelzine (*Nardil*)**

SUMMARY: Dextromethorphan may cause serotonin syndrome (agitation, confusion, hypomania, myoclonus, rigidity, hyperreflexia, tremor, incoordination, sweating, shivering, seizures, coma) when administered with monoamine oxidase (MAO) inhibitors.

RISK FACTORS: No specific risk factors are known.

RELATED DRUGS: In one case, a patient taking isocarboxazid (*Marplan*) 30 mg/day developed dizziness, muscle tremor, and urinary retention within 1 hour of ingesting 15 mg of dextromethorphan. Assume Tranylcypromine (*Parnate*) to produce serotonin syndrome with dextromethorphan.

MANAGEMENT OPTIONS:

➡ *AVOID COMBINATION.* Dextromethorphan is contraindicated in patients receiving nonselective MAO inhibitors. Remember that the effects of nonselective MAO inhibitors can persist for 2 weeks after they are discontinued.

REFERENCES:

Rivers N, et al. Possible lethal reaction between *Nardil* and dextromethorphan. *Can Med Assoc J.* 1970;103:85.

Sovner R, et al. Interaction between dextromethorphan and monoamine oxidase inhibitor therapy with isocarboxazid. *N Engl J Med.* 1988;319:1671.

Nierenberg DW, et al. The central nervous system serotonin syndrome. *Clin Pharmacol Ther.* 1993;53:84.

Dextromethorphan (eg, *Robitussin-DM*)

Quinidine

SUMMARY: Dextromethorphan concentrations may be increased to toxic levels during quinidine coadministration.

RISK FACTORS:

➡ ***Pharmacogenetics.*** Rapid metabolizers of dextromethorphan are at risk.

RELATED DRUGS: No information is available.

MANAGEMENT OPTIONS:

➡ ***Circumvent/Minimize.*** Caution patients taking quinidine to avoid dextromethorphan-containing medications. Consider dextromethorphan dosage reduction if it is administered with quinidine. Codeine may not be a suitable alternative since quinidine inhibits its conversion to morphine and may thus limit its antitussive effects.

➡ ***Monitor.*** If dextromethorphan is administered with quinidine, patients should be monitored for side effects (eg, nausea, headache, nervousness, insomnia, tremors, confusion).

REFERENCES:

Zhang Y, et al. Dextromethorphan: enhancing its systemic availability by way of low-dose quinidine-mediated inhibition of cytochrome P4502D6. *Clin Pharmacol Ther.* 1992;51:647.

Dextromethorphan (eg, *Robitussin-DM*)

Selegiline (eg, *Eldepryl*)

SUMMARY: Since dextromethorphan can cause serotonin syndrome when administered with nonselective monoamine oxidase inhibitors (MAOIs), selegiline (especially in large doses) theoretically could produce the same effect.

RISK FACTORS:

➡ ***Dosage Regimen.*** Selegiline doses of 10 mg/day can have some inhibitory effect on MAO-A, and this effect increases as the daily dose is increased.

RELATED DRUGS: Meperidine interacts similarly with selegiline. Other nonselective MAOIs also interact similarly with selegiline.

MANAGEMENT OPTIONS:

➡ ***Avoid Unless Benefit Outweighs Risk.*** Although dextromethorphan is contraindicated in patients receiving nonselective or type A MAO inhibitors, little is known about the use of type B MAO inhibitors such as selegiline with dextromethorphan. Nonetheless, it would be prudent to avoid concomitant use until more data are available.

➡ ***Monitor.*** If the combination is used, monitor for evidence of serotonin syndrome (eg, agitation, confusion, hypomania, myoclonus, rigidity, hyperreflexia, tremor, incoordination, sweating, shivering, seizures, coma).

REFERENCES:

Rivers N, et al. Possible lethal reaction between *Nardil* and dextromethorphan. *Can Med Assoc J.* 1970;103:85.

Sovner R, et al. Interaction between dextromethorphan and monoamine oxidase inhibitor therapy with isocarboxazid. *N Engl J Med.* 1988;319:1671.

Nierenberg DW, et al. The central nervous system serotonin syndrome. *Clin Pharmacol Ther.* 1993;53:84.

Zornberg GL, et al. Severe adverse interaction between pethidine and selegiline. *Lancet.* 1991;337:246.

2 Dextromethorphan (eg, *Robitussin-DM*)

Sibutramine (*Meridia*)

SUMMARY: The risk of serotonin syndrome would theoretically increase when sibutramine is combined with other serotonergic drugs such as dextromethorphan.

RISK FACTORS: No specific risk factors are known.

RELATED DRUGS: No information is available.

MANAGEMENT OPTIONS:

➡ ***Avoid Unless Benefit Outweighs Risk.*** The manufacturer states that sibutramine should not be used with meperidine (eg, *Demerol*). This is a prudent recommendation until more information is available.

➡ ***Monitor.*** Serotonin syndrome can result in neurotoxicity (eg, myoclonus, tremors, rigidity, incoordination, restlessness, hyperreflexia, seizures, coma), psychiatric symptoms (eg, agitation, confusion, hypomania), and temperature regulation abnormalities (eg, fever, sweating). Note that mild forms of serotonin syndrome have also been reported, so any combination of the above symptoms should be considered possibly related to excessive serotonin activity.

REFERENCES:

Product information. Sibutramine (*Meridia*). Knoll Pharmaceuticals. 1997.

Mills KC. Serotonin syndrome: a clinical update. *Crit Care Clin.* 1997;13:763.

3 Dextromethorphan (eg, *Robitussin-DM*)

Terbinafine (*Lamisil*)

SUMMARY: Terbinafine increases the concentration of dextromethorphan, a marker drug for CYP2D6 activity; the clearance of other CYP2D6 substrates is also likely to be reduced by terbinafine.

RISK FACTORS: Patients who are extensive CYP2D6 metabolizers (about 93% of the US population) will have a greater reduction in metabolic activity following terbinafine administration compared with poor CYP2D6 metabolizers.

RELATED DRUGS: Other drugs metabolized by CYP2D6 include amitriptyline (eg, *Elavil*), carvedilol (*Coreg*), codeine, haloperidol (eg, *Haldol*), metoprolol (eg, *Lopressor*), nortriptyline (eg, *Pamelor*), and timolol (eg, *Blocadren*). The magnitude of the effect of terbinafine on these drugs awaits further study.

MANAGEMENT OPTIONS:

➡ ***Monitor.*** Pending data on the effect of terbinafine on other CYP2D6 substrates, monitor carefully for altered effect if terbinafine is added to or discontinued from a patient's drug regimen.

REFERENCES:

Abdel-Rahman SM, et al. Investigation of terbinafine as a CYP2D6 inhibitor in vivo. *Clin Pharmacol Ther.* 1999;65:465.

Dextrothyroxine (*Choloxin*)
Warfarin (eg, *Coumadin*)

SUMMARY: Dextrothyroxine consistently increases the hypoprothrombinemic response to warfarin and probably other oral anticoagulants. Adjustments in oral anticoagulant dosage are likely to be needed when dextrothyroxine therapy is initiated or discontinued.

RISK FACTORS: No specific risk factors are known.

RELATED DRUGS: All combinations of thyroid and oral anticoagulants are likely to interact.

MANAGEMENT OPTIONS:

➡ *Avoid Unless Benefit Outweighs Risk.* Avoid concomitant therapy with dextrothyroxine and oral anticoagulants if possible. If oral anticoagulant therapy is begun in a patient receiving dextrothyroxine, use conservative doses until the maintenance dose is established.

➡ *Monitor.* Initiation or discontinuation of dextrothyroxine therapy in a patient stabilized on an oral anticoagulant is likely to necessitate a change in the maintenance anticoagulant dose.

REFERENCES:

Weintraub M, et al. The effects of dextrothyroxine on the kinetics of prothrombin activity: proposed mechanism of the potentiation of warfarin by D-thyroxine. *J Lab Clin Med*. 1973;81:273.

Loeliger EA, et al. The biological disappearance rate of prothrombin and factors VII, IX, and X from plasma in hypothyroidism, hyperthyroidism and during fever. *Thromb Diath Haemorrh*. 1964;10:267.

Schrogie JJ, et al. The anticoagulant response to bishydroxycoumarin II: the effect of D-thyroxine, clofibrate, and norethandrolone. *Clin Pharmacol Ther*. 1967;8:70.

Solomon HM, et al. Change in receptor site affinity: a proposed explanation for the potentiating effect of D-thyroxine on the anticoagulant response to warfarin. *Clin Pharmacol Ther*. 1967;8:797.

Owens JC, et al. Effect of sodium dextrothyroxine in patients receiving anticoagulants. *N Engl J Med*. 1962;266:76.

Diazepam (eg, *Valium*)
Disulfiram (*Antabuse*)

SUMMARY: Disulfiram may increase serum concentrations of diazepam and benzodiazepines that undergo oxidative metabolism, but the frequency of excessive benzodiazepine response is unknown.

RISK FACTORS: No specific risk factors are known.

RELATED DRUGS: Other benzodiazepines that undergo oxidative metabolism (eg, clonazepam [eg, *Klonopin*], clorazepate [eg, *Tranxene*], flurazepam [eg, *Dalmane*], halazepam [*Paxipam*], prazepam[+], and triazolam [eg, *Halcion*]) also might be affected by disulfiram treatment, but studies are not available. In 11 alcoholic patients undergoing withdrawal, disulfiram 0.5 g/day for 14 days did not appear to affect the pharmacokinetics of alprazolam (eg, *Xanax*); however, poor compliance with the disulfiram therapy and the alcohol withdrawal process may have affected the results of this study. Oxazepam (eg, *Serax*) and lorazepam (eg, *Ativan*) are converted to inactive glucuronides, a process that does not appear to be affected by disulfiram. Temazepam (eg, *Restoril*) also undergoes glucuronide conjugation and would not be expected to be affected by disulfiram.

MANAGEMENT OPTIONS:

➡ **Monitor.** Be alert for evidence of enhanced benzodiazepine response in patients receiving disulfiram. Some patients may require a reduction in benzodiazepine dosage during concurrent disulfiram use.

REFERENCES:

MacLeod SM, Sellers EM, Giles HG, et al. Interaction of disulfiram with benzodiazepines. *Clin Pharmacol Ther.* 1978;24:583-589.

Diquet B, Gujadhur L, Lamiable D, Warot D, Hayoun H, Choisy H. Lack of interaction between disulfiram and alprazolam in alcoholic patients. *Eur J Clin Pharmacol.* 1990;38:157.

Sellers EM, Giles HG, Greenblatt DJ, Naranjo CA. Differential effects of benzodiazepine disposition by disulfiram and ethanol. *Arzneimittelforschung.* 1980;30:882-886.

† Not available in the US.

 Diazepam (eg, *Valium*)

Ethanol (*Ethyl Alcohol*)

SUMMARY: Ethanol may enhance the adverse psychomotor effects of benzodiazepines like diazepam; combined use may be dangerous in patients performing tasks requiring alertness.

RISK FACTORS: No specific risk factors are known.

RELATED DRUGS: Nitrazepam, bromazepam, and lorazepam (eg, *Ativan*), appear to have a similar effect when given with ethanol. Chlordiazepoxide (eg, *Librium*) may be less likely and diazepam more likely to enhance the adverse psychomotor effects of alcohol. Ethanol seems less likely to affect the hepatic metabolism of oxazepam (eg, *Serax*) than diazepam, but additive CNS depression would be expected in either case. Expect all benzodiazepines to result in additive CNS depression with alcohol.

MANAGEMENT OPTIONS:

➡ **Circumvent/Minimize.** Warn patients receiving benzodiazepines against moderate to large amounts of ethanol ingestion. Occasional ingestion of small amounts of ethanol (especially if taken with food) probably causes little difficulty unless alertness is required (eg, driving) or the patient has a disease or condition that makes him sensitive to CNS depression.

➡ **Monitor.** Monitor for excessive CNS depression if the combination is used.

REFERENCES:

Linnoila M, et al. Effects of diazepam and codeine, alone and in combination with alcohol, on simulated driving. *Clin Pharmacol Ther.* 1974;15:368.

Reggiani G, et al. Some aspects of the experimental and clinical toxicology of chlordiazepoxide. In: Toxicity and Side-Effects of Psychotropic Drugs. Amsterdam: Excerpta Medica Foundation; 1968:79–97.

Rosinga WM. Interaction of drugs and alcohol in relation to traffic safety. In: Meyer L, Peck HM eds. Drug Induced Disease. Vol. 3. Amsterdam: Excerpta Medica Foundation; 1968:295–306.

Sarrio I, et al. Interaction of drugs with alcohol on human psychomotor skills related to driving: effect of sleep deprivation or two weeks' treatment with hypnotics. *J Clin Pharmacol.* 1975;15:52.

Hayes SL, et al. Ethanol and oral diazepam absorption. *N Engl J Med.* 1977;296:186.

Saario I. Psychomotor skills during subacute treatment with thioridazine and bromazepam, and their combined effects with alcohol. *Ann Clin Res.* 1976;8:117.

MacLeod SM, et al. Diazepam actions and plasma concentrations following ethanol ingestion. *Eur J Clin Pharmacol.* 1977;11:345.

Linnoila M. Effects of diazepam, chlordiazepoxide, thioridazine, haloperidol, flupenthixole and alcohol on psychomotor skills related to driving. *Ann Med Exp Biol Fenn.* 1973;51:125.

Linnoila M. Drug interaction on psychomotor skills related to driving: hypnotics and alcohol. *Ann Med Exp Biol Fenn.* 1973;51:118.

Linnoila M, et al. Drug interaction on psychomotor skills related to driving: diazepam and alcohol. *Eur J Clin Pharmacol.* 1973;5:186.

Morland J, et al. Combined effects of diazepam and ethanol on mental and psychomotor functions. *Acta Pharmacol Toxicol.* 1974;34:5.

Linnoila M, et al. Effect of treatment with diazepam or lithium and alcohol on psychomotor skills related to driving. *Eur J Clin Pharmacol.* 1974;7:337.

Hughes FW, et al. Comparative effect in human subjects of chlordiazepoxide, diazepam, and placebo on mental and physical performance. *Clin Pharmacol Ther.* 1965;6:139.

Hoffer A. Lack of potentiation by chlordiazepoxide (Librium) of depression or excitation due to alcohol. *Can Med Assoc J.* 1962;87:920.

Betts TA, et al. Effect of four commonly-used tranquilizers on lowspeed driving performance tests. *BMJ.* 1972;4:580.

Dundee JW, et al. Alcohol and the benzodiazepines. The interaction between intravenous ethanol and chlordiazepoxide and diazepam. *Q J Stud Alcohol.* 1971;32:960.

Goldberg L. Behavioral and physiological effects of alcohol on man. *Psychosom Med.* 1966;28:570.

Miller AI, et al. Effects of combined chlordiazepoxide and alcohol in man. *Q J Stud Alcohol.* 1963;24:9.

Sellers EM, et al. Intravenous diazepam and oral ethanol interaction. *Clin Pharmacol Ther.* 1980;28:638.

Sellers EM, et al. Different effects on benzodiazepine disposition by disulfiram and ethanol. *Arzneimittel-forschung.* 1980;30:882.

Juhl RP, et al. Alprazolam pharmacokinetics in alcoholic liver disease. *J Clin Pharmacol.* 1984;24:113.

Mattila MJ, et al. Acute effects of buspirone and alcohol on psychomotor skills. *J Clin Psychiatry.* 1982;43:56.

Linnoila M, et al. Effect of adinazolam and diazepam, alone and in combination with ethanol, on psychomotor and cognitive performance and on autonomic nervous system reactivity in healthy volunteers. *Eur J Clin Pharmacol.* 1990;38:371.

van Steveninck AL, et al. Pharmacodynamic interactions of diazepam and intravenous alcohol at pseudo steady-state. *Psychopharmacology.* 1993;110:471.

Diazepam (eg, *Valium*)

Fluoxetine (*Prozac*)

SUMMARY: A study in healthy subjects suggests that fluoxetine increases plasma diazepam concentrations and reduces the plasma concentration of its active metabolite, desmethyldiazepam. Fluoxetine may increase modestly the psychomotor impairment produced by diazepam in some patients, but the clinical importance of this effect is not established.

RISK FACTORS:

➡ *Effects of Age.* The elderly are known to be more sensitive to diazepam and may be more sensitive to this interaction.

RELATED DRUGS: Preliminary evidence suggests that sertraline (*Zoloft*) slightly reduces diazepam elimination. The effect of other selective serotonin reuptake inhibitors other than fluoxetine on diazepam is not established, but fluvoxamine (*Luvox*) is known to inhibit CYP3A4, an isozyme important in the metabolism of diazepam. Fluoxetine also inhibits the metabolism of alprazolam (eg, *Xanax*).

MANAGEMENT OPTIONS:

➡ *Circumvent/Minimize.* It would be prudent to use conservative doses of diazepam in the presence of fluoxetine until patient response is assessed. Advise patients receiving combined therapy to watch for excessive sedation.

➡ *Monitor.* Monitor for altered diazepam effect if fluoxetine is initiated, discontinued, or changed in dosage; adjust diazepam dose as needed.

REFERENCES:

Lemberger L, et al. The effect of fluoxetine on the pharmacokinetics and psychomotor responses of diazepam. *Clin Pharmacol Ther.* 1988;43:412.

Moskowitz H, et al. The effects on performance of two antidepressants, alone and in combination with diazepam. *Prog Neuropsychopharmacol Biol Psychiatry.* 1988;12:783.

Diazepam (eg, *Valium*)

Isoniazid (INH; eg, *Nydrazid*)

SUMMARY: Isoniazid may increase diazepam serum concentrations; the clinical significance is not known.

RISK FACTORS: No specific risk factors are known.

RELATED DRUGS: The effect of isoniazid on other benzodiazepines is unknown. Isoniazid may affect other benzodiazepines (eg, triazolam [eg, *Halcion*]) in a similar manner.

MANAGEMENT OPTIONS:

➡ *Monitor.* Watch for evidence of altered diazepam effects when isoniazid is initiated or discontinued.

REFERENCES:

Ochs HR, et al. Diazepam interaction with antituberculosis drugs. *Clin Pharmacol Ther.* 1981;29:671.

Diazepam (eg, *Valium*)

Itraconazole (*Sporanox*)

SUMMARY: Itraconazole administration increases the serum concentration of diazepam; diazepam toxicity could result.

RISK FACTORS: No specific risk factors are known.

RELATED DRUGS: Itraconazole is known to inhibit triazolam (eg, *Halcion*) and temazepam (eg, *Restoril*) metabolism. It also is likely to reduce the metabolism of chlordiazepoxide (eg, *Librium*) and midazolam (*Versed*). Lorazepam (eg, *Ativan*), a benzodiazepine not metabolized by CYP3A4, may be less likely to interact. Other antifungal agents such as ketoconazole (eg, *Nizoral*) and fluconazole (*Diflucan*) would be likely to inhibit the metabolism of diazepam.

MANAGEMENT OPTIONS:

➡ *Consider Alternative.* A benzodiazepine such as lorazepam that is not metabolized by CYP3A4 would be a potential alternative anxiolytic agent.

➥ ***Monitor.*** Monitor for increased diazepam effects (eg, sedation, ataxia, mental confusion) when itraconazole is coadministered with diazepam.

REFERENCES:

Ahonen J, et al. The effects of the antimycotic itraconazole on the pharmacokinetics and pharmacodynamics of diazepam. *Fundam Clin Pharmacol.* 1996;10:314.

Diazepam (eg, *Valium*)

Levodopa (eg, *Larodopa*)

SUMMARY: Diazepam appeared to exacerbate parkinsonism in a few patients receiving levodopa, but a causal relationship was not established.

RISK FACTORS: No specific risk factors are known.

RELATED DRUGS: Another patient well controlled on levodopa, benztropine (eg, *Cogentin*), and diphenhydramine (eg, *Antivert*) developed an acute exacerbation of parkinsonism following administration of chlordiazepoxide (eg, *Librium*); control returned 5 days after the chlordiazepoxide was discontinued. These case reports suggest that benzodiazepines are capable of inhibiting the antiparkinsonian effects of levodopa, but little is known regarding the incidence of the interaction between these drugs or the factors that make it more likely to occur. The effect of other benzodiazepines on levodopa is not established.

MANAGEMENT OPTIONS:

➥ ***Monitor.*** Monitor for evidence of a reduced antiparkinsonian effect of levodopa in the presence of benzodiazepine therapy. If this suspected interaction may be occurring, discontinue benzodiazepine and monitor the patient to determine whether improvement occurs.

REFERENCES:

Wodak J, et al. Review of 12 months' treatment with L-DOPA in Parkinson's disease, with remarks on unusual side effects. *Med J Aust.* 1972;2:1277.

Hunter KR, et al. Use of levodopa with other drugs. *Lancet.* 1970;2:1283.

Yosselson-Superstine S, et al. Chlordiazepoxide interaction with levodopa. *Ann Intern Med.* 1982;96:259.

Diazepam (eg, *Valium*)

Metoprolol (eg, *Lopressor*)

SUMMARY: Metoprolol may slightly reduce the metabolism of diazepam, but it does not affect the metabolism of lorazepam (eg, *Ativan*) or alprazolam (eg, *Xanax*). Metoprolol may increase the pharmacodynamic effects of some benzodiazepines.

RISK FACTORS: No specific risk factors are known.

RELATED DRUGS: Atenolol (eg, *Tenormin*) had no effect on diazepam pharmacokinetics or pharmacodynamics. Propranolol (eg, *Inderal*) and labetalol (eg, *Normodyne*) increased the pharmacodynamic effects of oxazepam (eg, *Serax*) without affecting its pharmacokinetics. Propranolol produces a small reduction in diazepam clearance. Metoprolol increased bromazepam[+] AUC 35%. Lorazepam (eg, *Ativan*) and alprazolam (eg, *Xanax*) metabolisms are unaffected by metoprolol.

MANAGEMENT OPTIONS:

➡️ *Monitor.* Monitor patients receiving diazepam and metoprolol or propranolol for increased central nervous system depression.

REFERENCES:

Scott AK, et al. Interaction of metoprolol with lorazepam and bromazepam. *Eur J Clin Pharmacol.* 1991;40:405.

Hawksorth G, et al. Diazepam/beta-adrenoceptor antagonist interactions. *Br J Clin Pharmacol.* 1984;17:69S.

Sonne J, et al. Single dose pharmacokinetics and pharmacodynamics of oral oxazepam during concomitant administration of propranolol and labetalol. *Br J Clin Pharmacol.* 1990;29:33.

† Not available in the US.

Diazepam (eg, *Valium*)

Omeprazole (*Prilosec*)

SUMMARY: Omeprazole increases plasma diazepam concentrations considerably after single doses of diazepam in healthy subjects; the effect of this interaction on diazepam response is not established.

RISK FACTORS: No specific risk factors are known.

RELATED DRUGS: The effect of omeprazole on other benzodiazepines is unknown, but it would be most likely to affect benzodiazepines that undergo phase I metabolism (eg, agents *other than* lorazepam [eg, *Ativan*], oxazepam [eg, *Serax*], and temazepam [eg, *Restoril*]). The effect of lansoprazole (*Prevacid*) on benzodiazepines needs further study, but it generally has less effect on hepatic drug metabolism than omeprazole.

MANAGEMENT OPTIONS:

➡️ *Monitor.* Until data on the pharmacodynamics of this interaction are available, monitor for enhanced diazepam response if omeprazole is given concurrently.

REFERENCES:

Henry DA, et al. Omeprazole: effects on oxidative drug metabolism. *Br J Clin Pharmacol.* 1984;18:195.

Jensen JC, et al. Inhibition of human liver cytochrome P-450 by omeprazole. *Br J Clin Pharmacol.* 1986;21:328.

Gugler R, et al. Omeprazole inhibits oxidative drug metabolism: studies with diazepam and phenytoin in vivo and 7-ethoxycoumarin in vitro. *Gastroenterology.* 1985;89:1235.

Diazepam (eg, *Valium*)

Rifampin (eg, *Rifadin*)

SUMMARY: Rifampin appears to reduce the serum concentration of diazepam and perhaps other benzodiazepines.

RISK FACTORS: No specific risk factors are known.

RELATED DRUGS: Rifampin did not significantly increase the clearance of temazepam (eg, *Restoril*). Rifampin increased nitrazepam clearance significantly. Rifampin also may reduce the effect of those benzodiazepines metabolized to desmethyldiazepam, such as halazepam (*Paxipam*), clorazepate (eg, *Tranxene*), and prazepam.

MANAGEMENT OPTIONS:

➡ *Monitor.* Monitor patients for evidence of reduced diazepam and nitrazepam effect when rifampin is given concurrently. The response to halazepam, clorazepate, and prazepam also may be reduced by rifampin.

REFERENCES:

Ochs HR, et al. Diazepam interaction with antituberculosis drugs. *Clin Pharmacol Ther.* 1981;29:671.

Ohnhaus EE, et al. The effect of antipyrine and rifampin on the metabolism of diazepam. *Clin Pharmacol Ther.* 1987;42:148.

Brockmeyer NH, et al. Comparative effects of rifampin or probenecid on the pharmacokinetics of temazepam and nitrazepam. *Int J Clin Pharmacol Ther Toxicol.* 1990;28:387.

† Not available in the US.

Diazoxide (*Hyperstat*)

Hydralazine (eg, *Apresoline*)

SUMMARY: Severe hypotensive reactions have occurred with combined use of diazoxide and parenteral hydralazine.

RISK FACTORS: No specific risk factors are known.

RELATED DRUGS: No information is available.

MANAGEMENT OPTIONS:

➡ *Monitor.* Undertake concomitant use of diazoxide and hydralazine with caution and with adequate monitoring for excessive hypotension.

REFERENCES:

Henrich WL, et al. Hypotensive sequelae of diazoxide and hydralazine therapy. *JAMA.* 1977;237:264.

Mizroch S, et al. Hypotension and bradycardia following diazoxide and hydralazine therapy. *JAMA.* 1977;237:2471.

Romberg GP, et al. Hypotensive sequelae of diazoxide and hydralazine therapy. *JAMA.* 1977;238:1025.

Diazoxide (*Hyperstat*)

Phenytoin (*Dilantin*)

SUMMARY: Diazoxide has been associated with markedly decreased serum phenytoin concentrations in several children.

RISK FACTORS: No specific risk factors are known.

RELATED DRUGS: No information is available.

MANAGEMENT OPTIONS:

➡ *Monitor.* Monitor patients receiving concomitant phenytoin and diazoxide for increased seizure activity and decreased phenytoin levels.

REFERENCES:

Petro DJ, et al. Diazoxide-diphenylhydantoin interaction. *J Pediatr.* 1976;89:331.

Roe TF, et al. Drug interaction—diazoxide and diphenylhydantoin. *J Pediatr.* 1975;87:480.

Diazoxide (*Hyperstat*)

Thiazides

SUMMARY: Combined use of thiazides and diazoxide may result in hyperglycemia.

RISK FACTORS: No specific risk factors are known.

RELATED DRUGS: No information is available.

MANAGEMENT OPTIONS:

➡ *Monitor.* Monitor blood glucose during combined therapy with thiazides and diazoxide.

REFERENCES:

Sellers EM, et al. Protein binding and vascular activity of diazoxide. *N Engl J Med.* 1969;281:1141.

Seltzer HS, et al. Hyperglycemia and inhibition of insulin secretion during administration of diazoxide and trichlormethiazide in man. *Diabetes.* 1969;18:19.

Wolff F. Diazoxide misunderstood. *N Engl J Med.* 1972;286:612.

Diclofenac (eg, *Voltaren*)

Lithium (eg, *Eskalith*)

SUMMARY: A study in healthy subjects suggests that diclofenac, like most nonsteroidal anti-inflammatory drugs (NSAIDs), increases plasma lithium concentrations; one would expect this to increase the risks of lithium toxicity.

RISK FACTORS: No specific risk factors are known.

RELATED DRUGS: Most NSAIDs increase lithium serum concentrations, but sulindac (eg, *Clinoril*) and aspirin appear to have minimal effects.

MANAGEMENT OPTIONS:

➡ *Consider Alternative.* If appropriate for the patient, consider using an anti-inflammatory agent that is less likely to affect lithium, such as sulindac or aspirin.

➡ *Monitor.* If diclofenac therapy is initiated in a patient taking lithium, monitor serum lithium concentrations for evidence of lithium toxicity (eg, nausea, vomiting, diarrhea, anorexia, coarse tremor, slurred speech, vertigo, confusion, lethargy; in severe cases, seizures, stupor, coma, and cardiovascular collapse). In a patient stabilized on lithium and an NSAID, discontinuation of the NSAID may result in inadequate serum lithium concentrations.

REFERENCES:

Reimann IW, et al. Effects of diclofenac on lithium kinetics. *Clin Pharmacol Ther.* 1981;30:348.

Ragheb M, et al. Ibuprofen can increase serum lithium level in lithium-treated patients. *J Clin Psychiatry.* 1987;48:161.

Diclofenac (eg, *Voltaren*)

Methotrexate (eg, *Rheumatrex*)

SUMMARY: One patient on high dose methotrexate developed severe methotrexate toxicity following the use of diclofenac.

RISK FACTORS:

➡ *Concurrent Diseases.* Particular caution is suggested in patients with pre-existing renal impairment (who may be more susceptible to nonsteroidal anti-inflammatory drug [NSAID]-induced renal failure).

➡ *Dosage Regimen.* The risk of adverse effects from this interaction is primarily in patients receiving antineoplastic doses of methotrexate, rather than the lower doses used to treat rheumatoid arthritis, psoriasis, and related diseases.

RELATED DRUGS: Other NSAIDS appear to interact similarly with methotrexate, but the relative risk of one NSAID versus another is not established.

MANAGEMENT OPTIONS:

➡ *Avoid Unless Benefit Outweighs Risk.* Until more information is available on this interaction, it would be prudent to avoid diclofenac (as well as other NSAIDs) in patients receiving antineoplastic doses of methotrexate. Particular caution is suggested in patients with pre-existing renal impairment, who may be more susceptible to NSAID-induced renal failure.

➡ *Monitor.* If the combination is used, monitor for methotrexate toxicity. Findings in methotrexate toxicity can include stomatitis, severe gastrointestinal symptoms (eg, nausea, diarrhea, vomiting), bone marrow suppression, fever, bleeding, skin rashes, nephrotoxicity, and hepatotoxicity. Although decreasing the methotrexate dosage would be expected to reduce the likelihood of toxicity, the magnitude of the required reduction in methotrexate dosage has not been established.

REFERENCES:

Aherne A, et al. Methotrexate kinetics in rheumatoid arthritis: is there an interaction with nonsteroidal antiinflammatory drugs? *J Rheumatol.* 1988;15:1356.

Furst DE, et al. Effect of aspirin and sulindac on methotrexate clearance. *J Pharm Sci.* 1990;79:782.

Dupuis LL, et al. Methotrexate-nonsteroidal anti-inflammatory drug interaction in children with arthritis. *J Rheumatol.* 1990;17:1469.

Liegler DG, et al. The effect of organic acids on renal clearance of methotrexate in man. *Clin Pharmacol Ther.* 1969;10:849.

Skeith KJ, et al. Lack of significant interaction between low dose methotrexate and ibuprofen or flurbiprofen in patients with arthritis. *J Rheumatol.* 1990;17:1008.

Stewart CF, et al. Effect of aspirin (ASA) on the disposition of methotrexate (MTX) in patients with rheumatoid arthritis (RA). *Clin Pharmacol Ther.* 1990;47:139. Abstract PP-56.

Taylor JR, et al. Effect of sodium salicylate and indomethacin on methotrexate-serum albumin binding. *Arch Dermatol.* 1977;113:588.

Tracy FS, et al. The effect of NSAIDS on methotrexate disposition in patients with rheumatoid arthritis. *Clin Pharmacol Ther.* 1990;47:138. Abstract PP-54.

Daly HM, et al. Methotrexate toxicity precipitated by azapropazone. *Br J Dermatol.* 1986;114:733.

Thyss A, et al. Clinical and pharmacokinetic evidence of a life-threatening interaction between methotrexate and ketoprofen. *Lancet.* 1986;1:256.

Boh LE, et al. Low-dose weekly oral methotrexate therapy for inflammatory arthritis. *Clin Pharm.* 1986;5:503.

Anderson PA, et al. Weekly pulse methotrexate in rheumatoid arthritis: clinical and immunologic effects in a randomized, double-blind study. *Ann Intern Med.* 1985;103:489.

Tugwell P, et al. Methotrexate in rheumatoid arthritis: indications, contraindications, efficacy, and safety. *Ann Intern Med.* 1987;107:358.

Adams JD, et al. Drug interactions in psoriasis. *Aust J Dermatol.* 1976;17:39.

Diclofenac (eg, *Voltaren*)

Verapamil (eg, *Calan*)

SUMMARY: Diclofenac reduces the plasma concentration of verapamil; the clinical significance is unknown.

RISK FACTORS: No specific risk factors are known.

RELATED DRUGS: Naproxen coadministration appears to have no effect on verapamil concentrations. The effects of other NSAIDs on verapamil are unknown. Diclofenac 50 mg administered once increased isradipine (*DynaCirc*) peak concentration by 20% but did not change its area under the concentration-time curve. The clinical effects of this change would be minimal.

MANAGEMENT OPTIONS:

➡ *Consider Alternative.* Consider naproxen for patients taking verapamil.

➡ *Monitor.* Until more information is available, monitor patients stabilized on verapamil for reduced efficacy during concomitant therapy with diclofenac.

REFERENCES:

Peterson MS, et al. Differential effects of naproxen and diclofenac on verapamil pharmacokinetics. *Clin Pharmacol Ther.* 1991;49:129.

Houston MC, et al. The effects of nonsteroidal anti-inflammatory drugs on blood pressures of patients with hypertension controlled by verapamil. *Arch Intern Med.* 1995;155:1049.

Sommers DK, et al. Effects of diclofenac on isradipine pharmacokinetics and platelet aggregation in volunteers. *Eur J Clin Pharmacol.* 1993;44:391.

 ## Diclofenac (eg, *Voltaren*)

Warfarin (eg, *Coumadin*)

SUMMARY: A preliminary study indicates that diclofenac does not affect the hypoprothrombinemic response to oral anticoagulants; nonetheless, cotherapy requires caution because of possible detrimental effects of diclofenac on the gastric mucosa and platelet function.

RISK FACTORS:

➡ *Concurrent Diseases.* Patients with peptic ulcer disease or a history of gastrointestinal (GI) bleeding are probably at greater risk.

RELATED DRUGS: All NSAIDs inhibit platelet function, cause gastric erosions, and appear to have an additive effect with oral anticoagulants in increasing the risk of GI bleeding.

MANAGEMENT OPTIONS:

➡ *Avoid Unless Benefit Outweighs Risk.* Since all NSAIDs probably increase the risk of GI bleeding in patients on oral anticoagulants, use the combination only after careful consideration of the benefit versus risk. If the diclofenac is being used as an analgesic or antipyretic, acetaminophen is probably safer to use with oral anticoagulants. Nonacetylated salicylates (eg, choline salicylate, magnesium salicylate, salsalate, sodium salicylate) also are probably safer with oral anticoagulants than diclofenac since they have minimal effects on platelet function and the gastric mucosa.

➠ **Monitor.** If any NSAID is used with an oral anticoagulant, carefully monitor the prothrombin time and watch for evidence of bleeding, especially from the GI tract.

REFERENCES:

Michot F, et al. A double-blind clinical trial to determine if an interaction exists between diclofenac sodium and the oral anticoagulant acenocoumarol (*Nicoamalone*). *J Int Med Res.* 1975;3:153.

Shorr RI, et al. Concurrent use of nonsteroidal anti-inflammatory drugs and oral anticoagulants places elderly persons at high risk for hemorrhagic peptic ulcer disease. *Arch Intern Med.* 1993;153:1665.

Dicumarol

Ethchlorvynol (*Placidyl*)

SUMMARY: Ethchlorvynol appears to inhibit the hypoprothrombinemic response to dicumarol and possibly warfarin.

RISK FACTORS: No specific risk factors are known.

RELATED DRUGS: In 1 patient receiving warfarin (eg, *Coumadin*), a marked decrease in hypoprothrombinemic response followed ethchlorvynol administration. Little is known about the effect of ethchlorvynol on the response to oral anticoagulants other than dicumarol or warfarin, but assume that they interact until it is proven otherwise. Benzodiazepines, such as diazepam (eg, *Valium*) or temazepam (eg, *Restoril*), are unlikely to affect oral anticoagulants.

MANAGEMENT OPTIONS:

➠ **Consider Alternative.** Consider using a benzodiazepine instead of ethchlorvynol as benzodiazepines are unlikely to affect oral anticoagulants.

➠ **Monitor.** Monitor for altered oral anticoagulant effect if ethchlorvynol is initiated, discontinued, or changed in dosage; adjustments of oral anticoagulant dosage may be needed.

REFERENCES:

Cullen SI, et al. Griseofulvin-warfarin antagonism. *JAMA.* 1967;199:582.

Johansson S. Apparent resistance to oral anticoagulant therapy and influence of hypnotics on some coagulation factors. *Acta Med Scand.* 1968;184:297.

Dicumarol

Tolbutamide (eg, *Orinase*)

SUMMARY: Dicumarol (but probably not warfarin) enhances the hypoglycemic response to tolbutamide. Most available evidence indicates that tolbutamide does not affect the hypoprothrombinemic response to oral anticoagulants.

RISK FACTORS: No specific risk factors are known.

RELATED DRUGS: Tolbutamide metabolism does not appear to be affected by warfarin (eg, *Coumadin*), phenindione,[†] or phenprocoumon.[†] Neither the half-life nor the plasma levels of phenprocoumon appear to be affected by tolbutamide, insulin, glyburide (eg, *DiaBeta*), or glibornuride[+] in diabetics, nondiabetic aged patients, or healthy young volunteers. Little is known regarding the effect of tolbutamide on warfarin response. It does not seem likely that oral anticoagulants would interact with insulin.

MANAGEMENT OPTIONS:

➡ *Consider Alternative.* Warfarin and phenprocoumon appear to be less likely than dicumarol to interact with tolbutamide.

➡ *Monitor.* If tolbutamide and dicumarol are used concurrently, monitor for altered hypoglycemic response if dicumarol is initiated, discontinued, or changed in dosage.

REFERENCES:

Solomon HM, et al. Effect of phenyramidol and bishydroxycoumarin on the metabolism of tolbutamide in human subjects. *Metabolism.* 1967;16:1029.

Kristensen M, et al. Potentiation of the tolbutamide effect of dicumarol. *Diabetes.* 1967;16:211.

Skovsted L, et al. The effect of different oral anticoagulants on diphenylhydantoin (DPH) and tolbutamide metabolism. *Acta Med Scand.* 1976;199:513.

Jahnschen E, et al. Pharmacokinetic analysis of the interaction between dicumarol and tolbutamide in man. *Eur J Clin Pharmacol.* 1976;10:349.

Spurney OM, et al. Protracted tolbutamide-induced hypoglycemia. *Arch Intern Med.* 1965;115:53.

Chaplin H Jr, et al. Studies on the possible relationship of tolbutamide to dicumarol in anticoagulant therapy. *Am J Med Sci.* 1958;235:706.

Poucher RL, et al. Absence of tolbutamide effect on anticoagulant therapy. *JAMA.* 1966;197:1069.

Heine P, et al. The influence of hypoglycaemic sulphonylureas on elimination and efficacy of phenprocoumon following a single oral dose in diabetic patients. *Eur J Clin Pharmacol.* 1976;10:31.

† Not available in the US.

Didanosine (*Videx*)

Food

SUMMARY: Didanosine plasma concentrations are reduced by administration with food; the clinical significance of this is unknown, but the magnitude of the interaction indicates that loss of efficacy may result.

RISK FACTORS: No specific risk factors are known.

RELATED DRUGS: No information is available.

MANAGEMENT OPTIONS:

➡ *Circumvent/Minimize.* Administer didanosine in the fasting state (approximately 0.5 hour before or greater than 2 hours after eating) to maximize its bioavailability.

➡ *Monitor.* If didanosine is coadministered with food, monitor patients for loss of antiviral efficacy.

REFERENCES:

Shyu WC, et al. Food-induced reduction in bioavailability of didanosine. *Clin Pharmacol Ther.* 1991;50:503.

Hartman NR, et al. Pharmacokinetics of 2′,3′-dideoxyinosine in patients with severe human immunodeficiency infection. II. The effects of different oral formulations and the presence of other medications. *Clin Pharmacol Ther.* 1991;50:278.

Knupp CA, et al. Effect of time of food administration on the bioavailability of didanosine from a chewable tablet formulation. *J Clin Pharmacol.* 1993;33:568.

Didanosine (eg, *Videx*)

Ganciclovir (*Cytovene*)

SUMMARY: Didanosine concentrations are increased during coadministration with ganciclovir; didanosine toxicity could occur in some patients.

RISK FACTORS: No specific risk factors are known.

RELATED DRUGS: No information is available.

MANAGEMENT OPTIONS:

➥ *Monitor.* Until further information regarding this interaction is available, monitor patients receiving didanosine carefully for toxicity, including peripheral neuropathy and pancreatitis, if ganciclovir is added.

REFERENCES:

Trapnell MD, et al. Altered didanosine pharmacokinetics with concomitant oral ganciclovir. *Clin Pharmacol Ther*. 1994;55:193.

Didanosine (eg, *Videx*)

Indinavir (*Crixivan*)

SUMMARY: Indinavir absorption can be reduced by coadministration of buffered didanosine; reduced antiviral efficacy is likely.

RISK FACTORS: No specific risk factors are known.

RELATED DRUGS: Other drugs that alkalinize the stomach will likely affect indinavir in a similar manner.

MANAGEMENT OPTIONS:

➥ *Circumvent/Minimize.* Administration of didanosine at least 1 hour before indinavir will minimize this interaction. Alternatively, the indinavir could be administered 2 hours prior to the didanosine. An enteric coated formulation of didanosine without buffers (*Videx EC*) does not affect indinavir absorption.

➥ *Monitor.* If indinavir and buffered didanosine are coadministered, watch the patient for reduced indinavir plasma concentrations or antiviral activity.

REFERENCES:

Product information. Didanosine (*Videx*). Bristol-Myers Squibb Company. 2000.

Shelton MJ, et al. If taken 1 hour before indinavir (IDV), didanosine does not affect IDV exposure, despite persistent buffering effects. *Antimicrob Agents Chemother*. 2001;45:298-300.

Damle BD, et al. Lack of effect of simultaneously administered didanosine encapsulated enteric bead formulation (*Videx EC*) on oral absorption of indinavir, ketoconazole, or ciprofloxacin. *Antimicrob Agents Chemother*. 2002;46:385-391.

Didanosine (eg, *Videx*)

Itraconazole (*Sporanox*)

SUMMARY: Didanosine administration can significantly reduce the absorption of itraconazole; loss of antifungal efficacy may result.

RISK FACTORS: No specific risk factors are known.

RELATED DRUGS: A similar effect of buffered didanosine on ketoconazole (eg, *Nizoral*) would be expected. Other drugs that alkalinize the stomach will affect itraconazole in a similar manner. Fluconazole (*Diflucan*) and voriconazole (*Vfend*) absorption does not appear to be affected by alkalinization of the stomach.

MANAGEMENT OPTIONS:

➡ *Circumvent/Minimize.* Administration of itraconazole at least 2 hours before didanosine will minimize this interaction. An enteric coated formulation of didanosine without buffers (*Videx EC*) would be unlikely to affect itraconazole absorption. Consider using an alternative antifungal such as fluconazole or voriconazole.

➡ *Monitor.* If itraconazole- and didanosine-containing buffers are coadministered, watch the patient for loss of antifungal activity.

REFERENCES:

May DB, et al. Effect of simultaneous didanosine administration on itraconazole absorption in healthy volunteers. *Pharmacotherapy.* 1994;14:509-518.

Moreno F, et al. Itraconazole-didanosine excipient interaction. *JAMA.* 1993;269:1508.

Damle BD, et al. Lack of effect of simultaneously administered didanosine encapsulated enteric bead formulation (*Videx EC*) on oral absorption of indinavir, ketoconazole, or ciprofloxacin. *Antimicrob Agents Chemother.* 2002;46:385-391.

Didanosine (eg, *Videx*)

Ketoconazole (eg, *Nizoral*)

SUMMARY: Didanosine administration can significantly reduce the absorption of ketoconazole; loss of antifungal efficacy may result.

RISK FACTORS: No specific risk factors are known.

RELATED DRUGS: Buffered didanosine has been reported to reduce the absorption of itraconazole (*Sporanox*). Other drugs that alkalinize the stomach will affect ketoconazole in a similar manner. Fluconazole (*Diflucan*) and voriconazole (*Vfend*) absorption does not appear to be affected by alkalinization of the stomach.

MANAGEMENT OPTIONS:

➡ *Circumvent/Minimize.* Administration of ketoconazole at least 2 hours before didanosine will minimize this interaction. An enteric coated formulation of didanosine without buffers (*Videx EC*) would be unlikely to affect ketoconazole absorption. Consider using an alternative antifungal such as fluconazole or voriconazole.

➡ **Monitor.** If ketoconazole and buffered didanosine are coadministered, watch the patient for loss of antifungal activity.

REFERENCES:

Knupp CA, et al. Pharmacokinetics of didanosine and ketoconazole after coadministration to patients seropositive for the human immunodeficiency virus. *J Clin Pharmacol.* 1993;33:912-917.

Damle BD, et al. Lack of effect of simultaneously administered didanosine encapsulated enteric bead formulation (*Videx EC*) on oral absorption of indinavir, ketoconazole, or ciprofloxacin. *Antimicrob Agents Chemother.* 2002;46:385-391.

Diflunisal (eg, *Dolobid*)
Warfarin (eg, *Coumadin*)

SUMMARY: Limited data indicate the diflunisal may enhance the hypoprothrombinemic response to oral anticoagulants in some patients; caution during cotherapy with these drugs also is required because of the detrimental effects of diflunisal on the gastric mucosa and platelet function.

RISK FACTORS:

➡ **Concurrent Diseases.** Patients with peptic ulcer disease or a history of gastrointestinal (GI) bleeding are probably at greater risk.

RELATED DRUGS: All NSAIDs inhibit platelet function, cause gastric erosions, and probably increase the risk of GI bleeding. Some NSAIDs, however, such as ibuprofen (eg, *Advil*), naproxen (eg, *Naprosyn*), or may be less likely to increase oral anticoagulant-induced hypoprothrombinemia than other NSAIDs. Acenocoumarol appears to interact with diflunisal similarly.

MANAGEMENT OPTIONS:

➡ **Avoid Unless Benefit Outweighs Risk.** Since all NSAIDs probably increase the risk of GI bleeding in patients on oral anticoagulants, use the combination only after careful consideration of the benefit versus risk. If an NSAID must be used with an oral anticoagulant, it would be prudent to use NSAIDs that are unlikely to affect the hypoprothrombinemic response to oral anticoagulants (see Related Drugs). If the NSAID is being used as an analgesic or antipyretic, acetaminophen is probably safer to use with oral anticoagulants. Nonacetylated salicylates (eg, choline salicylate, magnesium salicylate, salsalate, sodium salicylate) are probably also safer with oral anti coagulants than NSAIDs, since such salicylates have minimal effects on platelet function and the gastric mucosa.

➡ **Monitor.** If any NSAID is used with an oral anticoagulant, carefully monitor the prothrombin time and watch for evidence of bleeding, especially from the GI tract.

REFERENCES:

Serlin MJ, et al. Interaction between diflunisal and warfarin. *Clin Pharmacol Ther.* 1980;28:493.

Tempero KF, et al. Diflunisal. A review of pharmacokinetic and pharmacodynamic properties, drug interactions and special tolerability studies in humans. *Br J Clin Pharmacol.* 1977;4:31S.

Davies RO. Review of the animal and clinical pharmacology of diflunisal. *Pharmacotherapy.* 1983;2(Suppl. 1):9S.

Rider JA. Comparison of fecal blood loss after use of aspirin and diflunisal. *Pharmacotherapy.* 1983;3(Suppl. 1):61S.

Green D, et al. Effects of diflunisal on platelet function and fetal blood loss. *Clin Pharmacol Ther.* 1981;30:378.

Petrillo M. Diflunisal, aspirin, and gastric mucosa. *Lancet.* 1979;2:638.

Ghosh ML, et al. Platelet aggregation in patients treated with diflunisal. *Curr Med Res Opin.* 1980;6:510.

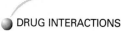

Admani AK, et al. Gastrointestinal haemorrhage associated with diflunisal. *Lancet*. 1979;1:1247.

Shorr RI, et al. Concurrent use of nonsteroidal anti-inflammatory drugs and oral anticoagulants places elderly persons at high risk for hemorrhagic peptic ulcer disease. *Arch Intern Med*. 1993;153:1665.

 Digitoxin†

Phenobarbital (eg, *Solfoton*)

SUMMARY: Phenobarbital administration may reduce digitoxin serum concentrations, but it is unknown how often this decreases the therapeutic response to digitoxin.

RISK FACTORS: No specific risk factors are known.

RELATED DRUGS: Digoxin (eg, *Lanoxin*) elimination is not likely to be affected by barbiturates to the same degree as digitoxin since it primarily is excreted renally.

MANAGEMENT OPTIONS:

➡ *Consider Alternative.* Digoxin would seem less likely to be affected by enzyme induction and may be preferable to digitoxin in patients taking chronic phenobarbital or other barbiturates.

➡ *Monitor.* Until further information is available, evaluate patients receiving digitoxin and a barbiturate for underdigitalization, and increase the digitoxin dose if necessary.

REFERENCES:

Jelliffe RW, et al. Effect of phenobarbital on digitoxin metabolism. *Clin Res*. 1966;14:160.

Solomon HM, et al. Interactions between digitoxin and other drugs in man. *Am Heart J*. 1972;83:277.

Kaldor A, et al. Interaction of heart glycosides and phenobarbital. *Int J Clin Pharmacol*. 1975;12:403.

† Not available in the US.

 Digitoxin†

Rifampin (eg, *Rifadin*)

SUMMARY: Rifampin reduces the serum concentration of digoxin and digitoxin.

RISK FACTORS: No specific risk factors are known.

RELATED DRUGS: Digoxin (eg, *Lanoxin*) is affected similarly by rifampin.

MANAGEMENT OPTIONS:

➡ *Circumvent/Minimize.* Dosage adjustments of digitalis glycosides (especially digitoxin) likely will be necessary when rifampin is added to or removed from a patient's regimen.

➡ *Monitor.* When rifampin and digitalis glycosides are used concomitantly, be alert for reduced digoxin and digitoxin efficacy.

REFERENCES:

Zilly W, et al. Pharmacokinetic interactions with rifampicin. *Clin Pharmacokinet*. 1977;2:61.

Boman G, et al. Acute cardiac failure during treatment with digitoxin, an interaction with rifampicin. *Br J Clin Pharmacol*. 1980;10:89.

Poor DM, et al. Interaction of rifampin and digitoxin. *Arch Intern Med*. 1983;143:599.

Gault H, et al. Digoxin-rifampin interaction. *Clin Pharmacol Ther*. 1984;35:750.

Novi C, et al. Rifampin and digoxin: possible drug interaction in a dialysis patient. *JAMA*. 1980;244:2521.

† Not available in the US.

Digoxin (eg, *Lanoxin*)

Diltiazem (eg, *Cardizem*)

SUMMARY: Diltiazem increases digoxin serum concentrations; digoxin toxicity may result.

RISK FACTORS: No specific risk factors are known.

RELATED DRUGS: Verapamil (eg, *Calan*), bepridil (*Vascor*), and nitrendipine (*Baypress*) appear to reduce digoxin elimination. Digitoxin (*Crystodigin*) is likely to be affected similarly. Nifedipine (eg, *Procardia*), isradipine (*DynaCirc*), nicardipine (eg, *Cardene*), felodipine (*Plendil*), and amlodipine (*Norvasc*) do not appear to increase digoxin concentration.

MANAGEMENT OPTIONS:

➡ ***Consider Alternative.*** Nifedipine, isradipine, nicardipine, felodipine, and amlodipine do not appear to increase digoxin concentration and may be possible alternatives.

➡ ***Circumvent/Minimize.*** Digoxin dosages may need to be reduced when diltiazem is added to a patient stabilized on digoxin.

➡ ***Monitor.*** Monitor patients for evidence of increased serum digitalis effects (eg, bradycardia, heart block, gastrointestinal upset, mental changes) in the presence of calcium channel blocker therapy.

REFERENCES:

Belz GG, et al. Digoxin plasma concentrations and nifedipine. *Lancet.* 1981;1:844.

Rameis H, et al. The diltiazem-digoxin interaction. *Clin Pharmacol Ther.* 1984;36:183.

Clarke WR, et al. Potentially serious drug interactions secondary to high-dose diltiazem used in the treatment of pulmonary hypertension. *Pharmacotherapy.* 1993;13:402.

Kuhlmann J. Effects of nifedipine and diltiazem on plasma levels and renal excretion of beta-acetyldigoxin. *Clin Pharmacol Ther.* 1985;37:150.

Schwartz JB, et al. Effect of nifedipine on serum digoxin concentration and renal digoxin clearance. *Clin Pharmacol Ther.* 1984;36:19.

Kirch W, et al. The felodipine/digoxin interaction. A placebo-controlled study in patients with heart failure. *Br J Clin Pharmacol.* 1988;26:644P.

Schwartz JB. Effects of amlodipine on steady-state digoxin concentrations and renal digoxin clearance. *J Cardiovasc Pharmacol.* 1988;12:1.

Hutt HJ, et al. Dose-dependence of the nifedipine/digoxin interaction? *Arch Toxicol.* 1986;9(Suppl.):209.

Boden WE, et al. No increase in serum digoxin concentration with high-dose diltiazem. *Am J Med.* 1986;81:425.

Andrejak M, et al. Diltiazem increases steady state digoxin serum levels in patients with cardiac disease. *J Clin Pharmacol.* 1987;27:967.

Rodin SM, et al. Comparative effects of verapamil and isradipine on steady-state digoxin kinetics. *Clin Pharmacol Ther.* 1988;43:668.

Debruyne D, et al. Nicardipine does not significantly affect serum digoxin concentrations at the steady state of patients with congestive heart failure. *Int J Clin Pharmacol.* 1989;9:15.

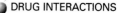

 Digoxin (eg, *Lanoxin*)

Erythromycin (eg, *E-Mycin*)

SUMMARY: Erythromycin administration increases the plasma concentration of digoxin. Digoxin toxicity, including nausea, malaise, visual changes, and arrhythmias, may occur.

RISK FACTORS: No specific risk factors are known.

RELATED DRUGS: Digitoxin[†] is likely affected in a similar manner by erythromycin. Clarithromycin also increases digoxin plasma concentrations. There is little data on the effect of other macrolides on digoxin.

MANAGEMENT OPTIONS:

➡ ***Consider Alternative.*** Select an antibiotic known to have no effect on digoxin concentrations in patients receiving chronic digoxin therapy. If azithromycin (*Zithromax*) or dirithromycin (*Dynabac*) are used, monitor for changes in digoxin concentrations.

➡ ***Monitor.*** In patients receiving digoxin, monitor for changes in digoxin concentrations when erythromycin is added or removed from the drug regimen.

REFERENCES:

Doherty JE. A digoxin-antibiotic drug interaction. *N Engl J Med.* 1981;305:827-828.

Morton MR, et al. Erythromycin-induced digoxin toxicity. *DICP.* 1989;23:668-670.

Marik PE, et al. A case series of hospitalized patients with elevated digoxin levels. *Am J Med.* 1998;105:110-115.

Sutton A, et al. Digoxin toxicity and erythromycin. *BMJ.* 1989;298:1101.

Maxwell DL, et al. Digoxin toxicity due to interaction of digoxin with erythromycin. *BMJ.* 1989;298:572.

Rengelshausen J, et al. Contribution of increased oral bioavailability and reduced nonglomerular renal clearance of digoxin to the digoxin-clarithromycin interaction. *Br J Clin Pharmacol.* 2003;56:32-38.

† Not available in the United States.

 Digoxin (eg, *Lanoxin*)

Furosemide (eg, *Lasix*)

SUMMARY: Diuretic-induced hypokalemia may increase the risk of digitalis toxicity.

RISK FACTORS: No specific risk factors are known.

RELATED DRUGS: Ethacrynic acid (*Edecrin*), bumetanide (eg, *Bumex*), chlorthalidone (eg, *Hygroton*), metolazone (eg, *Zaroxolyn*), and thiazides interact similarly. Torsemide (*Demadex*) may produce a similar increased risk of digoxin toxicity. Patients taking digitoxin[†] also would be at risk.

MANAGEMENT OPTIONS:

➡ ***Consider Alternative.*** Potassium-sparing diuretics can be considered as alternatives to potassium-wasting agents; however, note the interactions with amiloride (*Midamor*) and spironolactone (eg, *Aldactone*).

➡ ***Monitor.*** Monitor the potassium and magnesium status of patients on concomitant diuretic-digitalis therapy. Undertake replacement potassium or magnesium therapy if needed. Be alert for increased digoxin effects.

REFERENCES:

Steiness E. Suppression of renal excretion of digoxin in hypokalemic patients. *Clin Pharmacol Ther.* 1978;23:511-514.

Tsutsumi E, et al. Effect of furosemide on serum clearance and renal excretion of digoxin. *J Clin Pharmacol.* 1979;19:200-204.

Beller GA, et al. Correlation of serum magnesium levels and cardiac digitalis intoxication. *Am J Cardiol.* 1974;33:225-229.

Young IS, et al. Magnesium status and digoxin toxicity. *Br J Clin Pharmacol.* 1991;32:717-721.

Seller RH, et al. Digitalis toxicity and hypomagnesemia. *Am Heart J.* 1970;79:57-68.

Steiness E, et al. Cardiac arrhythmias induced by hypokalaemia and potassium loss during maintenance digoxin therapy. *Br Heart J.* 1976;38:167-172.

McAllister RG, et al. Effect of intravenous furosemide on the renal excretion of digoxin. *J Clin Pharmacol.* 1976;16:110-117.

Malcolm AD, et al. Digoxin kinetics during furosemide administration. *Clin Pharmacol Ther.* 1977;21:567-574.

† Not available in the United States.

Digoxin (eg, *Lanoxin*)

Hydroxychloroquine (eg, *Plaquenil*)

SUMMARY: Hydroxychloroquine may increase serum digoxin concentrations, but the degree to which this increases the risk of digoxin toxicity is unknown.

RISK FACTORS: No specific risk factors are known.

RELATED DRUGS: No information is available.

MANAGEMENT OPTIONS:

➡ ***Monitor.*** Monitor digoxin concentration and patients observed for toxicity (eg, nausea, arrhythmia) when hydroxychloroquine is started in a patient receiving digoxin. Digoxin dosage may need to be altered.

REFERENCES:

Leden I. Digoxin-hydroxychloroquine interaction? *Acta Med Scand.* 1982;211:411-412.

Digoxin (eg, *Lanoxin*)

Itraconazole (*Sporanox*)

SUMMARY: Itraconazole administration can result in elevated digoxin concentrations and symptoms of digoxin toxicity, including nausea, malaise, visual changes, and arrhythmias.

RISK FACTORS: No specific risk factors are known.

RELATED DRUGS: Ketoconazole (eg, *Nizoral*) is known to be an inhibitor of p-glycoprotein and would be expected to affect digoxin in a similar manner. It is likely that digitoxin† concentrations would also be increased by itraconazole administration. Voriconazole (*Vfend*) does not appear to alter digoxin plasma concentrations.

MANAGEMENT OPTIONS:

➥ *Consider Alternative.* Voriconazole does not affect digoxin concentrations and can be considered as an alternative.

➥ *Monitor.* Monitor patients stabilized on digoxin for changing digoxin concentrations and evidence of digoxin response if itraconazole is initiated, changed in dose, or discontinued from the regime.

REFERENCES:

Partanen J, et al. Itraconazole increases serum digoxin concentrations. *Pharmacol Toxicol.* 1996;79:274-276.

Jalava KM, et al. Itraconazole decreases renal clearance of digoxin. *Ther Drug Monit.* 1997;19:609-613.

Sachs MK, et al. Interaction of itraconazole and digoxin. *Clin Infect Dis.* 1993;16:400-403.

Alderman CP, et al. Digoxin-itraconazole interaction: possible mechanisms. *Ann Pharmacother.* 1997;31:438-440.

Lopez F, et al. Nausea and malaise during treatment of coccidioimycosis. *Hosp Pract.* 1997;32:21-22.

† Not available in the United States.

 Digoxin (eg, *Lanoxin*)

Kaolin-Pectin

SUMMARY: Kaolin-pectin appears to reduce the bioavailability of digoxin tablets, but digoxin capsules do not appear to be affected.

RISK FACTORS:

➥ *Dosage Form.* Digoxin tablets (but not capsules) appear to be affected by kaolin-pectin.

RELATED DRUGS: Kaolin-pectin may be expected to affect digitoxin† in a similar manner.

MANAGEMENT OPTIONS:

➥ *Circumvent/Minimize.* Administer digoxin 2 hours before the kaolin-pectin to minimize the interaction. The use of digoxin capsules may help minimize the interaction.

➥ *Monitor.* Monitor patients receiving digoxin and kaolin-pectin for reduced digoxin concentrations and effect.

REFERENCES:

Brown DD, et al. Decreased bioavailability of digoxin due to antacids and kaolin-pectin. *N Engl J Med.* 1976;295:1034-1037.

Albert KS, et al. Influence of kaolin-pectin suspension on digoxin bioavailability. *J Pharm Sci.* 1978;67:1582-1586.

Albert KS, et al. Influence of kaolin-pectin suspension on steady-state plasma digoxin levels. *J Clin Pharmacol.* 1981;21:449-455.

Allen MD, et al. Effect of magnesium-aluminum hydroxide and kaolin-pectin on absorption of digoxin from tablets and capsules. *J Clin Pharmacol.* 1981;21:26-30.

† Not available in the United States.

Digoxin (eg, *Lanoxin*)

Metoclopramide (eg, *Reglan*)

SUMMARY: Metoclopramide reduces the serum digoxin concentration when it is coadministered with slowly dissolving digoxin tablets.

RISK FACTORS:

➡ ***Dosage Form.*** Patients taking slow dissolving digoxin preparations will be at increased risk of this interaction.

RELATED DRUGS: Other drugs that increase GI motility (eg, cisapride [*Propulsid*]) also may affect digoxin absorption from slowly dissolving formulations.

MANAGEMENT OPTIONS:

➡ ***Monitor.*** In patients receiving chronic digoxin therapy, the addition of metoclopramide (or other drugs increasing GI motility) may result in decreased digoxin effect. The interaction probably can be minimized by using rapidly dissolving preparations such as Lanoxin tablets or digoxin capsules (eg, *Lanoxicaps*).

REFERENCES:

Johnson BF, et al. The influence of digoxin particle size on absorption of digoxin and the effect of propantheline and metoclopramide. *Br J Clin Pharmacol.* 1978;5:465.

Manninen V, et al. Altered absorption of digoxin in patients given propantheline and metoclopramide. *Lancet.* 1973;1:398.

Kirch W, et al. Effect of cisapride and metoclopramide on digoxin bioavailability. *Eur J Drug Metab Pharmacokin.* 1986;11:249.

Johnson BF, et al. Effect of metoclopramide on digoxin absorption from tablets and capsules. *Clin Pharmacol Ther.* 1984;36:745.

Digoxin (eg, *Lanoxin*)

Mibefradil

SUMMARY: Mibefradil produces a dose-dependent increase in digoxin concentrations; increased digoxin side effects may occur at high mibefradil doses.

RISK FACTORS:

➡ ***Dosage Regimen.*** Mibefradil doses greater than 100 mg/day may increase the risk of interaction.

RELATED DRUGS: Other calcium channel blockers including verapamil (eg, *Calan*) and diltiazem (eg, *Cardizem*) are known to increase digoxin concentrations and may produce similar effects on cardiac conduction.

MANAGEMENT OPTIONS:

➡ ***Monitor.*** Observe patients taking digoxin and mibefradil, particularly if mibefradil doses exceed 100 mg/day, for evidence of increased digoxin concentrations or heart block.

REFERENCES:

Siepmann M, et al. The interaction of the calcium antagonist RO 40–5967 with digoxin. *Br J Clin Pharmacol.* 1995;39:491.

Digoxin (eg, *Lanoxin*)

Nefazodone (*Serzone*)

SUMMARY: Nefazodone produces a modest increase in digoxin serum concentrations; some patients may experience an increase in digoxin side effects.

RISK FACTORS: No specific risk factors are known.

RELATED DRUGS: It is unknown if other antidepressants that inhibit serotonin uptake affect digoxin serum concentrations.

MANAGEMENT OPTIONS:

➡ ***Monitor.*** Monitor patients stabilized on digoxin for increased digoxin side effects or serum concentrations following the addition of nefazodone. Because of digoxin's long half-life, 5 to 10 days may be required to reach a new steady-state digoxin concentration following the addition of nefazodone.

REFERENCES:
Dockens RC, et al. Assessment of pharmacokinetic and pharmacodynamic drug interactions between nefazodone and digoxin in healthy male volunteers. *J Clin Pharmacol.* 1996;36:160-67.

 ## Digoxin (eg, *Lanoxin*)

Neomycin (eg, *Neo-Tabs*)

SUMMARY: Neomycin reduces digoxin serum concentrations.

RISK FACTORS: No specific risk factors are known.

RELATED DRUGS: The potential for other orally administered aminoglycosides to inhibit digoxin absorption is unknown.

MANAGEMENT OPTIONS:

➡ ***Circumvent/Minimize.*** Administration of digoxin IV will avoid the interaction.

➡ ***Monitor.*** Since separating the doses of digoxin and antibiotic will not avoid the interaction, monitor patients receiving both drugs for reduced digoxin effect and serum concentrations.

REFERENCES:
Lindenbaum J, et al. Inhibition of digoxin absorption by neomycin. *Gastroenterology.* 1976;71:399.

 ## Digoxin (eg, *Lanoxin*)

Omeprazole (*Prilosec*)

SUMMARY: Omeprazole increases the serum concentration of digoxin. Digoxin effects may be increased, but the clinical importance is not established.

RISK FACTORS: No specific risk factors are known.

RELATED DRUGS: Pentagastrin may reduce digoxin response. Lansoprazole (*Prevacid*) may produce similar effects on digoxin.

MANAGEMENT OPTIONS:

➡ *Monitor.* Until further information is available, monitor patients receiving digoxin for elevated digoxin concentrations and symptoms of toxicity if omeprazole is added and diminished effect if omeprazole is deleted from their regimen.

REFERENCES:

Cohen AF, et al. Influence of gastric acidity on the bioavailability of digoxin. *Ann Intern Med.* 1991;115:540.

Cohen AF, et al. Effects of gastric acidity on the bioavailability of digoxin. Evidence for a new mechanism for interactions with omeprazole. *Br J Clin Pharmacol.* 1991;31:565P.

Oosterhuis B, et al. Minor effect of multiple dose omeprazole on the pharmacokinetics of digoxin after a single oral dose. *Br J Clin Pharmacol.* 1991;32:569.

Digoxin (eg, *Lanoxin*)

Penicillamine (eg, *Cuprimine*)

SUMMARY: Penicillamine has been reported to reduce digoxin serum concentrations, but the clinical importance of the effect is not established.

RISK FACTORS: No specific risk factors are known.

RELATED DRUGS: No information is available.

MANAGEMENT OPTIONS:

➡ *Monitor.* Monitor patients for evidence of reduced digoxin concentration and effect when penicillamine is initiated. Adjust the digoxin dosage as necessary.

REFERENCES:

Moezzi B, et al. The effect of penicillamine on serum digoxin levels. *Jpn Heart J.* 1978;19:366.

Digoxin (eg, *Lanoxin*)

Propafenone (*Rythmol*)

SUMMARY: Propafenone increases digoxin serum concentrations and potentially can cause toxicity.

RISK FACTORS: No specific risk factors are known.

RELATED DRUGS: A similar effect may be seen with digitoxin (*Crystodigin*) but data are lacking.

MANAGEMENT OPTIONS:

➡ *Circumvent/Minimize.* The digoxin dosage may need to be reduced during propafenone coadministration.

➡ *Monitor.* Since propafenone may increase digoxin serum concentrations by 30% to 60%, some patients maintained on digoxin could develop toxicity following its addition. Monitor digoxin concentrations and response when propafenone is initiated or discontinued in a patient taking digoxin.

REFERENCES:

Salerno DM, et al. Controlled trial of propafenone for treatment of frequent and repetitive ventricular premature complexes. *Am J Cardiol.* 1984;53:77.

Nolan PE, et al. Effects of co-administration of propafenone on the pharmacokinetics of digoxin in healthy volunteer subjects. *J Clin Pharmacol.* 1989;29:46.

Cardaioli P, et al. Influence of propafenone on the pharmacokinetics of digoxin administered by the oral route:study on healthy volunteers. *G Ital Cardiol*. 1986;16:247.

Belz GG, et al. Interaction between digoxin and calcium antagonists and antiarrhythmic drugs. *Clin Pharmacol Ther*. 1983;33:410.

Hodges M, et al. Double-blind placebo-controlled evaluation of propafenone in suppressing ventricular ectopic activity. *Am J Cardiol*. 1984;54:45.

Calvo MV, et al. Interaction between digoxin and propafenone. *Ther Drug Monit*. 1989;11:10.

Bigot MC, et al. Serum digoxin levels related to plasma propafenone levels during concomitant treatment. *J Clin Pharmacol*. 1991;31:521.

Zalzstein E, et al. Interaction between digoxin and propafenone in children. *J Pediatr*. 1990;116:310.

Digoxin (eg, *Lanoxin*)

Propranolol (eg, *Inderal*)

SUMMARY: Bradycardia may be potentiated by the combination of digoxin and propranolol.

RISK FACTORS:

➡ **Concurrent Diseases.** Patients with concomitant myocardial conduction delays or those with renal dysfunction may be at greater risk.

RELATED DRUGS: Most beta-blockers would be expected to have the potential for bradycardia when used with digoxin. Although specific data are lacking, beta-blockers with partial agonist activity may be less likely to produce bradycardia at rest. A similar interaction would be expected with digitoxin.

MANAGEMENT OPTIONS:

➡ **Monitor.** Monitor patients receiving beta-blockers and digoxin for reduced heart rate and the occurrence of arrhythmias.

REFERENCES:

LeWinter MM, Crawford MH, O'Rourke RA, Karliner JS. The effects of oral propranolol, digoxin and combination therapy on the resting and exercise electrocardiogram. *Am Heart J*. 1977;93:202-209.

Kochiadakis GE, Kanoupakis EM, Kalebubas MD, et al. Sotalol vs metoprolol for ventricular rate control in patients with chronic atrial fibrillation who have undergone digitalization: a single-blinded crossover study. *Europace*. 2001;3:73-79.

Klein L, O'Connor CM, Gattis WA, et al. Pharmacologic therapy for patients with chronic heart failure and reduced systolic function: review of trials and practical considerations. *Am J Cardiol*. 2003;91:18F-40F.

Foody JM, Farrell MH, Krumholz HM. Beta-blocker therapy in heart failure: scientific review. *JAMA*. 2002;287:883-889.

Digoxin (eg, *Lanoxin*)

Quinidine

SUMMARY: Quinidine increases the serum concentration of digoxin and digitoxin sufficiently to lead to digitalis toxicity in some patients.

RISK FACTORS:

➡ **Dosage Regimen.** Quinidine doses above 500 mg/day may increase digoxin serum concentration.

RELATED DRUGS: The effect of quinidine on digitoxin disposition has been disputed, but the bulk of the evidence indicates that quinidine does increase serum digitoxin concentrations to a clinically significant degree. Quinidine appears to reduce digitoxin nonrenal clearance but causes less change in its renal clearance and no change in the volume of distribution of digitoxin.

MANAGEMENT OPTIONS:

➡ *Circumvent/Minimize.* A reduction in digoxin dose when quinidine is started will reduce the likelihood of digoxin toxicity. However, because the magnitude of the interaction varies considerably from patient to patient, further adjustments in digoxin dose are likely to be necessary.

➡ *Monitor.* During the first 7 to 10 days of combined therapy, monitor the patient carefully for symptoms and electrocardiogram evidence of digoxin toxicity. In general, these precautions also would apply to the concurrent use of quinidine and digitoxin, although it may take longer to achieve a new steady-state serum digitoxin level after starting quinidine therapy.

REFERENCES:

Angelin B, Arvidsson A, Dahlqvist R, Hedman A, Schenck-Gustafsson K. Quinidine reduces biliary clearance of digoxin in man. *Eur J Clin Invest.* 1987;17:262-265.

Fenster PE, Hager WD, Perrier D, Powell JR, Graves PE, Michael VF. Digoxin-quinidine interaction in patients with chronic renal failure. *Circulation.* 1982;66:1277-1280.

Mungall DR, Robichaux RP, Perry W, et al. Effects of quinidine on serum digoxin concentration. *Ann Intern Med.* 1980;93:689.

Leahey EB, Bigger JT, Butler VP, et al. Quinidine-digoxin interaction: time course and pharmacokinetics. *Am J Cardiol.* 1981;48:1141-1146.

Ochs HR, Bodem G, Greenblatt DJ, et al. Impairment of digoxin clearance by co-administration of quinidine. *J Clin Pharmacol.* 1981;21:396-400.

Belz GG, Doering W, Aust PE, Heinz M, Matthews J, Schneider B. Quinidine-digoxin interaction: cardiac efficacy of elevated serum digoxin concentration. *Clin Pharmacol Ther.* 1982;31:548-554.

Schenck-Gustafsson K, Jogestrand T, Nordlander R, Dahlqvist R. Effect of quinidine on digoxin concentration in skeletal muscle and serum in patients with atrial fibrillation. *N Engl J Med.* 1981;305:209-211.

Williams JF, Mathew B. Effect of quinidine on positive inotropic action of digoxin. *Am J Cardiol.* 1981;47:1052-1055.

Pedersen KE, Christiansen BD, Klitgaard NA, Nielsen-Kudsk F. Effect of quinidine on digoxin bioavailability. *Eur J Clin Pharmacol.* 1983;24:41-47.

Schenck-Gustafsson K, Dahlqvist R. Pharmacokinetics of digoxin in patients subjected to the quinidine-digoxin interaction. *Br J Clin Pharmacol.* 1981;11:181-186.

Ochs HR, Pabst J, Greenblatt DJ, Dengler HJ. Noninteraction of digitoxin and quinidine. *N Engl J Med.* 1980;303:672-674.

Kuhlmann J, Dohrmann M, Marcin S. Effects of quinidine on pharmacokinetics and pharmacodynamics of digitoxin achieving steady-state conditions. *Clin Pharmacol Ther.* 1986;39:288-294.

Kuhlmann J. Effects of quinidine, verapamil and nifedipine on the pharmacokinetics and pharmacodynamics of digitoxin during steady state conditions. *Arzneimittelforschung.* 1987;37:545-548.

Digoxin (eg, *Lanoxin*)

Quinine

SUMMARY: Quinine potentially could increase digoxin concentrations, particularly when it is administered in high doses.

RISK FACTORS:

➡ *Dosage Regimen.* Quinine doses of greater than or equal to 600 mg/day could increase digoxin concentrations.

RELATED DRUGS: Digitoxin also may be affected by large doses of quinine.

MANAGEMENT OPTIONS:

➡ **Monitor.** No digoxin dosage adjustment is likely to be required when quinine is administered in low doses. If large quinine doses are administered, monitor the patient for increased digoxin concentrations and signs of digoxin toxicity (eg, nausea, anorexia, arrhythmia).

REFERENCES:
Wandell M, Powell JR, Hager WD, et al. Effect of quinine on digoxin kinetics. *Clin Pharmacol Ther.* 1980;28:425-430.

Digoxin (eg, *Lanoxin*)

Ritonavir (*Norvir*)

SUMMARY: Ritonavir appears to increase serum digoxin concentrations; digoxin toxicity may occur.

RISK FACTORS: No specific risk factors are known.

RELATED DRUGS: Digitoxin is likely to be affected in a similar manner by ritonavir. The effect of other protease inhibitors on digoxin is unknown. However, indinavir (*Crixivan*) did not appear to affect digoxin elimination in this patient.

MANAGEMENT OPTIONS:

➡ **Monitor.** Pending further data regarding this interaction, monitor patients stabilized on digoxin for altered serum concentrations if ritonavir is added or removed from the drug regimen.

REFERENCES:
Phillips EJ, Rachlis AR, Ito S. Digoxin toxicity and ritonavir: a drug interaction mediated through p-glycoprotein? *AIDS.* 2003;17:1577-1578.

Digoxin (eg, *Lanoxin*)

Spironolactone (eg, *Aldactone*)

SUMMARY: Substantial evidence indicates that spironolactone may interfere with certain serum digoxin assays. More limited evidence suggests that spironolactone may produce a true increase in serum digoxin concentrations.

RISK FACTORS: No specific risk factors are known.

RELATED DRUGS: No information is available.

MANAGEMENT OPTIONS:

➡ **Monitor.** In patients receiving digoxin and spironolactone, monitor the digoxin response by means other than serum digoxin concentrations, unless the digoxin assay used has been proven not to be affected by spironolactone therapy. Because there is some evidence that spironolactone may produce a small increase in serum digoxin concentration, watch for evidence of enhanced digoxin effect, such as nausea or arrhythmia.

REFERENCES:
Thomas RW, et al. The interaction of spironolactone and digoxin: a review and evaluation. *Ther Drug Monit.* 1981;3:117.

Hedman A, et al. Digoxin-interactions in man: spironolactone reduced renal but not biliary digoxin clearance. *Eur J Clin Pharmacol.* 1992;42:481.

Morris RG, et al. Spironolactone as a source of interference in commercial digoxin immunoassays. *Ther Drug Monit.* 1987;9:208.

Steiness E. Renal tubular secretion of digoxin. *Circulation.* 1974;50:103.

Waldorff S, et al. Spironolactone-induced changes in digoxin kinetics. *Clin Pharmacol Ther.* 1978;24:162.

DiPiro JT, et al. Spironolactone interference with digoxin radioimmunoassay in cirrhotic patients. *Am J Hosp Pharm.* 1980;37:1518.

Silber B, et al. Spironolactone-associated digoxin radioimmunoassay interference. *Clin Chem.* 1979;25:48.

Muller H, et al. Cross reactivity of digitoxin and spironolactone in two radioimmunoassays for serum digoxin. *Clin Chem.* 1978;24:706.

Paladino JA, et al. Influence of spironolactone on serum digoxin concentration. *JAMA.* 1984;251:470.

Morris RG, et al. The effect of renal and hepatic impairment and of spironolactone on digoxin immunoassays. *Eur J Clin Pharmacol.* 1988;34:233.

Digoxin (eg, *Lanoxin*)

St. John's Wort

SUMMARY: The main component of St. John's wort, hypericum extract, appeared to reduce digoxin plasma concentrations. A reduction in digoxin effect may occur in some patients.

RISK FACTORS: No specific risk factors are known.

RELATED DRUGS: The effect of hypericum extract on digitoxin (*Crystodigin*) is unknown, but hypericum would be expected to produce some reduction in digitoxin concentrations.

MANAGEMENT OPTIONS:

➡ *Monitor.* Monitor patients stabilized on digoxin for changing digoxin plasma concentrations if St. John's wort is added to or removed from their daily drug regimen.

REFERENCES:
Johne A, et al. Pharmacokinetic interaction of digoxin with an herbal extract from St. John's wort (*hypericum perforatum*). *Clin Pharmacol Ther.* 1999;66:338-45.

Digoxin (eg, *Lanoxin*)

Succinylcholine (eg, *Anectine*)

SUMMARY: The administration of succinylcholine to digitalized patients may increase the risk of arrhythmias.

RISK FACTORS: No specific risk factors are known.

RELATED DRUGS: No information is available.

MANAGEMENT OPTIONS:

➡ *Monitor.* Cautiously use succinylcholine in digitalized patients. One succinylcholine manufacturer states that it should not be used in digitalized patients unless absolutely necessary.

REFERENCES:
Birch AA Jr, et al. Changes in serum potassium response to succinylcholine following trauma. *JAMA.* 1969;210:490.

Perez HR. Cardiac arrhythmia after succinylcholine. *Anesth Analg.* 1970;49:33.

Digoxin (eg, *Lanoxin*)

Sulfasalazine (*Azulfidine*)

SUMMARY: Sulfasalazine can reduce digoxin serum concentrations.

RISK FACTORS:

➡ **Dosage Regimen.** Sulfasalazine doses greater than 2 g/day can reduce digoxin serum concentrations.

RELATED DRUGS: Digitoxin (*Crystodigin*) may be less likely to interact with sulfasalazine.

MANAGEMENT OPTIONS:

➡ **Consider Alternative.** Digitoxin may be preferable in sulfasalazine-treated patients.

➡ **Monitor.** It does not seem necessary to avoid the concomitant use of digoxin and sulfasalazine, but monitor patients for a decreased or inadequate therapeutic response to digoxin. Based on the response of one patient, separation of the doses of digoxin and sulfasalazine did not circumvent the interaction.

REFERENCES:

Juhl RP, et al. Effect of sulfasalazine on digoxin bioavailability. *Clin Pharmacol Ther.* 1976;20:387.

Digoxin (eg, *Lanoxin*)

Telmisartan (*Micardis*)

SUMMARY: Digoxin concentrations were increased modestly during telmisartan administration.

RISK FACTORS: No specific risk factors are known.

RELATED DRUGS: The effects of telmisartan on digitoxin (*Crystodigin*) are unknown.

MANAGEMENT OPTIONS:

➡ **Monitor.** Monitor digoxin plasma concentrations and be alert for signs of digoxin toxicity when telmisartan is administered to patients taking digoxin.

REFERENCES:

Product information. Telmisartan (*Micardis*). Boehringer Ingelheim. 1998.

Digoxin (eg, *Lanoxin*)

Tetracycline (eg, *Sumycin*)

SUMMARY: Tetracycline can reduce bacterial gastrointestinal (GI) flora and increase digoxin concentrations in a minority of patients.

RISK FACTORS: No specific risk factors are known.

RELATED DRUGS: No information is available.

MANAGEMENT OPTIONS:

➡ **Monitor.** In the 1 patient in 10 who metabolizes substantial amounts of digoxin in the GI tract, concomitant tetracycline therapy can increase serum digoxin concentrations. Monitor for digoxin toxicity (eg, nausea, anorexia, arrhythmia) and reduce the dosage as needed.

REFERENCES:

Lindenbaum J, et al. Inactivation of digoxin by the gut flora: reversal by antibiotic therapy. *N Engl J Med.* 1981;305:789.

Norregaard-Hansen K, et al. The significance of the enterohepatic circulation on the metabolism of digoxin in patients with the ability of intestinal conversion of the drug. *Acta Med Scand.* 1986;220:89.

Digoxin (eg, *Lanoxin*)

Verapamil (eg, *Calan*)

SUMMARY: Verapamil increases digoxin serum concentrations; digoxin toxicity may result.

RISK FACTORS:

➡ **Dosage Regimen.** Verapamil doses greater than 160 mg/day produce larger increases in digoxin concentrations.

RELATED DRUGS: Diltiazem (eg, *Cardizem*), bepridil (*Vascor*), and nitrendipine (*Baypress*) appear to reduce digoxin elimination. Digitoxin (*Crystodigin*) is likely to be affected similarly. Nifedipine (eg, *Procardia*), isradipine (*DynaCirc*), nicardipine (eg, *Cardene*), felodipine (*Plendil*), and amlodipine (*Norvasc*) do not appear to increase digoxin concentrations.

MANAGEMENT OPTIONS:

➡ **Consider Alternative.** Nifedipine, isradipine, nicardipine, felodipine, and amlodipine do not appear to increase digoxin concentrations and may be suitable alternatives.

➡ **Circumvent/Minimize.** Digoxin dosages may need to be reduced when verapamil is added to a patient stabilized on digoxin.

➡ **Monitor.** Monitor patients for evidence of increased serum digitalis effects (eg, bradycardia, heart block, gastrointestinal upset, mental changes) in the presence of verapamil therapy.

REFERENCES:

Klein HO, et al. The influence of verapamil on serum digoxin concentration. *Circulation.* 1982;65:998.

Johnson BF, et al. The comparative effects of verapamil and a new dihydropyridine calcium channel blocker on digoxin pharmacokinetics. *Clin Pharmacol Ther.* 1987;42:66.

Hedman A. Inhibition by basic drugs of digoxin secretion into human bile. *Eur J Clin Pharmacol.* 1992;42:457.

Pedersen KE, et al. Digoxin-verapamil interaction. *Clin Pharmacol Ther.* 1981;30:311.

Klein HO, et al. Verapamil and digoxin: their respective effects on atrial fibrillation and their interaction. *Am J Cardiol.* 1982;50:894.

Belz GG, et al. Interaction between digoxin and calcium antagonists and antiarrhythmic drugs. *Clin Pharmacol Ther.* 1983;33:410.

Rodin SM, et al. Comparative effects of verapamil and isradipine on steady-state digoxin kinetics. *Clin Pharmacol Ther.* 1988;43:668.

Hedman A, et al. Digoxin-verapamil interaction: reduction of biliary but not renal digoxin clearance in humans. *Clin Pharmacol Ther.* 1991;49:256.

Belz GG, et al. Digoxin plasma concentrations and nifedipine. *Lancet.* 1981;1:844.

Kuhlmann J. Effects of nifedipine and diltiazem on plasma levels and renal excretion of beta-acetyldigoxin. *Clin Pharmacol Ther.* 1985;37:150.

Schwartz JB, et al. Effect of nifedipine on serum digoxin concentration and renal digoxin clearance. *Clin Pharmacol Ther.* 1984;36:19.

Hutt HJ, et al. Dose-dependence of the nifedipine/digoxin interaction? *Arch Toxicol Suppl*. 1986;9:209.

Debruyne D, et al. Nicardipine does not significantly affect serum digoxin concentrations at the steady state of patients with congestive heart failure. *Int J Clin Pharmacol Res*. 1989;9:15.

Kirch W, et al. The felodipine/digoxin interaction. A placebo-controlled study in patients with heart failure. *Br J Clin Pharmacol*. 1988;26:644P.

Schwartz JB. Effects of amlodipine on steady-state digoxin concentrations and renal digoxin clearance. *J Cardiovasc Pharmacol*. 1988;12:1.

② **Dihydroergotamine**

Sibutramine (*Meridia*)

SUMMARY: The risk of serotonin syndrome would theoretically increase when sibutramine is combined with other serotonergic drugs such as dihydroergotamine.

RISK FACTORS: No specific risk factors are known.

RELATED DRUGS: No information is available.

MANAGEMENT OPTIONS:

➡ *Avoid Unless Benefit Outweighs Risk.* The manufacturer states that sibutramine should not be used with dihydroergotamine. This is a prudent recommendation until more information is available.

➡ *Monitor.* Serotonin syndrome can result in neurotoxicity (eg, myoclonus, tremors, rigidity, incoordination, restlessness, hyperreflexia, seizures, coma), psychiatric symptoms (eg, agitation, confusion, hypomania), and temperature regulation abnormalities (eg, fever, sweating). Note that mild forms of serotonin syndrome have also been reported, so consider any combination of the above symptoms possibly related to excessive serotonin activity.

REFERENCES:

Product information. Sibutramine (*Meridia*). Knoll Pharmaceuticals. 1997.

Mills KC. Serotonin syndrome: a clinical update. *Crit Care Clin*. 1997;13:763.

③ **Diltiazem (eg, *Cardizem*)**

Encainide

SUMMARY: Diltiazem substantially increases serum encainide concentrations, but the clinical importance of this interaction is not established.

RISK FACTORS:

➡ *Pharmacogenetics.* Rapid encainide metabolizers are at risk.

RELATED DRUGS: The effect of other calcium channel blockers on encainide metabolism has not been studied; however, verapamil (eg, *Calan*) might produce similar effects because of its effects on drug metabolism.

MANAGEMENT OPTIONS:

➡ ***Monitor.*** Monitor patients maintained on encainide for possible toxicity (eg, arrhythmia, dizziness) or increased encainide concentrations when diltiazem is coadministered.

REFERENCES:

Kazierad DJ, et al. Effects of diltiazem on the disposition of encainide and its active metabolites. *Clin Pharmacol Ther.* 1989;46:668.

Diltiazem (eg, *Cardizem*)

Lovastatin (*Mevacor*)

SUMMARY: Diltiazem administration produces a marked increase in lovastatin concentrations; increased toxicity may result.

RISK FACTORS: No specific risk factors are known.

RELATED DRUGS: Simvastatin (*Zocor*) is likely to be affected by diltiazem in a similar manner. Verapamil (eg, *Isoptin*) and mibefradil would be likely to produce similar changes in lovastatin concentrations. Dihydropyridine calcium channel antagonists would be less likely to alter lovastatin pharmacokinetics, although isradipine (*DynaCirc*) was reported to decrease lovastatin concentrations. Pravastatin (*Pravachol*) metabolism is not altered by diltiazem. The effect of diltiazem on other HMG-CoA reductase inhibitors is unknown.

MANAGEMENT OPTIONS:

➡ ***Consider Alternative.*** Pravastatin would be a good alternative for patients taking calcium channel blockers that inhibit CYP3A4 activity (eg, diltiazem, verapamil, and mibefradil).

➡ ***Monitor.*** Carefully monitor Patients taking lovastatin or simvastatin who receive diltiazem, verapamil, or mibefradil for evidence of myositis.

REFERENCES:

Agbim NE, et al. Interaction of diltiazem with lovastatin and pravastatin. *Clin Pharmacol Ther.* 1997;61:201.

Zhou L-X, et al. Pharmacokinetic interaction between isradipine and lovastatin in normal, female and male volunteers. *J Pharmacol Exper Ther.* 1995;273:121.

Diltiazem (eg, *Cardizem*)

Methylprednisolone (eg, *Medrol*)

SUMMARY: Diltiazem administration increases the plasma concentration of methylprednisolone; increased glucocorticoid effects are likely to occur.

RISK FACTORS: No specific risk factors are known.

RELATED DRUGS: Verapamil (eg, *Calan*) may also inhibit methylprednisolone metabolism. Dihydropyridine calcium channel antagonists (eg, amlodipine [*Norvasc*], felodipine [*Plendil*]) would not be expected to alter methylprednisolone metabolism. It is likely that other glucocorticoids would be affected in a similar manner by diltiazem administration.

MANAGEMENT OPTIONS:

➡ *Consider Alternative.* Consider using a dihydropyridine calcium channel antagonist instead of diltiazem.

➡ *Monitor.* Monitor patients receiving diltiazem and methylprednisolone for signs and symptoms of excess glucocorticoid effects.

REFERENCES:

Varis T, et al. Diltiazem and mibefradil increase the plasma concentrations and greatly enhance the adrenal-suppressant effect of oral methylprednisolone. *Clin Pharmacol Ther.* 2000;67(3):215-21.

Diltiazem (eg, *Cardizem*)

Midazolam (*Versed*)

SUMMARY: Diltiazem increases midazolam plasma concentrations and may prolong sedation and respiratory depression.

RISK FACTORS: No specific risk factors are known.

RELATED DRUGS: Diltiazem has been noted to increase the concentrations of triazolam (eg, *Halcion*). Verapamil (eg, *Isoptin*) may affect midazolam in a similar manner. Mibefradil also would be expected to inhibit midazolam metabolism.

MANAGEMENT OPTIONS:

➡ *Consider Alternative.* The use of a dihydropyridine calcium channel blocker would probably avoid the interaction. Selection of a benzodiazepine such as lorazepam (*Ativan*) or temazepam (*Restoril*) that is not metabolized by CYP3A4 would prevent an interaction with diltiazem.

➡ *Monitor.* Monitor patients receiving diltiazem and midazolam for prolonged sedation and respiratory depression.

REFERENCES:

Ahonen J, et al. Effect of diltiazem on midazolam and alfentanil disposition in patients undergoing coronary artery bypass grafting. *Anesthesiology.* 1996;85:1246.

Backman JT, et al. Dose of midazolam should be reduced during diltiazem and verapamil treatments. *Br J Clin Pharmacol.* 1994;55:481.

Kosuge K, et al. Enhanced effect of triazolam with diltiazem. *Br J Clin Pharmacol.* 1997;43:367.

Varhe A, et al. Diltiazem enhances the effects of triazolam by inhibiting its metabolism. *Clin Pharmacol Ther.* 1996;59:369.

Diltiazem (eg, *Cardizem*)

Nifedipine (eg, *Procardia*)

SUMMARY: Diltiazem increases the serum concentration of nifedipine; nifedipine increases the serum concentration of diltiazem. Increased pharmacodynamic effects could occur.

RISK FACTORS:

➡ *Dosage Regimen.* Patients with daily diltiazem doses of greater than 270 mg are at particular risk.

RELATED DRUGS: The combination of nitrendipine (*Baypress*) and diltiazem produced greater hypotensive effects than each drug alone; no pharmacokinetic data were evaluated. The combination of amlodipine (*Norvasc*) and verapamil (eg, *Calan*) produced a greater increase in forearm blood flow than amlodipine alone. Since the drugs were infused into the brachial artery for 3 minutes, this effect is likely caused by combined vasodilation.

MANAGEMENT OPTIONS:

➡ *Monitor.* Monitor patients receiving nifedipine and diltiazem for increased nifedipine effects such as hypotension or headache and increased diltiazem effects including bradycardia.

REFERENCES:

Toyosaki N, et al. Combination therapy with diltiazem and nifedipine in patients with effort angina pectoris. *Circulation.* 1988;77:1370.

Tateishi T, et al. Dose dependent effect of diltiazem on the pharmacokinetics of nifedipine. *J Clin Pharmacol.* 1989;29:994.

Ohashi K, et al. Effects of diltiazem on the pharmacokinetics of nifedipine. *J Caradiovasc Pharmacol.* 1990;15:96.

Kiowski W, et al. Arterial vasodilator effects of the dihydropyridine calcium antagonist amlodipine alone and in combination with verapamil in systemic hypertension. *Am J Cardiol.* 1990;66:1469.

Ohashi K, et al. The influence of pretreatment periods with diltiazem on nifedipine kinetics. *J Clin Pharmacol.* 1993;33:222.

Tateishi T, et al. The effect of nifedipine on the pharmacokinetics and dynamics of diltiazem: the preliminary study in normal volunteers. *J Clin Pharmacol.* 1993;33:738.

Andreyev N, et al. Comparison of diltiazem, nitrendipine, and their combination for systemic hypertension and stable angina pectoris. *J Cardiovasc Pharmacol.* 1991;18(Suppl. 9):S73.

Diltiazem (eg, *Cardizem*)

Nitroprusside (*Nipride*)

SUMMARY: Diltiazem administration reduces the dose of nitroprusside required to produce hypotension and may enhance nitroprusside-induced hypotension.

RISK FACTORS: No specific risk factors are known.

RELATED DRUGS: Other calcium channel blockers may produce similar interactions with nitroprusside.

MANAGEMENT OPTIONS:

➡ *Monitor.* Patients stabilized on diltiazem may require reduced doses of nitroprusside to produce a controlled hypotension. This interaction could be advantageous in that the reduced thiocyanate formation could decrease the risk of cyanide toxicity in patients who require long-term infusions. Additional data are needed to assess this interaction over longer administration times.

REFERENCES:

Bernard J-M, et al. Diltiazem reduces the nitroprusside doses for deliberate hypotension. *Anesthesiology.* 1992;77:A427.

Diltiazem (eg, *Cardizem*)

Propranolol (eg, *Inderal*)

SUMMARY: Diltiazem increases the plasma concentrations of propranolol and metoprolol (eg, *Lopressor*). Although the interaction may be used to advantage, some predisposed patients may experience adverse effects.

RISK FACTORS: No specific risk factors are known.

RELATED DRUGS: Diltiazem had no effect on atenolol (eg, *Tenormin*) serum concentrations. Verapamil (eg, *Calan*) reduces the metabolism of several beta blockers, including metoprolol.

MANAGEMENT OPTIONS:

➡ *Circumvent/Minimize.* The use of beta blockers that are not metabolized (eg, atenolol) should minimize pharmacokinetic (but not pharmacodynamic) interactions with diltiazem.

➡ *Monitor.* Monitor patients receiving therapy with beta blockers and diltiazem for enhanced effects, particularly AV-conduction slowing, resulting from pharmacokinetic or pharmacodynamic interactions.

REFERENCES:

Dimmett DC, et al. Pharmacokinetics of cardizem and propranolol when administered alone and in combination. *Biopharm Drug Dispos.* 1991;12:515.

Tateishi T, et al. Effect of diltiazem on the pharmacokinetics of propranolol, metoprolol and atenolol. *Eur J Clin Pharmacol.* 1989;36:67.

Hunt BA, et al. Effects of calcium channel blockers on the pharmacokinetics of propranolol stereoisomers. *Clin Pharmacol Ther.* 1990;47:584.

Tateishi T, et al. The influence of diltiazem versus cimetidine on propranolol metabolism. *J Clin Pharmacol.* 1992;32:1099.

Diltiazem (eg, *Cardizem*)

Quinidine (eg, *Quinora*)

SUMMARY: Diltiazem increases the plasma concentration of quinidine at doses greater than 120 mg/day. Increased quinidine effect on myocardial conduction may occur.

RISK FACTORS: No specific risk factors are known.

RELATED DRUGS: Verapamil (eg, *Calan*) has been reported to inhibit the metabolism of quinidine. Dihydropyridine calcium channel antagonists (eg, amlodipine [*Norvasc*], felodipine [*Plendil*]) would not be expected to alter quinidine metabolism.

MANAGEMENT OPTIONS:

➡ *Circumvent/Minimize.* Patients taking quinidine could be treated with other calcium channel blockers such as amlodipine or felodipine that do not inhibit drug metabolism.

➡ *Monitor.* If quinidine and diltiazem are coadministered, monitor for increased quinidine effect such as prolonged QTc.

REFERENCES:

Matera MG, et al. Quinidine-Diltiazem: pharmacokinetic interaction in humans. *Curr Ther Res.* 1986;40:653-56.

Laganiere S, et al. Pharmacokinetic and pharmacodynamic interactions between diltiazem and quinidine. *Clin Pharmacol Ther.* 1996;60(3):255-64.

Diltiazem (eg, *Cardizem*)

Rifampin (eg, *Rifadin*)

SUMMARY: Rifampin decreases diltiazem plasma concentrations; loss of therapeutic effect may result.

RISK FACTORS:

➡ *Route of Administration.* Oral administration of diltiazem will lead to a greater effect.

RELATED DRUGS: Rifampin probably affects other calcium channel blockers in a similar manner.

MANAGEMENT OPTIONS:

➡ *Consider Alternative.* Because this interaction is likely to reduce the efficacy of diltiazem, consider an alternative to diltiazem. Other calcium channel blockers also may be affected. A therapeutic substitution to a different class of agent (noncalcium blocker) may be required.

➡ *Circumvent/Minimize.* Larger doses of calcium channel blocker (particularly those administered orally) may be required when rifampin is coadministered.

➡ *Monitor.* Monitor patients taking calcium channel blockers for a reduction in efficacy when rifampin is given.

REFERENCES:

Drda KD, et al. Effects of debrisoquine hydroxylation phenotype and enzyme induction with rifampin on diltiazem pharmacokinetics and pharmacodynamics. *Pharmacotherapy.* 1991;11:278.

Diltiazem (eg, *Cardizem*)

Sildenafil (*Viagra*)

SUMMARY: Diltiazem may increase the plasma concentrations of sildenafil; this could result in increased side effects, particularly if another vasodilator is administered.

RISK FACTORS: No specific risk factors are known.

RELATED DRUGS: Verapamil (eg, *Isoptin SR*) is another calcium channel blocker known to inhibit CYP3A4. It may inhibit sildenafil metabolism.

MANAGEMENT OPTIONS:

➡ *Circumvent/Minimize.* Avoid using calcium channel blockers that inhibit CYP3A4 in patients taking sildenafil. Minimal interference with the metabolism of sildenafil would be expected with dihydropyridine calcium channel blockers (eg, amlodipine [*Norvasc*] or felodipine [*Plendil*]). All calcium channel blockers may produce increased hypotensive effects when combined with sildenafil.

➡ *Monitor.* Be alert for hypotensive reactions if diltiazem is coadministered with sildenafil.

REFERENCES:

Khoury V, et al. Diltiazem-mediated inhibition of sildenafil metabolism may promote nitrate-induced hypotension. *Aust N Z J Med.* 2000;30:641-642.

Diltiazem (eg, *Cardizem*)

Sirolimus (*Rapamune*)

SUMMARY: Diltiazem administration increases sirolimus plasma concentrations; side effects are likely to occur in some patients.

RISK FACTORS: No specific risk factors are known.

RELATED DRUGS: Verapamil (eg, *Isoptin*) may affect sirolimus in a similar manner. Diltiazem is known to increase the concentrations of other immunosuppressants including cyclosporine (eg, *Neoral*) and tacrolimus (*Prograf*).

MANAGEMENT OPTIONS:

➡ *Monitor.* Pending studies of the effect of chronic diltiazem dosing on sirolimus plasma concentrations, carefully monitor patients receiving the drug combination.

REFERENCES:
Bottiger Y, et al. Pharmacokinetic interaction between single oral doses of diltiazem and sirolimus in healthy volunteers. *Clin Pharmacol Ther.* 2001;69:32-40.

 Diltiazem (eg, *Cardizem*)

Tacrolimus (eg, *Prograf*)

SUMMARY: Tacrolimus concentrations increased during diltiazem administration, resulting in tacrolimus toxicity.

RISK FACTORS: No specific risk factors are known.

RELATED DRUGS: Verapamil (eg, *Calan*) also may increase tacrolimus concentrations because it has been reported to inhibit CYP3A4.

MANAGEMENT OPTIONS:

➡ *Consider Alternative.* Consider patients taking tacrolimus who require treatment for atrial fibrillation for cardioversion, digoxin, quinidine (eg, *Quinora*), or procainamide (eg, *Pronestyl*). Dihydropyridine calcium blockers (eg, amlodipine [*Norvasc*], nifedipine [eg, *Procardia*]) could be used to treat hypertension in patients taking tacrolimus.

➡ *Monitor.* In patients taking tacrolimus who are treated with diltiazem, carefully monitor their tacrolimus concentrations. Adjust doses to keep the tacrolimus concentration within the therapeutic range (approximately 5 to 15 ng/mL).

REFERENCES:
Hebert MF, et al. Diltiazem increases tacrolimus concentrations. *Ann Pharmacother.* 1999;33:680-682.

 Diltiazem (eg, *Cardizem*)

Triazolam (eg, *Halcion*)

SUMMARY: Diltiazem increases triazolam serum concentrations; increased triazolam effects (sedation, ataxia) should be expected.

RISK FACTORS: No specific risk factors are known.

RELATED DRUGS: Verapamil (eg, *Calan*) would be expected to interact with triazolam in a similar manner. Other benzodiazepines that are metabolized by CYP3A4 such as alprazolam (eg, *Xanax*), midazolam (eg, *Versed*), or halazepam would likely interact with diltiazem.

MANAGEMENT OPTIONS:

➡ *Consider Alternative.* Other calcium channel blockers, except verapamil, are unlikely to interact with triazolam. Benzodiazepines that are not metabolized by CYP3A4 (eg, oxazepam [eg, *Serax*], temazepam [eg, *Restoril*]) are not be likely to be affected by diltiazem.

➡ *Monitor.* Monitor patients taking triazolam who are administered diltiazem for evidence of increased triazolam effect.

REFERENCES:

Varhe A, Olkkola KT, Neuvonen PJ. Diltiazem enhances the effects of triazolam by inhibiting its metabolism. *Clin Pharmacol Ther.* 1996;59:369-375.

Kosuge K, Nishimoto M, Kimura M, Umemura K, Nakashima M, Ohashi K. Enhanced effect of triazolam with diltiazem. *Br J Clin Pharmacol.* 1997;43:367-372.

Scharf MB, et al. The effects of a calcium channel blocker on the effects of temazepam and triazolam. *Curr Ther Res.* 1990;48:516.

Diphenhydramine (eg, *Benadryl*)

Metoprolol (eg, *Lopressor*)

SUMMARY: Diphenhydramine increased the plasma concentration of metoprolol in patients who have high intrinsic CYP2D6 activity. Because of metoprolol's wide therapeutic range, toxicity is not likely to occur in most patients.

RISK FACTORS:

➡ *Pharmacogenetics.* Patients who have high CYP2D6 activity experience a greater reduction in their metoprolol metabolism than those with low CYP2D6 activity.

RELATED DRUGS: Other beta blockers that undergo CYP2D6 metabolism (eg, timolol [*Blocadren*], carvedilol [*Coreg*], and propranolol [eg, *Inderal*]) will probably be affected by diphenhydramine in a similar manner. In vitro studies found that other classic antihistamines (eg, chlorpheniramine [eg, *Chlor-Trimeton*], tripelennamine [eg, *Di-Delamine*], promethazine [eg, *Phenergan*]) reduced the CYP2D6 metabolism of metoprolol.

MANAGEMENT OPTIONS:

➡ *Consider Alternative.* Newer antihistamines (eg, fexofenadine [*Allegra*], cetirizine [*Zyrtec*], loratadine [*Claritin*]) have not demonstrated any inhibitory action on CYP2D6. Beta blockers not metabolized by CYP2D6 could be used in place of metoprolol in patients chronically taking diphenhydramine. Atenolol (eg, *Tenormin*) is a beta-2 selective blocker that is not metabolized and would not be expected to interact with diphenhydramine.

➡ *Monitor.* Monitor patients receiving metoprolol for bradycardia and hypotension when they are given diphenhydramine.

REFERENCES:

Hamelin BA, et al. Metoprolol/diphenhydramine interaction in men with high and low CYP2D6 activity. *Clin Pharmacol Ther.* 1999;65:157.

Hamelin BA, et al. Classic antihistamines inhibit metoprolol hydroxylation in vitro. *Clin Pharmacol Ther.* 1999;65:157.

Diphenhydramine (eg, *Benadryl*)

Thioridazine (eg, *Mellaril*)

SUMMARY: Diphenhydramine may increase thioridazine serum concentrations, and thus may increase the risk of ventricular arrhythmias; avoid concurrent use.

RISK FACTORS:

➡ *Pharmacogenetics.* Only patients with the extensive metabolizer CYP2D6 phenotype (EMs) would be expected to experience this interaction. Poor metabolizers (PMs) do not have the gene for production of CYP2D6, and would likely already have high serum concentrations of thioridazine. Approximately 8% of whites are deficient in CYP2D6, but the deficiency is rare in Asians, usually 1% or less.

➡ *Hypokalemia.* The corrected QT interval (QTc) may be prolonged in patients with hypokalemia, thus increasing the risk of this interaction. Any other factor that may prolong the QTc interval would also increase the risk of this interaction.

RELATED DRUGS: Other antihistamines are not known to inhibit CYP2D6. Although a number of antipsychotic drugs, like thioridazine, have been shown to prolong the QT interval clinical evidence suggests that thioridazine may produce the greatest risk.

MANAGEMENT OPTIONS:

➡ *Use Alternative.* Although the risk of this combination is not well established, it would be prudent to use alternatives for 1 of the drugs (see Related Drugs).

➡ *Monitor.* If the combination must be used, monitor the ECG for evidence of QT prolongation and for clinical evidence of arrhythmias (eg, syncope).

REFERENCES:

Hartigan-Go K, et al. Concentration-related pharmacodynamic effects of thioridazine and its metabolites in humans. *Clin Pharmacol Ther.* 1996;60:543-53.

'Dear Doctor or Pharmacist' Letter, Novartis Pharmaceuticals, July 7, 2000.

Disopyramide (*Norpace*)

Clarithromycin (*Biaxin*)

SUMMARY: Clarithromycin administration increases disopyramide concentrations; toxicity including hypoglycemia or delayed cardiac repolarization may result.

RISK FACTORS: No specific risk factors are known.

RELATED DRUGS: Erythromycin (eg, *E-Mycin*) is known to inhibit the metabolism of disopyramide and troleandomycin (*Tao*) would be expected to inhibit disopyramide clearance as well. Erythromycin is also known to prolong the QTc interval, especially when administered IV.

MANAGEMENT OPTIONS:

➡ *Consider Alternative.* Azithromycin (*Zithromax*) and dirithromycin (*Dynabac*) would be unlikely to affect disopyramide metabolism. Consider alternative antiarrhythmic agents for patients who cannot avoid clarithromycin or erythromycin.

➡ *Monitor.* Carefully monitor patients taking disopyramide for prolonged QTc intervals and hypoglycemia if clarithromycin is coadministered.

REFERENCES:

Iida H, et al. Hypoglycemia induced by interaction between clarithromycin and disopyramide. *Jpn Heart J.* 1999;40:91.

Disopyramide (eg, *Norpace*)
Erythromycin (eg, *Erythrocin*)

SUMMARY: In isolated case reports, erythromycin administration appeared to increase the serum disopyramide concentration, resulting in cardiac arrhythmias.

RISK FACTORS: No specific risk factors are known.

RELATED DRUGS: Other macrolides (eg, troleandomycin [*Tao*], clarithromycin [*Biaxin*]) may affect disopyramide similarly. Azithromycin (*Zithromax*) and dirithromycin (*Dynabac*) would be unlikely to inhibit disopyramide elimination.

MANAGEMENT OPTIONS:

➡ *Consider Alternative.* Azithromycin (*Zithromax*) and dirithromycin (*Dynabac*) would be unlikely to affect disopyramide metabolism. Consider alternative antiarrhythmic agents for patients who cannot avoid clarithromycin or erythromycin.

➡ *Monitor.* Monitor patients taking disopyramide for the development of arrhythmias if erythromycin is added to their regimen.

REFERENCES:

Ragosta M, et al. Potentially fatal interaction between erythromycin and disopyramide. *Am J Med.* 1989;86:465.

Echizen H, et al. A potent inhibitory effect of erythromycin and other macrolide antibiotics on the mono-N-dealkylation metabolism of disopyramide with human liver microsomes. *J Pharmacol Exp Ther.* 1993;264:1425.

Disopyramide (eg, *Norpace*)
Lidocaine (eg, *Xylocaine*)

SUMMARY: Combined use of lidocaine and disopyramide can induce arrhythmias or heart failure in predisposed patients.

RISK FACTORS: No specific risk factors are known.

RELATED DRUGS: No information is available.

MANAGEMENT OPTIONS:

➡ *Monitor.* Closely monitor patients receiving combined therapy with disopyramide and lidocaine for arrhythmias and heart failure.

REFERENCES:

Ellrodt G, et al. Adverse effects of disopyramide (*Norpace*): toxic interactions with other antiarrhythmic agents. *Heart Lung.* 1980;9:469.

Disopyramide (eg, *Norpace*)

Phenobarbital (eg, *Solfoton*)

SUMMARY: Phenobarbital appears to reduce the serum concentrations of disopyramide, perhaps to subtherapeutic levels.

RISK FACTORS: No specific risk factors are known.

RELATED DRUGS: Other barbiturates probably have a similar effect on disopyramide, but little clinical evidence is available.

MANAGEMENT OPTIONS:

➡ ***Monitor.*** The changes in disopyramide clearance and half-life observed after phenobarbital administration could result in loss of arrhythmia control in some patients. Monitor disopyramide serum concentrations when phenobarbital is added to or removed from the drug regimen. Watch for dry mouth and urinary retention caused by increased metabolite serum concentrations.

REFERENCES:

Kapil RP, et al. Disopyramide pharmacokinetics and metabolism: effect of inducers. *Br J Clin Pharmacol.* 1987;24:781.

Disopyramide (eg, *Norpace*)

Phenytoin (*Dilantin*)

SUMMARY: Phenytoin increases the metabolism of disopyramide, potentially reducing its efficacy and increasing its toxicity to some extent.

RISK FACTORS: No specific risk factors are known.

RELATED DRUGS: No information is available.

MANAGEMENT OPTIONS:

➡ ***Monitor.*** Closely monitor disopyramide serum concentrations and patient response (eg, control of arrhythmia) when phenytoin therapy is added to or removed from disopyramide therapy. Be alert for reduced antiarrhythmic efficacy and increased anticholinergic side effects such as dry mouth or urinary retention.

REFERENCES:

Ellrodt G, et al. Adverse effects of disopyramide (*Norpace*): toxic interactions with other antiarrhythmic agents. *Heart Lung.* 1980;9:469.

Aitio ML, et al. Enhanced metabolism and diminished efficacy of disopyramide by enzyme induction? *Br J Clin Pharmacol.* 1980;9:149.

Aitio ML, et al. The effect of enzyme induction on the metabolism of disopyramide in man. *Br J Clin Pharmacol.* 1981;11:279.

Kessler JM, et al. Disopyramide and phenytoin interaction. *Clin Pharm.* 1982;1:263.

Matos JA, et al. Disopyramide-phenytoin interaction. *Clin Res.* 1981;29:655A.

Nightingale J, et al. Effect of phenytoin on serum disopyramide concentrations. *Clin Pharm.* 1987;6:46.

Disopyramide (eg, *Norpace*)

Potassium

SUMMARY: Increased serum concentrations of potassium can enhance disopyramide effects on myocardial conduction.

RISK FACTORS:

➡ *Concurrent Diseases.* Renal dysfunction increases the risk of the interaction.

RELATED DRUGS: The administration of potassium-sparing diuretics might cause a similar reaction with disopyramide.

MANAGEMENT OPTIONS:

➡ *Monitor.* Be alert for electrocardiographic evidence of disopyramide toxicity (eg, QRS widening) when potassium supplementation is given concurrently, especially if large doses of disopyramide and potassium are used or if renal function is impaired.

REFERENCES:

Maddux BD, et al. Toxic synergism of disopyramide and hyperkalemia. *Chest.* 1980;78:654.

Disopyramide (eg, *Norpace*)

Practolol

SUMMARY: Disopyramide and beta blockers may produce additive negative inotropic effects on the heart.

RISK FACTORS:

➡ *Route of Administration.* IV administration of both drugs may produce the interaction.

RELATED DRUGS: Atenolol appears to interact with disopyramide similarly. Propranolol does not appear to interact.

MANAGEMENT OPTIONS:

➡ *Monitor.* Until more clinical information is available, administer disopyramide (especially if given IV) only with caution to patients receiving beta blockers. Monitor for bradycardia and reduced cardiac output.

REFERENCES:

Cumming AD, et al. Interaction between disopyramide and practolol. *BMJ.* 1979;2:1204.

Cathcart-Rake WF, et al. The pharmacodynamics of concurrent disopyramide and propranolol. *Clin Pharmacol Ther.* 1979;25:217.

Karim A, et al. Clinical pharmacokinetics of disopyramide. *J Pharmacokinet Biopharm.* 1982;10:465.

Cathcart-Rake WF, et al. The effect of concurrent oral administration of propranolol and disopyramide on cardiac function in healthy men. *Circulation.* 1980;61:938.

Bonde J, et al. Haemodynamic effects and kinetics of concomitant intravenous disopyramide and atenolol in patients with ischaemic heart disease. *Eur J Clin Pharmacol.* 1986;30:161.

Bonde J, et al. Atenolol inhibits the elimination of disopyramide. *Eur J Clin Pharmacol.* 1985;28:41.

Disopyramide (eg, *Norpace*)

Rifampin (eg, *Rifadin*)

SUMMARY: Rifampin can lower serum disopyramide concentrations to subtherapeutic levels; loss of efficacy may result.

RISK FACTORS: No specific risk factors are known.

RELATED DRUGS: No information is available.

MANAGEMENT OPTIONS:

➡ *Monitor.* Monitor patients for re-emergence of arrhythmias when rifampin is added to disopyramide and disopyramide toxicity if rifampin is discontinued. Serum disopyramide concentrations would be useful to monitor this interaction.

REFERENCES:

Aitio ML, et al. The effect of enzyme induction on the metabolism of disopyramide in man. *Br J Clin Pharmacol.* 1981;11:279.

Staum JM, et al. Enzyme induction: rifampin-disopyramide interaction. *DICP.* 1990;24:701.

Disopyramide (eg, *Norpace*)

Thioridazine (eg, *Mellaril*)

SUMMARY: Disopyramide may produce additive prolongation of the QT interval with thioridazine, and thus may increase the risk of ventricular arrhythmias; avoid concurrent use.

RISK FACTORS:

➡ *Hypokalemia.* The corrected QT interval (QTc) may be prolonged in patients with hypokalemia, thus increasing the risk of this interaction. Any other factor that may prolong the QTc interval would also increase the risk of this interaction.

RELATED DRUGS: Other antiarrhythmics such as amiodarone (eg, *Cordarone*), procainamide (eg, *Procan SR*), and quinidine (*Quinora*) can also increase the QT interval, and may increase the risk of arrhythmias. Also, amiodarone, propafenone (*Rythmol*), and quinidine are know inhibitors of CYP2D6, and may increase thioridazine serum concentrations. Although a number of antipsychotic drugs, like thioridazine, have been shown to prolong the QT interval clinical evidence suggests that thioridazine may produce the greatest risk.

MANAGEMENT OPTIONS:

➡ *Use Alternative.* Although the risk of this combination is not well established, it would be prudent to use alternatives for 1 of the drugs (see Related Drugs).

➡ *Monitor.* If the combination must be used, monitor the ECG for evidence of QT prolongation and for clinical evidence of arrhythmias (eg, syncope).

REFERENCES:

Hartigan-Go K, et al. Concentration-related pharmacodynamic effects of thioridazine and its metabolites in humans. *Clin Pharmacol Ther.* 1996;60:543-53.

'Dear Doctor of Pharmacist' Letter, Novartis Pharmaceuticals, July 7, 2000.

Disulfiram (eg, *Antabuse*)

Ethanol (*Ethyl Alcohol*) `AVOID`

SUMMARY: Disulfiram results in severe ethanol intolerance; patients must be warned to avoid all forms of ethanol.

RISK FACTORS: No specific risk factors are known.

RELATED DRUGS: No information is available.

MANAGEMENT OPTIONS:

➡ *AVOID COMBINATION.* Warn patients about ethanol in foods and pharmaceuticals, as well as beverages. Advise patients receiving disulfiram to avoid oral liquid pharmaceuticals unless they are known to be ethanol-free.

REFERENCES:

Fernandez D. Another esophageal rupture after alcohol and disulfiram. *N Engl J Med*. 1972;286:610.

Elenbaas RM. Drug therapy reviews: management of the disulfiram/alcohol reaction. *Am J Hosp Pharm*. 1977;34:827.

Kitson TM. The disulfiram-ethanol reaction: a review. *J Stud Alcohol*. 1977;38:96.

Syed J, et al. An unusual presentation of a disulfiram-alcohol reaction. *Del Med J*. 1995;67:183.

Johansson B, et al. Dose-effect relationship of disulfiram in human volunteers. II. A study of the relation between the disulfiram-alcohol reaction and plasma concentrations of acetaldehyde, diethyldithiocarbamic acid methyl ester, and erythrocyte aldehyde dehydrogenase activity. *Pharmacol Toxicol*. 1991;68:166.

Disulfiram (eg, *Antabuse*)

Isoniazid (INH; eg, *Laniazid*)

SUMMARY: The combined use of disulfiram and INH may result in adverse CNS effects.

RISK FACTORS: No specific risk factors are known.

RELATED DRUGS: No information is available.

MANAGEMENT OPTIONS:

➡ *Avoid Unless Benefit Outweighs Risk.* Although evidence is somewhat limited, enough has been presented to warrant caution in the concomitant use of INH and disulfiram. It would be wise in most cases to avoid the use of disulfiram in patients receiving INH until more information is known about the interaction.

➡ *Monitor.* If combined use is necessary, monitor patients for adverse central nervous system effects (eg, altered mood, behavioral changes, ataxia).

REFERENCES:

Rothstein E. Rifampin with disulfiram. *JAMA*. 1972;219:1216.

Whittington HG, et al. Possible interaction between disulfiram and isoniazid. *Am J Psychiatry*. 1969;125:1725.

Disulfiram (eg, *Antabuse*)

Metronidazole (eg, *Flagyl*)

SUMMARY: The combined use of disulfiram and metronidazole may produce central nervous system toxicity.

RISK FACTORS: No specific risk factors are known.

RELATED DRUGS: No information is available.

MANAGEMENT OPTIONS:

➡ *Consider Alternative.* Until the potential interaction between metronidazole and disulfiram is better described, it would be wise to avoid concomitant use of these drugs.

➡ *Monitor.* If the drugs are coadministered, watch for behavioral toxicity and confusion.

REFERENCES:

Rothstein E, et al. Toxicity of disulfiram combined with metronidazole. *N Engl J Med.* 1969;280:1006.

Goodhue WW Jr. Disulfiram-metronidazole (well identified) toxicity. *N Engl J Med.* 1969;280:1482.

Scher JM. Psychotic reaction to disulfiram. *JAMA.* 1967;201:1051.

Disulfiram (eg, *Antabuse*)

Phenytoin (*Dilantin*)

SUMMARY: Disulfiram consistently increases serum phenytoin concentrations; symptoms of phenytoin toxicity have occurred in some patients.

RISK FACTORS: No specific risk factors are known.

RELATED DRUGS: No information is available.

MANAGEMENT OPTIONS:

➡ *Consider Alternative.* Consider using alternative treatment for alcohol abuse.

➡ *Circumvent/Minimize.* Reduction of the phenytoin dose may be necessary.

➡ *Monitor.* Monitor patients receiving phenytoin and disulfiram for evidence of phenytoin toxicity (eg, ataxia, nystagmus, mental impairment). Serum phenytoin determinations are useful to detect an interaction between these drugs. Monitor patients for a reduced phenytoin response when disulfiram therapy is discontinued.

REFERENCES:

Olesen OV. The influence of disulfiram and calcium carbamide on the serum diphenylhydantoin. *Arch Neurol.* 1967;16:642.

Olesen OV. Disulfiram (*Antabuse*) as inhibitor of phenytoin metabolism. *Acta Pharmacol Toxicol.* 1966;24:317.

Kiorboe E. Phenytoin intoxication during treatment with *Antabuse* (disulfiram). *Epilepsia.* 1966;7:246.

Svendsen TL, et al. The influence of disulfiram on the half-life and metabolic clearance rate of diphenyl-hydantoin and tolbutamide in man. *Eur J Clin Pharmacol.* 1976;9:439.

Taylor JW, et al. Mathematical analysis of a phenytoin-disulfiram interaction. *Am J Hosp Pharm.* 1981;38:93.

Disulfiram (eg, *Antabuse*)

Theophylline (eg, *Theolair*)

SUMMARY: Disulfiram increases serum theophylline concentrations; the magnitude of the effect appears sufficient to produce theophylline toxicity in at least some patients.

RISK FACTORS: No specific risk factors are known.

RELATED DRUGS: No information is available.

MANAGEMENT OPTIONS:

➡ ***Monitor.*** Monitor for altered theophylline effect if disulfiram therapy is initiated, discontinued, or if the disulfiram dosage is changed. Patients receiving disulfiram therapy may require lower theophylline dosages.

REFERENCES:
Loi CM, et al. Dose-dependent inhibition of theophylline metabolism by disulfiram in recovering alcoholics. *Clin Pharmacol Ther.* 1989;45:476.

Disulfiram (eg, *Antabuse*)

Tranylcypromine (*Parnate*)

SUMMARY: A patient on disulfiram developed delirium following the addition of tranylcypromine, but a causal relationship was not established.

RISK FACTORS: No specific risk factors are known.

RELATED DRUGS: The effect of combining other nonselective monoamine oxidase inhibitors (MAOIs) with disulfiram is not established; assume that they may interact until proven otherwise.

MANAGEMENT OPTIONS:

➡ ***Monitor.*** Although data are limited, monitor for evidence of delirium if tranylcypromine or other nonselective MAOIs are used with disulfiram.

REFERENCES:
Blansjaar BA, et al. Delirium in a patient treated with disulfiram and tranylcypromine. *Am J Psychiatry.* 1995;152:296.

Disulfiram (eg, *Antabuse*)

Warfarin (eg, *Coumadin*)

SUMMARY: Disulfiram increases the hypoprothrombinemic response to warfarin in most patients receiving both drugs concurrently.

RISK FACTORS: No specific risk factors are known.

RELATED DRUGS: Although little is known regarding the effect of disulfiram on oral anticoagulants other than warfarin, assume that they interact until evidence to the contrary is available.

MANAGEMENT OPTIONS:

➡ ***Avoid Unless Benefit Outweighs Risk.*** Avoid concomitant use of disulfiram and oral anticoagulants if possible. If oral anticoagulant therapy is begun in the patient receiving disulfiram, use conservative doses until the maintenance dose is established.

➡ ***Monitor.*** Monitor patients receiving oral anticoagulants for altered anticoagulant effect when disulfiram is started or stopped.

REFERENCES:
O'Reilly RA. Dynamic interaction between disulfiram and separated enantiomorphs of racemic warfarin. *Clin Pharmacol Ther.* 1981;29:332.

O'Reilly RA. Interaction of sodium warfarin and disulfiram (*Antabuse*) in man. *Ann Intern Med.* 1973;78:73.

Rothstein E. Warfarin effect enhanced by disulfiram. *JAMA.* 1968;206:1574.

Rothstein E. Warfarin effect enhanced by disulfiram (*Antabuse*). *JAMA.* 1972;22:1052.

O'Reilly RA. Potentiation of anticoagulant effect by disulfiram. *Clin Res.* 1971;19:180.

② Dofetilide (*Tikosyn*)

Ziprasidone (*Geodon*)

SUMMARY: Ziprasidone and dofetilide can prolong the corrected QT (QTc) interval on the electrocardiogram. Theoretically, this could increase the risk of ventricular arrhythmias such as torsades de pointes.

RISK FACTORS:

➡ **Hypokalemia.** The QTc on the ECG may be prolonged in patients with hypokalemia, thus increasing the risk of this interaction.

➡ **Miscellaneous.** Other factors that may prolong the QTc interval (eg, hypomagnesemia, bradycardia, impaired liver function, hypothyroidism) also may increase the risk of ventricular arrhythmias.

RELATED DRUGS: Available data suggest that ziprasidone produces less QTc prolongation than thioridazine (*Mellaril*), but about twice that of quetiapine (*Seroquel*), risperidone (*Risperdal*), haloperidol (*Haldol*), and olanzapine (*Zyprexa*).

MANAGEMENT OPTIONS:

➡ **Use Alternative.** Given the theoretical risk and the fact that dofetilide is listed in the ziprasidone product information as "contraindicated," it would be prudent to use an alternative to 1 of the drugs (see Related Drugs).

➡ **Monitor.** If dofetilide and ziprasidone are used concurrently, monitor for evidence of arrhythmias (eg, syncope) and for prolonged QT intervals.

REFERENCES:

De Ponti F, et al. QT-interval prolongation by non-cardiac drugs: lessons to be learned from recent experience. *Eur J Clin Pharmacol.* 2000;56:1-18.

Product information. Ziprasidone (*Geodon*). Pfizer Pharmaceuticals. 2001.

Briefing Information, Psychopharmacological Drugs Advisory Committee, U.S. Food and Drug Administration, July 19, 2000.

③ Dopamine (eg, *Intropin*)

Ergonovine

SUMMARY: A case of gangrene with concurrent use of ergonovine and dopamine has been reported.

RISK FACTORS: No specific risk factors are known.

RELATED DRUGS: The effect of other combinations of ergot alkaloids and vasoconstricting sympathomimetics is unknown, but excessive vasoconstriction might occur.

MANAGEMENT OPTIONS:

➡ *Monitor.* Undertake the concurrent use of dopamine and ergot alkaloids such as ergonovine with caution; monitor for evidence of excessive vasoconstriction in the extremities (eg, cold, pale skin, pain).

REFERENCES:

Buchanan N, et al. Symmetrical gangrene of the extremities associated with the use of dopamine subsequent to ergometrine administration. *Intensive Care Med.* 1977;3:55.

Dopamine (eg, *Intropin*)

Phenytoin (*Dilantin*)

SUMMARY: Case reports and animal studies indicate that patients receiving dopamine may be more susceptible to hypotension following IV phenytoin.

RISK FACTORS: No specific risk factors are known.

RELATED DRUGS: No information is available.

MANAGEMENT OPTIONS:

➡ *Monitor.* In patients receiving IV dopamine, administer IV phenytoin only with careful monitoring of the cardiovascular status.

REFERENCES:

Bivins BA, et al. Dopamine-phenytoin interaction. *Arch Surg.* 1978;113:245.

Doxazosin (*Cardura*)

Nifedipine (eg, *Procardia*)

SUMMARY: The combination of nifedipine with doxazosin can result in enhanced hypotensive effects.

RISK FACTORS: No specific risk factors are known.

RELATED DRUGS: Other calcium channel blockers may have additive hypotensive effects when administered with doxazosin or other alpha blockers.

MANAGEMENT OPTIONS:

➡ *Monitor.* The combination of nifedipine and doxazosin appears to produce an increased antihypertensive effect. Monitor patients stabilized on 1 of these drugs for hypotension during the institution of the second drug.

REFERENCES:

Donnelly R, et al. The pharmacodynamics and pharmacokinetics of the combination of nifedipine and doxazosin. *Eur J Clin Pharmacol.* 1993;44:279.

Doxepin (eg, *Sinequan*)

Propoxyphene (eg, *Darvocet-N*)

SUMMARY: Preliminary evidence suggests that propoxyphene increases serum concentrations of doxepin.

RISK FACTORS: No specific risk factors are known.

RELATED DRUGS: It is not known whether tricyclic antidepressants other than doxepin would be affected by propoxyphene, but it certainly seems possible. Propoxyphene impairs the hepatic metabolism of carbamazepine.

MANAGEMENT OPTIONS:

➡ **Monitor.** Monitor for altered doxepin effect if propoxyphene is initiated, discontinued, or changed in dosage; adjust doxepin dose as needed.

REFERENCES:

Abernethy DR, et al. Impairment of hepatic drug oxidation by propoxyphene. *Ann Intern Med.* 1982;97:223.

Doxepin (eg, *Sinequan*)

Tolazamide (eg, *Tolinase*)

SUMMARY: Doxepin may enhance the hypoglycemic effects of tolazamide or insulin.

RISK FACTORS: No specific risk factors are known.

RELATED DRUGS: A patient who had been maintained on chlorpropamide (eg, *Diabinese*) 250 mg/day was found to have a blood glucose of 50 mg/dL 4 days after the initiation of nortriptyline (eg, *Pamelor*). Chlorpropamide was discontinued, and the patient remained normoglycemic. Nortriptyline has been reported to increase insulin sensitivity and lower blood glucose. In other case reports, patients with diabetes developed hypoglycemia following the addition of amitriptyline (eg, *Elavil*), imipramine (eg, *Tofranil*), and maprotiline (eg, *Ludiomil*).

MANAGEMENT OPTIONS:

➡ **Monitor.** Pending prospective evaluation of this interaction, diabetic patients should monitor their blood glucose daily when cyclic antidepressants are initiated or discontinued.

REFERENCES:

True BL, et al. Profound hypoglycemia with the addition of tricyclic antidepressant to maintenance sulfonylurea therapy. *Am J Psychiatry.* 1987;144:1220.

Grof E, et al. Effects of lithium, nortriptyline and dexamethasone on insulin sensitivity. *Prog Neuropsychopharmacol Biol Psychiatry.* 1984;8:687.

Sherman KE, et al. Amitriptyline and asymptomatic hypoglycemia. *Ann Intern Med.* 1988;109:683.

Shrivastava RK, et al. Hypoglycemia associated with imipramine. *Biol Psychiatry.* 1983;18:1509.

Zogno MG, et al. Hypoglycemia caused by maprotiline in a patient taking oral antidiabetics. *Ann Pharmacother.* 1994;28:406.

Doxorubicin (eg, *Adriamycin*)

Verapamil (eg, *Calan*)

SUMMARY: Verapamil appears to increase doxorubicin serum concentrations.

RISK FACTORS: No specific risk factors are known.

RELATED DRUGS: The effect of calcium channel blockers other than verapamil on doxorubicin is not established.

MANAGEMENT OPTIONS:

➡ *Monitor.* Monitor for altered doxorubicin effect if verapamil is initiated, discontinued, or changed in dosage; adjust doxorubicin dose as needed.

REFERENCES:

Kerr DJ, et al. The effect of verapamil on the pharmacokinetics of Adriamycin. *Cancer Chemother Pharmacol.* 1986;18:239.

Doxycycline (eg, *Vibramycin*)

Ethanol (Ethyl Alcohol)

SUMMARY: Chronic alcohol ingestion may reduce the serum concentration of doxycycline.

RISK FACTORS: No specific risk factors are known.

RELATED DRUGS: Tetracycline does not appear to interact with ethanol.

MANAGEMENT OPTIONS:

➡ *Consider Alternative.* When a tetracycline is needed in an alcoholic patient, it may be preferable to use an agent other than doxycycline.

➡ *Monitor.* If doxycycline is used, be alert for diminished doxycycline effect.

REFERENCES:

Neuvonen PJ, et al. Effect of long-term alcohol consumption on the half-life of tetracycline and doxycycline in man. *Int J Clin Pharmacol.* 1976;14:303.

Doxycycline (eg, *Vibramycin*)

Methotrexate (eg, *Rheumatrex*)

SUMMARY: Doxycycline administration appears to increase methotrexate concentrations; methotrexate toxicity is likely.

RISK FACTORS: No specific risk factors are known.

RELATED DRUGS: Tetracycline (eg, *Sumycin*) may also increase methotrexate concentrations.

MANAGEMENT OPTIONS:

➡ *Consider Alternative.* Patients receiving high-dose methotrexate should avoid treatment with doxycycline. Select an alternative, non-tetracycline antibiotic. Note that some penicillins (eg, carbenicillin [eg, *Geocillin*]) have been reported to increase the plasma concentration of methotrexate.

➡ *Monitor.* If patients being treated with high-dose methotrexate are administered doxycycline, carefully monitor methotrexate concentrations. Methotrexate dosage reduction may be necessary.

REFERENCES:

Tortajada-Ituren JJ, et al. High-dose methotrexate-doxycycline interaction. *Ann Pharmacother.* 1999;33:804–8.

Doxycycline (eg, *Vibramycin*)

Phenobarbital (eg, *Solfoton*)

SUMMARY: Doxycycline serum concentrations may be reduced by the administration of phenobarbital.

RISK FACTORS: No specific risk factors are known.

RELATED DRUGS: Other barbiturates may affect doxycycline in a similar manner. Theoretically, other tetracyclines should not be affected by barbiturates like phenobarbital.

MANAGEMENT OPTIONS:

➥ ***Consider Alternative.*** Tetracyclines other than doxycycline, theoretically, should not be affected by barbiturates, because hepatic metabolism is not an important route of elimination.

➥ ***Monitor.*** If barbiturates cannot be avoided in patients receiving doxycycline, closely monitor the clinical response to doxycycline.

REFERENCES:

Neuvonen PJ, et al. Interaction between doxycycline and barbiturates. *BMJ.* 1974;1:535.

 Doxycycline (eg, *Vibramycin*)

Phenytoin (*Dilantin*)

SUMMARY: Phenytoin reduces doxycycline serum concentrations, but other tetracyclines do not appear to be affected.

RISK FACTORS: No specific risk factors are known.

RELATED DRUGS: Chlortetracycline (*Aureomycin*), demeclocycline (*Declomycin*), methacycline, and oxytetracycline (eg, *Terramycin*) do not appear to be affected by phenytoin administration. Theoretically, tetracycline also should be unaffected by phenytoin.

MANAGEMENT OPTIONS:

➥ ***Consider Alternative.*** If possible, use a tetracycline other than doxycycline in patients receiving phenytoin (see Related Drugs).

➥ ***Monitor.*** If doxycycline is used with phenytoin, watch for reduced doxycycline efficacy and consider using larger doses of doxycycline.

REFERENCES:

Penttila O, et al. Interaction between doxycycline and some antiepileptic drugs. *BMJ.* 1974;2:470.

Neuvonen PJ, et al. Interaction between doxycycline and barbiturates. *BMJ.* 1974;1:535.

Neuvonen PJ, et al. Effect of antiepileptic drugs on the elimination of various tetracycline derivatives. *Eur J Clin Pharmacol.* 1975;9:147.

Doxycycline (eg, *Vibramycin*)

Warfarin (eg, *Coumadin*)

SUMMARY: Although doxycycline theoretically may increase the hypoprothrombinemic response to oral anticoagulants like warfarin, clinical evidence is limited.

RISK FACTORS:

➡ *Concurrent Diseases.* The hypoprothrombinemic response to doxycycline may be larger in patients with deficient vitamin K intake.

RELATED DRUGS: Other tetracyclines may produce similar effects on oral anticoagulants.

MANAGEMENT OPTIONS:

➡ *Monitor.* Although the clinical evidence for an interaction between doxycycline and oral anticoagulants is limited, monitor patients for an enhanced anticoagulant effect when these drugs are used concurrently.

REFERENCES:

Searcy RL, et al. Blood clotting anomalies associated with intensive tetracycline therapy. *Clin Res.* 1964;12:230.

Westfall LK, et al. Potentiation of warfarin by tetracycline. *Am J Hosp Pharm.* 1980;37:1620.

Messinger WJ, et al. The effect of bowel sterilizing antibiotic on blood coagulation mechanism. *Angiology.* 1965;16:29.

Caraco Y, et al. Enhanced anticoagulant effect of coumarin derivatives induced by doxycycline coadministration. *Ann Pharmacother.* 1992;26:1084.

Dyphylline (eg, *Lufyllin*)

Probenecid (*Benemid*)

SUMMARY: Single-dose studies indicate that probenecid substantially increases serum dyphylline concentrations.

RISK FACTORS: No specific risk factors are known.

RELATED DRUGS: Unlike dyphylline, theophylline (eg, *Theolair*) does not appear to interact with probenecid. (Also see Allopurinol/Theophylline; consult index for page number.)

MANAGEMENT OPTIONS:

➡ *Consider Alternative.* Theophylline does not appear to interact with probenecid and may be a suitable alternative.

➡ *Monitor.* Monitor for evidence of altered dyphylline effect if probenecid therapy is initiated, discontinued, or changed in dosage.

REFERENCES:

May DC, et al. Effect of probenecid on dyphylline elimination. *Clin Pharmacol Ther.* 1983;33:822-825.

Chen TW, et al. Effect of probenecid on the pharmacokinetics of aminophylline. *Drug Intell Clin Pharm.* 1983;17:465-466.

Echothiophate Iodide (*Phosphate Iodide*)

Succinylcholine (eg, *Anectine*)

SUMMARY: Echothiophate prolongs the neuromuscular blocking effects of succinylcholine; avoid succinylcholine in patients on echothiophate if possible.

RISK FACTORS: No specific risk factors are known.

RELATED DRUGS: No information is available.

MANAGEMENT OPTIONS:

➥ ***Avoid Unless Benefit Outweighs Risk.*** A neuromuscular blocker other than succinylcholine is preferred in most patients on echothiophate.

➥ ***Monitor.*** If succinylcholine is used, monitor carefully for prolonged neuromuscular blockade. Serum pseudocholinesterase determinations would be useful to determine which patients are at highest risk.

REFERENCES:

Mone JG, et al. Qualitative defects of pseudocholinesterase activity. *Anaesthesia.* 1967;22:55-68.

Cavallaro RJ, et al. Effect of echothiophate therapy on metabolism of succinylcholine in man. *Anesth Analg.* 1968;47:570-574.

Kinyon GE. Anticholinesterase eye drops—need for caution. *N Engl J Med.* 1969;280:53.

Lipson ML, et al. Oral administration of pralidoxime chloride in echothiophate iodide therapy. *Arch Ophthalmol.* 1969;82:830-835.

Cohen PJ, et al. A simple test for abnormal pseudocholinesterase. *Anesthesiology.* 1970;32:281-282.

Kothary SP, et al. Plasma cholinesterase activity in relation to the safe use of succinylcholine in myasthenic patients on chronic anticholinesterase treatment. *Clin Pharmacol Ther.* 1977;21:108.

Eilderton TE, et al. Reduction in plasma cholinesterase levels after prolonged administration of echothiophate iodide eyedrops. *Can Anaesth Soc J.* 1968;15:291-296.

 Efavirenz (*Sustiva*)

Indinavir (*Crixivan*)

SUMMARY: Efavirenz administration reduces indinavir concentrations, even when ritonavir is being coadministered with indinavir to inhibit the metabolism of indinavir.

RISK FACTORS: No specific risk factors are known.

RELATED DRUGS: Efavirenz reduces the plasma concentration of ritonavir. Its effect on other protease inhibitors that are metabolized by CYP3A4 (eg, nelfinavir [*Viracept*], saquinavir [eg, *Fortovase*]) is likely to be similar.

MANAGEMENT OPTIONS:

➥ ***Circumvent/Minimize.*** It may be possible to circumvent the effects of efavirenz on indinavir by increasing the dose of ritonavir that is coadministered. The added inhibitory effect of ritonavir on CYP3A4 may lessen or reverse the induction effect of efavirenz.

➡ *Monitor.* Monitor patients taking indinavir and ritonavir who are prescribed efavirenz for reduced indinavir concentrations and possible loss of antiviral efficacy.

REFERENCES:

Aarnoutse RE, et al. The influence of efavirenz on the pharmacokinetics of a twice-daily combination of indinavir and low-dose ritonavir in healthy volunteers. *Clin Pharmacol Ther.* 2002;71:57-67.

Efavirenz (*Sustiva*)

Methadone (eg, *Dolophine*)

SUMMARY: Efavirenz reduces methadone plasma concentrations; methadone withdrawal or loss of analgesic effect may occur.

RISK FACTORS: No specific risk factors are known.

RELATED DRUGS: Nevirapine (*Viramune*) has also been reported to reduce methadone plasma concentrations and precipitate methadone withdrawal symptoms. Other narcotic analgesics metabolized by CYP3A4 (eg, fentanyl) may be similarly affected by efavirenz.

MANAGEMENT OPTIONS:

➡ *Consider Alternative.* The use of an analgesic that is not a substrate for CYP3A4 (eg, morphine, codeine) could be considered in patients taking efavirenz.

➡ *Monitor.* Be alert for symptoms of methadone withdrawal if efavirenz is initiated in patients on methadone maintenance regimens. Discontinuation of efavirenz may result in excessive methadone effects (sedation, respiratory depression). Methadone dosage adjustments may be necessary whenever efavirenz is added to or removed from the regimen of patients maintained on methadone.

REFERENCES:

Clarke SM, et al. The pharmacokinetics of methadone in HIV-positive patients receiving the nonnucleoside reverse transcriptase inhibitor efavirenz. *Br J Clin Pharmacol.* 2001;51:213-217.

Efavirenz (*Sustiva*)

Ritonavir (*Norvir*)

SUMMARY: Efavirenz administration reduces ritonavir concentrations; some loss of antiviral efficacy may result.

RISK FACTORS: No specific risk factors are known.

RELATED DRUGS: Efavirenz reduces the plasma concentration of indinavir. Its effect on other protease inhibitors that are metabolized by CYP3A4 (eg, nelfinavir [*Viracept*], saquinavir [eg, *Fortovase*]) is likely to be similar.

MANAGEMENT OPTIONS:

➡ *Monitor.* Monitor patients taking ritonavir who are prescribed efavirenz for reduced ritonavir concentrations and possible loss of efficacy.

REFERENCES:

Aarnoutse RE, et al. The influence of efavirenz on the pharmacokinetics of a twice-daily combination of indinavir and low-dose ritonavir in healthy volunteers. *Clin Pharmacol Ther.* 2002;71:57-67.

▼ Enalapril (*Vasotec*)

Furosemide (eg, *Lasix*)

SUMMARY: Initiation of angiotensin-converting enzyme (ACE) inhibitor therapy in the presence of intensive diuretic therapy, results in a precipitous fall in blood pressure in some patients. ACE inhibitors may induce renal insufficiency in the presence of diuretic-induced sodium depletion.

RISK FACTORS:

➡ ***Concurrent Diseases.*** Preexisting high blood pressure, secondary hypertension, high circulating levels of renin and angiotensin II, and CHF may increase the risk of acute hypotensive episodes.

➡ ***Dosage Regimen.*** Hypovolemia caused by diuretic therapy may predispose hypotensive reactions or acute renal failure.

RELATED DRUGS: Other loop diuretics (eg, bumetanide [eg, *Bumex*], torsemide [*Demadex*], ethacrynic acid [*Edecrin*]) probably interact with ACE inhibitors in the same way as furosemide. All ACE inhibitors most likely interact in a similar way with diuretics.

MANAGEMENT OPTIONS:

➡ ***Circumvent/Minimize.*** Some have recommended that CHF patients on furosemide should be kept supine for 3 hours after the first dose of ACE inhibitors; this especially refers to the elderly.

➡ ***Monitor.*** Undertake initiation of therapy with ACE inhibitors cautiously in patients receiving diuretics, especially if there is evidence of hypovolemia. Monitor blood pressure carefully for at least 3 hours after the ACE inhibitor is given. In some patients it may be desirable to withdraw the diuretic temporarily before starting the ACE inhibitor.

REFERENCES:

Hodsman GP, et al. Factors related to first dose hypotensive effect of captopril: prediction and treatment. *BMJ*. 1983;286:832-834.

Mandal AK, et al. Diuretics potentiate angiotensin converting enzyme inhibitor-induced acute renal failure. *Clin Nephrol*. 1994;42:170-174.

MacFayden RJ. The response to the first dose of an ACE inhibitor in essential hypertension: a placebo-controlled study utilizing ambulatory blood pressure recording. *Br J Clin Pharmacol*. 1991;31:568P.

Atkinson AB, et al. Captopril in a hyponatremic hypertensive: need for caution in initiating therapy. *Lancet*. 1979;1:557-558.

Vlasses PH, et al. Captopril: clinical pharmacology and benefit-to-risk ratio in hypertension and congestive heart failure. *Pharmacotherapy*. 1982;2:1-17.

Chalmers D, et al. Postmarketing surveillance of captopril for hypertension. *Br J Clin Pharmacol*. 1992;34:215-223.

Rakhit A, et al. Pharmacokinetics and pharmacodynamics of pentopril, a new angiotensin-converting-enzyme inhibitor in humans. *J Clin Pharmacol*. 1986;26:156-164.

Fujimura A, et al. Influence of captopril on urinary excretion of furosemide in hypertensive subjects. *J Clin Pharmacol*. 1990;30:538-542.

Van Hecken AM, et al. Absence of a pharmacokinetic interaction between enalapril and furosemide. *Br J Clin Pharmacol*. 1987;23:84-87.

Gluck Z, et al. Long-term effects of captopril on renal function in hypertensive patients. *Eur J Clin Pharmacol*. 1984;26:315-323.

Clementy J, et al. Comparative study of the efficacy and tolerance of capozide and moduretic administered in a single daily dose for the treatment of chronic moderate arterial hypertension. *Postgrad Med J.* 1986;62(suppl. 1):132-134.

Pandhi P, et al. Low-dose captopril alone and in combination with hydrochlorothiazide in treatment of mild to moderate essential hypertension. *Int J Clin Pharmacol Ther Toxicol.* 1986;24:294-297.

Toto RD, et al. Reversible renal insufficiency due to angiotensin converting enzyme inhibitors in hypertensive nephrosclerosis. *Ann Intern Med.* 1991;115:513-519.

Funck-Brentano C, et al. Reversible renal failure after combined treatment with enalapril and furosemide in a patient with congestive heart failure. *Br Heart J.* 1986;55:596-598.

Mets T, et al. First-dose hypotension, ACE inhibitors, and heart failure in the elderly. *Lancet.* 1992;339:1487.

Enalapril (eg, *Vasotec*)
Indomethacin (eg, *Indocin*)

SUMMARY: Indomethacin (and probably other nonsteroidal anti-inflammatory drugs [NSAIDs]) inhibits the antihypertensive effects of enalapril (and probably other angiotensin converting enzyme [ACE] inhibitors).

RISK FACTORS: No specific risk factors are known.

RELATED DRUGS: Theoretically, any combination of an ACE inhibitor and an NSAID would result in inhibition of the antihypertensive effect of the ACE inhibitor.

MANAGEMENT OPTIONS:

➡ *Consider Alternative.* Antihypertensive agents other than ACE inhibitors (eg, amlodipine [*Norvasc*]) may be less affected by NSAIDs.

➡ *Monitor.* If indomethacin or other NSAIDs are used with enalapril or other ACE inhibitors, monitor the blood pressure carefully.

REFERENCES:
Morgan TO, et al. Effect of indomethacin on blood pressure in elderly people with essential hypertension well controlled on amlodipine or enalapril. *Am J Hypertens.* 2000;13:1161-1167.

Enalapril (eg, *Vasotec*)
Iron

SUMMARY: Three patients on enalapril developed systemic reactions (GI symptoms, hypotension) following IV iron; more study is needed to establish a causal relationship.

RISK FACTORS:

➡ *Route of Administration.* IV administration of iron appears more likely to interact than oral.

RELATED DRUGS: Oral iron has not been associated with these reactions in patients receiving other ACE inhibitors.

MANAGEMENT OPTIONS:

➡ *Consider Alternative.* Although this potential interaction is not well established, given the severity of the reactions it would be prudent to consider alternatives to the IV iron or the ACE inhibitor.

➡ **Monitor.** If IV iron is given to a patient on an ACE inhibitor, monitor for systemic reactions and be prepared to treat anaphylaxis.

REFERENCES:

Rolla G, et al. Systemic reactions to intravenous iron therapy in patients receiving angiotension converting enzyme inhibitor. *J Allergy Clin Immunol*. 1994;93:1074-1075.

Enalapril (eg, *Vasotec*)
Rofecoxib (*Vioxx*)

SUMMARY: A patient on enalapril developed hyperkalemia after starting rofecoxib, but it is not known how often this problem occurs.

RISK FACTORS: No specific risk factors are known, but it seems likely that renal impairment or diabetes would increase the risk of hyperkalemia.

RELATED DRUGS: It is likely that rofecoxib could also increase the risk of hyperkalemia in patients receiving other ACE inhibitors such as benazepril (*Lotensin*), captopril (eg, *Capoten*), fosinopril (*Monopril*), lisinopril (eg, *Prinivil*), moexipril (eg, *Univasc*), quinapril (*Accupril*), ramipril (*Altace*), and trandolapril (*Mavik*).

MANAGEMENT OPTIONS:

➡ **Monitor.** In patients receiving rofecoxib and an ACE inhibitor, monitor serum potassium and renal function, particularly if the patient has one or more risk factors such as diabetes or renal impairment.

REFERENCES:

Hay H, et al. Fatal hyperkalemia related to combined therapy with a COX-2 inhibitor, ACE inhibitor and potassium rich diet. *J Emerg Med*. 2002;22:349-352.

Enalapril (eg, *Vasotec*)
Trimethoprim-Sulfamethoxazole (eg, *Bactrim*)

SUMMARY: A patient on enalapril developed severe hyperkalemia after receiving trimethoprim-sulfamethoxazole.

RISK FACTORS: No specific risk factors are known, but it seems likely that renal impairment or diabetes would increase the risk of hyperkalemia.

RELATED DRUGS: Other ACE inhibitors would also be expected to interact, including benazepril (*Lotensin*), captopril (eg, *Capoten*), fosinopril (*Monopril*), lisinopril (eg, *Prinivil*), moexipril (eg, *Univasc*), quinapril (*Accupril*), ramipril (*Altace*), and trandolapril (*Mavik*).

MANAGEMENT OPTIONS:

➡ **Monitor.** In patients receiving trimethoprim and an ACE inhibitor, monitor serum potassium and renal function, particularly if the patient has 1 or more risk factors such as diabetes or renal impairment.

REFERENCES:

Bugge JF. Severe hyperkalaemia induced by trimethoprim in combination with an angiotensin-converting enzyme inhibitor in a patient with transplanted lungs. *J Intern Med*. 1996;240:249-251.

Encainide[†]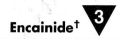

Quinidine

SUMMARY: Quinidine can substantially increase encainide serum concentrations in patients who are extensive (rapid) encainide metabolizers. However, because of the opposing effects of quinidine on the serum concentrations of encainide and its active metabolites, the clinical outcome is likely to be limited.

RISK FACTORS:

➥ **Pharmacogenetics.** Rapid encainide metabolizers are at greater risk.

RELATED DRUGS: No information is available.

MANAGEMENT OPTIONS:

➥ **Monitor.** Monitor patients maintained on encainide for changes in antiarrhythmic efficacy when quinidine is added or deleted.

REFERENCES:

Funck-Brentano C, et al. Effect of low dose quinidine on encainide pharmacokinetics and pharmacodynamics. Influence of genetic polymorphism. *J Pharmacol Exp Ther.* 1989;249:134-142.

Turgeon J, et al. Genetically determined steady-state interaction between encainide and quinidine in patients with arrhythmias. *J Pharmacol Exp Ther.* 1990;255:642-649.

Turgeon J, et al. Genetically determined stereoselective excretion of encainide in humans and electrophysiologic effects of its enantiomers in canine cardiac Purkinje fibers. *Clin Pharmacol Ther.* 1991;49:488-496.

† Not available in the United States.

Enoxacin[†]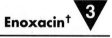

Fenbufen[†]

SUMMARY: The combination of enoxacin and fenbufen has been reported to produce seizures.

RISK FACTORS:

➥ **Concurrent Diseases.** Patients with epilepsy or a history of convulsions are at greater risk.

RELATED DRUGS: Ciprofloxacin (eg, *Cipro*) and diclofenac (eg, *Cataflam*) do not appear to interact nor do ketoprofen (eg, *Orudis*) and pefloxacin or ofloxacin (eg, *Floxin*).

MANAGEMENT OPTIONS:

➥ **Consider Alternative.** Consider using a quinolone, which is less likely to interact (eg, ciprofloxacin, ketoprofen, pefloxacin, ofloxacin, diclofenac).

➥ **Monitor.** Until more data are available, carefully observe patients with a history of convulsions when prescribed quinolones and NSAIDs. Special precautions are not necessary for most patients.

REFERENCES:

Akahane K, et al. Possible intermolecular interaction between quinolones and biphenylacetic acid inhibits gamma-aminobutyric acid receptor sites. *Antimicrob Agents Chemother.* 1994;38:2323-2329.

Halliwell RF, et al. Antagonism of GABA$_A$ receptors by 4-quinolones. *J Antimicrob Chemother.* 1993;31:457-462.

Christ W, et al. Interactions of quinolones with opioids and fenbufen, a NSAID: involvement of dopaminergic neurotransmission. *Rev Infect Dis.* 1989;11(suppl 5):S1393.

Davies BI, et al. Drug interactions with quinolones. *Rev Infect Dis.* 1989;11(suppl 5):S1083-S1090.

Hori, et al. A study on enhanced epileptogenicity of new quinolones in the presence of anti-inflammatory drugs. In: Abstracts of the 26th Interscience Conference on Antimicrobial Agents and Chemotherapy. Washington, DC: American Society for Microbiology; 1986.

Segev S, et al. Quinolones, theophylline, and diclofenac interactions with the gamma-aminobutyric acid receptor. *Antimicrob Agents Chemother.* 1988;32:1624-1626.

Fillastre JP, et al. Lack of effect of ketoprofen on the pharmacokinetics of pefloxacin and ofloxacin. *J Antimicrob Chemother.* 1993;31:805-806.

† Not available in the US.

Enoxacin (*Penetrex*)

Ranitidine (eg, *Zantac*)

SUMMARY: Ranitidine administration reduces the plasma concentrations of enoxacin; failure of antibiotic efficacy could result.

RISK FACTORS: No specific risk factors are known.

RELATED DRUGS: The effects of other H_2-receptor antagonists (eg, cimetidine [eg, *Tagamet*], famotidine [eg, *Pepcid*], nizatidine [*Axid*]) or proton pump inhibitors (eg, lansoprazole [*Prevacid*], omeprazole [*Prilosec*]) on orally administered enoxacin are unknown but would be expected to be similar to those of ranitidine.

MANAGEMENT OPTIONS:

➡ **Consider Alternative.** Separation of the doses of ranitidine and oral enoxacin will probably have little effect on this interaction since the pH tends to stay somewhat elevated during therapy with H_2-receptor antagonists or omeprazole. The administration of IV enoxacin or an alternative antibiotic may be necessary in patients requiring gastric acid suppression.

➡ **Monitor.** Observe patients receiving enoxacin and drugs that alkalinize the gut for loss of antibiotic efficacy.

REFERENCES:
Lebsack ME, et al. Effect of gastric acidity on enoxacin absorption. *Clin Pharmacol Ther.* 1992;52:252.

Grasela TH, et al. Inhibition of enoxacin absorption by antacids or ranitidine. *Antimicrob Agents Chemother.* 1989;33:615.

Enoxacin (*Penetrex*)

Tacrine (*Cognex*)

SUMMARY: In vitro studies suggest that enoxacin is a potent inhibitor of tacrine metabolism. Given the major effect that enoxacin has on theophylline metabolism (which is metabolized by the same enzyme [CYP1A2] as tacrine), it seems likely that enoxacin has a similar effect on tacrine.

RISK FACTORS: No specific risk factors are known.

RELATED DRUGS: Expect the various quinolones to affect tacrine metabolism in a manner similar to their effects on theophylline. If that proves to be true, enoxacin would have a marked effect on tacrine metabolism, ciprofloxacin (*Cipro*) a moderate effect, and norfloxacin (*Noroxin*) a small effect. Theoretically, quinolones such as lomefloxacin (*Maxaquin*) and ofloxacin (*Floxin*) would be less likely to interact with tacrine.

MANAGEMENT OPTIONS:

➡ *Consider Alternative.* Consider using a quinolone, which is less likely to interact (eg, lomefloxacin, ofloxacin).

➡ *Monitor.* If quinolones and tacrine are used together, monitor for tacrine toxicity (eg, nausea, vomiting, anorexia, diarrhea, abdominal pain). However, some evidence suggests that tacrine hepatotoxicity results from reactive tacrine metabolites. Thus, if quinolones are found to inhibit tacrine metabolism clinically, possibly expect the effect to reduce the risk of hepatotoxicity.

REFERENCES:

Madden S, et al. An investigation into the formation of stable, proteinreactive, and cytotoxic metabolites from tacrine in vitro. Studies with human and rat liver microsomes. *Biochem Pharmacol.* 1993;46:13.

Enoxacin (*Penetrex*)

Theophylline (eg, *Theolair*)

SUMMARY: Enoxacin markedly increases the serum concentrations of theophylline and may result in the development of theophylline toxicity.

RISK FACTORS:

➡ *Dosage Regimen.* Higher doses of enoxacin produce a greater risk.

RELATED DRUGS: Quinolones reported to inhibit the metabolism of drugs include ciprofloxacin (*Cipro*), enoxacin, norfloxacin (*Noroxin*), pipemidic acid, and pefloxacin.[†] Quinolones reported to produce no or minor changes in theophylline pharmacokinetics include fleroxacin,[†] lomefloxacin (*Maxaquin*), ofloxacin (*Floxin*), rufloxacin,[†] and sparfloxacin (eg, *Zagam*).

MANAGEMENT OPTIONS:

➡ *Use Alternative.* Enoxacin should not be administered with theophylline. Use a quinolone known to have no or minor effect on theophylline pharmacokinetics (eg, fleroxacin, lomefloxacin, ofloxacin, rufloxacin, sparfloxacin).

REFERENCES:

Wijnands WJA, et al. Enoxacin raises plasma theophylline concentrations. *Lancet.* 1984;2:108.

Wijnands WJA, et al. The effect of the 4-quinolone enoxacin on plasma theophylline concentrations. *Pharm Weekly [Sci].* 1986;8:42.

Wijnands WJA, et al. The influence of quinolone derivatives on theophylline clearance. *Br J Clin Pharmacol.* 1986;22:677.

Koup JR, et al. Theophylline dosage adjustment during enoxacin coadministration. *Anitmicrob Agents Chemother.* 1990;34:803.

Beckmann EW, et al. Enoxacin—a potent inhibitor of theophylline metabolism. *Eur J Clin Pharmacol.* 1987;33:227.

Rogge MC, et al. The theophylline-enoxacin interaction: I. Effect of enoxacin dose size on theophylline disposition. *Clin Pharmacol Ther.* 1988;44:579.

Sano M, et al. Effects of enoxacin, ofloxacin, and norfloxacin on theophylline disposition in humans. *Eur J Clin Pharmacol.* 1988;35:161.

Sarkar M, et al. In vitro effect of fluoroquinolones of theophylline metabolism in human liver microsomes. *Antimicrob Agents Chemother.* 1990;34:594.

Wijnands WJA, et al. Steady-state kinetics of the quinolone derivatives ofloxacin, enoxacin, ciprofloxacin, and pefloxacin during maintenance treatment with theophylline. *Drugs.* 1987;34(Suppl. 1):159.

† Not available in the US.

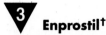

 Enprostil†

Ethanol (Ethyl Alcohol)

SUMMARY: Enprostil appears to increase instead of decrease the gastric mucosal damage produced by ethanol.

RISK FACTORS: No specific risk factors are known.

RELATED DRUGS: The effect of ethanol combined with prostaglandins other than enprostil is not established.

MANAGEMENT OPTIONS:

➡ *Circumvent/Minimize.* Until more information is available, it would be prudent for patients taking enprostil (and possibly other prostaglandins) to minimize their alcohol intake.

➡ *Monitor.* Monitor for evidence of GI intolerance if the combination is used.

REFERENCES:

Cohen MM, et al. Human antral damage induced by alcohol is potentiated by enprostil. *Gastroenterology.* 1990;99:45.

† Not available in the US.

 Ephedrine

Guanethidine (*Ismelin*)

SUMMARY: Preliminary evidence indicates that ephedrine inhibits the antihypertensive response to guanethidine.

RISK FACTORS: No specific risk factors are known.

RELATED DRUGS: Theoretically, one would expect guanadrel (eg, *Hylorel*), a drug pharmacologically similar to guanethidine, to be similarly affected by ephedrine.

MANAGEMENT OPTIONS:

➡ *Monitor.* If ephedrine must be used in a patient receiving guanethidine, closely watch the patient for rising blood pressure. If the guanethidine dosage is increased to compensate for this effect, watch for hypotension when ephedrine is discontinued.

REFERENCES:

Starr KJ, et al. Drug interactions in patients on long-term oral anticoagulant and antihypertensive adrenergic neuron-blocking drugs. *BMJ.* 1972;4:133-135.

Day MD, et al. Antagonism of guanethidine and bretylium by various agents. *Lancet.* 1962;2:1282.

Gulati OD, et al. Antagonism of adrenergic neuron blockade in hypertensive subjects. *Clin Pharmacol Ther.* 1966;7:510-514.

 Ephedrine

Moclobemide†

SUMMARY: Moclobemide substantially enhances the pressor response to ephedrine, and increases the risk of palpitations, headache, and lightheadedness.

RISK FACTORS: No specific risk factors are known.

RELATED DRUGS: Theoretically, the pressor response to other sympathomimetics with significant indirect activity (eg, pseudoephedrine [eg, *Sudafed*]) also would be increased in patients receiving moclobemide.

MANAGEMENT OPTIONS:

➡ *Use Alternative.* Based upon available data, avoid ephedrine in patients receiving moclobemide. Until safety data are available, avoid other indirect acting sympathomimetics (eg, pseudoephedrine) with agents that inhibit MAO-A.

REFERENCES:

Dingemanse J. An update of recent moclobemide interaction data. *Int Clin Psychopharmacol.* 1993;7:167-180.

† Not available in the US.

Epinephrine (eg, *Adrenalin*)
Imipramine (eg, *Tofranil*)

SUMMARY: The pressor response to IV epinephrine may be markedly enhanced in patients receiving tricyclic antidepressants (TCAs) like imipramine.

RISK FACTORS: No specific risk factors are known.

RELATED DRUGS: Little is known about the use of epinephrine with other TCAs; assume they interact until proved otherwise.

MANAGEMENT OPTIONS:

➡ *Avoid Unless Benefit Outweighs Risk.* Give patients receiving TCAs IV epinephrine only with close monitoring of blood pressure. Some caution should also be exercised if the epinephrine is administered by other routes. However, when epinephrine is used to prevent or treat anaphylaxis, consider the real possibility that the benefit of giving epinephrine will outweigh the risks in such patients.

➡ *Monitor.* If IV epinephrine is given to patients receiving TCAs, monitor blood pressure carefully and adjust epinephrine dose as needed.

REFERENCES:

Boakes AJ, et al. Interactions between sympathomimetic amines and antidepressant agents in man. *BMJ.* 1973;1:311.

Svedmyr N. The influence of a tricyclic antidepressant agent (protriptyline) on some of the circulatory effects of noradrenaline and adrenaline in man. *Life Sci.* 1968;7:77.

Boakes AJ. Sympathomimetic amines and antidepressant agents. *BMJ.* 1973;2:114.

Epinephrine (eg, *Adrenalin*)
Propranolol (eg, *Inderal*)

SUMMARY: Noncardioselective beta-blockers enhance the pressor response to epinephrine, resulting in hypertension and bradycardia.

RISK FACTORS: No specific risk factors are known.

RELATED DRUGS: Other nonspecific beta-blockers (eg, alprenolol,† nadolol [eg, *Corgard*], pindolol [eg, *Visken*], timolol [eg, *Blocadren*]) would produce a similar effect. Labetalol (eg, *Trandate*, which is a nonspecific beta-blocker as well as an alpha$_1$-blocker) increases the diastolic pressure and slows the heart rate during epinephrine infusions, but acute hypertensive reactions appear unlikely. Metoprolol (eg, *Lopressor*), and perhaps other cardioselective beta-blockers, have minimal effects on the pressor response to epinephrine even at doses of 200 to 300 mg/day.

MANAGEMENT OPTIONS:

➥ *Consider Alternative.* Selective $beta_1$-blockers (eg, metoprolol) may be less likely than propranolol to result in hypertension and bradycardia when epinephrine is administered or when endogenous epinephrine is released.

➥ *Monitor.* Administer epinephrine with caution in patients receiving propranolol or other nonselective beta-blockers, and monitor blood pressure carefully. If the epinephrine is used to treat anaphylaxis, the response to epinephrine may be poor and vigorous supportive care (eg, volume replacement) may be needed.

REFERENCES:

Gandy W. Severe epinephrine-propranolol interaction. *Ann Emerg Med.* 1989;18:98-99.

Houben H, et al. Effect of low-dose epinephrine infusion on hemodynamics after selective and nonselective beta-blockade in hypertension. *Clin Pharmacol Ther.* 1982;31:685-690.

Houben H, et al. Influence of selective and non-selective beta-adrenoreceptor blockade on the haemodynamic effect of adrenaline during combined antihypertensive drug therapy. *Clin Sci.* 1979;57(suppl 5):397s-399s.

van Herwaarden CL, et al. Haemodynamic effects of adrenaline during treatment of hypertensive patients with propranolol and metoprolol. *Eur J Clin Pharmacol.* 1977;12:397-402.

Hansbrough JF. Propranolol-epinephrine antagonism with hypertension and stroke. *Ann Intern Med.* 1980;92:717.

Lampman RM, et al. Cardiac arrhythmias during epinephrine-propranolol infusions for measurement of in vivo insulin resistance. *Diabetes.* 1981;30:618-620.

Foster CA, et al. Propranolol-epinephrine interaction: a potential disaster. *Plast Reconstr Surg.* 1983;72:74-78.

Newman BR, et al. Epinephrine-resistant anaphylaxis in a patient taking propranolol hydrochloride. *Ann Allergy.* 1981;47:35-37.

Jacobs RL, et al. Potentiated anaphylaxis in patients with drug-induced beta-adrenergic blockade. *J Allergy Clin Immunol.* 1981;68:125-127.

Hannaway PJ, et al. Severe anaphylaxis and drug-induced beta-blockade. *N Engl J Med.* 1983;308:1536.

Richards DA, et al. Circulatory effects of noradrenaline and adrenaline before and after labetalol. *Br J Clin Pharmacol.* 1979;7:371-378.

Doshi BS, et al. Effects of labetalol and propranolol on responses to adrenaline infusion in healthy volunteers. *Int J Clin Pharmacol Res.* 1984;4:29-33.

† Not available in the US.

Eplerenone (*Inspra*)

Candesartan (*Atacand*)

SUMMARY: Combining eplerenone with candesartan or other angiotensin II receptor blockers (ARBs) may increase the risk of hyperkalemia, especially in patients with 1 or more risk factors.

RISK FACTORS:

➡ ***Other Drugs.*** CYP3A4 inhibitors such as itraconazole, ketoconazole, erythromycin, clarithromycin, diltiazem, verapamil, and protease inhibitors may increase eplerenone serum concentrations and may increase the risk of hyperkalemia. Also, the addition of other hyperkalemic drugs may increase the risk of hyperkalemia in patients on eplerenone and ARBs. Hyperkalemic drugs include ACE inhibitors, potassium supplements, cyclosporine, tacrolimus, NSAIDs, COX-2 inhibitors, non-selective beta-adrenergic blockers, trimethoprim, and pentamidine.

➡ ***Concurrent Diseases.*** Diseases that increase the risk of hyperkalemia for this interaction include diabetes and significant renal impairment.

➡ ***Diet/Food.*** A diet high in potassium may increase the risk of hyperkalemia from this interaction. Salt substitutes may contain potassium.

RELATED DRUGS: Eplerenone can be expected to increase the risk of hyperkalemia when combined with other ARBs, including eprosartan (*Teveten*), irbesartan (*Avapro*), losartan (*Cozaar*), telmisartan (*Micardis*), and valsartan (*Diovan*).

MANAGEMENT OPTIONS:

➡ ***Monitor.*** In patients receiving eplerenone and an ARB, monitor serum potassium and renal function, particularly if the patient has 1 or more of the risk factors listed above.

REFERENCES:

Wrenger E, et al. Interaction of spironolactone with ACE inhibitors or antiogensin receptor blockers: analysis of 44 cases. *BMJ*. 2003;327:147-149.

Eplerenone (*Inspra*)

Enalapril (eg, *Vasotec*)

SUMMARY: Combining eplerenone with enalapril or other ACE inhibitors may increase the risk of hyperkalemia, especially in patients with 1 or more risk factors.

RISK FACTORS:

➡ ***Other Drugs.*** In patients on eplerenone and ACE inhibitors, the addition of other hyperkalemic drugs can increase the risk. Such drugs include potassium supplements, nonselective beta-adrenergic blockers, cyclosporine, tacrolimus, NSAIDs, COX-2 inhibitors, trimethoprim, and pentamidine.

➡ ***Concurrent Diseases.*** Diseases that increase the risk of hyperkalemia for this interaction include diabetes and significant renal impairment.

➡ ***Diet/Food.*** A diet high in potassium may increase the risk of hyperkalemia from this interaction. Some salt substitutes contain potassium.

RELATED DRUGS: Eplerenone would also be expected to interact with other ACE inhibitors, including benazepril (*Lotensin*), captopril (eg, *Capoten*), fosinopril (*Monopril*), lisinopril (eg, *Prinivil*), moexipril (eg, *Univasc*), quinapril (*Accupril*), ramipril (*Altace*), and trandolapril (*Mavik*).

MANAGEMENT OPTIONS:

➡ ***Monitor.*** In patients receiving eplerenone and an ACE inhibitor, monitor serum potassium and renal function, particularly if the patient has 1 or more of the risk factors listed above.

REFERENCES:

Pitt B, Zannad F, Remme WJ, et al. The effect of spironolactone on morbidity and mortality in patients with severe heart failure. Randomized Aldactone Evaluation Study Investigators. *New Engl J Med.* 1999;341:709-717.

Schepkens H, et al. Life-threatening hyperkalemia during combined therapy with angiotensin-converting enzyme inhibitors and spironolactone. *Am J Med.* 2001;110:438-441.

Berry C, McMurray J. Life-threatening hyperkalemia during combined therapy with angiotensin-converting enzyme inhibitors and spironolactone. *Am J Med.* 2001;111:587.

Blaustein DA, et al. Estimation of glomerular filtration rate to prevent life-threatening hyperkalemia due to combined therapy with spironolactone and antiotensin-converting enzyme inhibition or antiotensin receptor blockade. *Am J Cardiol.* 2002;90:662-663.

Wrenger E, et al. Interaction of spironolactone with ACE inhibitors or antiogensin receptor blockers: analysis of 44 cases. *BMJ.* 2003;327:147-149.

Weber EW, et al. Incidence of hyperkalemia in chronic heart failure patients taking spironolactone in a VA medical center. *Pharmacotherapy.* 2003;23:391.

 ## Ergotamine (*Ergomar*)

Indinavir (*Crixivan*)

SUMMARY: Indinavir is likely to increase the plasma concentrations of ergotamine, possibly leading to toxicity including vasospasm and cyanosis.

RISK FACTORS: No specific risk factors are known.

RELATED DRUGS: Other protease inhibitors such as ritonavir (*Norvir*), amprenavir (*Agenerase*), nelfinavir (*Viracept*), and saquinavir (eg, *Fortovase*) would be expected to affect ergotamine in a similar manner.

MANAGEMENT OPTIONS:

➡ ***Use Alternative.*** If possible, avoid ergot derivatives in patients taking protease inhibitors.

➡ ***Monitor.*** If ergotamine is administered to a patient taking a protease inhibitor, start the patient on low doses of ergotamine and monitor carefully for any signs of ergotism.

REFERENCES:

Rosenthal E, et al. Ergotism related to concurrent administration of ergotamine tartrate and indinavir. *JAMA.* 1999;281:987.

Ergotamine (*Ergostat*) 2

Nitroglycerin

SUMMARY: Ergotamine may oppose the coronary vasodilation of nitrates.

RISK FACTORS: No specific risk factors are known.

RELATED DRUGS: No information is available.

MANAGEMENT OPTIONS:

➡ *Avoid Unless Benefit Outweighs Risk.* Patients receiving nitroglycerin for angina pectoris should avoid ergotamine if at all possible.

➡ *Monitor.* If the combination is used, monitor patients for enhanced ergotamine effect, the ergot dosage lowered as needed.

REFERENCES:

Bobik A, et al. Low oral bioavailability of dihydroergotamine and firstpass extraction in patients with orthostatic hypotension. *Clin Pharmacol Ther*. 1981;30:673.

Ergotamine (*Ergostat*) 2

Ritonavir (*Norvir*)

SUMMARY: Ritonavir is likely to increase the plasma concentrations of ergotamine possibly leading to toxicity including vasospasm and cyanosis.

RISK FACTORS: No specific risk factors are known.

RELATED DRUGS: Other protease inhibitors such as indinavir (*Crixivan*), amprenavir (*Agenerase*), nelfinavir (*Viracept*), and saquinavir (*Invirase*) would be expected to affect ergotamine in a similar manner.

MANAGEMENT OPTIONS:

➡ *Use Alternative.* If possible, avoid ergot derivatives in patients taking protease inhibitors.

➡ *Monitor.* If ergotamine is administered to a patient taking a protease inhibitor, start the patient on low doses of ergotamine and monitor carefully for any signs of ergotism.

REFERENCES:

Caballero-Granado FJ, et al. Ergotism related to concurrent administration of ergotamine tartrate and ritonavir in an AIDS patient. *Antimicrob Agents Chemother*. 1997;41:1207.

Erythromycin

Clopidogrel (*Plavix*)

SUMMARY: Erythromycin appears to inhibit the antiplatelet effects of clopidogrel, but the extent to which the therapeutic effects of clopidogrel are reduced is not known.

RISK FACTORS: No specific risk factors are known.

RELATED DRUGS: Troleandomycin (*TAO*) also appears to inhibit the antiplatelet effects of clopidogrel. Clarithromycin (Biaxin) is also an inhibitor of CYP3A4 and would theoretically interact with clopidogrel in a similar manner.

MANAGEMENT OPTIONS:

➡ *Consider Alternative.* Theoretically, azithromycin (*Zithromax*) and dirithromycin (*Dynabac*) would be unlikely to interact with clopidogrel since they do not inhibit CYP3A4.

➡ *Monitor.* Consider monitoring platelet function if erythromycin is initiated or discontinued. Adjustments in clopidogrel dose may be needed.

REFERENCES:

Clarke TA, et al. The metabolism of clopidogrel is catalyzed by human cytochrome P450 3A and is inhibited by atorvastatin. *Drug Metab Dispos.* 2003;31:53-59.

Lau WC, et al. Atorvastatin reduces the ability of clopidogrel to inhibit platelet aggregation: a new drug-drug interaction. *Circulation.* 2003;107:32-37.

Erythromycin (eg, *EryPed*)

Ethanol (*Ethyl Alcohol*)

SUMMARY: Erythromycin ethylsuccinate plasma concentrations are reduced by ethanol coadministration; clinically significant changes are unlikely.

RISK FACTORS: No specific risk factors are known.

RELATED DRUGS: No information is available.

MANAGEMENT OPTIONS:

➡ *Circumvent/Minimize.* Counsel patients taking erythromycin ethylsuccinate to avoid ingesting alcoholic beverages with the antibiotic. An increase in ethanol effects may be noted in some patients.

➡ *Monitor.* Alert patients for enhanced ethanol effects during coadministration of erythromycin.

REFERENCES:

Morasso MI, et al. Influence of alcohol consumption on erythromycin ethylsuccinate kinetics. *Int J Clin Pharmacol Ther Toxicol.* 1990;28:426-429.

Min DI, et al. Effect of erythromycin on ethanol's pharmacokinetics and perception of intoxication. *Pharmacotherapy.* 1995;15:164-169.

Edelbroek MA, et al. Effects of erythromycin on gastric emptying, alcohol absorption and small intestinal transit in normal subjects. *J Nucl Med.* 1993;34:582-188.

Erythromycin (eg, *E-Mycin*)

Felodipine (*Plendil*)

SUMMARY: Erythromycin administration resulted in elevated felodipine concentrations accompanied by flushing, edema, and tachycardia. More information is needed to establish a causal relationship.

RISK FACTORS: No specific risk factors are known.

RELATED DRUGS: Troleandomycin (*TAO*) also may inhibit the metabolism of calcium channel blockers. Because other calcium channel blockers are metabolized similarly to felodipine, erythromycin also may affect their metabolism.

MANAGEMENT OPTIONS:

➡ *Monitor.* Until further information is available, observe patients taking felodipine, and perhaps other calcium channel blockers, for adverse effects (eg, hypotension, headache, arrythmias) during the coadministration of erythromycin.

REFERENCES:

Liedholm H, et al. Erythromycin-felodipine interaction. *DICP.* 1991;25:1007-1008.

Erythromycin (eg, *E-Mycin*)

Food

SUMMARY: Food has variable effects on erythromycin bioavailability; some formulations increase, decrease, or have no change in bioavailability when administered with food.

RISK FACTORS: No specific risk factors are known.

MANAGEMENT OPTIONS:

➡ *Circumvent/Minimize.* Because the results of studies on the effects of food on erythromycin bioavailability are variable, follow the manufacturer's recommendations concerning the timing of specific erythromycin products in relationship to meals.

➡ *Monitor.* Counsel patients to follow label directions carefully when taking erythromycin.

REFERENCES:

Thompson PJ, et al. Influence of food on absorption of erythromycin ethyl succinate. *Antimicrob Agents Chemother.* 1980;18:829.

Coyne TC, et al. Bioavailability of erythromycin ethylsuccinate in pediatric patients. *J Clin Pharmacol.* 1987;18:194.

Bechtol LD, et al. The influence of food on the absorption of erythromycin esters and enteric-coated erythromycin in single-dose studies. *Curr Ther Res.* 1979;25:618.

Malmborg AS. Effect of food on absorption of erythromycin: a study of two derivatives, the stearate and the base. *J Antimicrob Chemother.* 1979;5:591.

Clayton D, et al. The bioavailability of erythromycin stearate vs enteric-coated erythromycin base when taken immediately before and after food. *J Int Med Res.* 1981;9:470.

Hovi T, et al. Effect of concomitant food intake on absorption kinetics of erythromycin in healthy volunteers. *Eur J Clin Pharmacol.* 1985;28:231.

Randinitis EJ, et al. Effect of a high-fat meal on the bioavailability of a polymer-coated erythromycin particle tablet formulation. *J Clin Pharmacol.* 1989;29:79.

Erythromycin (eg, *E-Mycin*)

Lovastatin (*Mevacor*)

SUMMARY: Erythromycin administration with lovastatin may produce rhabdomyolysis.

RISK FACTORS: No specific risk factors are known.

RELATED DRUGS: Other macrolides (eg, troleandomycin [*TAO*], clarithromycin [*Biaxin*]) could affect lovastatin in a similar manner. Azithromycin (*Zithromax*) and dirithromycin (*Dynabac*) would not likely inhibit the metabolism of lovastatin.

MANAGEMENT OPTIONS:

➥ *Monitor.* Until further information is available, watch patients maintained on lovastatin for symptoms of rhabdomyolysis (eg, muscle pain and myoglobinuria) when erythromycin is coadministered.

REFERENCES:

Ayanian JZ, et al. Lovastatin and rhabdomyolysis. *Ann Intern Med.* 1988;109:682.

East C, et al. Rhabdomyolysis in patients receiving lovastatin after cardiac transplantation. *N Engl J Med.* 1988;318:47.

Erythromycin (eg, *E-Mycin*)

Midazolam (*Versed*)

SUMMARY: Erythromycin administration appears to increase the plasma concentrations and effect of midazolam.

RISK FACTORS:

➥ *Route of Administration.* Oral midazolam is much more affected than parenteral.

RELATED DRUGS: Three days erythromycin administration reduced the clearance of triazolam (eg, *Halcion*) 52%. Triazolam is metabolized by the same cytochrome P450 isozyme as midazolam. Troleandomycin (*TAO*) and clarithromycin (*Biaxin*) also may inhibit the metabolism of midazolam and triazolam. Other benzodiazepines also may be affected by erythromycin, clarithromycin, or troleandomycin. Azithromycin (*Zithromax*) and dirithromycin (*Dynabac*) would be less likely to affect midazolam metabolism.

MANAGEMENT OPTIONS:

➥ *Monitor.* Until further information is available, monitor patients taking erythromycin for increased response (eg, sedation, drowsiness) to midazolam and triazolam.

REFERENCES:

Hiller A, et al. Unconsciousness associated with midazolam and erythromycin. *Br J Anaesth.* 1990;65:826.

Philips JP, et al. A pharmacokinetic drug interaction between erythromycin and triazolam. *J Clin Psychopharmacol.* 1986;6:297.

Olkkola KT, et al. A potentially hazardous interaction between erythromycin and midazolam. *Clin Pharmacol Ther.* 1993;53:298.

Kronbach T, et al. Oxidation of midazolam and triazolam by human liver cytochrome P450IIIA4. *Mol Pharmacol.* 1989;36:89.

Mattila MJ, et al. Oral single doses of erythromycin and roxithromycin may increase the effects of midazolam on human performance. *Pharmacol Toxicol.* 1993;73:180.

Erythromycin (eg, *E-Mycin*)

Penicillin G

SUMMARY: Erythromycin may inhibit the antibacterial activity of penicillins.

RISK FACTORS:

➡ *Dosage Regimen.* Low doses of both agents may interfere with antibacterial activity.

RELATED DRUGS: Other macrolides (eg, clarithromycin [*Biaxin*], azithromycin [*Zithromax*]) might interact in a similar manner.

MANAGEMENT OPTIONS:

➡ *Monitor.* Use combination therapy with antibiotics only when necessary. Indications for the concomitant use of penicillin and erythromycin should be rare. If a penicillin is used with erythromycin, it would be prudent to observe the following points: 1) Be sure that appropriate doses of each agent are given; antagonism is most likely when small doses of each are given. 2) Begin administration of the penicillin at least a few hours before the erythromycin.

REFERENCES:

Kabins SA. Interactions among antibiotics and other drugs. *JAMA.* 1972;219:206.

Jawetz E. The use of combinations of antimicrobial drugs. *Ann Rev Pharmacol.* 1968;8:151.

Mills J, et al. Clinical use of antimicrobials. In: Katzung BG. *Basic and Clinical Pharmacology.* Los Altos: Lange Medical Publications; 1982:538–52.

Jawetz E. Synergism and antagonism among antimicrobial drugs, a personal perspective. *West J Med.* 1975;123:87.

Bach MC, et al. Pulmonary nocardiosis: therapy with minocycline and with erythromycin plus ampicillin. *JAMA.* 1973;224:1378.

Erythromycin (eg, *E-Mycin*)

Quinidine (eg, *Quinora*)

SUMMARY: Erythromycin increased quinidine concentrations; cardiac arrhythmias could result.

RISK FACTORS:

➡ *Concurrent Diseases.* Patients with preexisting cardiac disease are at greater risk.

RELATED DRUGS: Other macrolides that inhibit CYP3A4 (eg, troleandomycin [*TAO*], clarithromycin [*Biaxin*]) also may inhibit quinidine metabolism. Azithromycin (*Zithromax*) and dirithromycin (*Dynabac*) are unlikely to affect quinidine concentrations.

MANAGEMENT OPTIONS:

➡ *Consider Alternative.* The use of azithromycin or a nonmacrolide antibiotic would likely avoid the interaction with quinidine.

➡ *Monitor.* If quinidine and erythromycin are coadministered, monitor for signs of quinidine cardiac toxicity (prolonged QRS and QT intervals).

REFERENCES:

Spinler SA, et al. Possible inhibition of hepatic metabolism of quinidine by erythromycin. *Clin Pharmacol Ther.* 1995;57:89.

Erythromycin (eg, *E-Mycin*)

Ritonavir (*Norvir*)

SUMMARY: Ritonavir may inhibit erythromycin metabolism; erythromycin may inhibit ritonavir metabolism. The clinical significance of this potential interaction is unknown.

RISK FACTORS: No specific risk factors are known.

RELATED DRUGS: Clarithromycin (*Biaxin*) serum concentrations are increased by ritonavir and clarithromycin produces a small increase in ritonavir concentrations. Other protease inhibitors such as indinavir (*Crixivan*), saquinavir (eg, *Invirase*), and nelfinavir (*Viracept*) may affect erythromycin in a similar manner. Since azithromycin (*Zithromax*) is not metabolized and is not a CYP3A4 inhibitor, ritonavir would not be expected to interact with azithromycin. Ritonavir concentrations are increased by clarithromycin, and troleandomycin (*TAO*) would be expected to have a similar effect. Dirithromycin (*Dynabac*) would not be expected to have much effect on ritonavir although it could reduce ritonavir concentrations. The effect of ritonavir on dirithromycin concentrations is unknown.

MANAGEMENT OPTIONS:

➡ ***Consider Alternative.*** Azithromycin would probably be a noninteracting alternative to erythromycin for patients receiving ritonavir.

➡ ***Monitor.*** Monitor for evidence of erythromycin or ritonavir toxicity when the 2 drugs are coadministered.

REFERENCES:

Product information. Ritonavir (*Norvir*). Abbott Laboratories. 1996.

 Erythromycin (eg, *E-Mycin*)

Sertraline (*Zoloft*)

SUMMARY: A patient developed an apparent serotonin syndrome following the addition of erythromycin to a chronic dose of sertraline.

RISK FACTORS: No specific risk factors are known.

RELATED DRUGS: Clarithromycin (*Biaxin*) and troleandomycin (*TAO*) are other macrolide antibiotics known to inhibit CYP3A4 metabolism and could affect sertraline similarly. Azithromycin (*Zithromax*) and dirithromycin (*Dynabac*) would not be expected to interact with sertraline. It is likely that other SSRIs that are metabolized by CYP3A4 (eg, citalopram [*Celexa*], nefazodone [*Serzone*]) would be affected in a similar manner by erythromycin, clarithromycin, and troleandomycin. Paroxetine (*Paxil*) is primarily metabolized by CYP2D6 and would be unlikely to be affected by erythromycin.

MANAGEMENT OPTIONS:

➡ ***Consider Alternative.*** The use of a non-CYP3A4-inhibiting macrolide such as azithromycin or dirithromycin would probably avoid any potential to induce the serotonin syndrome in patients taking SSRIs.

➧ *Monitor.* Monitor patients taking any SSRI metabolized by CYP3A4 for signs of excess serotonin effect if CYP3A4 inhibitors are coadministered.

REFERENCES:
Lee DO, et al. Serotonin syndrome in a child associated with erythromycin and sertraline. *Pharmacotherapy.* 1999;19:894–96.

Erythromycin (eg, *E-Mycin*)

Sildenafil (*Viagra*)

SUMMARY: Erythromycin administration produces a large increase in sildenafil plasma concentrations; increased side effects are possible.

RISK FACTORS: No specific risk factors are known.

RELATED DRUGS: Other macrolides that inhibit CYP3A4 [eg, clarithromycin (*Biaxin*), troleandomycin (*TAO*) would be likely to affect sildenafil in a similar manner. Noninhibiting macrolides such as azithromycin (*Zithromax*) or dirithromycin (*Dynabac*) would be unlikely to alter the plasma concentration of sildenafil.

MANAGEMENT OPTIONS:

➧ *Circumvent/Minimize.* Use small doses of sildenafil (eg, 25 mg) when patients are taking macrolides that inhibit CYP3A4 metabolism. Noninhibiting macrolides (eg, azithromycin, dirithromycin) would be unlikely to alter sildenafil concentrations.

➧ *Monitor.* Counsel patients to use a low dose of sildenafil during the administration of erythromycin or other macrolides that inhibit CYP3A4 metabolism. Be alert for increased side effects including headache, abnormal vision, or flushing.

REFERENCES:
Product information. Sildenafil (*Viagra*). Pfizer Pharmaceuticals. 1998.

Erythromycin (eg, *E-Mycin*)

Simvastatin (*Zocor*)

SUMMARY: Erythromycin administration may markedly increase simvastatin concentrations; avoid using the drugs together to avoid the risk of increased side effects.

RISK FACTORS: No specific risk factors are known.

RELATED DRUGS: Erythromycin will likely affect lovastatin (*Mevacor*) plasma concentrations in a similar manner. Atorvastatin (*Lipitor*) plasma concentrations are increased to a lesser degree by erythromycin administration. While no data are available, erythromycin may also increase the plasma concentrations of cerivastatin (*Baycol*). Clarithromycin (*Biaxin*) and troleandomycin (*TAO*) would probably reduce the metabolism of simvastatin. Azithromycin (*Zithromax*) and dirithromycin (*Dynabac*) would not likely inhibit the metabolism of simvastatin. The metabolism of pravastatin (*Pravachol*) and fluvastatin (*Lescol*) would not be expected to be affected by erythromycin.

MANAGEMENT OPTIONS:

➧ *Use Alternative.* Consider the use of a HMG-CoA reductase inhibitor other than simvastatin or lovastatin for patients receiving erythromycin. Atorvastatin and cerivastatin plasma concentrations are likely to be increased by a smaller amount during erythromycin coadministration. Pravastatin and fluvastatin metabolism should not be altered by erythromycin. Azithromycin or dirithromycin are macrolides that will not affect simvastatin metabolism.

REFERENCES:

Kantola T, et al. Erythromycin and verapamil considerably increase serum simvastatin and simvastatin acid concentrations. *Clin Pharmacol Ther.* 1988;64:177.

 Erythromycin (eg, E-Mycin)

Tacrolimus (*Prograf*)

SUMMARY: Patients receiving tacrolimus developed increased concentrations and nephrotoxicity following coadministration with erythromycin.

RISK FACTORS: No specific risk factors are known.

RELATED DRUGS: Erythromycin also is known to inhibit cyclosporine (eg, *Sandimmune*) metabolism. The effects of other macrolides on tacrolimus concentration are unknown, but troleandomycin (*TAO*) and clarithromycin (*Biaxin*) might produce similar changes in tacrolimus. While no data is available, azithromycin (*Zithromax*) would appear to be less likely to interact with tacrolimus.

MANAGEMENT OPTIONS:

➥ *Monitor.* Pending further investigation of this interaction, patients should have their tacrolimus and creatinine serum concentrations monitored if they are coadministered erythromycin.

REFERENCES:

Shaeffer MS, et al. Interaction between FK506 and erythromycin. *Ann Pharmacother.* 1994;28:280.

Jensen C, et al. Interaction between tacrolimus and erythromycin. *Lancet.* 1994;344:825.

Furlan V, et al. Interactions between FK506 and rifampicin or erythromycin in pediatric liver recipients. *Transplantation.* 1995;59:1217.

 Erythromycin (eg, E-Mycin)

Terfenadine (*Seldane*)

SUMMARY: Erythromycin administration may cause cardiac arrythmias in patients taking terfenadine.

RISK FACTORS: No specific risk factors are known.

RELATED DRUGS: The manufacturer of terfenadine has received case reports of an interaction between troleandomycin (*TAO*) and terfenadine that resulted in cardiac arrhythmias.

MANAGEMENT OPTIONS:

➥ *AVOID COMBINATION.* Patients taking terfenadine should avoid concomitant use of erythromycin or troleandomycin. Until further data are available, careful observation is warranted during the administration of terfenadine and other macrolides.

Loratadine (*Claritin*) or cetirizine (*Zyrtec*) may be acceptable alternatives for terfenadine.

REFERENCES:

Honig PK, et al. Erythromycin changes terfenadine pharmacokinetics and electrocardiographic pharmacodynamics. *Clin Pharmacol Ther*. 1992;51:156.

Mathews DR, et al. Torsades de pointes occurring in association with terfenadine use. *JAMA*. 1991;266:2375.

Biglin KE, et al. Drug-induced torsades de pointes: a possible interaction of terfenadine and erythromycin. *Ann Pharmacother*. 1994;28:282.

Eller M, et al. Effect of erythromycin on terfenadine metabolite pharmacokinetics. *Clin Pharmacol Ther*. 1993;53:161.

Honig PK, et al. Comparison of the effect of the macrolide antibiotics erythromycin, clarithromycin and azithromycin on terfenadine steady-state pharmacokinetics and electrocardiographic parameters. *Drug Invest*. 1994;7:148.

Erythromycin (eg, *E-Mycin*)
Theophylline (eg, *Theolair*)

SUMMARY: Erythromycin can increase theophylline serum concentrations and may produce toxicity; theophylline can reduce the concentration of erythromycin.

RISK FACTORS: No specific risk factors are known.

RELATED DRUGS: Troleandomycin (*TAO*) and clarithromycin (*Biaxin*) also may inhibit the metabolism of theophylline.

MANAGEMENT OPTIONS:

➡ *Consider Alternative.* Azithromycin (*Zithromax*) does not appear to alter theophylline concentrations.

➡ *Monitor.* Closely monitor patients when erythromycin therapy is initiated. Although some clinicians suggest lowering the dose of theophylline 25% when erythromycin is initiated, this precaution may excessively complicate the management of low-risk patients (ie, those likely to have a low serum theophylline concentration). Be aware that a reduction in erythromycin serum concentration by theophylline may also be observed.

REFERENCES:

Pasic J, et al. The interaction between chronic oral slow-release theophylline and single-dose intravenous erythromycin. *Xenobiotica*. 1987;17:493.

Branigan TA, et al. The effect of erythromycin on the absorption and disposition kinetics of theophylline. *Eur J Clin Pharmacol*. 1981;21:115.

Zarowitz BJM, et al. Effect of erythromycin base on the theophylline kinetics. *Clin Pharmacol Ther*. 1981;29:601.

Renton KW, et al. Depression of theophylline elimination by erythromycin. *Clin Pharmacol Ther*. 1981;30:422.

LaForce CF, et al. Effect of erythromycin on theophylline clearance in asthmatic children. *J Pediatr*. 1981;99:153.

Iliopoulou A, et al. Pharmacokinetic interaction between theophylline and erythromycin. *Br J Clin Pharmacol*. 1982;14:495.

Paulsen O, et al. The interaction of erythromycin with theophylline. *Eur J Clin Pharmacol*. 1987;32:493.

Reisz G, et al. The effect of erythromycin on theophylline pharmacokinetics in chronic bronchitis. *Am Rev Resp Dis*. 1982;127:581.

Paulsen O, et al. The interaction of erythromycin with theophylline. *Eur J Clin Pharmacol*. 1987;32:493.

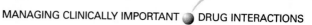

Melethil S, et al. Steady state urinary excretion of theophylline and its metabolites in the presence of erythromycin. *Res Commun Chem Pathol Pharmacol*. 1982;35:341.

Hildebrandt R, et al. Lack of clinically important interaction between erythromycin and theophylline. *Eur J Clin Pharmacol*. 1984;26:485.

Erythromycin (eg, E-Mycin)

Triazolam (eg, *Halcion*)

SUMMARY: Erythromycin causes considerable increases in triazolam plasma concentrations.

RISK FACTORS: No specific risk factors are known.

RELATED DRUGS: Troleandomycin (*TAO*) and clarithromycin (*Biaxin*) also may inhibit the metabolism of triazolam; theoretically, azithromycin (*Zithromax*) would be unlikely to interact. Other benzodiazepines that undergo oxidative metabolism are likely to be affected similarly.

MANAGEMENT OPTIONS:

➡ *Monitor.* Carefully observe patients receiving triazolam who are prescribed erythromycin for enhanced triazolam effects. Several days may be required for the maximum effect of erythromycin to become evident, and triazolam dosages may require adjustment after addition of the antibiotic and again when it is discontinued.

REFERENCES:

Philips JP, et al. A pharmacokinetic drug interaction between erythromycin and triazolam. *J Clin Psychopharmacol*. 1986;6:297.

Erythromycin (eg, E-Mycin)

Valproic Acid (eg, *Depakene*)

SUMMARY: In 1 patient, valproic acid plasma concentrations increased after the addition of erythromycin resulting in symptoms of valproic acid toxicity.

RISK FACTORS: No specific risk factors are known.

RELATED DRUGS: Troleandomycin (*TAO*) and clarithromycin (*Biaxin*) also may inhibit the metabolism of valproic acid.

MANAGEMENT OPTIONS:

➡ *Monitor.* Monitor patients for altered responses to valproic acid when erythromycin is initiated, discontinued, or changed in dosage.

REFERENCES:

Redington K. Erythromycin and valproate interaction. *Ann Intern Med*. 1992;116:877-878.

Erythromycin (eg, *E-Mycin*)

Warfarin (eg, *Coumadin*)

SUMMARY: Erythromycin markedly increases the hypoprothrombinemic response to warfarin in some patients, but the incidence of the interaction in patients receiving both drugs is unknown.

RISK FACTORS:

➥ *Concurrent Diseases.* Fever may enhance the catabolism of clotting factors.

➥ *Diet/Food.* A diet low in vitamin K may contribute to the risk of this interaction.

RELATED DRUGS: Little is known regarding the effect of erythromycin on oral anticoagulants other than warfarin. A study in 6 healthy subjects found no effect of ponsinomycin[†] on the pharmacokinetics of a single dose of acenocoumarol.[†] Troleandomycin (*TAO*) or clarithromycin (*Biaxin*) may alter warfarin elimination, but specific information is not available.

MANAGEMENT OPTIONS:

➥ *Consider Alternative.* Early evidence suggests that azithromycin (*Zithromax*) is not likely to be an enzyme inhibitor, and the manufacturer states that it did not affect the hypoprothrombinemic response to a single dose of warfarin.

➥ *Monitor.* Be alert for evidence of an increased response to oral anticoagulants when erythromycin therapy is initiated and the converse when erythromycin is discontinued. The anticoagulant dose may need to be adjusted.

REFERENCES:

Loeliger EA, et al. The biological disappearance rate of prothrombin and factors VII, IX, and X from plasma in hypothyroidism, hyperthyroidism, and during fever. *Thromb Diath Haemorrh.* 1964;10:267.

Schwartz J, et al. Interaction between warfarin and erythromycin. *South Med J.* 1983;76:91-93.

Bartle WR. Possible warfarin-erythromycin interaction. *Arch Intern Med.* 1980;140:985-987.

Husserl FE. Erythromycin-warfarin interaction. *Arch Intern Med.* 1983;143:1831, 1836.

Sato RI, et al. Warfarin interaction with erythromycin. *Arch Intern Med.* 1984;144:2413-2414.

Grau E, et al. Erythromycin-oral anticoagulant interaction. *Arch Intern Med.* 1986;146:1639.

Bussey HI, et al. Warfarin-erythromycin interaction. *Arch Intern Med.* 1985;145:1736-1737.

Bachmann K, et al. The effect of erythromycin on the disposition kinetics of warfarin. *Pharmacology.* 1984;28:171-176.

Couet W, et al. Lack of effect of ponsinomycin on the pharmacokinetics of nicoumalone enantiomers. *Br J Clin Pharmacol.* 1990;30:616-620.

Weibert RT, et al. Effect of erythromycin in patients receiving long-term warfarin therapy. *Clin Pharm.* 1989;8:210-214.

† Not available in the US.

Erythromycin (eg, *E-Mycin*)

Zafirlukast (*Accolate*)

SUMMARY: Erythromycin coadministration reduces the plasma concentrations of zafirlukast; reduced efficacy may result.

RISK FACTORS: No specific risk factors are known.

RELATED DRUGS: The effect of other macrolides on zafirlukast is unknown.

MANAGEMENT OPTIONS:

➡ *Monitor.* Be alert for reduced zafirlukast efficacy when it is administered with erythromycin.

REFERENCES:

Product information. Zafirlukast (*Accolate*). Zeneca Pharmaceuticals. 1997.

▼③ Erythromycin (eg, *E-Mycin*)

Zopiclone†

SUMMARY: The administration of erythromycin with zopiclone resulted in increased plasma concentrations and pharmacodynamic effects.

RISK FACTORS: No specific risk factors are known.

RELATED DRUGS: Other macrolides (eg, clarithromycin [*Biaxin*], troleandomycin [*TAO*]) may affect zopiclone in a similar manner.

MANAGEMENT OPTIONS:

➡ *Monitor.* Patients receiving zopiclone may experience increased sedation following the addition of erythromycin therapy. Zopiclone dosage adjustment may be required to avoid morning sedation.

REFERENCES:

Aranko K, et al. The effect of erythromycin on the pharmacokinetics and pharmacodynamics of zopiclone. *Br J Clin Pharmacol.* 1994;38:363-367.

† Not available in the US.

▼③ Estramustine (*Emcyt*)

Food

SUMMARY: Food and milk cause significant reductions in estramustine serum concentrations; loss of efficacy could result.

RISK FACTORS: No specific risk factors are known.

RELATED DRUGS: No information is available.

MANAGEMENT OPTIONS:

➡ *Circumvent/Minimize.* Administer estramustine in a fasting state.

➡ *Monitor.* Monitor for reduced estramustine effect if the patient takes it with food or milk.

REFERENCES:

Gunnarsson PO, et al. Impairment of estramustine phosphate absorption by concurrent intake of milk and food. *Eur J Clin Pharmacol.* 1990;38:189.

Ethacrynic Acid (*Edecrin*)

Gentamicin (eg, *Garamycin*)

SUMMARY: The risk of ototoxicity increases when ethacrynic acid and aminoglycosides are coadministered.

RISK FACTORS:

➥ *Concurrent Diseases.* Impaired renal function increases the risk of interaction.

RELATED DRUGS: Furosemide (*Lasix*), torsemide (*Demadex*), or bumetanide (eg, *Bumex*) are less likely to produce an increase in nephrotoxicity when used with an aminoglycoside. Other aminoglycosides, such as kanamycin, neomycin, and streptomycin, are likely to produce ototoxicity with ethacrynic acid.

MANAGEMENT OPTIONS:

➥ *Use Alternative.* Select an alternative diuretic such as furosemide, torsemide, or bumetanide, which are less likely to produce increased nephrotoxicity when coadministered with an aminoglycoside.

REFERENCES:

Mathog RH, et al. Ototoxicity of ethacrynic acid and aminoglycoside antibiotics in uremia. *N Engl J Med.* 1969;280:1223.

Pillay VKG, et al. Transient and permanent deafness following treatment with ethacrynic acid in renal failure. *Lancet.* 1969;1:77.

Meriwether WD, et al. Deafness following standard intravenous dose of ethacrynic acid. *JAMA.* 1971;216:795.

Ethanol (Ethyl Alcohol)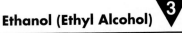

Furazolidone (*Furoxone*)

SUMMARY: A disulfiram-like reaction may occur when patients taking furazolidone ingest alcohol.

RISK FACTORS: No specific risk factors are known.

RELATED DRUGS: No information is available.

MANAGEMENT OPTIONS:

➥ *Monitor.* Warn patients on furazolidone that a disulfiram-like reaction (eg, flushing, nausea, sweating) may occur following ethanol ingestion.

REFERENCES:

Todd RG, ed. Extra Pharmacopoeia-Martindale. 25th ed. London: The Pharmaceutical Press; 1967:844–45.

Kolodny AL. Side-effects produced by alcohol in a patient receiving furazolidone. *Maryland State Med J.* 1962;11:248.

Calesnick B. Antihypertensive action of the antimicrobial agent furazolidone. *Am J Med Sci.* 1958;236:736.

Ethanol (Ethyl Alcohol)

Glutethimide

SUMMARY: The combined use of ethanol and glutethimide may cause excessive central nervous system (CNS) depression and impaired psychomotor performance.

RISK FACTORS: No specific risk factors are known.

RELATED DRUGS: Alcohol would be expected to increase the CNS depression of all sedative-hypnotic drugs.

MANAGEMENT OPTIONS:

➥ **Circumvent/Minimize.** Patients on glutethimide should limit their intake of ethanol to avoid excessive CNS depression.

➥ **Monitor.** Monitor for excessive CNS depression if the combination is used.

REFERENCES:

Mould GP, et al. Interaction of glutethimide and phenobarbitone with ethanol in man. *J Pharm Pharmacol.* 1972;24:894.

Ethanol (Ethyl Alcohol)

Isoniazid (INH)

SUMMARY: Alcoholics have a higher incidence of INH-induced hepatitis.

RISK FACTORS:

➥ **Dosage Regimen.** Daily alcohol consumption can increase the risk of interaction.

RELATED DRUGS: No information is available.

MANAGEMENT OPTIONS:

➥ **Circumvent/Minimize.** Avoiding the combination of alcohol and isoniazid would be prudent, but because alcoholism and tuberculosis often coexist, it may not be possible in some cases.

➥ **Monitor.** Monitor alcoholic patients carefully for INH hepatitis if they are administered isoniazid.

REFERENCES:

Isoniazid [package insert]. Princeton, NJ: Apothecon, Inc.; 1996.

Ethanol (Ethyl Alcohol)

Ketoconazole (eg, *Nizoral*)

SUMMARY: Ethanol consumption during ketoconazole therapy may result in a disulfiram-like reaction.

RISK FACTORS: No specific risk factors are known.

RELATED DRUGS: No information is available.

MANAGEMENT OPTIONS:

➡ *Circumvent/Minimize.* Advise patients taking ketoconazole to minimize their alcohol intake.

➡ *Monitor.* Counsel patients taking ketoconazole that ethanol consumption might cause flushing, nausea, and headache and should avoid ethanol while taking ketoconazole.

REFERENCES:

Magnasco AJ, et al. Interaction of ketoconazole and ethanol. *Clin Pharm*. 1986;5:522.

Ethanol (Ethyl Alcohol)

Meperidine (eg, *Demerol*)

SUMMARY: Ethanol and narcotic analgesics are likely to exhibit additive central nervous system (CNS) depressant effects. Ethanol also may affect the distribution of meperidine, but the clinical importance of this effect is not established.

RISK FACTORS: No specific risk factors are known.

RELATED DRUGS: Ethanol also would be expected to add to the CNS depressant effects of narcotic analgesics other than meperidine.

MANAGEMENT OPTIONS:

➡ *Circumvent/Minimize.* Patients taking narcotic analgesics should limit their use of alcohol, especially if performing tasks requiring alertness.

➡ *Monitor.* Monitor for excessive CNS depression in patients receiving the combination.

REFERENCES:

Linnoila M, et al. Effects of diazepam and codeine, alone and in combination with alcohol, on simulated driving. *Clin Pharmacol Ther*. 1974;15:368.

Mather LE, et al. Meperidine kinetics in man. Intravenous injection in surgical patients and volunteers. *Clin Pharmacol Ther*. 1975;17:21.

Ethanol (Ethyl Alcohol)

Meprobamate (eg, *Equanil*)

SUMMARY: Concurrent use of ethanol and meprobamate results in enhanced CNS depression.

RISK FACTORS: No specific risk factors are known.

RELATED DRUGS: Alcohol would be expected to increase the CNS depression of all sedative-hypnotics.

MANAGEMENT OPTIONS:

➡ *Circumvent/Minimize.* Make patients aware that the combined use of ethanol and meprobamate can cause excessive CNS depression. Patients on meprobamate should avoid ingesting moderate to large amounts of ethanol.

➥ *Monitor.* Monitor for excessive CNS depression in patients receiving the combination.

REFERENCES:

Misra PS, et al. Increase of ethanol, meprobamate and pentobarbital metabolism after chronic ethanol administration in man and in rats. *Am J Med.* 1971;41:346.

Valsrub S. Alcohol-induced sensitivity and tolerance. *JAMA.* 1972;219:508. Editorial.

Rubin E, et al. Inhibition of drug metabolism by acute ethanol intoxication: a hepatic microsomal mechanism. *Am J Med.* 1970;49:801.

Ashford JR, et al. Drug interactions. The effects of alcohol and meprobamate applied singly and jointly in human subjects. III. *J Stud Alcohol.* 1975;7(Suppl.):140.

Cobby JM, et al. Drug interactions. The effect of alcohol and meprobamate applied singly and jointly in human subjects. IV. *J Stud Alcohol.* 1975;7(Suppl.):162.

Ashford JR, et al. Drug interactions. The effects of alcohol and meprobamate applied singly and jointly in human subjects. V. *J Stud Alcohol.* 1975;7(Suppl.):177.

 Ethanol (Ethyl Alcohol)

AVOID **Methotrexate (eg, *Rheumatrex*)**

SUMMARY: Some evidence indicates that ethanol may increase the likelihood of methotrexate-induced liver injury, but a causal relationship has not been established.

RISK FACTORS: No specific risk factors are known.

RELATED DRUGS: No information is available.

MANAGEMENT OPTIONS:

➥ *AVOID COMBINATION.* Avoid ethanol in patients receiving methotrexate. The manufacturer of methotrexate also recommends the avoidance of ethanol. Even though the evidence for additive hepatotoxic effects is not conclusive, alcohol restriction probably is appropriate for most patients receiving methotrexate.

REFERENCES:

Tobias H, et al. Hepatotoxicity of long-term methotrexate therapy for psoriasis. *Arch Intern Med.* 1973;132:391.

Pai SH, et al. Severe liver damage caused by treatment of psoriasis with methotrexate. *NY State J Med.* 1973;73:2585.

Methotrexate. Product Information. Wayne, NJ: Lederle Laboratories; 1988.

Glassner J. Methotrexate and psoriasis. *JAMA.* 1970;210:1925.

 Ethanol (Ethyl Alcohol)

Metoclopramide (eg, *Reglan*)

SUMMARY: Metoclopramide may enhance the sedative effects of ethanol, but the clinical importance of this effect is not established.

RISK FACTORS: No specific risk factors are known.

RELATED DRUGS: No information is available.

MANAGEMENT OPTIONS:

➥ *Circumvent/Minimize.* Until more is known about this purported interaction, advise patients taking metoclopramide that alcohol may have a greater than expected effect.

➡ *Monitor.* Monitor for excessive central nervous system depression in patients receiving the combination.

REFERENCES:
Bateman DN, et al. Pharmacokinetic and concentration-effect studies with intravenous metoclopramide. *Br J Clin Pharmacol.* 1978;6:401.

Gibbons DO, et al. Effects of intravenous and oral propantheline and metoclopramide on ethanol absorption. *Clin Pharmacol Ther.* 1975;17:578.

Ethanol (Ethyl Alcohol)

Metronidazole (eg, *Flagyl*)

SUMMARY: Alcohol ingestion during metronidazole therapy may lead to a disulfiram-like reaction in some patients.

RISK FACTORS: No specific risk factors are known.

RELATED DRUGS: The coadministration of metronidazole and other IV drugs containing ethanol (eg, phenytoin [eg, *Dilantin*], trimethoprim-sulfamethoxazole, phenobarbital [eg, *Solfoton*], diazepam [eg, *Valium*], and nitroglycerin [eg, *Tridil*]) may result in flushing and vomiting.

MANAGEMENT OPTIONS:

➡ *Circumvent/Minimize.* Warn patients receiving metronidazole about the possibility of reactions following ethanol ingestion and avoid ethanol or ethanol-containing drugs.

➡ *Monitor.* If ethanol is taken by a patient receiving metronidazole, watch for flushing, nausea, and vomiting.

REFERENCES:
Edwards DL, et al. Disulfiram-like reaction associated with intravenous trimethoprim-sulfamethoxazole and metronidazole. *Clin Pharm.* 1986;5:999.

Ethanol (Ethyl Alcohol)

Nitroglycerin

SUMMARY: Additive vasodilation could cause hypotension when ethanol is consumed by patients taking nitroglycerin.

RISK FACTORS: No specific risk factors are known.

RELATED DRUGS: No information is available.

MANAGEMENT OPTIONS:

➡ *Circumvent/Minimize.* Until further information is available, advise patients receiving nitroglycerin to limit their alcohol intake.

➡ *Monitor.* Be alert for evidence of hypotension (eg, lightheadedness, fainting) in patients receiving the combination.

REFERENCES:
Shafer N. Hypotension due to nitroglycerin combined with alcohol. *N Engl J Med.* 1965;273:1169.

Allison RD, et al. Effects of alcohol and nitroglycerin on vascular responses in man. *Angiology.* 1971;22:211.

① Ethanol (Ethyl Alcohol)

AVOID Phenelzine (*Nardil*)

SUMMARY: Alcoholic beverages containing tyramine may induce a severe hypertensive response in patients taking nonselective monoamine oxidase inhibitors (MAOIs).

RISK FACTORS: No specific risk factors are known.

RELATED DRUGS: All nonselective MAOIs including isocarboxazid (*Marplan*) and tranylcypromine (*Parnate*) interact with tyramine-containing alcoholic beverages.

MANAGEMENT OPTIONS:

➡ **AVOID COMBINATION.** Because it is difficult to assess the tyramine content of a given drink (especially drinks with many ingredients), advise patients receiving MAOIs to avoid all alcoholic beverages. If alcohol is ingested, the patient should use products that are unlikely to contain significant amounts of tyramine (eg, vodka, white wine) and ingest small amounts initially. Assume that the effects of nonselective monoamine oxidase inhibitors to persist for 2 weeks after they are discontinued.

REFERENCES:

Sjoqvist F. Psychotropic drugs (2). Interaction between monoamine oxidase (MAO) inhibitors and other substances. *Proc R Soc Med.* 1965;58:967.

Ellis J, et al. Modification by monoamine oxidase inhibitors of the effect of some sympathomimetics on blood pressure. *BMJ.* 1967;2:75.

MacLeod I. Fatal reaction to phenelzine. *BMJ.* 1965;1:1554.

Shulman KI, et al. Dietary restriction, tyramine, and the use of monoamine oxidase inhibitors. *J Clin Psychopharmacol.* 1989;9:397.

③ Ethanol (Ethyl Alcohol)

Phenobarbital (eg, *Solfoton*)

SUMMARY: Ethanol and barbiturates like phenobarbital have additive depressant effects on the CNS; combined use is dangerous in patients performing tasks requiring alertness and may be fatal in overdose.

RISK FACTORS: No specific risk factors are known.

RELATED DRUGS: All barbiturates are likely to result in additive CNS depressant effects with ethanol. Acute ethanol intoxication appears to inhibit pentobarbital (eg, *nembutal*) metabolism.

MANAGEMENT OPTIONS:

➡ **Circumvent/Minimize.** Warn patients receiving barbiturates that the combined use of ethanol can lead to excessive CNS depression.

➡ **Monitor.** Monitor for excessive CNS depression in patients receiving the combination.

REFERENCES:

Mould GP, et al. Interaction of glutethimide and phenobarbitone with ethanol in man. *J Pharm Pharmacol.* 1972;24:894.

Lieber CS. Hepatic and metabolic effects of alcohol (1966 to 1973). *Gastroenterology.* 1973;65:821.

Misra PS, et al. Increase of ethanol, meprobamate and pentobarbital metabolism after chronic ethanol administration in man and in rats. *Am J Med*. 1971;43:346.

Valsrub S. Alcohol-induced sensitivity and tolerance. *JAMA*. 1972;219:508. Editorial.

Rubin E, et al. Inhibition of drug metabolism by acute ethanol intoxication: a hepatic microsomal mechanism. *Am J Med*. 1970;49:801.

Mezey E, et al. Effects of phenobarbital administration on rates of ethanol clearance and on ethanol-oxidizing enzymes in man. *Gastroenterology*. 1974;66:248.

Johnstone RE, et al. Respiratory interaction of alcohol. *JAMA*. 1975;233:770.

Mezey E. Effect of phenobarbital administration on ethanol oxidizing enzymes and on rates of ethanol degradation. *Biochem Pharmacol*. 1971;20:508.

Milner G. Interaction between barbiturates, alcohol and some psychotropic drugs. *Med J Aust*. 1970;1:1204.

Stead AH, et al. Quantification of the interaction between barbiturates and alcohol and interpretation of fatal blood concentrations. *Hum Toxicol*. 1983;2:5.

Ethanol (Ethyl Alcohol)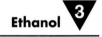

Phenytoin (eg, *Dilantin*)

SUMMARY: Chronic ethanol abuse may reduce serum phenytoin concentrations, but the clinical importance of this effect is not established.

RISK FACTORS: No specific risk factors are known.

RELATED DRUGS: No information is available.

MANAGEMENT OPTIONS:

➡ ***Monitor.*** Monitor epileptic patients receiving phenytoin who also drink heavily for a decreased anticonvulsant effect.

REFERENCES:

Kater RMH, et al. Increased rate of clearance of drugs from the circulation of alcoholics. *Am J Med Sci*. 1969;258:35.

Finer MJ. Diphenylhydantoin in alcohol withdrawal. *JAMA*. 1971;217:211.

Ethanol

Prazosin (*Minipress*)

SUMMARY: Prazosin enhanced alcohol-induced hypotension in Asian hypertensive patients; limit alcohol intake in such patients.

RISK FACTORS:

➡ ***Pharmacogenetics.*** Japanese and other Asians may be more susceptible to this interaction because Asians are more likely than Whites to be deficient in aldehyde dehydrogenase. When such patients ingest alcohol, the vasodilatory alcohol metabolite, acetaldehyde, accumulates and reduces the blood pressure. Thus, patients who develop flushing with alcohol ingestion may be more susceptible to the interaction with prazosin.

RELATED DRUGS: Theoretically, one would expect a similar interaction with alcohol with other α_1-adrenergic blockers, such as doxazosin (eg, *Cardura*) and terazosin (eg, *Hytrin*).

MANAGEMENT OPTIONS:

➡ *Circumvent/Minimize.* Patients (especially those who flush after alcohol ingestion) should limit their alcohol intake while on prazosin or other alpha$_1$-adrenergic blockers.

REFERENCES:

Kawano Y, et al. Interaction of alcohol and an α_1-blocker on ambulatory blood pressure in patients with essential hypertension. *Am J Hypertens.* 2000;13:307.

 Ethanol (Ethyl Alcohol)

AVOID **Procarbazine (*Matulane*)**

SUMMARY: Ingestion of ethanol by patients receiving procarbazine may result in a disulfiram-like reaction: flushing, headache, nausea, and hypotension.

RISK FACTORS: No specific risk factors are known.

RELATED DRUGS: No information is available.

MANAGEMENT OPTIONS:

➡ *AVOID COMBINATION.* Advise patients receiving procarbazine to avoid alcohol.

REFERENCES:

Vasiliou V, et al. The mechanism of alcohol intolerance produced by various therapeutic agents. *Acta Pharmacol et Toxicol.* 1986;58:305.

Brul G, et al. N-isopropyl-a-(2-methylhydrazino)-p-toluamide, hydrochloride (NSC-77213) in treatment of solid tumors. *Cancer Chemother Rep.* 1965;44:31.

Math G, et al. Methyl-hydrazine in treatment of Hodgkin's disease and various forms of haematosarcoma and leukaemia. *Lancet.* 1963;2:1077.

Todd IDH. Natulan in management of late Hodgkin's disease, other lymphoreticular neoplasms, and malignant melanoma. *BMJ.* 1965;628.

 Ethanol (Ethyl Alcohol)

Propoxyphene (eg, *Darvocet-N*)

SUMMARY: Overdoses of propoxyphene combined with ethanol have been associated with fatal reactions, but there is little evidence of danger when alcohol is combined with therapeutic doses of propoxyphene.

RISK FACTORS:

➡ *Dosage Regimen.* The danger of this interaction occurs primarily when large amounts of alcohol are ingested.

RELATED DRUGS: No information is available.

MANAGEMENT OPTIONS:

➡ *Circumvent/Minimize.* It does not appear that patients taking propoxyphene need to abstain from alcohol, but warn them to avoid acute alcohol intoxication.

➡ *Monitor.* Monitor for excessive central nervous system depression in patients receiving the combination.

REFERENCES:

Girre C, et al. Enhancement of propoxyphene bioavailability by ethanol: relation to psychomotor and cognitive function in healthy volunteers. *Eur J Clin Pharmacol.* 1991;41:147.

Sellers EM, et al. Pharmacokinetic interaction of propoxyphene with ethanol. *Br J Clin Pharmacol.* 1985;19:398.

Finkle BS, et al. A national assessment of propoxyphene in postmortem medicolegal investigation 1972–1975. *J Forensic Sci.* 1976;21:706.

Ethanol (Ethyl Alcohol)

Quetiapine (*Seroquel*)

SUMMARY: Patients on quetiapine who ingest alcohol may develop excessive impairment of cognitive and motor function; the manufacturer advises against the use of alcohol in patients on quetiapine.

RISK FACTORS: No specific risk factors are known.

RELATED DRUGS: No information is available.

MANAGEMENT OPTIONS:

➡ *Circumvent/Minimize.* Advise patients on quetiapine to avoid alcohol. If alcohol is ingested, it should be in small amounts and the patient should avoid operating automobiles or machinery.

REFERENCES:

Product information. Quetiapine (*Seroquel*). Zeneca Pharmaceuticals. Wilmington, DE. 1997.

Ethanol (Ethyl Alcohol)

Tolbutamide (eg, *Orinase*) AVOID

SUMMARY: Excessive ethanol intake may lead to altered glycemic control, most commonly hypoglycemia. An "*Antabuse*-like" reaction may occur in patients taking sulfonylureas.

RISK FACTORS: No specific risk factors are known.

RELATED DRUGS: Excessive ethanol produce hypoglycemia in patients taking insulin or other oral hypoglycemic agents. Two patients receiving chlorpropamide (eg, *Diabinese*) for diabetes insipidus developed polyuria and polydipsia following ethanol intake, presumably caused by ethanol inhibition of chlorpropamide-induced antidiuresis. Ethanol ingestion may contribute to lactic acidosis in patients receiving phenformin.,

MANAGEMENT OPTIONS:

➡ *AVOID COMBINATION.* Since an "*Antabuse* reaction" may occur following ethanol ingestion in patients receiving sulfonylureas, inform patients of this possibility when therapy is initiated. Advise patients on antidiabetics to avoid ingestion of moderate to large amounts of ethanol because of the possible adverse effects of alcohol on diabetic control.

REFERENCES:

Arky RA, et al. Irreversible hypoglycemia, a complication of alcohol and insulin. *JAMA.* 1968;206:575.

Hartling SG, et al. Interaction of ethanol and glipizide in humans. *Diabetes Care.* 1987;10:263.

Kater RMH, et al. Increased rate of tolbutamide metabolism in alcoholic patients. *JAMA.* 1969;207:363.

Johnson HK, et al. Relationship of alcohol and hyperlactatemia in diabetic subjects treated with phenformin. *Am J Med.* 1968;45:98.

Kreisberg RA, et al. Hyperlacticacidemia in man: ethanol-phenformin synergism. *J Clin Endocrinol.* 1972;34:29.

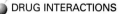

Carulli N, et al. Alcohol-drugs interaction in man: alcohol and tolbutamide. *Eur J Clin Invest.* 1971;1:421.

Baruh S, et al. Fasting hypoglycemia. *Med Clin North Am.* 1973;57:1441.

Yamamoto LT. Diabetes insipidus and drinking alcohol. *N Engl J Med.* 1976;294:55.

Sotaniemi EA, et al. Half-life of intravenous tolbutamide in the serum of patients in medical wards. *Ann Clin Res.* 1974;6:146.

Asaad MM, et al. Studies on the biochemical aspects of the "disulfiram like" reaction induced by oral hypoglycemics. *Eur Pharmacol.* 1976;35:301.

Wardle EN, et al. Alcohol and glibenclamide. *BMJ.* 1971;3:309.

 Ethanol (Ethyl Alcohol)

Verapamil (eg, *Calan*)

SUMMARY: Consumption of ethanol following the chronic administration of verapamil results in increased ethanol concentrations with the possibility of prolonged and increased levels of intoxication.

RISK FACTORS: No specific risk factors are known.

RELATED DRUGS: Ethanol was reported to increase the hypotensive response of a 5 mg dose of felodipine (*Plendil*) in 10 hypertensive patients. The ethanol was administered in doublestrength grapefruit juice which has been demonstrated to increase felodipine concentrations. Therefore, it is uncertain whether ethanol affects felodipine or if the changes were caused by an interaction between grapefruit juice and felodipine. Ethanol administration resulted in a 53% increase in nifedipine (eg, *Procardia*) area under the concentration-time curve in healthy subjects; nifedipine-induced blood pressure changes were not affected by ethanol.

MANAGEMENT OPTIONS:

➡ *Avoid Unless Benefit Outweighs Risk.* Avoid or reduce ethanol intake while taking verapamil. Verapamil may enhance the psychomotor effects of ethanol.

➡ *Monitor.* Caution patients taking verapamil regarding the consumption of ethanol. Serum ethanol concentrations may be higher than normally experienced when the patient is not taking verapamil.

REFERENCES:

Bauer LA, et al. Verapamil inhibits ethanol elimination and prolongs the perception of intoxication. *Clin Pharmacol Ther.* 1992;52:6.

Bailey DG, et al. Ethanol enhances the hemodynamic effect of felodipine. *Clin Invest Med.* 1989;12:357.

Bailey DG, et al. Interaction of citrus juices with felodipine and nifedipine. *Lancet.* 1991;337:268.

Perez-Reyes M, et al. Interaction between ethanol and calcium channel blockers in humans. *Alcohol Clin Exp Res.* 1992;16:769.

Qureshi S, et al. Effect of an acute dose of alcohol on the pharmacokinetics of oral nifedipine in humans. *Pharm Res.* 1992;9:683.

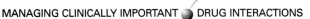

Ethanol (Ethyl Alcohol)

Warfarin (eg *Coumadin*)

SUMMARY: Enhanced hypoprothrombinemic response to oral anticoagulants has been reported following acute ethanol intoxication.

RISK FACTORS:

➡ ***Dosage Regimen.*** Enhanced anticoagulant effect appears to occur primarily with acute alcohol intoxication; small amounts of ethanol (eg, 2 drinks or fewer per day) seem to have little effect on most patients.

RELATED DRUGS: Until we have evidence to the contrary, expect all oral anticoagulants to be affected by alcohol intoxication. In another study, 80 g of ethanol did not affect the hypoprothrombinemic response in healthy subjects maintained on phenprocoumon.[†] Additional study in patients with coronary disease indicated a slight increase in hypoprothrombinemic response to phenprocoumon in some patients following administration of moderate amounts of ethanol.

MANAGEMENT OPTIONS:

➡ ***Circumvent/Minimize.*** Patients on oral anticoagulants should avoid large amounts of ethanol, but 2 or 3 drinks/day or less are unlikely to affect warfarin response.

➡ ***Monitor.*** Monitor for altered hypoprothrombinemic response if a patient takes greater than 3 drinks per day or if alcohol intake changes considerably.

REFERENCES:

Kater RHM, et al. Increased rate of clearance of drugs from the circulation of alcoholics. *Am J Med Sci.* 1969;258:35.

Udall JA. Drug interference with warfarin therapy. *Clin Med.* 1970;77:20.

Waris E. Effect of ethyl alcohol on some coagulation factors in man during anticoagulant therapy. *Ann Med Exp Biol Fenn.* 1963;41:45.

O'Reilly RA. Lack of effect of mealtime wine on the hypoprothrombinemia of oral anticoagulants. *Am J Med Sci.* 1979;277:189.

O'Reilly RA. Lack of effect of fortified wine ingested during fasting and anticoagulant therapy. *Arch Intern Med.* 1981;141:458.

Breckenridge A. Pathophysiological factors influencing drug kinetics. *Acta Pharmacol Toxicol.* 1971;29(Suppl. 3):225.

† Not available in the US.

Ethinyl Estradiol (eg, *Ortho-Novum 1/35*)

Grapefruit Juice

SUMMARY: Grapefruit juice appears to increase ethinyl estradiol serum concentrations somewhat, but the clinical importance of this effect is not established.

RISK FACTORS:

➡ ***Route of Administration.*** This interaction probably only occurs with oral administration of ethinyl estradiol.

RELATED DRUGS: The effect of grapefruit juice on other estrogens is not established, but since many hormonal steroids undergo metabolism by CYP3A4, it is possible that other estrogens (given orally) would be similarly affected. Nonoral administration of estrogens (eg, transdermal patches) theoretically would not be affected by grapefruit juice.

MANAGEMENT OPTIONS:

➡ **Consider Alternative.** Orange juice does not appear to inhibit CYP3A4 and would not be expected to interact with ethinyl estradiol.

➡ **Circumvent/Minimize.** Although it is not known how often this interaction would cause adverse effects, it would be prudent for patients taking ethinyl estradiol (and perhaps other estrogens) to avoid taking the estrogen with or within several hours after grapefruit products. If grapefruit juice is used, it would be prudent to keep the dosing interval between the ethinyl estradiol and the grapefruit juice about the same from day to day.

REFERENCES:

Schubert W, et al. Flavonoids in grapefruit juice inhibit the in vitro hepatic metabolism of 17b-estradiol. *Eur J Drug Metab Pharmacokinet.* 1995;20:219.

Weber A, et al. Can grapefruit juice influence ethinylestradiol bioavailability? *Contraception.* 1996;53:41.

Etintidine†

Propranolol (eg, *Inderal*)

SUMMARY: Serum concentrations of propranolol and probably of other beta blockers that undergo significant hepatic metabolism may be increased by etintidine administration.

RISK FACTORS: No specific risk factors are known.

RELATED DRUGS: Cimetidine (eg, *Tagamet*) is known to inhibit the metabolism of propranolol and other beta blockers (eg, metoprolol [eg, *Lopressor*], labetalol [eg, *Normodyne*]) that undergo hepatic metabolism. Etintidine might affect them similarly. Other H_2-receptor antagonists (ranitidine [eg, *Zantac*], famotidine [eg, *Pepcid*], nizatidine [*Axid*]) would have little effect on propranolol.

MANAGEMENT OPTIONS:

➡ **Consider Alternative.** Possibly administer atenolol (eg, *Tenormin*) or nadolol (eg, *Corgard*) instead of hepatically metabolized beta blockers. Ranitidine, famotidine, nizatidine, antacids, or sucralfate (eg, *Carafate*) also may be suitable alternatives to etintidine, although separate beta blocker doses from antacids or sucralfate to minimize the possibility of impaired absorption of the beta blocker.

➡ **Monitor.** Etintidine administration may result in large increases in propranolol serum concentrations. Monitor patients stabilized on propranolol for altered response to beta blockade if etintidine is instituted or discontinued.

REFERENCES:

Huang S-M, et al. Etintidine-propranolol interaction study in humans. *J Pharmacokinet Biopharm.* 1987;15:557.

† Not available in the US.

Etodolac (eg, *Lodine*) 2

Warfarin (eg, *Coumadin*)

SUMMARY: Preliminary data suggest that etodolac does not affect the hypoprothrombinemic response to warfarin, but cotherapy requires caution because of possible detrimental effects of etodolac on the gastric mucosa and platelet function.

RISK FACTORS:

➡ **Concurrent Diseases.** Patients with peptic ulcer disease (PUD) or a history of GI bleeding probably are at greater risk.

RELATED DRUGS: All NSAIDs inhibit platelet function, cause gastric erosions, and probably increase the risk of GI bleeding.

MANAGEMENT OPTIONS:

➡ **Avoid Unless Benefit Outweighs Risk.** Because all NSAIDs probably increase the risk of GI bleeding in patients on oral anticoagulants, use the combination only after careful consideration of the benefit vs risk. If the NSAID is being used as an analgesic or antipyretic, acetaminophen (eg, *Tylenol*) probably is safer to use with oral anticoagulants. Nonacetylated salicylates (eg, choline salicylate, magnesium salicylate, salsalate, sodium salicylate) probably also are safer with oral anticoagulants than NSAIDs since they have minimal effects on platelet function and the gastric mucosa.

➡ **Monitor.** If any NSAID is used with an oral anticoagulant, carefully monitor the prothrombin time and watch for evidence of bleeding, especially from the GI tract.

REFERENCES:

Ermer JC, et al. Concomitant etodolac affects neither the unbound clearance nor the pharmacologic effect of warfarin. *Clin Pharmacol Ther*. 1994;55:305.

Shorr RI, et al. Concurrent use of nonsteroidal anti-inflammatory drugs and oral anticoagulants places elderly persons at high risk for hemorrhagic peptic ulcer disease. *Arch Intern Med*. 1993;153:1665.

▼ Felbamate (*Felbatol*)

Phenobarbital (eg, *Solfoton*)

SUMMARY: Felbamate increases phenobarbital concentrations and may result in toxicity.

RISK FACTORS: No specific risk factors are known.

RELATED DRUGS: No information is available.

MANAGEMENT OPTIONS:

➡ *Consider Alternative.* Given the serious toxicity that has been reported with felbamate, it is reserved for carefully selected patients. Thus, use alternatives to felbamate if possible, whether or not the patient is on interacting drugs.

➡ *Circumvent/Minimize.* Since patients may manifest an increase in serum phenobarbital concentrations when felbamate therapy is added, consider reducing the phenobarbital dose 20% to 25% when felbamate is added. Conversely, an increase in phenobarbital dosage may be required if felbamate is discontinued. It is not clear whether an alteration in felbamate dosage is needed when phenobarbital therapy is initiated or discontinued.

➡ *Monitor.* Monitor symptoms of phenobarbital toxicity for at least 1 month after felbamate is added.

REFERENCES:

Gidal B, et al. Potential pharmacokinetic interaction between felbamate and phenobarbital. *Ann Pharmacother.* 1994;28:455.

Reidenberg P, et al. Effects of felbamate on the pharmacokinetics of phenobarbital. *Clin Pharmacol Ther.* 1995;58:279.

▼ Felbamate (*Felbatol*)

Phenytoin (eg, *Dilantin*)

SUMMARY: Felbamate consistently increases serum phenytoin concentrations; phenytoin toxicity may occur in some patients. Phenytoin appears to decrease serum felbamate concentrations, but the clinical importance of this effect is not established.

RISK FACTORS: No specific risk factors are known.

RELATED DRUGS: No information is available.

MANAGEMENT OPTIONS:

➡ *Consider Alternative.* Given the serious toxicity that has been reported with felbamate, it is reserved for carefully selected patients. Thus, use alternatives to felbamate if possible, whether or not the patient is on interacting drugs.

➡ *Circumvent/Minimize.* Since almost all patients appear to manifest an increase in serum phenytoin concentrations when felbamate therapy is added, consider reducing the phenytoin dose by 25% when felbamate is added. Conversely, an increase in phenytoin dosage may be required if felbamate is discontinued. It is not clear whether an alteration in felbamate dosage is needed when phenytoin therapy is initiated or discontinued.

➡ *Monitor.* When the 2 agents are used together, monitor for symptoms of phenytoin toxicity.

REFERENCES:

Graves NM, et al. Effects of felbamate on phenytoin and carbamazepine serum concentrations. *Epilepsia.* 1989;30:488.

Fuerst RH, et al. Felbamate increases phenytoin and decreases carbamazepine concentrations. *Epilepsia.* 1988;29:488.

Wilensky AJ, et al. Pharmacokinetics of W-544 (ADD03055) in epileptic patients. *Epilepsia.* 1985;26:602.

Wagner ML, et al. Discontinuation of phenytoin and carbamazepine in patients receiving felbamate. *Epilepsia.* 1991;32:398.

Felbamate (*Felbatol*)

Valproic Acid (eg, *Depakene*)

SUMMARY: Preliminary evidence suggests that felbamate consistently increases serum valproic acid concentrations, but the magnitude of the effect varies from patient to patient.

RISK FACTORS: No specific risk factors are known.

RELATED DRUGS: No information is available.

MANAGEMENT OPTIONS:

➡ *Consider Alternative.* Given the serious toxicity that has been reported with felbamate, it is reserved for carefully selected patients. Thus, use alternatives to felbamate if possible, whether or not the patient is on interacting drugs.

➡ *Circumvent/Minimize.* In patients stabilized on valproic acid, titrating felbamate slowly may reduce the risk of adverse effects. If felbamate is rapidly added to valproic acid, it may be necessary to reduce valproic acid doses. Also be aware that *discontinuing* felbamate may affect valproic acid requirements.

➡ *Monitor.* Monitor for symptoms of valproic toxicity such as tremor, confusion, irritability, and restlessness.

REFERENCES:

Wagner ML, et al. The effect of felbamate on valproic acid disposition. *Clin Pharmacol Ther.* 1994;56:494.

Felodipine (*Plendil*)

Itraconazole (*Sporanox*)

SUMMARY: Itraconazole increases felodipine concentrations and enhances its vasodilatory effects; excessive hypotensive response could result.

RISK FACTORS: No specific risk factors are known.

RELATED DRUGS: The bioavailability and metabolism of other calcium channel blockers that undergo CYP3A4 metabolism are likely to be affected by itraconazole. Other azole antifungal agents such as ketoconazole (eg, *Nizoral*), miconazole (eg, *Monistat*), and fluconazole (*Diflucan*) would also be expected to reduce the metabolism of felodipine. Terbinafine (*Lamisil*) may be less likely to affect felodipine clearance.

MANAGEMENT OPTIONS:

➡ *Consider Alternative.* Although there are no specific data, terbinafine may be less likely to affect felodipine clearance. Since most calcium channel blockers will likely be affected to some extent, the use of a noncalcium blocker may be appropriate during treatment with an azole antifungal agent.

➡ *Circumvent/Minimize.* A reduction in the dose of felodipine may be necessary to avoid excessive pharmacologic effects.

➡ *Monitor.* Monitor patients receiving the combination of itraconazole and felodipine carefully for excessive hypotension.

REFERENCES:

Jalava K-M, et al. Itraconazole greatly increases plasma concentrations and effects of felodipine. *Clin Pharmacol Ther*. 1997;61:410.

 Fenfluramine (*Pondimin*)

Fluoxetine (*Prozac*)

SUMMARY: Cotherapy with fenfluramine and selective serotonin reuptake inhibitors (SSRIs) such as fluoxetine theoretically could result in serotonin syndrome.

RISK FACTORS: No specific risk factors are known.

RELATED DRUGS: Avoid dexfenfluramine (*Redux*) in combination with other SSRIs such as paroxetine (*Paxil*), sertraline (*Zoloft*), and fluvoxamine (*Luvox*).

MANAGEMENT OPTIONS:

➡ *Avoid Unless Benefit Outweighs Risk.* Patients should avoid the use of SSRIs with fenfluramine or dexfenfluramine, unless the combinations are found to be safe in well-controlled clinical trials. There is also a medicolegal risk in using the combinations, since the manufacturer's information states that cotherapy should be avoided.

➡ *Monitor.* If the combination is used, be alert for evidence of serotonin syndrome, which can result in neurotoxicity (eg, myoclonus, tremors, rigidity, incoordination, restlessness, hyperreflexia, seizures, coma); psychiatric symptoms (eg, agitation, confusion, hypomania); and temperature regulation abnormalities (eg, fever, sweating).

REFERENCES:

Gross AS, et al. The influence of the sparteine/debrisoquine genetic polymorphism on the disposition of dexfenfluramine. *Br J Clin Pharmacol*. 1996;41:311.

Product information. Dexfenfluramine (*Redux*). Wyeth-Ayerst Laboratories. 1996.

 Fenfluramine†

AVOID Phenelzine (eg, *Nardil*)

SUMMARY: Cotherapy with fenfluramine and nonselective monamine oxidase (MAO) inhibitors such as phenelzine theoretically could result in serotonin syndrome.

RISK FACTORS: No specific risk factors are known.

RELATED DRUGS: Fenfluramine also is contraindicated with other nonselective MAO inhibitors such as tranylcypromine (eg, *Parnate*) and isocarboxazid (*Marplan*).

Given that selegiline (eg, *Eldepryl*) also can act as a nonselective MAO inhibitors (especially if given in large doses), it also might interact adversely with fenfluramine. Dexfenfluramine is the S-enantiomer of the racemate fenfluramine, so the 2 drugs probably interact in a similar way with nonselective MAO inhibitors.

MANAGEMENT OPTIONS:

➡ **AVOID COMBINATION.** Patients should avoid any combination of a nonselective MAO inhibitors with fenfluramine or dexfenfluramine.

REFERENCES:

Product information. Fenfluramine (*Pondimin*). A. H. Robins Company, 1996.

Gross AS, et al. The influence of the sparteine/debrisoquine genetic polymorphism on the disposition of dexfenfluramine. *Br J Clin Pharmacol.* 1996;41:311-317.

† Not available in the US.

Fenofibrate (eg, *Tricor*)

Warfarin (eg, *Coumadin*)

SUMMARY: Based on case reports, it appears that fenofibrate increases the anticoagulant effect of warfarin.

RISK FACTORS: No specific risk factors are known.

RELATED DRUGS: Clofibrate (*Atromid-S*) and gemfibrozil (eg, *Lopid*) have also been reported to increase the hypoprothrombinemic response of warfarin.

MANAGEMENT OPTIONS:

➡ **Monitor.** Closely monitor the hypoprothrombinemic response to warfarin if fenofibrate is initiated, discontinued, or changed in dosage.

REFERENCES:

Ascah KJ, Rock GA, Wells PS. Interaction between fenofibrate and warfarin. *Ann Pharmacother.* 1998;32:765-768.

Fenoprofen (eg, *Nalfon*)

Warfarin (eg, *Coumadin*)

SUMMARY: Although little is known regarding the effect of fenoprofen on the hypoprothrombinemic response to oral anticoagulants, cotherapy requires caution because of possible detrimental effects of fenoprofen on the gastric mucosa and platelet function.

RISK FACTORS:

➡ **Concurrent Diseases.** Patients with peptic ulcer disease (PUD) or a history of GI bleeding probably are at greater risk.

RELATED DRUGS: All NSAIDs inhibit platelet function, cause gastric erosions, and probably increase the risk of GI bleeding. However, some NSAIDs such as ibuprofen (eg, *Advil*), naproxen (eg, *Anaprox*), or diclofenac (eg, *Voltaren*) may be less likely to increase oral anticoagulant-induced hypoprothrombinemia than other NSAIDs.

MANAGEMENT OPTIONS:

➡ **Avoid Unless Benefit Outweighs Risk.** Because all NSAIDs probably increase the risk of GI bleeding in patients on oral anticoagulants, use the combination only after careful consideration of the benefit vs risk. If an NSAID must be used with an oral anticoagulant, it would be prudent to use NSAIDs that are unlikely to affect the hypoprothrombinemic response to oral anticoagulants. If the NSAID is being used as an analgesic or antipyretic, acetaminophen is probably safer to use with oral anticoagulants. Nonacetylated salicylates (eg, choline salicylate, magnesium salicylate, salsalate, sodium salicylate) probably also are safer with oral anticoagulants than NSAIDs, because such salicylates have minimal effects on platelet function and the gastric mucosa.

➡ *Monitor.* If any NSAID is used with an oral anticoagulant, carefully monitor the prothrombin time and watch for evidence of bleeding, especially from the GI tract.

REFERENCES:

Rubin A, Warrick P, Wolen RL, Chernish SM, Ridolfo AS, Gruber CM. Physiological disposition of fenoprofen in man 3. Metabolism and protein binding of fenoprofen. *J Pharmacol Exp Ther.* 1972;183:449-457.

Shorr RI, Ray WA, Daugherty JR, Griffin MR. Concurrent use of nonsteroidal anti-inflammatory drugs and oral anticoagulants places elderly persons at high risk for hemorrhagic peptic ulcer disease. *Arch Intern Med.* 1993;153:1665-1670.

Fentanyl (eg, *Sublimaze*)

Lidocaine (eg, *Xylocaine*)

SUMMARY: A patient who received fentanyl and morphine (eg, *Duramorph*) during anesthetic induction developed respiratory depression and lost consciousness after receiving IV lidocaine; carefully monitor patients receiving opioids and lidocaine for excessive opioid effects.

RISK FACTORS:

➡ *Route of Administration.* The observed reaction occurred following IV use of lidocaine. Theoretically, an interaction with opioids would be unlikely to occur with lidocaine administration routes that do not result in lidocaine reaching the CNS.

RELATED DRUGS: Theoretically, lidocaine would enhance the effect of any opioid.

MANAGEMENT OPTIONS:

➡ *Monitor.* If lidocaine is used concurrently with opioids, monitor for excessive opioid effects (eg, respiratory depression, CNS depression). Based on the case reported, administration of an opioid antagonist such as naloxone may be effective in reversing the reaction.

REFERENCES:

Jensen E, et al. Potentiation of narcosis after intravenous lidocaine in a patient given spinal opioids. *Anesth Analg.* 1999;89:758-61.

Fentanyl (eg, *Sublimaze*)

Ritonavir (*Norvir*)

SUMMARY: Ritonavir administration results in large increases in fentanyl concentrations; increased analgesic effects and side effects may occur during concurrent therapy.

RISK FACTORS: No specific risk factors are known.

RELATED DRUGS: Other protease inhibitors such as indinavir (*Crixivan*), saquinavir (eg, *Invirase*), and nelfinavir (*Viracept*) may affect fentanyl in a similar manner. Alfentanil (*Alfenta*) may be affected in a similar manner by ritonavir. Ritonavir has been reported to reduce methadone effects following 1 week of concurrent therapy.

MANAGEMENT OPTIONS:

➡ *Monitor.* Monitor patients taking ritonavir for increased narcotic effects (eg, sedation, respiratory depression) following the administration of fentanyl.

REFERENCES:

Olkkola KT, et al. Ritonavir's role in reducing fentanyl clearance and prolonging its half-life. *Anesthesiology.* 1999;91:681-85.

Ferrous Sulfate (eg, *Feosol*)

Trovafloxacin (*Trovan*)

SUMMARY: Ferrous sulfate reduces the bioavailability of trovafloxacin; a loss of therapeutic efficacy may occur in some patients.

RISK FACTORS: No specific risk factors are known.

RELATED DRUGS: Ferrous sulfate affects other quinolones similarly (eg, ciprofloxacin [*Cipro*], ofloxacin [*Floxin*]).

MANAGEMENT OPTIONS:

➡ *Circumvent/Minimize.* Administer the antibiotic at least 2 hours before the ferrous sulfate. If possible, avoid iron products in patients during trovafloxacin administration. If indicated, administer parenteral iron.

➡ *Monitor.* Observe patients receiving trovafloxacin who take iron products for a potential reduction in antibiotic effect.

REFERENCES:

Product information. Trovafloxacin (*Trovan*). Pfizer Inc. 1998.

Flecainide (*Tambocor*)

Propranolol (eg, *Inderal*)

SUMMARY: Flecainide increases the serum concentration of propranolol; propranolol increases the concentration of flecainide. Coadministration of these drugs produces additive negative inotropic effects.

RISK FACTORS: No specific risk factors are known.

RELATED DRUGS: It is probable that other beta blockers will exert additive negative inotropic effects with flecainide, but little is known regarding a pharmacokinetic interaction between flecainide and other beta blockers.

MANAGEMENT OPTIONS:

➡ *Monitor.* Monitor patients taking propranolol and flecainide for increased effects of both drugs and additive negative inotropic effects on the heart.

REFERENCES:

Holtzman JL, et al. The pharmacodynamic and pharmacokinetic interaction of flecainide acetate with propranolol: effects on cardiac function and drug clearance. *Eur J Clin Pharmacol.* 1987;33:97-99.

▼ Flecainide (*Tambocor*)

Sodium Bicarbonate

SUMMARY: Increases in urine pH will increase the serum concentrations of flecainide; the clinical significance of this interaction is unclear.

RISK FACTORS: No specific risk factors are known.

RELATED DRUGS: Drugs that alter urinary pH such as sodium bicarbonate, acetazolamide (eg, *Diamox*), ammonium chloride, or large doses of antacids will be likely to affect flecainide clearance.

MANAGEMENT OPTIONS:

➡ *Monitor.* Monitor flecainide concentrations in patients receiving drugs likely to alter their urinary pH such as sodium bicarbonate, acetazolamide (*Diamox*), ammonium chloride, or large doses of antacids.

REFERENCES:

Johnston A, et al. Flecainide pharmacokinetics in healthy volunteers: the influence of urinary pH. *Br J Clin Pharmacol.* 1985;20:333.

Hertrampf R, et al. Elimination of flecainide as a function of urinary flow rate and pH. *Eur J Clin Pharmacol.* 1991;41:61.

Muhiddin KA, et al. The influence of urinary pH on flecainide excretion and its serum pharmacokinetics. *Br J Clin Pharmacol.* 1984;17:447.

▼ Flecainide (*Tambocor*)

Sotalol (*Betapace*)

SUMMARY: A case report notes sinus bradycardia, atrioventricular (AV) block, and cardiac arrest following a switch from flecainide to sotalol therapy for ventricular arrhythmia, but a causal relationship was not established.

RISK FACTORS: No specific risk factors are known.

RELATED DRUGS: Propranolol (eg, *Inderal*) and other beta blockers may cause similar reactions with flecainide.

MANAGEMENT OPTIONS:

➡ *Circumvent/Minimize.* It may be prudent to avoid the administration of sotalol for several days to patients previously receiving drugs that depress myocardial conduction.

➡ *Monitor.* Until further information is available, carefully monitor patients receiving sotalol and flecainide for reduced myocardial conduction (eg, bradycardia).

REFERENCES:

Warren R, et al. Serious interactions of sotalol with amiodarone and flecainide. *Med J Aust.* 1990;152:227.

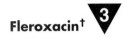

Fleroxacin[†]

Sucralfate (eg, *Carafate*)

SUMMARY: Sucralfate administration moderately reduces the bioavailability of fleroxacin; some reduction of antibiotic efficacy could result.

RISK FACTORS: No specific risk factors are known.

RELATED DRUGS: Sucralfate inhibits the absorption of ciprofloxacin (*Cipro*), fleroxacin, norfloxacin (*Noroxin*), and ofloxacin (*Floxin*).

MANAGEMENT OPTIONS:

➡ *Consider Alternative.* If dosage separation is not possible, consider an alternative to sucralfate (eg, H_2-receptor antagonist, proton-pump inhibitor), but *not* an antacid.

➡ *Circumvent/Minimize.* Administer fleroxacin at least 2 hours before or 6 hours after a sucralfate dose to maximize its absorption. Because fleroxacin can be administered once daily, minimize the clinical significance of this interaction by adjusting the dose administration times.

➡ *Monitor.* If sucralfate and a quinolone are coadministered, monitor the patient for reduced antibiotic efficacy.

REFERENCES:

Lubowski TJ, et al. Effect of sucralfate on pharmacokinetics of fleroxacin in healthy volunteers. *Antimicrob Agents Chemother.* 1992;36:2758-2768.

Shiba K, et al. Interactions of fleroxacin with dried aluminum hydroxide gel and probenecid. *Rev Infect Dis.* 1989;11(suppl 5):S1097.

† Not available in the US.

Fluconazole (*Diflucan*)

Fluvastatin (*Lescol*)

SUMMARY: Fluconazole administration increases the plasma concentration of fluvastatin. An increased risk of toxicity may occur.

RISK FACTORS: No specific risk factors are known.

RELATED DRUGS: The effect of fluconazole on other HMG-CoA reductase inhibitors is unknown. However, because of the ability of fluconazole to inhibit CYP3A4, other HMG-CoA reductase inhibitors (eg, simvastatin [*Zocor*], lovastatin [eg, *Mevacor*], atorvastatin [*Lipitor*]) may be affected to some extent. Fluconazole administration produced a nonsignificant (36%) increase in pravastatin (*Pravachol*) AUC. No other antifungal agents are known to inhibit CYP2C9 and would not be expected to interact with fluvastatin.

MANAGEMENT OPTIONS:

➡ *Circumvent/Minimize.* Temporarily discontinue fluvastatin in patients taking fluvastatin during fluconazole administration. Because fluconazole has a long half-life, hold fluvastatin for several days after fluconazole is discontinued.

➡️ *Monitor.* Monitor patients taking fluvastatin who are prescribed fluconazole for fluvastatin side effects including muscle pain.

REFERENCES:

Kantola T, et al. Effect of fluconazole on plasma fluvastatin and pravastatin concentrations. *Eur J Clin Pharmacol.* 2000;56:225-229.

 Fluconazole (*Diflucan*)

Glimepiride (*Amaryl*)

SUMMARY: Fluconazole increases plasma concentrations of glimepiride.

RISK FACTORS: No specific risk factors are known.

RELATED DRUGS: Fluconazole has been noted to reduce the metabolism of tolbutamide (eg, *Orinase*) resulting in increased tolbutamide plasma concentrations. Other hypoglycemic drugs that are substrates for CYP2C9, such as glipizide (eg, *Glucotrol*) and glyburide (eg, *DiaBeta*), may be similarly affected by fluconazole but with limited effect on plasma glucose concentrations.

MANAGEMENT OPTIONS:

➡️ *Monitor.* Until more information is available, monitor patients stabilized on glimepiride in whom fluconazole is initiated or discontinued.

REFERENCES:

Niemi M, et al. Effects of fluconazole and fluvoxamine on the pharmacokinetics and pharmacodynamics of glimepiride. *Clin Pharmacol Ther.* 2001;69:194-200.

Rowe BR, et al. Safety of fluconazole in women taking oral hypoglycemic agents. *Lancet.* 1992;339:255-256.

 Fluconazole (*Diflucan*)

Losartan (*Cozaar*)

SUMMARY: Fluconazole reduces the concentration of losartan's active metabolite; reduction of losartan's antihypertensive efficacy may result.

RISK FACTORS: No specific risk factors are known.

RELATED DRUGS: Antifungal agents that do not inhibit CYP2C9 (eg, terbinafine [*Lamisil*]) are unlikely to interact. The effect of other antifungal agents on losartan is unknown but is likely to be less than the effect seen with fluconazole. The effects of fluconazole on other angiotensin receptor antagonists are unknown.

MANAGEMENT OPTIONS:

➡️ *Consider Alternative.* An antifungal agent that does not inhibit CYP2C9 could be selected for patients stabilized on losartan. Patients taking fluconazole could be treated with an angiotensin-converting enzyme inhibitor.

➡️ *Monitor.* Monitor patients stabilized on losartan for a reduction in blood pressure control if fluconazole is administered.

REFERENCES:

Kazierad DJ, et al. Fluconazole significantly alters the pharmacokinetics of losartan but not eprosartan. *Clin Pharmacol Ther.* 1997;61:203.

Fluconazole (*Diflucan*)

Methadone (eg, *Dolophine*)

SUMMARY: Fluconazole administration increases the plasma concentration of methadone; some patients may experience increased narcotic effects.

RISK FACTORS: No specific risk factors are known.

RELATED DRUGS: Other azole antifungal agents including ketoconazole (eg, *Nizoral*) and itraconazole (*Sporanox*) may affect methadone in a similar manner. Since terbinafine (*Lamisil*) does not inhibit CYP3A4 metabolism, it would not be expected to affect the metabolism of methadone. Narcotic analgesics that are not metabolized by CYP3A4 such as morphine (eg, *MSIR*) or codeine derivatives are not likely to interact with fluconazole.

MANAGEMENT OPTIONS:

➡ *Consider Alternative.* Consider an antifungal agent that does not inhibit CYP3A4 (eg, terbinafine) for patients receiving methadone. Consider alternative analgesics such as codeine or morphine in patients receiving fluconazole.

➡ *Monitor.* Monitor patients receiving methadone and fluconazole for enhanced narcotic effects including sedation.

REFERENCES:

Cobb MN, Desai J, Brown LS, Zannikos PN, Rainey PM. The effect of fluconazole on the clinical pharmacokinetics of methadone. *Clin Pharmacol Ther.* 1998;63:655-662.

Fluconazole (*Diflucan*)

Midazolam (eg, *Versed*)

SUMMARY: Fluconazole administration appears to increase the concentrations and effects of midazolam.

RISK FACTORS: No specific risk factors are known.

RELATED DRUGS: Ketoconazole (eg, *Nizoral*) and itraconazole (*Sporanox*) also may inhibit midazolam metabolism. Other benzodiazepines including diazepam (eg, *Valium*) and triazolam (eg, *Halcion*) are likely to be affected in a similar manner by fluconazole.

MANAGEMENT OPTIONS:

➡ *Monitor.* Monitor patients requiring midazolam and fluconazole for increased sedation.

REFERENCES:

Mattila MJ, et al. Fluconazole moderately increases midazolam effects on performance. *Br J Clin Pharmacol.* 1995;39:567P.

Fluconazole (*Diflucan*)

Nateglinide (*Starlix*)

SUMMARY: Fluconazole increases the serum concentration of nateglinide; some diabetic patients may be at increased risk for hypoglycemic episodes.

RISK FACTORS: No specific risk factors are known.

RELATED DRUGS: Voriconazole (*Vfend*) also inhibits both CYPC9 and CYP3A4 and may produce a similar interaction with nateglinide. Itraconazole (*Sporanox*) and keto-conazole (eg, *Nizoral*) are CYP3A4 inhibitors and may produce some inhibition of nateglinide. Other oral hypoglycemics that are metabolized by CYP2C9 or CYP3A4 (eg, tolbutamide [eg, *Orinase*], glipizide [eg, *Glucotrol*], glyburide [*Dia-Beta*]) may interact similarly with fluconazole.

MANAGEMENT OPTIONS:

➡ *Monitor.* Carefully observe patients taking nateglinide for altered blood glucose control when fluconazole is added or removed from the drug regimen.

REFERENCES:

Niemi M, Neuvonen M, Juntti-Patinen L, Backman JT, Neuvonen PJ. Effect of fluconazole on the pharma-cokinetics and pharmacodynamics of nateglinide. *Clin Pharmacol Ther.* 2003;74:25-31.

Fluconazole (*Diflucan*)

Phenytoin (eg, *Dilantin*)

SUMMARY: Fluconazole may increase plasma phenytoin concentrations substantially, resulting in phenytoin toxicity in some patients.

RISK FACTORS: No specific risk factors are known.

RELATED DRUGS: Available evidence suggests that ketoconazole (eg, *Nizoral*) does not affect phenytoin pharmacokinetics.

MANAGEMENT OPTIONS:

➡ *Monitor.* Monitor patients carefully for phenytoin toxicity (eg, nystagmus, ataxia, confusion, dizziness, slurred speech, involuntary muscular movements) when flu-conazole is started in the presence of phenytoin therapy. Serum phenytoin deter-minations would also be useful. When fluconazole therapy is stopped in the presence of phenytoin therapy, monitor the patient for a reduced phenytoin effect.

REFERENCES:

Lazar JD, Wilner KD. Drug interactions with fluconazole. *Rev Infect Dis.* 1990;12(suppl 3):S327-S333.

Howitt KM, Oziemski MA. Phenytoin toxicity induced by fluconazole. *Med J Aust.* 1989;151:603-604.

Mitchell AS, Holland JT. Fluconazole and phenytoin: a predictable interaction. *BMJ.* 1989;298:1315.

Cadle RM, Zenon GJ, Rodriguez-Barradas MC, Hamill RJ. Fluconazole induced symptomatic phenytoin toxicity. *Ann Pharmacother.* 1994;28:191-195.

Blum RA, Wilton JH, Hilligoss DM, et al. Effect of fluconazole on the disposition of phenytoin. *Clin Phar-macol Ther.* 1991;49:420-425.

Touchette M, Chandrasekar PH, Milad MA, Edwards DJ. Contrasting effects of fluconazole and ketocona-zole on phenytoin and testosterone disposition in man. *Br J Clin Pharmacol.* 1992;34:75.

Fluconazole (*Diflucan*)

Rifampin (eg, *Rifadin*)

SUMMARY: Chronic rifampin administration reduces fluconazole plasma concentrations; the clinical significance of this interaction is unknown.

RISK FACTORS: No specific risk factors are known.

RELATED DRUGS: Rifampin reduces the concentration of fluconazole, itraconazole (*Sporanox*), and ketoconazole (eg, *Nizoral*). Rifabutin (*Mycobutin*) does not affect fluconazole.

MANAGEMENT OPTIONS:

➡ *Circumvent/Minimize.* A limited increase in fluconazole dose may be warranted in patients requiring high fluconazole concentrations.

➡ *Monitor.* Until further information is available, be aware of potentially reduced fluconazole plasma concentrations when rifampin is coadministered.

REFERENCES:

Apseloff G, et al. Induction of fluconazole metabolism by rifampin: *in vivo* study in humans. *J Clin Pharmacol*. 1991;31:358.

Coker RJ, et al. Interaction between fluconazole and rifampicin. *BMJ*. 1990;301:818.

Fluconazole (*Diflucan*)

Tacrolimus (*Prograf*)

SUMMARY: Fluconazole administration significantly increases tacrolimus concentrations and can increase the risk of nephrotoxicity.

RISK FACTORS:

➡ *Dosage Regimen.* Fluconazole doses greater than 100 mg/day will increase the risk of an interaction.

RELATED DRUGS: Fluconazole also inhibits cyclosporine (eg, *Sandimmune*) metabolism. Other oral antifungal agents (eg, ketoconazole [eg, *Nizoral*], itraconazole [*Sporanox*]) also may inhibit tacrolimus metabolism.

MANAGEMENT OPTIONS:

➡ *Monitor.* Patients receiving tacrolimus should have their plasma concentrations monitored during the coadministration of fluconazole. A reduction in the dose of tacrolimus is likely to be necessary to avoid nephrotoxicity.

REFERENCES:

Manez R, et al. Fluconazole therapy in transplant recipients receiving FK506. *Transplantation*. 1994;57:1521.

Assan R, et al. FK 506/ fluconazole interaction enhances FK 506 nephrotoxicity. *Diabetes Metab*. 1994;20:49.

Fluconazole (*Diflucan*)

Terfenadine (*Seldane*)

SUMMARY: The plasma concentration of terfenadine is increased by large doses of fluconazole; the concentration of the active, carboxylic acid metabolite of terfenadine is increased, but this is without apparent significance.

RISK FACTORS:

➡ *Dosage Regimen.* Fluconazole doses above 200 mg/day may lead to terfenadine accumulation.

RELATED DRUGS: Ketoconazole (eg, *Nizoral*) and itraconazole (*Sporanox*) also inhibit the metabolism of terfenadine. Loratadine (*Claritin*), fexofenadine (eg, *Allegra*), and cetirizine (*Zyrtec*) would be less likely to interact with fluconazole and cause toxicity.

MANAGEMENT OPTIONS:

➡ *Circumvent/Minimize.* Until additional studies of the interaction between fluconazole and terfenadine are available, it would be prudent to avoid giving the 2 drugs together. The use of sedating antihistamines or perhaps loratadine or cetirizine instead of terfenadine would seem to be preferred in patients taking fluconazole or other oral antifungal agents.

➡ *Monitor.* Watch for cardiotoxicity in patients receiving terfenadine and fluconazole.

REFERENCES:

Honig PK, et al. The effect of fluconazole on the steady-state pharmacokinetics and electrocardiographic pharmacodynamics of terfenadine in humans. *Clin Pharmacol Ther.* 1993;53:630.

Cantilena LR, et al. Fluconazole alters terfenadine pharmacokinetics and electrocardiographic pharmacodynamics. *Clin Pharmacol Ther.* 1995;57:185.

Fluconazole (*Diflucan*)

Tolbutamide (eg, *Orinase*)

SUMMARY: Fluconazole increases the plasma concentration of tolbutamide; the clinical significance of this interaction in diabetic patients is unknown.

RISK FACTORS: No specific risk factors are known.

RELATED DRUGS: Fluconazole 50 mg/day for 14 days did not affect the glycosylated hemoglobin or fructosamine concentrations in 14 diabetic women taking glipizide (eg, *Glurotrol*) or glyburide (eg, *DiaBeta*). Although glycosylated hemoglobin concentrations may not reflect short-term changes in blood glucose, no patient had symptoms of hypoglycemia. No pharmacokinetic data were presented; higher fluconazole doses may alter glipizide or glyburide pharmacokinetics. Other azole antifungal agents (eg, ketoconazole [eg, *Nizoral*], miconazole [eg, *Monistat*], itraconazole [*Sporanox*]) may inhibit the metabolism of tolbutamide.

MANAGEMENT OPTIONS:

➡ ***Monitor.*** Until further information is available, observe patients maintained on tolbutamide for reduced glucose concentrations when fluconazole is started or increased glucose when fluconazole is discontinued.

REFERENCES:
Lazar J, et al. Drug interactions with fluconazole. *Rev Infect Dis*. 1990;12(Suppl. 3):S327.

Rowe BR, et al. Safety of fluconazole in women taking oral hypoglycemic agents. *Lancet*. 1992;339:255.

Fluconazole (*Diflucan*)
Triazolam (eg, *Halcion*)

SUMMARY: Fluconazole increases the serum concentration of triazolam and may increase its pharmacodynamic effects such as sedation.

RISK FACTORS:

➡ ***Dosage Regimen.*** While the authors did not do a dose response study, fluconazole is known to produce a greater magnitude of metabolic inhibition when administered in doses above 100 mg/day.

RELATED DRUGS: Fluconazole inhibits the metabolism of midazolam (*Versed*) (also see Fluconazole/Midazolam monograph) and could affect diazepam (eg, *Valium*) in a similar manner. A benzodiazepine such as lorazepam (eg, *Ativan*), which is not metabolized by CYP3A4 may be less likely to interact. Other antifungal agents such as ketoconazole (eg, *Nizoral*) or itraconazole (*Sporanox*) similarly inhibit the metabolism of triazolam; however, terbinafine does not appear to inhibit triazolam metabolism.

MANAGEMENT OPTIONS:

➡ ***Use Alternative.*** Avoid the combination of fluconazole and triazolam. A benzodiazepine such as lorazepam that is not metabolized by CYP3A4 would be a potential alternative anxiolytic agent. The antifungal agent terbinafine does not appear to inhibit the metabolism of triazolam.

REFERENCES:
Varhe A, et al. Fluconazole, but not terbinafine, enhances the effects of triazolam by inhibiting its metabolism. *Br J Clin Pharmacol*. 1996;41:319.

Fluconazole (*Diflucan*)
Warfarin (eg, *Coumadin*)

SUMMARY: Case reports and clinical studies show that fluconazole enhances the hypoprothrombinemic response to warfarin; adjustments in warfarin dose may be needed.

RISK FACTORS:

➡ ***Dosage Regimen.*** Although the ability of fluconazole to inhibit drug metabolism by CYP3A4 has been shown to require large doses of fluconazole, doses of 100 mg/day can inhibit warfarin metabolism (metabolized by CYP2C9).

RELATED DRUGS: The effect of fluconazole on oral anticoagulants other than warfarin is unknown, but consider the possibility. However, phenprocoumon[+] is metabolized primarily by glucuronidation and, theoretically, would be less likely to interact with cytochrome P450 inhibitors such as fluconazole. Ketoconazole (eg, *Nizoral*) and itraconazole (*Sporanox*) also may increase the effect of oral anticoagulants.

MANAGEMENT OPTIONS:

➡ ***Monitor.*** Monitor for altered oral anticoagulant effect if fluconazole is initiated, discontinued, or changed in dosage. Adjust the anticoagulant dose as needed.

REFERENCES:

Lazar JD, et al. Drug interactions with fluconazole. *Rev Infect Dis.* 1990;12(Suppl. 3):S327.

Seaton TL, et al. Possible potentiation of warfarin by fluconazole. *DICP.* 1990;24:1177.

Black DJ, et al. An evaluation of the effect of fluconazole (F) on the stereoselective metabolism of warfarin (W). *Clin Pharmacol Ther.* 1992;51:184.

Gericke KR. Possible interaction between warfarin and fluconazole. *Pharmacotherapy.* 1993;13:508.

Baciewicz AM, et al. Fluconazole-warfarin interaction. *Ann Pharmacother.* 1994.28:1111.

Kerr HD. Case report: potentiation of warfarin by fluconazole. *Am J Med Sci.* 1993;305:164.

Tett S, et al. Drug interactions with fluconazole. *Med J Aust.* 1992;156:365.

Crussel-Porter LL, et al. Low-dose fluconazole therapy potentiates the hypoprothrombinemic response of warfarin sodium. *Arch Intern Med.* 1993;153:102.

† Not available in the US.

 Fluorouracil (5-FU)

Metronidazole (eg, *Flagyl*)

SUMMARY: Metronidazole enhances the toxicity of fluorouracil without increasing its efficacy.

RISK FACTORS: No specific risk factors are known.

RELATED DRUGS: No information is available.

MANAGEMENT OPTIONS:

➡ ***Avoid Unless Benefit Outweighs Risk.*** Patients taking fluorouracil should generally avoid metronidazole administration.

➡ ***Monitor.*** Monitor patients for enhanced toxicity when metronidazole is coadministered.

REFERENCES:

Bardakji Z, et al. 5-fluorouracil-metronidazole combination therapy in metastatic colorectal cancer. *Cancer Chemother Pharmacol.* 1986;18:140-144.

 Fluorouracil (5-FU)

Phenytoin (eg, *Dilantin*)

SUMMARY: Limited clinical evidence suggest that fluorouracil can increase phenytoin serum concentrations.

RISK FACTORS: No specific risk factors are known.

RELATED DRUGS: No information available.

MANAGEMENT OPTIONS:

➡ ***Monitor.*** In patients given phenytoin and fluorouracil, monitor phenytoin serum concentrations and be alert for evidence of phenytoin toxicity. Adjustments in phenytoin dose may be needed if fluorouracil is initiated, discontinued, or changed in dosage.

REFERENCES:

Gilbar PJ, et al. Phenytoin and fluorouracil interaction. *Ann Pharmacother.* 2001;35:1367-1370.

Fluorouracil (5-FU)

Warfarin (eg, *Coumadin*)

SUMMARY: Case reports suggest that fluorouracil may increase the hypoprothrombinemic response to warfarin; more study is needed to establish a causal relationship.

RISK FACTORS: No specific risk factors are known.

RELATED DRUGS: The effect of fluorouracil on oral anticoagulants other than warfarin is not established, but assume that they interact until proven otherwise.

MANAGEMENT OPTIONS:

➡ *Monitor.* Monitor for altered warfarin effect if fluorouracil is initiated, discontinued, or changed in dosage; adjustments of warfarin dosage may be needed. If warfarin is initiated in the presence of fluorouracil therapy, it would be prudent to begin with conservative doses of warfarin.

REFERENCES:

Scarfe MA, et al. Possible drug interaction between warfarin and combination of levamisole and fluorouracil. *Ann Pharmacother.* 1994;28:464-467.

Wajima T, et al. Possible interactions between warfarin and 5-fluorouracil. *Am J Hematol.* 1992;40:238.

Fluoxetine (*Prozac*)

Furosemide (eg, *Lasix*)

SUMMARY: Two patients receiving fluoxetine and furosemide died unexpectedly, and it was proposed that the combination of these 2 drugs may have contributed to their deaths. However, a causal relationship was not established.

RISK FACTORS: No specific risk factors are known.

RELATED DRUGS: If the furosemide-fluoxetine combination did, in fact, contribute to the fatal reactions, expect other loop diuretics such as bumetanide (eg, *Bumex*) and torsemide (*Demadex*) to produce the same effect. Little is known regarding the ability of other selective serotonin reuptake inhibitors (SSRIs) to produce SIADH. Sertraline (*Zoloft*) has been reported to produce hyponatremia caused by SIADH in one 73-year-old man, and cases of paroxetine (*Paxil*)-induced hyponatremia have been reported to the manufacturer. It is possible that other SSRIs have a similar effect.

MANAGEMENT OPTIONS:

➡ *Monitor.* Monitor for evidence of hyponatremia if fluoxetine is used in patients undergoing vigorous diuresis or others at risk of hyponatremia. The relative likelihood of SIADH in patients receiving fluoxetine vs other SSRIs or tricyclic antidepressants is not established. Thus, it is not known if any of them would be preferable to fluoxetine in a patient prone to hyponatremia.

REFERENCES:

Spier SA, et al. Unexpected deaths in depressed medical inpatients treated with fluoxetine. *J Clin Psychiatry.* 1991;52:377.

Hwang AS, et al. Syndrome of inappropriate secretion of antidiuretic hormone due to fluoxetine. *Am J Psychiatry.* 1989;146:399.

Cohen BJ, et al. More cases of SIADH with fluoxetine. *Am J Psychiatry.* 1990;147:948.

Crews JR, et al. Hyponatremia in a patient treated with sertraline. *Am J Psychiatry.* 1993;150:1564.

Product Information. Paroxetine (*Paxil*). SmithKline Beecham. 1993.

Fluoxetine (eg, *Prozac*)

Haloperidol (eg, *Haldol*)

SUMMARY: A woman on haloperidol developed severe extrapyramidal symptoms after starting fluoxetine, but a causal relationship was not established.

RISK FACTORS: No specific risk factors are known.

RELATED DRUGS: The effect of fluoxetine on other neuroleptics is not established. Paroxetine (*Paxil*) also is a potent inhibitor of CYP2D6 and also might inhibit haloperidol metabolism. Sertraline (*Zoloft*) appears to be a less potent CYP2D6 inhibitor, but it may have some effect.

MANAGEMENT OPTIONS:

➡ *Monitor.* Until more information is available, monitor patients for extrapyramidal symptoms if fluoxetine is used concomitantly with haloperidol (and possibly other neuroleptics).

REFERENCES:

Tate JL. Extrapyramidal symptoms in a patient taking haloperidol and fluoxetine. *Am J Psychiatry.* 1989;146:399-400.

Fluoxetine (eg, *Prozac*)

Ibuprofen (eg, *Motrin*)

SUMMARY: The combined use of fluoxetine (or other selective serotonin reuptake inhibitors [SSRIs]) with ibuprofen (or other nonsteroidal anti-inflammatory drugs [NSAIDs]) appears to increase the risk of upper gastrointestinal bleeding.

RISK FACTORS: No specific risk factors are known.

RELATED DRUGS: Assume that all other drugs that inhibit serotonin reuptake (citalopram [*Effexor*], clomipramine [*Anafranil*], fluvoxamine [*Luvox*], nefazodone [*Serzone*], paroxetine [*Paxil*], sertraline [*Zoloft*], and venlafaxine [*Effexor*]) would interact with all NSAIDs: diclofenac (*Voltaren*), diflunisal (*Dolobid*), etodolac (*Lodine*), fenoprofen (*Nalfon*), flurbiprofen (*Ansaid*), ibuprofen (*Motrin*), indomethacin (*Indocin*), ketoprofen (*Orudis*), ketorolac (*Toradol*), meclofenamate (*Meclomen*), mefenamic acid (*Ponstel*), meloxicam (*Mobic*), nabumetone (*Relafen*), naproxen (*Aleve*), oxaprozin (*Daypro*), piroxicam (*Feldene*), sulindac (*Clinoril*), tolmetin (*Tolectin*).

MANAGEMENT OPTIONS:

➥ **Consider Alternative.** Consider using a non-NSAID analgesic such as acetaminophen. If an NSAID is needed, consider a non-acetylated salicylate such as choline magnesium trisalicylate (*Trilisate*), salsalate (*Disalcid*), or magnesium salicylate (*Doan's*) since these products have minimal effects on platelets and the gastric mucosa. It is not known whether COX-2 inhibitors such as celecoxib (*Celebrex*), rofecoxib (*Vioxx*), or valdecoxib (*Bextra*) would be less likely to cause GI bleeding with SSRIs. Antidepressants with less effect on serotonin may reduce the risk of GI bleeding when combined with NSAIDs.

➥ **Monitor.** Patients receiving both a SSRI and NSAID should be alert for evidence of GI bleeding.

REFERENCES:

de Abajo FJ, et al. Association between selective serotonin reuptake inhibitors and upper gastrointestinal bleeding: population based case-control study. *BMJ.* 1999;319:1106-1109.

Dalton SO, et al. Use of selective serotonin reuptake inhibitors and risk of upper gastrointestinal tract bleeding: a population-based cohort study. *Arch Intern Med.* 2003;163:59-64.

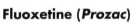

Fluoxetine (*Prozac*)

Lithium (eg, *Eskalith*)

SUMMARY: Some patients receiving lithium and fluoxetine have developed neurotoxicity, but the incidence of this reaction is unknown.

RISK FACTORS: No specific risk factors are known.

RELATED DRUGS: Theoretically, other selective serotonin reuptake inhibitors would interact with lithium in a similar manner.

MANAGEMENT OPTIONS:

➥ **Monitor.** Until additional information is available, monitor for evidence of neurotoxicity in patients receiving lithium and fluoxetine. Symptoms have included tremor, confusion, ataxia, dizziness, dysarthria, and absence seizures. If symptoms occur, consider trying a tricyclic antidepressant (eg, nortriptyline, imipramine [eg, *Tofranil*]) with the lithium.

REFERENCES:

Sacristan JA, et al. Absence seizures induced by lithium: possible interaction with fluoxetine. *Am J Psychiatry.* 1991;148:146.

Austin LS, et al. Toxicity resulting from lithium augmentation of antidepressant treatment in elderly patients. *J Clin Psychiatry.* 1990;51:344.

Noveske FG, et al. Possible toxicity of combined fluoxetine and lithium. *Am J Psychiatry.* 1989;146:1515.

Salama AA, et al. A case of severe lithium toxicity induced by combined fluoxetine and lithium carbonate. *Am J Psychiatry.* 1989;146:278.

Pope HG, et al. Possible synergism between fluoxetine and lithium in refractory depression. *Am J Psychiatry.* 1988;145:1292.

Fluoxetine (eg, *Prozac*)

Nefazodone (*Serzone*)

SUMMARY: A patient on fluoxetine developed serotonin syndrome after nefazodone was added without discontinuation of the fluoxetine.

RISK FACTORS: No specific risk factors are known.

RELATED DRUGS: Serotonin syndrome also has been reported in a patient receiving paroxetine (*Paxil*) plus nefazodone. All selective serotonin reuptake inhibitors (SSRIs) can be expected to have additive serotonergic effects with nefazodone.

MANAGEMENT OPTIONS:

➥ *Circumvent/Minimize.* When switching from fluoxetine to another serotonergic drug, be aware that the serotonergic effects of fluoxetine and its active metabolite can last for several weeks.

➥ *Monitor.* Be alert for evidence of serotonin syndrome when nefazodone is used concurrently or sequentially with SSRIs. Serotonin syndrome can result in neurotoxicity (myoclonus, tremors, rigidity, incoordination, hyperreflexia, seizures, coma), psychiatric symptoms (agitation, confusion, hypomania, restlessness), and autonomic dysfunction (fever, sweating, tachycardia, hypertension).

REFERENCES:

Smith DL, Wenegrat BG. A case report of serotonin syndrome associated with combined nefazodone and fluoxetine. *J Clin Psychiatry.* 2000;61:146.

Fluoxetine (eg, *Prozac*)

Phenytoin (eg, *Dilantin*)

SUMMARY: Several case reports have been published describing phenytoin toxicity with concurrent use of fluoxetine.

RISK FACTORS: No specific risk factors are known.

RELATED DRUGS: The effect of selective serotonin reuptake inhibitors other than fluoxetine on phenytoin is not established.

MANAGEMENT OPTIONS:

➥ *Monitor.* Carefully monitor patients for phenytoin toxicity (eg, nystagmus, ataxia, confusion, dizziness, slurred speech, involuntary muscular movements) when fluoxetine is started. Serum phenytoin determinations would be useful. Monitor the patient for a reduced phenytoin effect when fluoxetine therapy is stopped during phenytoin therapy.

REFERENCES:

Woods DJ, et al. Interaction of phenytoin and fluoxetine. *N Z Med J.* 1994;107:19.

Jalil P. Toxic reaction following the combined administration of fluoxetine and phenytoin: two case reports. *J Neurol Neurosurg Psychiatry.* 1992;55:412.

Fluoxetine (eg, *Prozac*)

Propafenone (eg, *Rythmol*)

SUMMARY: Fluoxetine increases the plasma concentration of propafenone; increased effect on myocardial conduction may occur including the induction of arrhythmias.

RISK FACTORS:

➡ **Pharmacogenetics.** Patients who are rapid metabolizers (CYP2D6) of propafenone are more susceptible to this interaction than poor CYP2D6 metabolizers.

RELATED DRUGS: Paroxetine (*Paxil*) is another antidepressant with significant CYP2D6 inhibitory activity; it would be expected to interact in a similar manner as fluoxetine. Sertraline (*Zoloft*) is a weaker inhibitor of CYP2D6 but may affect the metabolism of propafenone at daily doses greater than 150 mg.

MANAGEMENT OPTIONS:

➡ **Consider Alternative.** Selecting antidepressants that do not inhibit CYP2D6 (eg, citalopram [*Celexa*], nefazodone [*Serzone*], venlafaxine [*Effexor*]) would avoid the interaction.

➡ **Monitor.** If fluoxetine is coadministered, carefully monitor patients taking propafenone for increased effect on myocardial conduction.

REFERENCES:
Cai WM, et al. Fluoxetine impairs the CYP2D6-mediated metabolism of propafenone enantiomers in healthy Chinese volunteers. *Clin Pharmacol Ther.* 1999;66:516.

Fluoxetine (eg, *Prozac*)

Propranolol (eg, *Inderal*)

SUMMARY: Fluoxetine increases the beta-adrenergic blocking effects of some beta blockers; cardiac toxicity may result.

RISK FACTORS: No specific risk factors are known.

RELATED DRUGS: Metoprolol interacts similarly with fluoxetine, while sotalol appears unaffected. While the effects of other selective serotonin reuptake inhibitors on beta blocker clearance is not known, fluvoxamine (eg, *Luvox*) and sertraline (*Zoloft*) appear to be less potent inhibitors of CYP2D6 than fluoxetine.

MANAGEMENT OPTIONS:

➡ **Consider Alternative.** Although specific data are lacking, beta blockers that are renally eliminated (eg, atenolol [eg, *Tenormin*]) may be a safer choice.

➡ **Monitor.** Monitor patients stabilized on propranolol or metoprolol for toxicity (eg, bradycardia, conduction defects, hypotension, heart failure, CNS disturbances) if fluoxetine is coadministered. The long half-life of fluoxetine (24 hours) and its metabolite norfluoxetine (half-life 7 days and also known to be a metabolic inhibitor) explains why this interaction may take several weeks to reach its maximum effect. Exercise caution when administering a beta blocker to a patient who has stopped taking fluoxetine within the past 2 weeks.

REFERENCES:
Otton SV, et al. Inhibition by fluoxetine of cytochrome P450 2D6 activity. *Clin Pharmacol Ther.* 1993;53:401.

Drake WM, et al. Heart block in a patient on propranolol and fluoxetine. *Lancet.* 1994;343:425.

Walley T, et al. Interaction of metoprolol and fluoxetine. *Lancet.* 1993;341:967.

Fluoxetine (*Prozac*)

Selegiline (eg, *Eldepryl*)

SUMMARY: Isolated cases suggest that combined therapy with selegiline and fluoxetine may result in mania or hypertension, but a causal relationship has not been established.

RISK FACTORS: No specific risk factors are known.

RELATED DRUGS: The manufacturer of selegiline recommends that it not be used with SSRIs, including fluoxetine, paroxetine (*Paxil*), sertraline (*Zoloft*), and fluvoxamine (*Luvox*).

MANAGEMENT OPTIONS:

➡ *Avoid Unless Benefit Outweighs Risk.* Although the risk of combined use is not established, the potential adverse effects are severe.

➡ *Monitor.* Monitor for evidence of hypertension or mania if the combination is used.

REFERENCES:

Suchowersky O, et al. Interaction of fluoxetine and selegiline. *Can J Psychiatry.* 1990;35:571.

Product information. Selegiline (*Eldepryl*). Solvay Pharmaceuticals. 1996.

Fluoxetine (*Prozac*)

Sibutramine (*Meridia*)

SUMMARY: The risk of serotonin syndrome would theoretically increase when sibutramine is combined with other serotonergic drugs such as fluoxetine.

RISK FACTORS: No specific risk factors are known.

RELATED DRUGS: Other selective serotonin reuptake inhibitors such as paroxetine(*Paxil*), sertraline (*Zoloft*), and fluvoxamine (*Luvox*) would be expected to interact with sibutramine as well.

MANAGEMENT OPTIONS:

➡ *Avoid Unless Benefit Outweighs Risk.* The manufacturer states that sibutramine should not be used with fluoxetine. This is a prudent recommendation until more information is available.

➡ *Monitor.* Serotonin syndrome can result in neurotoxicity (eg, myoclonus, tremors, rigidity, incoordination, restlessness, hyperreflexia, seizures, coma), psychiatric symptoms (eg, agitation, confusion, hypomania), and temperature regulation abnormalities (eg, fever, sweating). Note that mild forms of serotonin syndrome have also been reported, so consider any combination of the above symptoms possibly related to excessive serotonin activity.

REFERENCES:

Product information. Sibutramine (*Meridia*). Knoll Pharmaceuticals. 1997.

Mills KC. Serotonin syndrome: a clinical update. *Crit Care Clin.* 1997;13:763.

Fluoxetine (*Prozac*)

Terfenadine (*Seldane*)

SUMMARY: A patient receiving fluoxetine and terfenadine developed possible cardiac rhythm disturbances, but a causal relationship was not established.

RISK FACTORS: No specific risk factors are known.

RELATED DRUGS: Astemizole (*Hismanal*), like terfenadine, is metabolized by CYP3A4 and can cause ventricular arrhythmias; its interactions appear similar to terfenadine. Loratadine (*Claritin*), fexofenadine (*Allegra*), and *cetirizine* (*Zyrtec*) do not appear to produce cardiotoxicity and thus probably would be safer in patients on fluoxetine. Fluvoxamine (*Luvox*) is known to inhibit CYP3A4 and is contraindicated with terfenadine or astemizole.

MANAGEMENT OPTIONS:

➡ ***Avoid Unless Benefit Outweighs Risk.*** Although evidence for an interaction between terfenadine and fluoxetine is scanty, it would be prudent to avoid concurrent use until more information is available.

➡ ***Monitor.*** If the combination is used, monitor for evidence of cardiac arrhythmias (eg, palpitations, fainting, shortness of breath).

REFERENCES:
Swims MP. Potential terfenadine-fluoxetine interaction. *Ann Pharmacother.* 1993;27:1404.

Fluoxetine (eg, *Prozac*)

Thioridazine (eg, *Mellaril*)

SUMMARY: Fluoxetine may increase thioridazine serum concentrations, and thus may increase the risk of ventricular arrhythmias; avoid concurrent use.

RISK FACTORS:

➡ ***Pharmacogenetics.*** Patients with the extensive metabolizer CYP2D6 phenotype (EMs) would be expected to experience this interaction to a greater extent than poor metabolizers (PMs) who do not have the gene for production of CYP2D6. PMs would likely already have high serum concentrations of thioridazine, but theoretically, inhibition of CYP2C19 by fluoxetine might increase levels further. Approximately 8% of whites are deficient in CYP2D6, but the deficiency is rare in Asians, usually 1% or fewer.

➡ ***Hypokalemia.*** The corrected QT interval (QTc) on the ECG may be prolonged in patients with hypokalemia, thus increasing the risk of this interaction. Any other factor that may prolong the QTc interval would also increase the risk of this interaction.

RELATED DRUGS: Paroxetine (*Paxil*), like fluoxetine, is a potent inhibitor of CYP2D6, and would also be expected to increase the risk of arrhythmias. Fluvoxamine (*Luvox*), although not a significant CYP2D6 inhibitor, also increases thioridazine serum concentrations, possibly by inhibiting CYP2C19 and CYP1A2. Other SSRIs such as citalopram (*Celexa*) and sertraline (*Zoloft*) are less likely to significantly inhibit CYP2D6, CYP2C19, or CYP1A2. Theoretically, they would be less likely to interact with thioridazine, but little clinical information is available. Although a number of antipsychotic drugs have, like thioridazine, been shown to prolong the QT interval, clinical evidence suggests that thioridazine may produce the greatest risk.

MANAGEMENT OPTIONS:

➡ *Use Alternative.* Although the risk of this combination is not well established, it would be prudent to use alternatives for 1 of the drugs (see Related Drugs).

➡ *Monitor.* If the combination must be used, monitor the ECG for evidence of QT prolongation and for clinical evidence of arrhythmias (eg, syncope).

REFERENCES:

Hartigan-Go K, et al. Concentration-related pharmacodynamic effects of thioridazine and its metabolites in humans. *Clin Pharmacol Ther*. 1996;60:543-53.

'Dear Doctor or Pharmacist' Letter, Novartis Pharmaceuticals, July 7, 2000.

 Fluoxetine (eg, *Prozac*)

AVOID **Tranylcypromine (*Parnate*)**

SUMMARY: Severe or fatal reactions have been reported when nonselective monoamine oxidase inhibitors (MAOIs) are coadministered with selective serotonin reuptake inhibitors (SSRIs) such as fluoxetine; avoid the combination.

RISK FACTORS: No specific risk factors are known.

RELATED DRUGS: All combinations of nonselective MAOIs (eg, phenelzine [*Nardil*], isocarboxazid) and SSRIs (eg, fluvoxamine [eg, *Luvox*], paroxetine [*Paxil*], sertraline [*Zoloft*]) are contraindicated.

MANAGEMENT OPTIONS:

➡ *AVOID COMBINATION.* Avoid the combined use of fluoxetine and MAOIs. Wait at least 2 weeks after stopping an MAOI before starting fluoxetine or any other SSRI; wait 5 weeks after stopping fluoxetine before starting an MAOI.

REFERENCES:

Feighner JP, et al. Adverse consequences of fluoxetine-MAOI combination therapy. *J Clin Psychiatry*. 1990;51:222.

Kline SS, et al. Serotonin syndrome versus neuroleptic malignant syndrome as a cause of death. *Clin Pharm*. 1989;8:510.

Sternbach H. Danger of MAOI therapy after fluoxetine withdrawal. *Lancet*. 1988;2:850.

 Fluoxetine (eg, *Prozac*)

Tryptophan

SUMMARY: Several patients on fluoxetine developed symptoms of agitation, restlessness, poor concentration, and nausea when tryptophan was added to their therapy; the symptoms resolved when the tryptophan was discontinued.

RISK FACTORS: No specific risk factors are known.

RELATED DRUGS: Pending additional study, assume that all selective serotonin reuptake inhibitors (SSRIs) interact with tryptophan.

MANAGEMENT OPTIONS:

➡ ***Avoid Unless Benefit Outweighs Risk.*** Until more information on safety and efficacy is available, it would be prudent to avoid concurrent use of fluoxetine or other SSRIs with tryptophan.

➡ ***Monitor.*** If the combination is used, monitor patients for the symptoms previously described and for a reduced therapeutic response to fluoxetine. It may be necessary to discontinue tryptophan if the reaction occurs.

REFERENCES:

Steiner W, et al. Toxic reaction following the combined administration of fluoxetine and L-tryptophan: five case reports. *Biol Psychiatry*. 1986;21:1067-1091.

Fluoxetine (*Prozac*)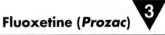

Warfarin (eg, *Coumadin*)

SUMMARY: Limited clinical evidence suggests fluoxetine does not affect the hypoprothrombinemic response to warfarin, but more study is needed. Isolated reports suggest that fluoxetine alone can increase the risk of bleeding in some patients.

RISK FACTORS: No specific risk factors are known.

RELATED DRUGS: Although little is known regarding the use of fluoxetine with oral anticoagulants other than warfarin, the same precautions would apply until data are available. Based on limited data, other selective serotonin reuptake inhibitors also may increase the risk of bleeding in patients receiving oral anticoagulants.

MANAGEMENT OPTIONS:

➡ ***Monitor.*** Although evidence for a fluoxetine-induced increase in the hypoprothrombinemic response to warfarin is scanty, monitor for altered warfarin effect if fluoxetine is initiated, discontinued, or changed in dosage. Adjust warfarin dose as needed. Keep in mind that the risk of bleeding might be increased even if the hypoprothrombinemic response is in the desired range.

REFERENCES:

Alderman CP, et al. Abnormal platelet aggregation associated with fluoxetine therapy. *Ann Pharmacother*. 1992;26:1517-1519.

Rowe H, et al. The effects of fluoxetine on warfarin metabolism in the rat and man. *Life Sci*. 1978;23:807-811.

Claire RJ, et al. Potential interaction between warfarin sodium and fluoxetine. *Am J Psychiatry*. 1991;148:1604.

Aranth J, et al. Bleeding, a side effect of fluoxetine. *Am J Psychiatry*. 1992;149:412.

Yaryura-Tobias JA, et al. Fluoxetine and bleeding in obsessive-compulsive disorder. *Am J Psychiatry*. 1991;148:949.

Fluphenazine Decanoate (eg, *Prolixin*)

Imipramine (eg, *Tofranil*)

SUMMARY: Phenothiazines may increase serum concentrations of some tricyclic antidepressants (TCAs), and TCAs may increase neuroleptic serum concentrations. These changes would be expected to increase both the therapeutic and toxic effects of each drug, but the degree to which these interactions alter the therapeutic and toxic responses to each drug is not well established.

RISK FACTORS: No specific risk factors are known.

RELATED DRUGS: No information is available.

MANAGEMENT OPTIONS:

➡ *Monitor.* In patients receiving combined therapy with neuroleptics and TCAs, be alert for evidence of increased toxicity and altered therapeutic response.

REFERENCES:

Gram LF, et al. Drug interaction: inhibitory effect of neuroleptics on metabolism of tricyclic antidepressants in man. *Br Med J.* 1972;1:463.

Gram LF, et al. Influence of neuroleptics and benzodiazepines on metabolism of tricyclic antidepressants in man. *Am J Psychiatry.* 1974;131:863.

El-yousef MK, et al. Tricyclic antidepressants and phenothiazines. *JAMA.* 1974;229:1419.

Loga S, et al. Interaction of chlorpromazine and nortriptyline in patients with schizophrenia. *Clin Pharmacokinet.* 1981;6:454.

Siris SG, et al. Plasma imipramine concentrations in patients receiving concomitant fluphenazine decanoate. *Am J Psychiatry.* 1982;139:104.

Overo KF, et al. Interaction of perphenazine with the kinetics of nortriptyline. *Acta Pharmacol Toxicol.* 1977;40:97.

Conrad CD, et al. Symptom exacerbation in psychotically depressed adolescents due to high desipramine plasma concentrations. *J Clin Psychopharmacol.* 1986;6:161.

Bock JL, et al. Desipramine hydroxylation: variability and effect of antipsychotic drugs. *Clin Pharmacol Ther.* 1983;33:322.

Wilens TE, et al. Adverse cardiac effects of combined neuroleptic ingestion and tricyclic antidepressant overdose. *J Clin Psychopharmacol.* 1990;10:51.

Flurbiprofen (eg, *Ansaid*)

Methotrexate (*Mexate*)

SUMMARY: A case report suggested flurbiprofen increased methotrexate toxicity; prospective study failed to demonstrate an interaction.

RISK FACTORS: No specific risk factors are known.

RELATED DRUGS: Several nonsteroidal anti-inflammatory drugs and aspirin have been shown to increase methotrexate plasma concentrations. Acetaminophen (eg, *Tylenol*) has not been shown to affect methotrexate response.

MANAGEMENT OPTIONS:

➡ *Consider Alternative.* Until more information is available on this interaction, it is preferable to avoid flurbiprofen (as well as other NSAIDs) in patients receiving antineoplastic doses of methotrexate. If possible, use a nonNSAID analgesic instead.

➡ **Monitor.** If the combination is used, observe the patient for signs of methotrexate toxicity including mucosal ulceration, renal dysfunction, and blood dyscrasias. Decreasing the methotrexate dosage may be required.

REFERENCES:

Frenia ML, et al. Methotrexate and nonsteroidal anti-inflammatory drug interactions. *Ann Pharmacother.* 1992;26:234.

Skeith KJ, et al. Lack of significant interaction between low dose methotrexate and ibuprofen or flurbiprofen in patients with arthritis. *J Rheumatol.* 1990;17:1008.

Flurbiprofen (eg, *Ansaid*)

Phenprocoumon†

SUMMARY: Some patients receiving oral anticoagulants have developed excessive hypoprothrombinemia and bleeding after flurbiprofen was initiated.

RISK FACTORS:

➡ **Concurrent Diseases.** Patients with peptic ulcer disease (PUD) or a history of GI bleeding are probably at greater risk.

RELATED DRUGS: All nonsteroidal anti-inflammatory drugs inhibit platelet function, cause gastric erosions, and probably increase the risk of GI bleeding. Some NSAIDs, however, such as ibuprofen (eg, *Advil*), naproxen (eg, *Naprosyn*), or diclofenac (eg, *Voltaren*) may be less likely to increase oral anticoagulant-induced hypoprothrombinemia than other NSAIDs. The degree to which warfarin interacts with flurbiprofen has not been established, but assume that an interaction will occur until evidence to the contrary is available. In a retrospective cohort study, hospitalizations for hemorrhagic PUD were about 13 times higher in patients receiving warfarin plus an NSAID than in patients receiving neither drug. Acenocoumarol interacts similarly.

MANAGEMENT OPTIONS:

➡ **Avoid Unless Benefit Outweighs Risk.** Since all NSAIDs probably increase the risk of GI bleeding in patients on oral anticoagulants, use the combination only after careful consideration of the benefit vs risk. If an NSAID must be used with an oral anticoagulant, it would be prudent to use NSAIDs that are unlikely to affect the hypoprothrombinemic response to oral anticoagulants (see Related Drugs). If the NSAID is being used as an analgesic or antipyretic, acetaminophen is probably safer to use with oral anticoagulants. Non-acetylated salicylates (eg, choline salicylate, magnesium salicylate, salsalate, sodium salicylate) also are probably safer with oral anticoagulants than NSAIDs, since such salicylates have minimal effects on platelet function and the gastric mucosa.

➡ **Monitor.** If any NSAID is used with an oral anticoagulant, monitor carefully the prothrombin time and watch for evidence of bleeding, especially from the GI tract.

REFERENCES:

Marbet GA, et al. Interaction study between phenoprocoumon and flurbiprofen. *Curr Med Res Opin.* 1977;5:26.

Stricker BHC, et al. Interaction between flurbiprofen and coumarins. *Br Med J.* 1982;285:812.

Shorr RI, et al. Concurrent use of nonsteroidal anti-inflammatory drugs and oral anticoagulants places elderly persons at high risk for hemorrhagic peptic ulcer disease. *Arch Intern Med.* 1993;153:1665.

† Not available in the US.

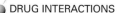

 Fluvastatin (*Lescol*)

Rifampin (eg, *Rifadin*)

SUMMARY: Rifampin administration reduces fluvastatin plasma concentrations; reduction of fluvastatin's cholesterol-lowering effect is likely.

RISK FACTORS: No specific risk factors are known.

RELATED DRUGS: Rifampin is known to reduce the plasma concentrations of other cholesterol lowering drugs, especially those that are CYP3A4 substrates (eg, simvastatin, [*Zocor*], lovastatin [*Mevacor*]). Other statins that are metabolized by CYP3A4 (cerivastatin [*Baycol*], atorvastatin [*Lipitor*]) probably would be affected by rifampin but perhaps to a lesser extent. Because pravastatin (*Pravachol*) is not a CYP3A4 substrate, rifampin may have limited effect on its pharmacokinetics.

MANAGEMENT OPTIONS:

➡ **Consider Alternative.** For patients taking rifampin, select cholesterol-lowering drugs that are not dependent on CYP3A4 or CYP2C9 for their metabolism.

➡ **Monitor.** Monitor serum cholesterol in patients taking fluvastatin when rifampin is administered for more than a few weeks.

REFERENCES:

Jokubaitis, LA. Updated clinical safety experience with fluvastatin. *Am J Cardiol.* 1994;73:18D. Review.

Product information. Fluvastatin (*Lescol*). Novartis Pharmaceuticals. 1999.

 Fluvoxamine (*Luvox*)

Lithium (eg, *Eskalith*)

SUMMARY: Isolated cases of adverse neurological effects have been reported in patients receiving fluvoxamine and lithium, but a causal relationship is not established.

RISK FACTORS: No specific risk factors are known.

RELATED DRUGS: Other SSRIs may interact with lithium in a similar manner.

MANAGEMENT OPTIONS:

➡ **Monitor.** Until more information is available, monitor patients for adverse neurologic effects if fluvoxamine and lithium are used concurrently.

REFERENCES:

Evans M, et al. Fluvoxamine and lithium: an unusual interaction. *Br J Psychiatry.* 1990;156:286.

 Fluvoxamine (*Luvox*)

Methadone (eg, *Dolophine*)

SUMMARY: Fluvoxamine may increase methadone serum concentrations, increasing the risk of methadone toxicity.

RISK FACTORS: No specific risk factors are known.

RELATED DRUGS: Fluvoxamine is the only selective serotonin reuptake inhibitor that inhibits CYP1A2 and CYP3A4, although fluoxetine (*Prozac*) inhibits CYP2C19 and is a weak CYP3A4 inhibitor. Other selective serotonin reuptake inhibitors, such as paroxetine (*Paxil*) sertraline (*Zoloft*), and citalopram (*Celexa*), do not appear to have much effect on CYP1A2 or CYP3A4, although paroxetine is a potent CYP2D6 inhibitor. Because the isozyme(s) involved in this interaction are not known, sertraline and citalopram would probably be the least likely to interact with methadone.

MANAGEMENT OPTIONS:

➡ *Consider Alternative.* Sertraline and citalopram may be less likely to interact with methadone.

➡ *Monitor.* If fluvoxamine and methadone are used concurrently, monitor the patient for evidence of excessive methadone effect (eg, respiratory depression).

REFERENCES:

Bertschy G, et al. Probable metabolic interaction between methadone and fluvoxamine in addict patients. *Ther Drug Monit.* 1994;16:42-45.

Alderman CP, et al. Fluvoxamine-methadone interaction. *Aust NZ J Psychiatry.* 1999;33:99-101.

Fluvoxamine (*Luvox*)
Mexiletine (*Mexitil*)

SUMMARY: Fluvoxamine administration increases the plasma concentrations of mexiletine; increased side effects could occur.

RISK FACTORS:

➡ *Pharmacogenetics.* Slow metabolizers of CYP2D6. Since mexiletine is mainly metabolized by CYP2D6, patients who are deficient in this enzyme are dependent on CYP1A2 for mexiletine metabolism. If CYP1A2 activity is inhibited, a large increase in mexiletine concentration is likely to occur.

RELATED DRUGS: While no data are currently available, fluoxetine (eg, *Prozac*) and paroxetine (*Paxil*) are CYP2D6 inhibitors and would be expected to increase mexiletine plasma concentrations.

MANAGEMENT OPTIONS:

➡ *Monitor.* Monitor patients stabilized on mexiletine for altered plasma concentrations if fluvoxamine is initiated or discontinued.

REFERENCES:

Kusumoto M, et al. Effect of fluvoxamine on the pharmacokinetics of mexiletine in healthy Japanese men. *Clin Pharmacol Ther.* 2001;69:104-107.

Fluvoxamine (*Luvox*)
Olanzapine (*Zyprexa*)

SUMMARY: Fluvoxamine may substantially increase olanzapine serum concentrations.

RISK FACTORS: No specific risk factors are known.

RELATED DRUGS: Fluvoxamine is the only selective serotonin reuptake inhibitor (SSRI) that is a potent inhibitor of CYP1A2, so other selective serotonin reuptake inhibitors such as fluoxetine (*Prozac*), paroxetine (*Paxil*), sertraline (*Zoloft*), and citalopram (*Celexa*) would not be expected to interact to the same degree. Indeed, sertraline (n = 21) was not associated with increased olanzapine serum concentrations in the current study.

MANAGEMENT OPTIONS:

➥ *Consider Alternative.* SSRIs other than fluvoxamine are probably less likely to interact with olanzapine.

➥ *Monitor.* If fluvoxamine is used with olanzapine, monitor for evidence of excessive olanzapine serum concentrations.

REFERENCES:

Weigmann H, et al. Fluvoxamine, but not sertraline, inhibits the metabolism of olanzapine: evidence from a therapeutic drug monitoring service. *Ther Drug Monit.* 2001;23:410-413.

Fluvoxamine (*Luvox*)

Phenytoin (*Dilantin*)

SUMMARY: A patient developed phenytoin toxicity after starting fluvoxamine therapy.

RISK FACTORS: No specific risk factors are known.

RELATED DRUGS: In vitro studies suggest that fluvoxamine is the most potent inhibitor of phenytoin hydroxylation among SSRIs. Nonetheless, fluoxetine (*Prozac*) appears to increase phenytoin serum concentrations, at least in some patients; numerous cases of phenytoin toxicity have been reported. Isolated cases of sertraline (*Zoloft*)-induced phenytoin toxicity have been reported but a causal relationship was not established.

MANAGEMENT OPTIONS:

➥ *Consider Alternative.* Consider using an SSRI other than fluvoxamine or fluoxetine (see Related Drugs).

➥ *Monitor.* If fluvoxamine is added to phenytoin therapy, monitor phenytoin serum concentrations and monitor for clinical evidence of phenytoin toxicity.

REFERENCES:

Mamiya K, et al. Phenytoin intoxication induced by fluvoxamine. *Ther Drug Monit.* 2001;23:75-77.

Fluvoxamine (*Luvox*)

Quinidine (eg, *Quinora*)

SUMMARY: Fluvoxamine administration produces a modest increase in quinidine concentrations; increased quinidine effect or toxicity could result.

RISK FACTORS: No specific risk factors are known.

RELATED DRUGS: Nefazodone (*Serzone*) is also known to inhibit CYP3A4 and would be expected to interact with quinidine, perhaps to an even greater extent than fluvoxamine.

MANAGEMENT OPTIONS:

➥ *Consider Alternative.* Consider alternative antidepressants that do not affect CYP3A4 metabolism, such as paroxetine (*Paxil*) or venlafaxine (*Effexor*), for patients taking quinidine. Other antiarrhythmics not metabolized by CYP3A4, such as procainamide (eg, *Procan SR*), could be considered, depending on the arrhythmia.

➡ ***Monitor.*** If fluvoxamine is administered to patients taking quinidine, monitor the electrocardiogram for evidence of increased quinidine concentrations (eg, prolonged QRS) and monitor quinidine serum concentrations.

REFERENCES:

Damkier P, et al. Effect of fluvoxamine on the pharmacokinetics of quinidine. *Eur J Clin Pharmacol.* 1999;55:451-456.

Fluvoxamine (*Luvox*)

Tacrine (*Cognex*)

SUMMARY: Fluvoxamine markedly increases tacrine serum concentrations and may increase tacrine adverse effects; avoid the combination if possible.

RISK FACTORS: No specific risk factors are known.

RELATED DRUGS: The effect of other selective serotonin reuptake inhibitors such as fluoxetine (*Prozac*), paroxetine (*Paxil*), and sertraline (*Zoloft*) on tacrine is not established, but none of these drugs is known to inhibit CYP1A2. The effect of fluvoxamine on donepezil (*Aricept*) is not established.

MANAGEMENT OPTIONS:

➡ ***Use Alternative.*** Until more data are available, it would be preferable to use an alternative selective serotonin reuptake inhibitor such as fluoxetine, paroxetine, or sertraline in patients on tacrine. If the combination is used, monitor for adverse tacrine GI effects and for tacrine-induced hepatotoxicity.

REFERENCES:

Becquemont L, et al. Influence of the CYP1A2 inhibitor fluvoxamine on tacrine pharmacokinetics in humans. *Clin Pharmacol Ther.* 1997;61:619.

Fluvoxamine (*Luvox*)

Terfenadine (*Seldane*) AVOID

SUMMARY: Fluvoxamine appears to inhibit the enzyme that metabolizes terfenadine, which theoretically could result in increased unchanged serum terfenadine concentrations and cardiac arrhythmias; avoid the combination.

RISK FACTORS: No specific risk factors are known.

RELATED DRUGS: Astemizole (*Hismanal*) also is metabolized by CYP3A4 and can cause the same types of cardiac arrhythmias when combined with CYP3A4 inhibitors; thus, it also may interact adversely with fluvoxamine. Loratadine (*Claritin*) also may be metabolized by CYP3A4, but it does not appear to produce cardiotoxicity when given with drugs that inhibit its metabolism.

MANAGEMENT OPTIONS:

➡ ***AVOID COMBINATION.*** Although this interaction is based largely upon theoretical considerations, generally avoid the combination of terfenadine and fluvoxamine. The potential adverse effects of the interaction can be life-threatening, and terfenadine is generally used for symptomatic relief of allergic disorders. Theoretically, lorata-dine would be a safer nonsedating antihistamine in the presence of fluvoxamine.

REFERENCES:

Fleishaker JC, et al. A pharmacokinetic and pharmacodynamic evaluation of the combined administration of alprazolam and fluvoxamine. *Eur J Clin Pharmacol*. 1994;46:35.

Product information. Fluvoxamine (*Luvox*). Solvay Pharmaceuticals. 1996.

② Fluvoxamine (*Luvox*)

Theophylline (eg, *Theolair*)

SUMMARY: Several cases of theophylline toxicity caused by fluvoxamine have been reported. Although more study is needed to establish a causal relationship, the interaction is consistent with the interactive properties of the 2 drugs.

RISK FACTORS: No specific risk factors are known.

RELATED DRUGS: Based on in vitro studies in human hepatic microsomes, other selective serotonin reuptake inhibitors (SSRIs) such as citalopram (*Celexa*), fluoxetine (*Prozac*), paroxetine (*Paxil*), and sertraline (*Zoloft*) would be less likely to interact with theophylline.

MANAGEMENT OPTIONS:

➡ ***Use Alternative.*** Given the magnitude of the interaction, and the potential toxicity of theophylline, it would be prudent to use an alternative to fluvoxamine, (eg, cita-lopram, fluoxetine, paroxetine, sertraline). Until clinical evidence is available, however, be alert for evidence of theophylline toxicity when therapy with any SSRI is started. If the combination is used, monitor for altered serum theophylline concentrations and clinical evidence of theophylline toxicity if fluvoxamine is ini-tiated, discontinued, or changed in dosage. Evidence of theophylline toxicity includes nausea, vomiting, diarrhea, restlessness, irritability, and insomnia. Higher serum concentrations can result in cardiac arrhythmias or seizures. Permanent brain damage and death have been reported in severe cases. Note that nausea is also a common side effect of fluvoxamine, so measuring the theophylline serum concentration may be needed to determine whether nausea is caused by fluvox-amine or theophylline toxicity.

REFERENCES:

Brosen K, et al. Fluvoxamine is a potent inhibitor of cytochrome P4501A2. *Biochem Pharmacol*. 1993;45:1211.

Sperber AD. Toxic interaction between fluvoxamine and sustained release theophylline in an 11-year-old boy. *Drug Safety*. 1991;6:460.

Thomson AH, et al. Interaction between fluvoxamine and theophylline. *Pharmaceutical J*. 1992;249:137.

Diot P, et al. Possible interaction between theophylline and fluvoxamine. *Therapie*. 1991;46:470.

Benfield P, et al. Fluvoxamine: a review of its pharmacodynamic and pharmacokinetic properties, and therapeutic efficacy in depressive illness. *Drugs*. 1986;32:313.

Fluvoxamine (*Luvox*)

Thioridazine (eg, *Mellaril*)

SUMMARY: Fluvoxamine increases thioridazine serum concentrations, and thus may increase the risk of ventricular arrhythmias; avoid concurrent use.

RISK FACTORS:

➥ *Hypokalemia.* The corrected QT interval (QTc) may be prolonged in patients with hypokalemia, thus increasing the risk of this interaction. Any other factor that may prolong the QTc interval would also increase the risk of this interaction.

RELATED DRUGS: Fluoxetine (eg, *Prozac*) and paroxetine (*Paxil*) are potent inhibitors of CYP2D6, and would be expected to increase the risk of arrhythmias. Other SSRIs such as citalopram (*Celexa*) and sertraline (*Zoloft*) are less likely to significantly inhibit CYP2D6, CYP2C19, or CYP1A2. Theoretically, they would be less likely to interact with thioridazine, but little clinical information is available. Although a number of antipsychotic drugs have been shown to prolong the QT interval, clinical evidence suggests that thioridazine may produce the greatest risk.

MANAGEMENT OPTIONS:

➥ *Use Alternative.* Although the risk of this combination is not well established, it would be prudent to use alternatives for 1 of the drugs (see Related Drugs).

➥ *Monitor.* If the combination must be used, monitor the ECG for evidence of QT prolongation and for clinical evidence of arrhythmias (eg, syncope).

REFERENCES:

Carrillo JA, et al. Pharmacokinetic interaction of fluvoxamine and thioridazine in schizophrenic patients. *J Clin Psychopharmacol.* 1999;19:494-99.

Hartigan-Go K, et al. Concentration-related pharmacodynamic effects of thioridazine and its metabolites in humans. *Clin Pharmacol Ther.* 1996;60:543-53.

'Dear Doctor or Pharmacist' Letter, Novartis Pharmaceuticals, July 7, 2000.

Fluvoxamine (*Luvox*)

Warfarin (eg, *Coumadin*)

SUMMARY: Preliminary data suggest that fluvoxamine increases the hypoprothrombinemic response to warfarin; more study is needed.

RISK FACTORS: No specific risk factors are known.

RELATED DRUGS: The effect of fluvoxamine on the response to other oral anticoagulants is not established. Some evidence suggests that other selective serotonin reuptake inhibitors (SSRIs) also may increase the bleeding risk from warfarin, in some cases without affecting the hypoprothrombinemic response.

MANAGEMENT OPTIONS:

➥ *Monitor.* Although data are scanty, be alert for evidence of altered hypoprothrombinemic response to warfarin (or other anticoagulants) if fluvoxamine is initiated, discontinued, or changed in dosage. Although not reported for fluvoxamine, some

SSRIs may impair hemostasis; be alert for evidence of bleeding even if the hypo-prothrombinemic response is in the desired range.

REFERENCES:

Benfield P, et al. Fluvoxamine: a review of its pharmacodynamic and pharmacokinetic properties, and therapeutic efficacy in depressive illness. *Drugs*. 1986;32:313.

Folic Acid (eg, *Folvite*)

Phenytoin (eg, *Dilantin*)

SUMMARY: Folic acid may decrease serum phenytoin concentrations to a clinically significant degree in an occasional patient. Whether folic acid is capable of directly antagonizing the anticonvulsant effects of phenytoin is not established.

RISK FACTORS:

➡ ***Dosage Regimen.*** Small amounts of folic acid found in multiple vitamins are not likely to have much effect.

RELATED DRUGS: No information is available.

MANAGEMENT OPTIONS:

➡ ***Monitor.*** When folic acid is given to patients receiving phenytoin, watch for decreased seizure control (although most patients are probably not significantly affected).

REFERENCES:

Reynolds EH. Anticonvulsants, folic acid and epilepsy. *Lancet*. 1973;1:1376.

Smith DB, et al. Folate metabolism and the anticonvulsant efficacy of phenobarbital. *Arch Neurol*. 1973;28:18.

Jensen ON, et al. Subnormal serum folate due to anticonvulsive therapy. A double-blind study of the effect of folic acid treatment in patients with drug-induced subnormal serum folates. *Arch Neurol*. 1970;22:181.

Norris JW, et al. A controlled study of folic acid in epilepsy. *Neurology*. 1971;21:659.

Spaans F. No effect of folic acid supplement on CSF folate and serum vitamin B in patients on anticonvulsants. *Epilepsia*. 1970;11:403.   ·

Ralston AJ, et al. Effects of folic acid on fit frequency and behavior of epileptics on anticonvulsants. *Lancet*. 1970;1:867.

Scott RB, et al. Reduced absorption of vitamin B 12 in two patients with folic acid deficiency. *Ann Intern Med*. 1968;69:111.

Baylis EM, et al. Influence of folic acid on blood-phenytoin levels. *Lancet*. 1971;1:62.

Houben PFM, et al. Anticonvulsant drugs and folic acid in young mentally retarded epileptic patients. *Epilepsia*. 1971;12:235.

Kariks J, et al. Serum folic acid and phenytoin levels in permanently hospitalized epileptic patients receiving anticonvulsant drug therapy. *Med J Aust*. 1971;2:368.

Glazko AJ. Antiepileptic drugs: biotransformation, metabolism, and serum half-life. *Epilepsia*. 1975;16:367.

Reynolds EH. Folate metabolism and anticonvulsant therapy. *Proc R Soc Med*. 1974;67:68.

Chien LT, et al. Harmful effect of megadoses of vitamins: electroencephalogram abnormalities and seizures induced by intravenous folate in drug-treated epileptics. *Am J Clin Nutr*. 1975;28:51.

Strauss RG, et al. Folic acid and Dilantin antagonism in pregnancy. *Obstet Gynecol*. 1974;44:345.

Furlanut M, et al. Effects of folic acid on phenytoin kinetics in healthy subjects. *Clin Pharmacol Ther*. 1978;24:294.

Poppell TD, et al. Effect of folic acid on recurrence of phenytoin-induced gingival overgrowth following gingivectomy. *J Clin Periodontol*. 1991;18:134.

Inoue F. Clinical implications of anticonvulsant-induced folate deficiency. *Clin Pharm*. 1982;1:372.

MacCosbe PE, et al. Interaction of phenytoin and folic acid. *Clin Pharm*. 1983;2:362.

Folic Acid (eg, *Folvite*)

Pyrimethamine (*Daraprim*)

SUMMARY: Folic acid potentially can interfere with the efficacy of pyrimethamine.

RISK FACTORS: No specific risk factors are known.

RELATED DRUGS: No information is available.

MANAGEMENT OPTIONS:

➡ *Avoid Unless Benefit Outweighs Risk.* Until more information is available, folic acid should not be administered to patients receiving pyrimethamine for treatment of toxoplasmosis or in patients with leukemia.

➡ *Monitor.* If folic acid is used, monitor for loss of efficacy of pyrimethamine.

REFERENCES:

Tong MJ, et al. Supplemental folates in the therapy of Plasmodium falciparum malaria. *JAMA.* 1970;214:2330.

Food

Indinavir (*Crixivan*)

SUMMARY: The administration of indinavir with food reduces the serum concentration; loss of efficacy may result.

RISK FACTORS: No specific risk factors are known.

RELATED DRUGS: Food produces a small (15%) increase in ritonavir (*Norvir*) serum concentrations and a large increase (2- to 5-fold) in saquinavir (eg, *Invirase*) concentrations.

MANAGEMENT OPTIONS:

➡ *Circumvent/Minimize.* Administer indinavir on an empty stomach or after a small snack.

➡ *Monitor.* for reduced indinavir effect in patients taking the drug with meals.

REFERENCES:

Product information. Indinavir (*Crixivan*). Merck and Company, Inc. 1996.

Product information. Ritonavir (*Norvir*). Abbott Laboratories. 1996.

Product information. Saquinavir (*Invirase*). Roche Laboratories. 1995.

Food

Isoniazid (INH)

SUMMARY: Food may reduce INH concentrations, and some cheeses may cause a reaction in patients taking INH.

RISK FACTORS: No specific risk factors are known.

RELATED DRUGS: No information is available.

MANAGEMENT OPTIONS:

➡ *Circumvent/Minimize.* For optimal absorption, give INH on an empty stomach.

➡ **Monitor.** Watch for "cheese reactions" (eg, flushing, chills, headache, tachycardia, hypertension) in patients on INH.

REFERENCES:

Melander A, et al. Reduction of isoniazid bioavailability in normal men by concomitant intake of food. *Acta Med Scand.* 1976;200:93.

Smith CK, et al. Isoniazid and reaction to cheese. *Ann Intern Med.* 1978;88:520.

Lejonc JL, et al. Isoniazid and reaction to cheese. *Ann Intern Med.* 1979;91:793.

▼ 3 Food

Itraconazole (*Sporanox*)

SUMMARY: The administration of itraconazole following a meal greatly enhances its bioavailability.

RISK FACTORS: No specific risk factors are known.

RELATED DRUGS: Food also increases the serum concentration of griseofulvin (eg, *Grisactin*).

MANAGEMENT OPTIONS:

➡ **Monitor.** Administer itraconazole capsules following a meal to obtain maximum serum concentration.

REFERENCES:

Van Peer A, et al. The effects of food and dose on the oral systemic availability of itraconazole in healthy subjects. *Eur J Clin Pharmacol.* 1989;36:423.

Zimmerman T, et al. Influence of concomitant food intake on the oral absorption of two triazole antifungal agents, itraconazole and fluconazole. *Eur J Clin Pharmacol.* 1994;46:147.

Barone JA, et al. Food interaction and steady-state pharmacokinetics of itraconazole capsules in healthy male volunteers. *Antimicrob Agents Chemother.* 1993;37:778.

▼ 3 Food

Levodopa (eg, *Larodopa*)

SUMMARY: Some evidence suggests that high-protein diets inhibit the efficacy of levodopa in parkinsonism.

RISK FACTORS: No specific risk factors are known.

RELATED DRUGS: No information is available.

MANAGEMENT OPTIONS:

➡ **Circumvent/Minimize.** Although it is usually recommended that levodopa be taken with meals to slow absorption and thus reduce the central emetic effect, patients on levodopa should probably avoid high-protein diets as well as diets with widely fluctuating protein content.

➡ **Monitor.** Monitor for reduced levodopa effect if high-protein foods are taken.

REFERENCES:

Mena I, et al. Protein treatment of Parkinson's disease with levodopa. *N Engl J Med.* 1975;292:181.

Morgan JP, et al. Metabolism of levodopa in patients with Parkinson's disease. *Arch Neurol.* 1971;25:39.

Gillespie NG, et al. Diets affecting treatment of parkinsonism with levodopa. *J Am Diet Assoc.* 1973;62:525.

Robertson DRC, et al. The influence of protein on the absorption of levodopa. *Br J Clin Pharmacol.* 1990;29:608P.

Food

Lincomycin (eg, *Lincocin*)

SUMMARY: Food significantly reduced lincomycin serum concentrations.

RISK FACTORS: No specific risk factors are known.

RELATED DRUGS: Diet foods or drinks with sodium cyclamate decrease the serum concentrations of clindamycin (eg, *Cleocin*) by up to 80%.

MANAGEMENT OPTIONS:

➥ *Circumvent/Minimize.* For optimal absorption, nothing should be given by mouth except water for 1 to 2 hours before and after oral lincomycin.

➥ *Monitor.* Monitor patients receiving lincomycin with food for loss of antibiotic effect.

REFERENCES:

DeHaan RM, et al. Clindamycin serum concentrations after administration of clindamycin palmitate with food. *J Clin Pharmacol.* 1972;12:205.

McCall CE, et al. Lincomycin: activity *in vitro* and absorption and excretion in normal young men. *Am J Med Sci.* 1967;254:144.

Kaplan K, et al. Microbiological, pharmacological and clinical studies of lincomycin. *Am J Med Sci.* 1965;250:137.

McGehee RF, et al. Comparative studies of antibacterial activity *in vitro* and absorption and excretion of lincomycin and clindamycin. *Am J Med Sci.* 1968;256:279.

Food

Melphalan (*Alkeran*)

SUMMARY: Food markedly reduces the bioavailability and plasma concentrations of melphalan.

RISK FACTORS: No specific risk factors are known.

RELATED DRUGS: No information is available.

MANAGEMENT OPTIONS:

➥ *Circumvent/Minimize.* Melphalan should not be administered with food. The marked reduction in its bioavailability could result in loss of efficacy.

➥ *Monitor.* Monitor patients receiving multiple courses of melphalan who are switched from postprandial to fasting administration for increased toxicity.

REFERENCES:

Bosanquet AG, et al. Comparison of the fed and fasting states on the absorption of melphalan in multiple myeloma. *Cancer Chemother Pharmacol.* 1984;12:183.

Reece PA, et al. The effect of food on oral melphalan absorption. *Cancer Chemother Pharmacol.* 1986;16:194.

Food

Nifedipine (eg, *Procardia*)

SUMMARY: Food reduces the peak plasma concentration of immediate release nifedipine; concentrations of sustained release nifedipine may be increased by food.

RISK FACTORS: No specific risk factors are known.

RELATED DRUGS: No information is available.

MANAGEMENT OPTIONS:

➡ *Circumvent/Minimize.* The absorption of sustained-release nifedipine appears to be *increased* by food. Thus, administer sustained-release dosage forms in the fasting state to avoid altering the release characteristics of the formulation. However, controlled-release nifedipine (*Procardia XL*) appears to be affected by food minimally and can be taken without regard for meals.

➡ *Monitor.* Patients taking immediate-release nifedipine capsules will have *reduced* peak concentrations when taking doses with food. This may help minimize side effects associated with elevated peak serum concentrations of nifedipine.

REFERENCES:

Reitberg DP, et al. Effect of food on nifedipine pharmacokinetics. *Clin Pharmacol Ther*. 1987;42:72.

Ueno K, et al. Effect of food on nifedipine sustained-release preparation. *DICP*. 1989;23:662.

Chung M, et al. Clinical pharmacokinetics of nifedipine GI therapeutic system. *Am J Med*. 1987;83(Suppl. 6B):10.

Food

Propafenone (*Rythmol*)

SUMMARY: Meals can substantially increase the peak serum concentrations of propafenone.

RISK FACTORS:

➡ *Pharmacogenetics.* Rapid propafenone metabolizers tend to have a greater increase in propafenone bioavailability if it is taken with food.

RELATED DRUGS: No information is available.

MANAGEMENT OPTIONS:

➡ *Monitor.* Until data are available describing the effect of food on multiple-dose propafenone administration, counsel patients to maintain a consistent relationship between their propafenone administration and meals.

REFERENCES:

Axelson JE, et al. Food increases the bioavailability of propafenone. *Br J Clin Pharmacol*. 1987;23:735.

Food

Tetracycline (eg, *Sumycin*)

SUMMARY: Food and dairy products containing high concentrations of cations may reduce the serum concentration of tetracycline; reduced clinical efficacy may result.

RISK FACTORS: No specific risk factors are known.

RELATED DRUGS: Food and dairy products seem to affect doxycycline (eg, *Vibramycin*) and minocycline (eg, *Minocin*) absorption minimally. Food reduces tetracycline, oxytetracycline, methacycline, and demeclocycline serum concentrations.

MANAGEMENT OPTIONS:

➡ ***Consider Alternative.*** Doxycycline and minocycline appear to be minimally affected and may be possible alternatives.

➡ ***Circumvent/Minimize.*** For optimal absorption, administer tetracycline as far apart as possible from milk and other dairy products high in cation content.

➡ ***Monitor.*** If tetracycline and food or dairy products containing large amounts of cations are coadministered, be alert for reduced antibiotic effects.

REFERENCES:

Scheiner J, et al. Experimental study of factors inhibiting absorption and effective therapeutic levels of declomycin. *Surg Gynecol Obstet.* 1962;114:9.

Neuvonen PJ. Interactions with the absorption of tetracyclines. *Drugs.* 1976;11:45.

Mattila MJ, et al. Interference of iron preparations and milk with the absorption of tetracyclines. In: International Congress Series No. 254: Toxological Problems of Drug Combinations. Amsterdam: Exerpta Medica; 1972:129–33.

Product Information. Minocycline (*Minocin*). Lederle. 1993.

Rosenblatt JE, et al. Comparison of *in vitro* activity and clinical pharmacology of doxycycline with other tetracyclines. *Antimicrob Agents Chemother.* 1966:134.

Welling PG, et al. Bioavailability of tetracycline and doxycycline in fasted and nonfasted subjects. *Antimicrob Agents Chemother.* 1977;11:462.

Cook HJ, et al. Influence of the diet on bioavailability of tetracycline. *Biopharm Drug Disposition.* 1993;14:549.

Food

Zidovudine (*Retrovir*)

SUMMARY: Taking zidovudine with meals lowers its plasma concentrations and could result in loss of efficacy.

RISK FACTORS:

➡ ***Diet/Food.*** High-fat meals may increase the bioavailability of a sustained release formulation of zidovudine.

RELATED DRUGS: No information is available.

MANAGEMENT OPTIONS:

➡ ***Circumvent/Minimize.*** Administer zidovudine 1 to 2 hours before a meal and taken in a consistent manner in relationship to meals.

➡ *Monitor.* If immediate release zidovudine is administered with meals, monitor for loss of efficacy.

REFERENCES:

Unadkat JD, et al. Pharmacokinetics of oral zidovudine (ZDV) when administered with and without a high-fat meal. *Clin Pharmacol Ther.* 1989;45:165.

Lotterer E, et al. Decreased and variable systemic availability of zidovudine in patients with AIDS if administered with a meal. *Eur J Clin Pharmacol.* 1991;40:305.

Ruhnke M, et al. Effects of standard breakfast on pharmacokinetics of oral zidovudine in patients with AIDS. *Antimicrob Agents Chemother.* 1993;37:2153.

Hollister AS, et al. The effects of a high fat meal on the serum pharmacokinetics of sustained-release zidovudine. *Clin Pharmacol Ther.* 1994;55:193.

Shelton MJ, et al. Prolonged, but not diminished, zidovudine absorption induced by a high-fat breakfast. *Pharmacotherapy.* 1994;14:671.

Sahai J, et al. The effect of a protein meal on zidovudine pharmacokinetics in HIV-infected patients. *Br J Clin Pharmacol.* 1992;33:657.

Furosemide (eg, *Lasix*)

Indomethacin (eg, *Indocin*)

SUMMARY: Indomethacin administration reduces the diuretic and antihypertensive efficacy of furosemide.

RISK FACTORS:

➡ *Concurrent Diseases.* Patients with hyponatremia may be at greatest risk for reduced glomerular filtration when nonsteroidal anti-inflammatory drugs (NSAIDs) are administered.

RELATED DRUGS: Some evidence indicates that other NSAIDs, including naproxen (eg, *Naprosyn*), ibuprofen (eg, *Advil*), piroxicam (eg, *Feldene*), flurbiprofen (eg, *Ansaid*), sulindac (eg, *Clinoril*), and large doses of salicylates have similar effects. Some clinical evidence suggests that sulindac may be less likely than other NSAIDs to interfere with the response to furosemide, but the difference may be only relative.

MANAGEMENT OPTIONS:

➡ *Monitor.* Monitor patients for evidence of reduced response to furosemide when indomethacin or another NSAID is coadministered. If increasing the dose of furosemide does not achieve the desired response, consider a different NSAID such as sulindac or salicylates, which may not affect furosemide to the same degree.

REFERENCES:

Davis A, et al. Interactions between non-steroidal anti-inflammatory drugs and antihypertensive and diuretics. *Aust NZ J Med.* 1986;16:537.

Brooks PM, et al. The effect of furosemide on indomethacin plasma levels. *Br J Clin Pharmacol.* 1974;1:485.

Dzau VJ, et al. Prostaglandins in severe congestive heart failure in relation to activation of the renin-angiotensin system and hyponatremia. *N Engl J Med.* 1984;310:347.

Allan SG, et al. Interaction between diuretics and indomethacin. *Br Med J.* 1981;283:1611.

Poe TE, et al. Interaction of indomethacin with furosemide. *J Fam Pract.* 1983;16:610.

Brater DC. Analysis of the effect of indomethacin on the response to furosemide in man: effect of dose of furosemide. *J Pharmacol Exp Ther.* 1979;210:386.

Smith DE, et al. Attenuation of furosemide's diuretic effect by indomethacin: pharmacokinetic evaluation. *J Pharmacokinet Biopharm.* 1979;7:265.

Patak RV, et al. Antagonism of the effects of furosemide by indomethacin in normal and hypertensive man. *Prostaglandins.* 1975;10:649.

Rawles JM. Antagonism between non-steroidal anti-inflammatory drugs and diuretics. *Scott Med J.* 1982;27:37.

Ciabattoni G, et al. Renal effects of anti-inflammatory drugs. *Eur J Rheumatol Inflamm.* 1980;3:210.

Bunning RD, et al. Sulindac: a potentially renal-sparing nonsteroidal anti-inflammatory drug. *JAMA.* 1982;248:2864.

Wong DG, et al. Non-steroidal antiinflammatory drugs (NSAIDs) vs placebo in hypertension treated with diuretic and beta-blocker. *Clin Pharmacol Ther.* 1984;35:284.

Roberts DG, et al. Comparative effects of sulindac and indomethacin in humans. *Clin Pharmacol Ther.* 1984;35:269.

Wilkins MR, et al. The effects of selective and nonselective inhibition of cyclo-oxygenase on furosemide-stimulated natriuresis. *Int J Clin Pharmacol Ther Toxicol.* 1986;24:55.

Brater DC, et al. Sulindac does not spare the kidney. *Clin Pharmacol Ther.* 1984;35:258.

Eriksson L-O, et al. Renal function and tubular transport effects of sulindac and naproxen in chronic heart failure. *Clin Pharmacol Ther.* 1987;42:646.

Furosemide (eg, *Lasix*)

Phenytoin (eg, *Dilantin*)

SUMMARY: Studies in patients and healthy subjects indicate that phenytoin may reduce the diuretic response to furosemide.

RISK FACTORS: No specific risk factors are known.

RELATED DRUGS: The effect of phenytoin on other loop diuretics is not established. Phenobarbital affects furosemide similarly.

MANAGEMENT OPTIONS:

➡ *Monitor.* In patients taking phenytoin, be alert for an impaired diuretic response to furosemide; larger furosemide doses may be required. It is not known if separating the doses of the drugs would minimize the interaction.

REFERENCES:
Ahmad S. Renal insensitivity to furosemide caused by chronic anticonvulsant therapy. *Br Med J.* 1974;3:657.

Fine A, et al. Malabsorption of furosemide caused by phenytoin. *Br Med J.* 1977;4:1061.

Furosemide (eg, *Lasix*)

Terbutaline (eg, *Brethaire*)

SUMMARY: The administration of furosemide and terbutaline produces additive hypokalemia; the clinical significance of this interaction is not well defined.

RISK FACTORS:

➡ *Other Drugs.* Patients taking potassium-depleting corticosteroids may be more prone to hypokalemia from this interaction.

➡ *Concurrent Diseases.* Patients with low basal serum potassium may be at increased risk for arrhythmia when treated with combinations of furosemide and terbutaline.

RELATED DRUGS: It is likely that other combinations of potassium-wasting diuretics and beta$_2$-agonists also would tend to reduce serum potassium concentrations.

MANAGEMENT OPTIONS:

➡ *Circumvent/Minimize.* In patients who appear predisposed to hypokalemia, triamterene or potassium supplementation may be given to prevent excessive reduction in serum potassium concentrations.

➡ *Monitor.* Monitor patients treated with combinations of potassium-wasting diuretics and beta$_2$-agonists for signs of hypokalemia including ECG changes, fatigue, and muscle pains.

REFERENCES:

Newnham DM, et al. The effects of furosemide and terbutaline on the hypokalemic and electrocardiographic responses to inhaled terbutaline. *Br J Clin Pharmacol.* 1991;32:630.

Furosemide (eg, *Lasix*)

Tubocurarine

SUMMARY: Furosemide appears to prolong the neuromuscular blockade following tubocurarine.

RISK FACTORS: No specific risk factors are known.

RELATED DRUGS: No information is available.

MANAGEMENT OPTIONS:

➡ *Monitor.* Monitor patients for altered dosage requirements for neuromuscular blocking agents when receiving furosemide.

REFERENCES:

Miller RD, et al. Enhancement of d-tubocurarine neuromuscular blockade by diuretics in man. *Anesthesiology.* 1976;45:442.

Scappaticci KA, et al. Effects of furosemide on the neuromuscular junction. *Anesthesiology.* 1982;57:381.

Gamma Globulin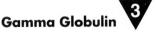

Phenytoin (eg, *Dilantin*)

SUMMARY: A patient on phenytoin therapy developed a hypersensitivity myocarditis (HM) and died after receiving gamma globulin, but a causal relationship was not established.

RISK FACTORS: No specific risk factors are known.

RELATED DRUGS: No information is available.

MANAGEMENT OPTIONS:

➥ *Consider Alternative.* Although a causal relationship between HM and combined phenytoin-gamma globulin therapy is not established, the severity of the reaction dictates that the benefit-risk of using this combination be considered carefully.

➥ *Monitor.* If gamma globulin is given in the presence of phenytoin therapy, be alert for evidence of hypersensitivity (eg, fever, skin rash, eosinophilia) and cardiac findings (eg, tachycardia, ECG changes, enzyme elevations).

REFERENCES:

Koehler PJ, et al. Lethal hypersensitivity myocarditis associated with the use of intravenous gamma globulin for Guillain-Barré syndrome, in combination with phenytoin. *J Neurol*. 1996;243:366-367.

Ganciclovir (eg, *Cytovene*)

Zidovudine (*Retrovir*) AVOID

SUMMARY: Combination therapy with ganciclovir and zidovudine in the treatment of cytomegalovirus (CMV) disease increases hematological toxicity.

RISK FACTORS: No specific risk factors are known.

RELATED DRUGS: No information is available.

MANAGEMENT OPTIONS:

➥ *AVOID COMBINATION.* Until more information is available, avoid this combination of drugs. Foscarnet (*Foscavir*) may be a reasonable alternative to ganciclovir for the treatment of CMV retinitis in patients treated with zidovudine.

REFERENCES:

Hochster H, et al. Toxicity of combined ganciclovir and zidovudine for cytomegalovirus disease associated with AIDS. *Ann Intern Med*. 1990;113:111-117.

Burger DM, et al. Pharmacokinetic variability of zidovudine in HIV-infected individuals: subgroup analysis and drug interactions. *AIDS*. 1994;8:1683-1689.

Jacobson MA, et al. Foscarnet therapy for ganciclovir-resistant cytomegalovirus retinitis in patients with AIDS. *J Infect Dis*. 1991;163:1348-1351.

Garlic

Saquinavir (eg, *Fortovase*)

SUMMARY: Garlic administration reduces saquinavir plasma concentrations; reduction in antiviral effect may occur.

RISK FACTORS: No specific risk factors are known.

RELATED DRUGS: Garlic administration for 4 days produced an insignificant reduction in ritonavir (*Norvir*) concentrations. The effect of garlic on other protease inhibitors is unknown.

MANAGEMENT OPTIONS:

➡ *Circumvent/Minimize.* Patients taking saquinavir should avoid chronic, high-dose garlic administration.

➡ *Monitor.* Observe patients taking saquinavir, and perhaps other protease inhibitors, for reduced antiviral plasma concentrations if garlic is ingested chronically.

REFERENCES:

Piscitelli SC, et al. The effect of garlic supplements on the pharmacokinetics of saquinavir. *Clin Infect Dis.* 2002;34:234-238.

 Gatifloxacin (*Tequin*)

Glyburide (eg, *Diabeta*)

SUMMARY: The administration of gatifloxacin to patients with diabetes may result in episodes of hypoglycemia.

RISK FACTORS: No specific risk factors are known.

RELATED DRUGS: Ciprofloxacin (eg, *Cipro*) has been associated with hypoglycemia in patients taking oral hypoglycemic agents. If gatifloxacin stimulates insulin secretion, any hypoglycemic agent could produce additive hypoglycemia.

MANAGEMENT OPTIONS:

➡ *Monitor.* Pending further data, monitor blood glucose concentrations carefully during gatifloxacin administration to patients with diabetes.

REFERENCES:

Gajjar DA, et al. Effect of multiple-dose gatifloxacin or ciprofloxacin on glucose homeostasis and insulin production in patients with noninsulin-dependent diabetes mellitus maintained with diet and exercise. *Pharmacotherapy.* 2000;20(6 pt 2):76S-86S.

Hussein G, et al. Gatifloxacin-induced hypoglycemia: a case report and review of the literature. *Clin Res Regul Aff.* 2002;19:333-339.

Baker SE, et al. Possible gatifloxacin-induced hypoglycemia. *Ann Pharmacother.* 2002;36:1722-1726.

Menzies DJ, et al. Severe and persistent hypoglycemia due to gatifloxacin interaction with oral hypoglycemic agents. *Am J Med.* 2002;113:232-234.

Product Information. Gatifloxacin (*Tequin*). Bristol-Meyers Squibb Company. 2000.

 Gemcitabine (*Gemzar*)

Warfarin (eg, *Coumadin*)

SUMMARY: A patient on warfarin developed increased anticoagulant effect when gemcitabine was given concurrently. A causal effect appears likely in this patient, but the general incidence and magnitude of this interaction are not established.

RISK FACTORS: No specific risk factors are known.

RELATED DRUGS: The effect of gemcitabine on other oral anticoagulants is not known. Nonetheless, if the mechanism is pharmacodynamic, one would expect all oral anticoagulants to interact in a similar manner.

MANAGEMENT OPTIONS:

➡ *Monitor.* Monitor the hypoprothrombinemic response more frequently in patients taking warfarin or other oral anticoagulants if gemcitabine is given concurrently. Weekly INR measurements should be sufficient.

REFERENCES:

Kinikar SA, et al. Identification of a gemcitabine-warfarin interaction. *Pharmacotherapy*. 1999;19:1331-1333.

Gemfibrozil (eg, *Lopid*)

Glyburide (eg, *DiaBeta*)

SUMMARY: Gemfibrozil appeared to cause hypoglycemia in a patient receiving glyburide; a causal relationship is likely in this patient, but more study is needed.

RISK FACTORS: No specific risk factors are known.

RELATED DRUGS: It is possible that other sulfonylureas would be affected similarly by gemfibrozil.

MANAGEMENT OPTIONS:

➡ *Circumvent/Minimize.* The glyburide dose may need to be reduced during concomitant gemfibrozil and glyburide therapy.

➡ *Monitor.* Monitor patients receiving gemfibrozil and glyburide for symptoms of hypoglycemia (eg, tachycardia, sweating, tremor).

REFERENCES:

Ahmad S. Gemfibrozil: interaction with glyburide. *South Med J.* 1991;84:102.

Gemfibrozil (eg, *Lopid*)

Lovastatin (eg, *Mevacor*)

SUMMARY: Case reports suggest that gemfibrozil increases the likelihood of lovastatin-induced myopathy, but the incidence of the reaction is not established.

RISK FACTORS: No specific risk factors are known.

RELATED DRUGS: Available evidence suggests that pravastatin (*Pravachol*) is less likely to cause myopathy than lovastatin, either when given alone or when combined with other drugs such as gemfibrozil. Nonetheless, comparative "head-to-head" studies will be required to confirm these findings. Little is known regarding the likelihood of myopathy with simvastatin (*Zocor*) plus gemfibrozil (or clofibrate), but assume that it is similar to lovastatin plus gemfibrozil until information is available. Although little is known regarding the safety of combined use of lovastatin and clofibrate, apply the same precautions as with lovastatin plus gemfibrozil.

MANAGEMENT OPTIONS:

➡ *Avoid Unless Benefit Outweighs Risk.* Some experts recommend against using combined therapy with lovastatin and gemfibrozil. The manufacturer suggests that the benefits of combined therapy are not likely to outweigh the risk of myopathy and rhabdomyolysis.

➡ *Monitor.* If the combination is used, alert patients to muscular symptoms such as pain, tenderness, or weakness; measure CK in patients with such symptoms. Early recognition of this disorder is important because it may progress to acute renal failure in some patients if the drugs are not discontinued promptly. The same precautions should apply to combined use of lovastatin and clofibrate.

REFERENCES:

Pierce LR, et al. Myopathy and rhabdomyolysis associated with lovastatin-gemfibrozil combination therapy. *JAMA.* 1990;264:71.

East C, et al. Rhabdomyolysis in patients receiving lovastatin after cardiac transplantation. *N Engl J Med.* 1988;318:47.

Tobert JA. Rhabdomyolysis in patients receiving lovastatin after cardiac transplantation. *N Engl J Med.* 1988;318:47.

Marais GE, et al. Rhabdomyolysis and acute renal failure induced by combination lovastatin and gemfibrozil therapy. *Ann Intern Med.* 1990;112:228-230.

Kogan AD, et al. Lovastatin-induced acute rhabdomyolysis. *Postgrad Med J.* 1990;66:294-296.

Manoukian AA, et al. Rhabdomyolysis secondary to lovastatin therapy. *Clin Chem.* 1990;36:2145-2147.

Goldman JA, et al. The role of cholesterol-lowering agents in drug-induced rhabdomyolysis and polymyositis. *Arthritis Rheum.* 1989;32:358-359.

East C, et al. Combination drug therapy for familial combined hyperlipidemia. *Ann Intern Med.* 1988;109:25-32.

Wirebaugh SR, et al. A retrospective review of the use of lipid-lowering agents in combination, specifically, gemfibrozil and lovastatin. *Pharmacotherapy.* 1992;12:445-450.

Product Information. Lovastatin (*Mevacor*). Merck Sharp & Dohme. 1993.

 Gemfibrozil (eg, *Lopid*)

Pravastatin (*Pravachol*)

SUMMARY: Most patients appear to tolerate the combined use of pravastatin and gemfibrozil well, but it is possible that an occasional patient might develop myopathy (as has been reported with lovastatin and gemfibrozil).

RISK FACTORS: No specific risk factors are known.

RELATED DRUGS: Available evidence suggests that pravastatin is less likely to cause myopathy than lovastatin (eg, *Mevacor*), either when given alone or when combined with other drugs such as gemfibrozil. Nonetheless, comparative "head-to-head" studies will be required to confirm these findings. Little is known regarding the likelihood of myopathy with simvastatin (*Zocor*) plus gemfibrozil, but assume that it is similar to lovastatin plus gemfibrozil until information is available. One patient developed myopathy when clofibrate was added to well-tolerated pravastatin therapy; the myopathy resolved when the clofibrate was discontinued with continued pravastatin therapy.

MANAGEMENT OPTIONS:

➡ *Consider Alternative.* Although the combination of pravastatin and gemfibrozil is well tolerated in most patients, generally avoid the routine use of this combination until more evidence of safety is available.

➡ **Monitor.** If the combination is used, alert patients for muscular symptoms such as pain, tenderness, or weakness; measure creatine kinase in patients with such symptoms.

REFERENCES:

Wiklund O, et al. Pravastatin and gemfibrozil alone and in combination for the treatment of hypercholesterolemia. *Am J Med.* 1993;94:13-20.

Jungnickel PW, et al. Pravastatin: a new drug for the treatment of hypercholesterolemia. *Clin Pharm.* 1992;11:677-689.

Product Information. Pravastatin (*Pravachol*). Bristol-Myers Squibb. 1993.

Gemfibrozil (eg, *Lopid*)
Repaglinide (*Prandin*)

SUMMARY: Gemfibrozil markedly increases serum concentrations of repaglinide; enhanced hypoglycemic effects are likely to result.

RISK FACTORS: No specific risk factors are known.

RELATED DRUGS: No information is available; however, the elimination of other oral hypoglycemic agents (eg, pioglitazone [*Actos*], rosiglitazone [*Avandia*]) metabolized by CYP2C8 may be reduced by gemfibrozil coadministration.

MANAGEMENT OPTIONS:

➡ **Consider Alternative.** Consider using alternative lipid-lowering drugs (eg, HMG-CoA reductase inhibitors) in patients stabilized on repaglinide. Alternative oral hypoglycemic agents not metabolized by CYP2C8 (eg, glipizide [eg, *Glucotrol*], tolbutamide [eg, *Orinase*]) could be considered for use in patients requiring gemfibrozil.

➡ **Monitor.** Monitor patients taking repaglinide for changes in blood glucose concentrations if gemfibrozil is added to or discontinued from the drug regimen.

REFERENCES:

Niemi M et al. Effects of gemfibrozil, itraconazole, and their combination on the pharmacokinetics and pharmacodynamics of repaglinide: potentially hazardous interaction between gemfibrozil and repaglinide. *Diabetologia.* 2003;46:347-351.

Gemfibrozil (eg, *Lopid*)
Warfarin (eg, *Coumadin*)

SUMMARY: Gemfibrozil appeared to increase the hypoprothrombinemic response to warfarin in 1 patient, but more study is needed to confirm this effect.

RISK FACTORS: No specific risk factors are known.

RELATED DRUGS: The effect of gemfibrozil on oral anticoagulants other than warfarin is not established, but consider the possibility of an interaction until clinical studies are performed. Clofibrate, lovastatin (eg, *Mevacor*), and simvastatin (*Zocor*) also may increase the effect of oral anticoagulants, while cholestyramine (eg, *Questran*) and colestipol (*Colestid*) may reduce their effect.

MANAGEMENT OPTIONS:

➡ **Avoid Unless Benefit Outweighs Risk.** Avoid concomitant therapy with gemfibrozil and oral anticoagulants if possible. If oral anticoagulant therapy is begun in a patient receiving gemfibrozil, anticoagulant doses probably should be conservatively administered until the maintenance dose is established.

➡ **Monitor.** Monitor patients for altered oral anticoagulant effect if gemfibrozil is initiated, discontinued, or dosage changed.

REFERENCES:

Ahmad S. Gemfibrozil interaction with warfarin sodium (*Coumadin*). *Chest.* 1990;98:1041-1042.

Product information. Gemfibrozil (*Lopid*). Parke-Davis. 1993.

Gentamicin (eg, *Garamycin*)

Indomethacin (eg, *Indocin*)

SUMMARY: Indomethacin appears to reduce the renal clearance of gentamicin and amikacin in premature infants, resulting in increased gentamicin serum concentrations.

RISK FACTORS:

➡ **Effects of Age.** The glomerular filtration rate for preterm newborns is only 0.7 to 0.8 mL/min compared to 2 to 4 mL/min or 10 to 20 mL/min/1.73 m^2 for full-term newborns.

RELATED DRUGS: Amikacin interacts similarly. Other aminoglycosides may be affected by indomethacin. Other nonsteroidal anti-inflammatory drugs also may reduce the renal clearance of aminoglycosides.

MANAGEMENT OPTIONS:

➡ **Monitor.** If aminoglycosides and indomethacin are administered to infants, monitor plasma antibiotic concentrations and renal function. The potential for this interaction in adults is unknown.

REFERENCES:

Gagliardi L. Possible indomethacin-aminoglycoside interaction in preterm infants. *J Pediatr.* 1985;106:991.

Zarfin Y, et al. Possible indomethacin-aminoglycoside interaction in preterm infants. *J Pediatr.* 1985;106:511.

Gentamicin (eg, *Garamycin*)

Methoxyflurane (*Penthrane*)

SUMMARY: Methoxyflurane appears to enhance the renal toxicity of aminoglycoside antibiotics.

RISK FACTORS: No specific risk factors known.

RELATED DRUGS: The nephrotoxicity of other aminoglycosides including kanamycin also may be enhanced by methoxyflurane.

MANAGEMENT OPTIONS:

➡ **Consider Alternative.** Avoid nephrotoxic antibiotics such as aminoglycosides in patients who have recently received methoxyflurane.

➡ **Monitor.** If aminoglycosides are administered with methoxyflurane, monitor for renal dysfunction.

REFERENCES:

Churchill D. Persisting renal insufficiency after methoxyflurane anesthesia. Report of two cases and review of literature. *Am J Med.* 1974;56:575.

Gentamicin (eg, *Garamycin*)

Vancomycin (eg, *Vancocin*)

SUMMARY: The combination of vancomycin and aminoglycosides may lead to increased nephrotoxicity in some patients.

RISK FACTORS:

➡ **Concurrent Diseases.** Individuals with pre-existing renal failure are at risk.

➡ **Dosage Regimen.** Individuals with increased antibiotic concentrations, undergoing prolonged therapy, or receiving other nephrotoxic drugs are at increased risk.

RELATED DRUGS: Other aminoglycosides administered with vancomycin may increase the risk of nephrotoxicity.

MANAGEMENT OPTIONS:

➡ **Monitor.** If aminoglycosides and vancomycin are coadministered, monitor renal function and maintain antibiotic concentrations in the normal range.

REFERENCES:

Farber BF, et al. Retrospective study of the toxicity of preparations of vancomycin from 1974 to 1981. *Antimicrob Agents Chemother.* 1983;23:138.

Rybak MJ, et al. Alanine aminopeptidase and beta$_2$ microglobulin excretion in patients receiving vancomycin and gentamicin. *Antimicrob Agents Chemother.* 1987;31:1461.

Cimino MA, et al. Relationship of serum antibiotic concentrations to nephrotoxicity in cancer patients receiving concurrent aminoglycoside and vancomycin therapy. *Am J Med.* 1987;83:1091.

Downs NJ, et al. Mild nephrotoxicity associated with vancomycin use. *Arch Intern Med.* 1989;149:1777.

Pauly DJ, et al. Risk of nephrotoxicity with combination vancomycinaminoglycoside therapy. *Pharmacotherapy.* 1990;10:378.

Rybak MJ, et al. Nephrotoxicity of vancomycin, alone and with an aminoglycoside. *J Antimicrob Chemother.* 1990;25:679.

Munar MY, et al. The effect of tobramycin on the renal handling of vancomycin. *J Clin Pharmacol.* 1991;31:618.

Ginkgo Biloba

Warfarin (eg, *Coumadin*)

SUMMARY: Isolated cases of bleeding have been reported following use of ginkgo biloba, with and without concurrent warfarin therapy, but the contribution of ginkgo to the bleeding was not established.

RISK FACTORS: No specific risk factors are known.

RELATED DRUGS: If ginkgo proves to increase the risk of bleeding in patients receiving warfarin because of inhibition of platelet function, it will probably have the same effect with all other oral anticoagulants.

MANAGEMENT OPTIONS:

➡ *Use Alternative.* Although the risk of serious bleeding associated with the addition of ginkgo to warfarin therapy is not established, generally avoid the combination because a) the benefit of ginkgo as a "memory aid" is questionable and b) the potential adverse outcome of the interaction is life-threatening.

REFERENCES:

Matthews MK Jr. Association of ginkgo biloba with intracerebral hemmorrhage. *Neurology.* 1998;50:1933-1934.

Rosenblatt M, et al. Spontaneous hyphema associated with ingestion of ginkgo biloba extract. *N Engl J Med.* 1997;336:1108.

Glipizide (eg, *Glucotrol*)

Ranitidine (eg, *Zantac*)

SUMMARY: Ranitidine may increase the serum concentration of glipizide and enhance its hypoglycemic effects. Ranitidine may have independent effects on serum glucose.

RISK FACTORS: No specific risk factors are known.

RELATED DRUGS: Ranitidine does not alter tolbutamide (eg, *Orinase*), or glyburide (eg, *DiaBeta*) pharmacokinetics. Cimetidine (eg, *Tagamet*) increases the concentrations of tolbutamide, glipizide, and glyburide. The effect of famotidine (eg, *Pepcid*) and nizatidine (*Axid*) on sulfonylurea pharmacokinetics is unknown, but they may interact if increased gastric pH is involved in the observed changes with cimetidine and ranitidine. Proton pump inhibitors (eg, omeprazole [*Prilosec*], lansoprazole [*Prevacid*]) may affect glipizide in a similar manner.

MANAGEMENT OPTIONS:

➡ *Consider Alternative.* Sucralfate (eg, *Carafate*) may be a good alternative therapy for the treatment of ulcer disease in diabetic patients because it appears unlikely to alter glycemic control to a clinically significant degree.

➡ *Monitor.* Observe diabetic patients stabilized on any hypoglycemic therapy (and especially glipizide) in whom H_2-receptor antagonist therapy is initiated or discontinued for altered glycemic responses.

REFERENCES:

Feely J, et al. Potentiation of the hypoglycaemic response to glipizide in diabetic patients by histamine H_2-receptor antagonists. *Br J Clin Pharmacol.* 1993;35:321.

MacWalter RS, et al. Potentiation by ranitidine of the hypoglycaemic response to glipizide in diabetic patients. *Br J Clin Pharmacol.* 1985;19:121P.

Cate EW, et al. Inhibition of tolbutamide elimination by cimetidine but not ranitidine. *J Clin Pharmacol.* 1986;26:372.

Toon S, et al. Effects of cimetidine, ranitidine and omeprazole on tolbutamide pharmacokinetics. *J Pharm Pharmacol.* 1995;47:85.

Kubacka RT, et al. The paradoxical effect of cimetidine and ranitidine on glibenclamide pharmacokinetics and pharmacodynamics. *Br J Clin Pharmacol.* 1987;23:743.

Adebayo GI, et al. Lack of efficacy of cimetidine and ranitidine as inhibitors of tolbutamide metabolism. *Eur J Clin Pharmacol.* 1988;34:653.

Letendre PW, et al. Effect of sucralfate on the absorption and pharmacokinetics of chlorpropamide. *J Clin Pharmacol.* 1986;26:622.

Glucagon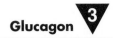

Warfarin (eg, *Coumadin*)

SUMMARY: Glucagon appears to enhance the hypoprothrombinemic response to warfarin, and possibly other oral anticoagulants, causing bleeding in some patients. Adjustment of the oral anticoagulant dose may be needed in patients receiving both drugs.

RISK FACTORS: No specific risk factors are known.

RELATED DRUGS: Little is known regarding the effect of glucagon on oral anticoagulants other than warfarin. Assume that an interaction occurs until information to the contrary appears. A potentiating effect of acenocoumarol[†] by glucagon has been demonstrated in animals.

MANAGEMENT OPTIONS:

➡ ***Monitor.*** Monitor for altered oral anticoagulant effect if glucagon is given concurrently. Adjust the anticoagulant dose as needed.

REFERENCES:

Koch-Weser J. Potentiation by glucagon of the hypoprothrombinemic action of warfarin. *Ann Intern Med.* 1970;72:331-335.

Weiner M, et al. The effect of glucagon and insulin on the prothrombin response to coumarin anticoagulants. *Proc Soc Exp Biol Med.* 1968;127:761-763.

† Not available in the US.

Glutethimide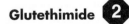

Warfarin (eg, *Coumadin*)

SUMMARY: Glutethimide inhibits the hypoprothrombinemic response to warfarin, and probably other oral anticoagulants; the dose of the oral anticoagulant may have to be increased during coadministration of these drugs.

RISK FACTORS:

➡ ***Dosage Regimen.*** Since the onset and offset of enzyme induction is gradual, this interaction would be expected to take place over a week or more and to continue for a week or more after glutethimide is stopped.

RELATED DRUGS: Although little is known regarding the effect of glutethimide on oral anticoagulants other than warfarin, assume that an interaction exists until information to the contrary appears.

MANAGEMENT OPTIONS:

➡ ***Use Alternative.*** Benzodiazepines such as flurazepam (eg, *Dalmane*), temazepam (eg, *Restoril*), and triazolam (eg, *Halcion*) are preferable to glutethimide in patients on oral anticoagulants. If glutethimide is used, monitor for altered oral anticoagulant effect if glutethimide is initiated, discontinued, or changed in dosage. Adjust the anticoagulant dose as needed. Note that it may take up to 2 weeks or more for the maximal effect of glutethimide on warfarin to develop, and a similar time for the effect to fully dissipate.

REFERENCES:

Corn M. Effect of phenobarbital and glutethimide on biological halflife of warfarin. *Thromb Diath Haemorrh.* 1966;16:606-612.

MacDonald MG, et al. The effects of phenobarbital, chloral betaine, and glutethimide administration on warfarin plasma levels and hypoprothrombinemic responses in man. *Clin Pharmacol Ther*. 1969;10:80-84.

Udall JA. Clinical implications of warfarin interactions with five sedatives. *Am J Cardiol*. 1975;35:67-71.

Glyburide (eg, *DiaBeta*)

Rifampin (eg, *Rifadin*)

SUMMARY: Rifampin reduces glyburide concentrations; reduction in hypoglycemic response is likely to occur.

RISK FACTORS: No specific risk factors are known.

RELATED DRUGS: The hypoglycemic efficacy of tolbutamide (*Orinase*) and glipizide (*Glucotrol*) may be reduced by rifampin. Rifabutin (*Mycobutin*) might affect glyburide in a similar manner.

MANAGEMENT OPTIONS:

➡ **Monitor.** When rifampin is coadministered with glyburide and possibly other sulfonylureas, watch for reduced hypoglycemic efficacy. Discontinuation of rifampin could result in hypoglycemia in a patient stabilized on glyburide and rifampin therapy.

REFERENCES:

Niemi M, et al. Effects of rifampin on the pharmacokinetics and pharmacodynamics of glyburide and glipizide. *Clin Pharmacol Ther*. 2001;69:400-406.

Self TH, et al. Interaction of rifampin and glyburide. *Chest*. 1989;96:1443-1444.

Surekha V, et al. Drug interaction: rifampicin and glibenclamide. *Natl Med J India*. 1997;10:11-12.

Glyburide (eg, *DiaBeta*)

Warfarin (eg, *Coumadin*)

SUMMARY: A patient on warfarin developed a marked increase in warfarin response and bleeding after starting glyburide, but a causal relationship was not established.

RISK FACTORS: No specific risk factors are known.

RELATED DRUGS: It does not seem likely that oral anticoagulants would interact with insulin.

MANAGEMENT OPTIONS:

➡ **Monitor.** Although this interaction is poorly documented, the potential severity of the adverse outcome suggests that warfarin response should be monitored if glyburide is initiated, discontinued, or changed in dosage.

REFERENCES:

Warfarin potentiated by proguanil. *BMJ*. 1991;303:789.

Heine P, et al. The influence of hypoglycaemic sulphonylureas on elimination and efficacy of phenprocoumon following a single oral dose in diabetic patients. *Eur J Clin Pharmacol*. 1976;10:31.

Grapefruit Juice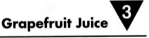

Felodipine (*Plendil*)

SUMMARY: Grapefruit juice increases felodipine plasma concentrations; increased hypotensive effects or headaches may occur.

RISK FACTORS: No specific risk factors are known.

RELATED DRUGS: Grapefruit juice has been demonstrated to inhibit the intestinal metabolism of most calcium channel blockers.

MANAGEMENT OPTIONS:

➡ *Circumvent/Minimize.* The use of calcium channel blockers with less first-pass metabolism (eg, amlodipine [*Norvasc*]) would be less affected by grapefruit juice. Other fruit juices may be substituted for grapefruit juice to avoid the interaction with calcium channel blockers.

➡ *Monitor.* Monitor patients stabilized on felodipine for orthostatic hypotension and tachycardia if grapefruit juice is administered, particularly if the juice consumption is daily.

REFERENCES:

Lundahl J, et al. Effects of grapefruit juice ingestion—pharmacokinetics and haemodynamics of intravenously and orally administered felodipine in healthy men. *Eur J Clin Pharmacol.* 1997;52:139-145.

Bailey DG, et al. Erythromycin-felodipine interaction: magnitude, mechanism, and comparison with grapefruit juice. *Clin Pharmacol Ther.* 1996;60:25-33.

Lown KS, et al. Grapefruit juice increases felodipine oral availability in humans by decreasing intestinal CYP3A4 protein expression. *J Clin Invest.* 1997;99:2545-2553.

Bailey DG, et al. Grapefruit juice-felodipine interaction: reproducibility and characterization with the extended release drug formulation. *Br J Clin Pharmacol.* 1995;40:135-140.

Dresser GK, et al. Grapefruit juice—felodipine interaction in the elderly. *Clin Pharmacol Ther.* 2000;68:28-34.

Grapefruit Juice

Fexofenadine (*Allegra*)

SUMMARY: Ingestion of large amounts of grapefruit juice reduces the absorption of fexofenadine, and may reduce fexofenadine efficacy.

RISK FACTORS: No specific risk factors are known.

RELATED DRUGS: Apple juice and orange juice also appear to reduce fexofenadine bioavailability.

MANAGEMENT OPTIONS:

➡ *Circumvent/Minimize.* Until more data are available, it would be prudent to take fexofenadine with water rather than with grapefruit juice or other fruit juices.

REFERENCES:

Dresser GK, et al. Fruit juices inhibit organic anion transporting polypeptide-mediated drug uptake to decrease the oral availability of fexofenadine. *Clin Pharmacol Ther.* 2002;71:11-20.

Grapefruit Juice

Itraconazole (*Sporanox*)

SUMMARY: Grapefruit juice administered with itraconazole reduces itraconazole plasma concentrations; antifungal efficacy may be reduced.

RISK FACTORS: No specific risk factors are known.

RELATED DRUGS: Although no data exist, grapefruit juice may also affect ketoconazole (eg, *Nizoral*) in a similar manner. Orange juice reduced itraconazole bioavailability in 1 study.

MANAGEMENT OPTIONS:

➡ *Consider Alternative.* Counsel patients taking itraconazole to avoid drinking grapefruit juice.

➡ *Monitor.* Monitor patients who take itraconazole and grapefruit juice for subtherapeutic itraconazole concentrations and possible loss of efficacy.

REFERENCES:
Penzak SR, et al. Grapefruit juice decreases the systemic availability of itraconazole capsules in healthy volunteers. *Ther Drug Monit.* 1999;21:304-309.

Kawakami M, et al. Effect of grapefruit juice on pharmacokinetics of itraconazole in healthy subjects. *Int J Clin Pharmacol Ther.* 1998;36:306-308.

 ## Grapefruit Juice

Lovastatin (*Mevacor*)

SUMMARY: Repeated doses of grapefruit juice markedly increased lovastatin serum concentrations in healthy subjects.

RISK FACTORS: No specific risk factors are known.

RELATED DRUGS: Simvastatin (*Zocor*), like lovastatin, undergoes extensive first-pass metabolism in the gut wall and liver; it is similarly affected by grapefruit juice. Atorvastatin (*Lipitor*) is also metabolized by CYP3A4, and would be expected to interact with grapefruit juice (but to a lesser extent than lovastatin and simvastatin). Pravastatin (*Pravachol*) and fluvastatin (*Lescol*) are not metabolized by CYP3A4 and are not likely to be affected by grapefruit juice.

MANAGEMENT OPTIONS:

➡ *Consider Alternative.* Orange juice does not inhibit CYP3A4, and would not be expected to interact with lovastatin.

➡ *Circumvent/Minimize.* Patients taking lovastatin should ingest grapefruit juice only occasionally.

REFERENCES:
Kantola T, et al. Grapefruit juice greatly increases serum concentrations of lovastatin and lovastatin acid. *Clin Pharmacol Ther.* 1998;63:397-402.

Lilja JJ, et al. Grapefruit juice-simvastatin interaction: effect on serum concentrations of simvastatin, simvastatin acid, and HMG-CoA reductase inhibitors. *Clin Pharmacol Ther.* 1998;64:477-483.

Grapefruit Juice

Methylprednisolone (eg, *Medrol*)

SUMMARY: Grapefruit juice increases methylprednisolone plasma concentrations; the extent to which this increases the risk of methylprednisolone toxicity is not established.

RISK FACTORS: No specific risk factors are known.

RELATED DRUGS: Theoretically, dexamethasone (eg, *Decadron*) would interact with grapefruit juice in a manner similar to methylprednisolone, but prednisone does not appear to be affected.

MANAGEMENT OPTIONS:

➥ *Circumvent/Minimize.* Because grapefruit juice is a mechanism-based (suicide) inhibitor, this interaction cannot be completely avoided by separating the doses of methylprednisolone from grapefruit juice. But, it seems unlikely that eating a fresh grapefruit half would have enough juice to interact with methylprednisolone in a clinically important way.

➥ *Monitor.* If a patient on methylprednisolone drinks grapefruit juice, monitor for methylprednisolone toxicity.

REFERENCES:

Varis T, et al. Grapefruit juice can increase the plasma concentrations of oral methylprednisolone. *Eur J Clin Pharmacol.* 2000;56:489.

Hollander AA, et al. The effect of grapefruit juice on cyclosporine and prednisone metabolism in transplant patients. *Clin Pharmacol Ther.* 1995;57:318.

Grapefruit Juice

Midazolam (*Versed*)

SUMMARY: Grapefruit juice increases oral midazolam serum concentrations and pharmacodynamic effects, but does not appear to affect intravenous midazolam. Although the clinical importance of this effect is not established, it seems likely that some patients would be adversely affected when oral midazolam is taken with grapefruit juice.

RISK FACTORS:

➥ *Route of Administration.* Only oral midazolam would be expected to interact with grapefruit juice, since the effect of grapefruit juice is primarily on intestinal CYP3A4.

RELATED DRUGS: Alprazolam (*Xanax*) and triazolam (*Halcion*) are also metabolized by CYP3A4. When given orally, they would also be expected to interact with grapefruit juice. Diazepam (*Valium*) is partially metabolized by CYP3A4, but would not be expected to interact to the same degree. Most other benzodiazepines are metabolized primarily by enzymes other than CYP3A4 and would not be expected to interact.

MANAGEMENT OPTIONS:

➥ *Consider Alternative.* Orange juice does not appear to inhibit CYP3A4 and would not be expected to interact with midazolam. Also, one could use a benzodiazepine other than midazolam, alprazolam, or triazolam such as diazepam.

➥ **Circumvent/Minimize.** Warn patients taking oral midazolam to avoid taking it with or within several hours after grapefruit products.

➥ **Monitor.** If the combination is used, be alert for evidence of excessive midazolam effect (eg, drowsiness).

REFERENCES:

Ha HR, et al. In vitro inhibition of midazolam and quinidine metabolism by flavonoids. *Eur J Clin Pharmacol.* 1995;48:367-371.

Kupferschmidt HH, et al. Interaction between grapefruit juice and midazolam in humans. *Clin Pharmacol Ther.* 1995;58:20-28.

Vanakoski J, et al. Grapefruit juice does not enhance the effects of midazolam and triazolam in man. *Eur J Clin Pharmacol.* 1996;50:501-508.

Grapefruit Juice

Nifedipine (eg, *Procardia*)

SUMMARY: Grapefruit juice increases the serum concentrations of several dihydropyridine calcium channel blockers; increased toxicity could occur in some patients.

RISK FACTORS:

➥ **Dosage Regimen.** Double-strength grapefruit juice (ie, diluted with half the usual amount of water) increased the risk of toxicity.

RELATED DRUGS: Grapefruit juice increases felodipine's AUC. Orange juice had no effect on felodipine. A single dose of grapefruit juice caused a 40% increase in the AUC of nitrendipine (*Baypress*), while multiple doses produced a 106% increase in the AUC. The combination of nisoldipine (*Sular*) and grapefruit juice produced a 2-fold increase in nisoldipine AUC and about a 4-fold increase in its peak concentration. Other dihydropyridine calcium channel blockers may be affected similarly by grapefruit juice.

MANAGEMENT OPTIONS:

➥ **Consider Alternative.** Patients should avoid taking calcium channel blockers with grapefruit juice. Orange juice does not affect calcium channel blocker metabolism.

➥ **Monitor.** Monitor patients who drink grapefruit juice while taking calcium channel blockers for increased response to the calcium channel blocker.

REFERENCES:

Bailey DG, et al. Interaction of citrus juices with felodipine and nifedipine. *Lancet.* 1991;337:268-269.

Chayen R, et al. Interaction of citrus juices with felodipine and nifedipine. *Lancet.* 1991;337:854.

Rashid TJ, et al. Factors affecting the absolute bioavailability of nifedipine. *Br J Clin Pharmacol.* 1995;40:51-58.

Rashid J, et al. Quercetin, an *in vitro* inhibitor of CYP3A4, does not contribute to the interaction between nifedipine and grapefruit juice. *Br J Clin Pharmacol.* 1993;36:460.

Bailey DG, et al. Formulation dependent interaction between felodipine and grapefruit juice. *Clin Pharmacol Ther.* 1990;47:181.

Bailey DG, et al. Grapefruit juice—felodipine interaction: mechanism, predictability, and effect of naringin. *Clin Pharmacol Ther.* 1993;53:637-642.

Edgar B, et al. Acute effects of drinking grapefruit juice on the pharmacokinetics and dynamics of felodipine–and its potential clinical relevance. *Eur J Clin Pharmacol.* 1992;42:313-317.

Lundahl J, et al. Relationship between time of intake of grapefruit juice and its effect on pharmacokinetics and pharmacodynamics of felodipine in healthy subjects. *Eur J Clin Pharmacol.* 1995;49:61-67.

Bailey DG, et al. Grapefruit juice and naringin interaction with nitrendipine. *Clin Pharmacol Ther.* 1992;51:156.

Soons PA, et al. Grapefruit juice and cimetidine inhibit stereoselective metabolism of nitrendipine in humans. *Clin Pharmacol Ther.* 1991;50:394-403.

Bailey DG, et al. Effect of grapefruit juice and naringin on nisoldipine pharmacokinetics. *Clin Pharmacol Ther.* 1993;54:589-594.

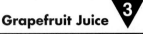

Grapefruit Juice

Nimodipine (*Nimotop*)

SUMMARY: Grapefruit juice increases the plasma concentration of nimodipine; increased pharmacodynamic effects may occur.

RISK FACTORS: No specific risk factors are known.

RELATED DRUGS: Other calcium channel blockers including felodipine (*Plendil*), nitrendipine (*Baypress*), and nifedipine (eg, *Procardia*) are similarly affected by grapefruit juice. Orange juice does not affect CYP3A4 activity in the intestinal wall. Grapefruit juice has little effect on amlodipine (eg, *Norvasc*).

MANAGEMENT OPTIONS:

➡ *Consider Alternative.* Advise patients receiving nimodipine to avoid drinking grapefruit juice. Substitute with orange juice or another fruit juice.

➡ *Monitor.* Monitor patients who are taking nimodipine and ingest grapefruit juice for increased hypotensive effects and possible side effects such as headache.

REFERENCES:

Fuhr U, et al. Grapefruit juice increases oral nimodipine bioavailability. *Int J Clin Pharmacol Ther.* 1998;36:126.

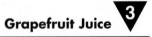

Grapefruit Juice

Nisoldipine (*Sular*)

SUMMARY: Grapefruit juice administered just before or with nisoldipine increases the plasma concentration and pharmacodynamic effect of nisoldipine.

RISK FACTORS: No specific risk factors are known.

RELATED DRUGS: Other calcium channel blockers are likely to be affected by grapefruit juice in a similar manner.

MANAGEMENT OPTIONS:

➡ *Consider Alternative.* Orange juice could be substituted for grapefruit juice to avoid the interaction. Calcium channel blockers with low first-pass metabolism such as amlodipine (*Norvasc*) will be less affected by grapefruit juice.

➡ *Monitor.* Watch for increased hypotensive effects or side effects (eg, headache, hypotension) when patients taking calcium channel blockers consume grapefruit juice.

REFERENCES:

Azuma J, et al. Effects of grapefruit juice on the pharmacokinetics of the calcium channel blockers nifedipine and nisoldipine. *Curr Ther Res.* 1998;59:619.

Grapefruit Juice

Sildenafil (*Viagra*)

SUMMARY: Study in healthy subjects suggests that grapefruit juice modestly increases sildenafil plasma concentrations, but large increases may be seen in some patients. Grapefruit juice also may slow the onset of sildenafil effect.

RISK FACTORS: No specific risk factors are known.

RELATED DRUGS: No information is available.

MANAGEMENT OPTIONS:

➡ ***Circumvent/Minimize.*** Patients who take sildenafil should probably avoid grapefruit juice completely.

REFERENCES:

Jetter A, et al. Effects of grapefruit juice on the pharmacokinetics of sildenafil. *Clin Pharmacol Ther.* 2002;71:21-29.

Grapefruit Juice

Simvastatin (*Zocor*)

SUMMARY: Repeated doses of grapefruit juice markedly increased simvastatin serum concentrations in healthy subjects.

RISK FACTORS: No specific risk factors are known.

RELATED DRUGS: Lovastatin (eg, *Mevacor*), like simvastatin, undergoes extensive first-pass metabolism in the gut wall and liver; it is similarly affected by grapefruit juice. Atorvastatin (*Lipitor*) is also metabolized by CYP3A4, and would be expected to interact with grapefruit juice (but to a lesser extent than lovastatin and simvastatin). Pravastatin (*Pravachol*) and fluvastatin (*Lescol*) are not metabolized by CYP3A4 and are not likely to be affected by grapefruit juice.

MANAGEMENT OPTIONS:

➡ ***Consider Alternative.*** Orange juice does not inhibit CYP3A4, and would not be expected to interact with simvastatin.

➡ ***Circumvent/Minimize.*** Patients taking simvastatin should ingest grapefruit juice only occasionally.

REFERENCES:

Lilja JJ, et al. Grapefruit juice-simvastatin interaction: effect on serum concentrations of simvastatin, simvastatin acid, and HMG-CoA reductase inhibitors. *Clin Pharmacol Ther.* 1998;64:477-483.

Kantola T, et al. Grapefruit juice greatly increases serum concentrations of lovastatin and lovastatin acid. *Clin Pharmacol Ther.* 1998;63:397-402.

Grapefruit Juice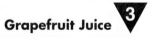

Terfenadine†

SUMMARY: Grapefruit juice increases the amount of oral terfenadine reaching the systemic circulation intact. Although the clinical importance of this effect is not established, it is possible that the risk of cardiac arrhythmias is increased in predisposed individuals.

RISK FACTORS: No specific risk factors are known.

RELATED DRUGS: Astemizole† is likely to interact with grapefruit juice in a similar manner, but one would not expect adverse effects with grapefruit juice given with the nonsedating antihistamines, loratadine (*Claritin*), and fexofenadine (*Allegra*), or the low-sedating agent, cetirizine (*Zyrtec*).

MANAGEMENT OPTIONS:

➡ *Circumvent/Minimize.* Although the clinical significance of this interaction is not established, given the potentially serious nature of the adverse effect, it would be prudent to warn patients to avoid grapefruit products while taking terfenadine or astemizole.

➡ *Monitor.* If terfenadine or astemizole is taken with grapefruit, monitor for evidence of ventricular arrhythmias (eg, syncope, palpitations).

REFERENCES:

Benton RE, et al. Grapefruit juice alters terfenadine pharmacokinetics, resulting in prolongation of repolarization on the electrocardiogram. *Clin Pharmacol Ther.* 1996;59:383-388.

Honig PK, et al. Grapefruit juice alters the systemic bioavailability and cardiac repolarization of terfenadine in poor metabolizers of terfenadine. *J Clin Pharmacol.* 1996;36:345-351.

† Not available in the US.

Grapefruit Juice

Triazolam (eg, *Halcion*)

SUMMARY: Grapefruit juice increases triazolam serum concentrations. Although the clinical importance of this effect is not established, it seems likely that some patients would be adversely affected.

RISK FACTORS:

➡ *Effects of Age.* The elderly are known to be more sensitive to triazolam and are likely to be at greater risk from this interaction.

RELATED DRUGS: Alprazolam (*Xanax*) and midazolam (*Versed*) are metabolized by CYP3A4. When given orally, they would be expected to interact with grapefruit juice. Diazepam (*Valium*) is partially metabolized by CYP3A4, but would not be expected to interact to the same degree. Most other benzodiazepines are metabolized primarily by enzymes other than CYP3A4 and would not be expected to interact.

MANAGEMENT OPTIONS:

➡ *Consider Alternative.* Orange juice does not appear to inhibit CYP3A4 and would not be expected to interact with triazolam. Also, one could use a benzodiazepine other than triazolam, alprazolam, or midazolam such as diazepam.

➡ *Circumvent/Minimize.* Warn patients on triazolam to avoid taking it with or within several hours after grapefruit. Ingesting grapefruit in the morning and taking the triazolam in the evening theoretically would minimize the interaction, but there may still be a small effect.

➡ *Monitor.* If the combination is used, be alert for excessive triazolam effect (eg, drowsiness).

REFERENCES:

Hukkinen SK, et al. Plasma concentrations of triazolam are increased by concomitant ingestion of grapefruit juice. *Clin Pharmacol Ther.* 1995;58:127-131.

Vanakoski J, et al. Grapefruit juice does not enhance the effects of midazolam and triazolam in man. *Eur J Clin Pharmacol.* 1996;50:501-508.

Griseofulvin (eg, *Grisactin*)

Contraceptives, Oral (eg, *Ortho-Novum*)

SUMMARY: Griseofulvin may induce menstrual irregularities or increase the risk of pregnancy in women taking oral contraceptives.

RISK FACTORS: No specific risk factors are known.

RELATED DRUGS: Other antifungal agents may affect oral contraceptives similarly.

MANAGEMENT OPTIONS:

➡ *Circumvent/Minimize.* Patients on low-estrogen oral contraceptives may need a contraceptive with a higher estrogen dose when taking griseofulvin.

➡ *Monitor.* Women taking oral contraceptives should consider using additional contraceptives during and for 1 cycle after griseofulvin therapy. The development of menstrual irregularities (eg, spotting, breakthrough bleeding) may indicate that the interaction is occurring and warrants particular caution.

REFERENCES:

Van Dijke CPH, et al. Interaction between oral contraceptives and griseofulvin. *Br Med J.* 1984;228:1125.

McDaniel PA, et al. Oral contraceptives and griseofulvin interaction. *Drug Intell Clin Pharm.* 1986;20:384.

Griseofulvin (eg, *Grisactin*)

Phenobarbital (eg, *Solfoton*)

SUMMARY: Phenobarbital may reduce the serum concentration of griseofulvin, but the clinical significance of this effect is not established.

RISK FACTORS: No specific risk factors are known.

RELATED DRUGS: Other barbiturates may produce a similar reaction with griseofulvin or other antifungal agents.

MANAGEMENT OPTIONS:

➡ *Circumvent/Minimize.* It has been suggested that divided griseofulvin doses (eg, 3 times/day) may be absorbed better than larger doses taken less often.

➡ *Monitor.* Until further information is available, monitor patients for lack of griseo-fulvin efficacy. Whether an increase in the daily dosage of griseofulvin is warranted when phenobarbital is coadministered requires further study.

REFERENCES:

Riegelman S, et al. Griseofulvin-phenobarbital interaction in man. *JAMA.* 1970;213:426.

Busfield D, et al. An effect of phenobarbitone on blood levels of griseofulvin in man. *Lancet.* 1963;2:1042.

Lorenc E. A new factor in griseofulvin treatment failures. *Missouri Med.* 1967;64:32.

Griseofulvin (eg, *Grisactin*)

Warfarin (eg, *Coumadin*)

SUMMARY: Griseofulvin appears to inhibit the hypoprothrombinemic response to warfarin and possibly other oral anti-coagulants. An adjustment in the oral anticoagulant dose may be required in patients receiving both drugs.

RISK FACTORS:

➡ *Dosage Regimen.* Some evidence suggests that the effect of griseofulvin on warfarin is very gradual, so it may take several weeks or longer for the maximal effect to be seen.

RELATED DRUGS: Little is known regarding the effect of griseofulvin on oral anticoagulants other than warfarin; however, assume that an interaction exists until information to the contrary appears.

MANAGEMENT OPTIONS:

➡ *Monitor.* Monitor for altered oral anticoagulant effect if griseofulvin is initiated, discontinued, or changed in dosage. Since the effect of griseofulvin may be very gradual, monitor the hypoprothrombinemic response until it is stable, adjusting the anticoagulant dose as needed.

REFERENCES:

Cullen SI, et al. Griseofulvin-warfarin antagonism. *JAMA.* 1967;199:582.

Okino K, et al. Warfarin-griseofulvin interaction. *Drug Intell Clin Pharm.* 1986;20:291.

Udall JA. Drug interference with warfarin therapy. *Clin Med.* 1970;77:20.

Guanethidine (*Ismelin*)

Haloperidol (eg, *Haldol*)

SUMMARY: Haloperidol has been associated with inhibition of the antihypertensive effect of guanethidine in a few patients.

RISK FACTORS: No specific risk factors are known.

RELATED DRUGS: Guanadrel (*Hylorel*) is pharmacologically similar to guanethidine and also may be inhibited by haloperidol.

MANAGEMENT OPTIONS:

➡ *Consider Alternative.* Consider using an antihypertensive other than guanethidine (or drugs related to guanethidine such as guanadrel).

➡ **Monitor.** If the combination is used, monitor blood pressure for inhibition of antihypertensive effect. Increasing the guanethidine dose may overcome the interaction.

REFERENCES:

Janowsky DS, et al. Antagonism of guanethidine by chlorpromazine. *Am J Psychiatry*. 1973;130:808.

Guanethidine (*Ismelin*)

Methylphenidate (eg, *Ritalin*)

SUMMARY: Methylphenidate appears to inhibit the antihypertensive effect of guanethidine.

RISK FACTORS: No specific risk factors are known.

RELATED DRUGS: Guanadrel (*Hylorel*) is pharmacologically similar to guanethidine and also may be inhibited by methylphenidate.

MANAGEMENT OPTIONS:

➡ **Consider Alternative.** Consider using antihypertensive agents other than guanethidine or guanadrel in patients who require methylphenidate therapy.

➡ **Monitor.** If the combination is used, monitor blood pressure and heart rate.

REFERENCES:

Day MD, et al. Antagonism of guanethidine and bretylium by various agents. *Lancet*. 1962;2:1282.

Gulati OD, et al. Antagonism of adrenergic neuron blockade in hypertensive subjects. *Clin Pharmacol Ther*. 1966;7:510.

Deshmankar BS, et al. Ventricular tachycardia associated with the administration of methylphenidate during guanethidine therapy. *Can Med Assoc J*. 1967;97:1166.

Guanethidine (eg, *Ismelin*)

Norepinephrine (*Levophed*)

SUMMARY: Patients on guanethidine have an exaggerated pressor response to norepinephrine.

RISK FACTORS: No specific risk factors are known.

RELATED DRUGS: Guanadrel (*Hylorel*) is pharmacologically similar to guanethidine and also may enhance the pressor response to norepinephrine.

MANAGEMENT OPTIONS:

➡ **Monitor.** In patients receiving guanethidine or guanadrel, use conservative doses of norepinephrine (and other sympathomimetics); monitor blood pressure carefully.

REFERENCES:

Muelheims GH, et al. Increased sensitivity of the heart to catecholamine-induced arrhythmias following guanethidine. *Clin Pharmacol Ther*. 1965;6:757.

Dollery CT. Physiological and pharmacological interactions of antihypertensive drugs. *Proc R Soc Med*. 1965;58:983.

Guanethidine (*Ismelin*)

Phenelzine (*Nardil*)

SUMMARY: Monoamine oxidase inhibitors (MAOIs) may inhibit the antihypertensive response to guanethidine.

RISK FACTORS: No specific risk factors known.

RELATED DRUGS: All nonselective MAOIs including isocarboxazid (*Marplan*) and tranylcypromine (*Parnate*) would be expected to inhibit guanethidine effect. Guanadrel (*Hylorel*) is pharmacologically similar to guanethidine and also may be inhibited by MAOIs.

MANAGEMENT OPTIONS:

➡ **Monitor.** Until more information is available, watch patients receiving guanethidine for hypertension if an MAOI is administered. Watch patients receiving MAOI therapy for a pressor response upon initiation of guanethidine therapy. Assume the effects of nonselective MAOIs to persist for 2 weeks after they are discontinued.

REFERENCES:

Day MD, et al. Antagonism of guanethidine and bretylium by various agents. *Lancet*. 1962;2:1282.

Gulati OD, et al. Antagonism of adrenergic neuron blockade in hypertensive subjects. *Clin Pharmacol Ther*. 1966;7:510.

Goldberg LI. Monoamine oxidase inhibitors: adverse reactions and possible mechanisms. *JAMA*. 1964;190:456.

Esbenshade JH Jr, et al. A long-term evaluation of pargyline hydrochloride in hypertension. *Am J Med Sci*. 1966;251:119.

Guanethidine (*Ismelin*)

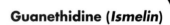

Phenylephrine (*Neo-Synephrine*)

SUMMARY: Guanethidine enhances the pupillary response to phenylephrine; other phenylephrine effects also might be enhanced.

RISK FACTORS: No specific risk factors known.

RELATED DRUGS: Guanadrel (*Hylorel*) is pharmacologically similar to guanethidine and also may interact with phenylephrine.

MANAGEMENT OPTIONS:

➡ **Monitor.** Monitor for excessive phenylephrine response in patients receiving guanethidine; adjust phenylephrine dose as needed.

REFERENCES:

Jablonski J. Guanethidine (*Ismelin*) as an adjuvant in pharmacological mydriasis. *Ophthalmologica*. 1974;168:27.

Sneddon JM, et al. The interactions of local guanethidine and sympathomimetic amines in the human eye. *Arch Ophthamol*. 1969;81:622.

Cooper B. Neo-Synephrine (10%) eye drops. *Med J Aust*. 1968;2:420.

▼ Guanethidine (*Ismelin*)

Thiothixene (eg, *Navane*)

SUMMARY: Thiothixene appeared to substantially inhibit the antihypertensive response to guanethidine in one patient; other neuroleptics may have a similar effect.

RISK FACTORS: No specific risk factors are known.

RELATED DRUGS: The effect of another thioxanthine, chlorprothixene[†], on guanethidine is not established, but it may interact in a similar way. Guanadrel (*Hylorel*) is pharmacologically similar to guanethidine and also may be inhibited by thiothixene.

MANAGEMENT OPTIONS:

➡ *Monitor.* Although evidence for an interaction is scanty at present, patients on guanethidine therapy might be watched more closely for a decreased antihypertensive response if thioxanthines also are prescribed.

REFERENCES:

Janowsky DS, et al. Antagonism of guanethidine by chlorpromazine. *Am J Psychiatry*. 1973;130:808.

† Not available in the US.

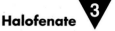

Halofenate

Tolbutamide (eg, *Orinase*)

SUMMARY: Halofenate appears to increase the serum concentrations of tolbutamide and reduce blood glucose concentrations.

RISK FACTORS: No specific risk factors are known.

RELATED DRUGS: Chlorpropamide interacts similarly.

MANAGEMENT OPTIONS:

➡ ***Monitor.*** Concomitant use of halofenate and oral hypoglycemics need not be avoided; however, alert patients to the need for blood glucose monitoring and the possible necessity of altering dosages of hypoglycemic agents when halofenate is taken concurrently.

REFERENCES:

Jain AK, et al. Potentiation of hypoglycemic effect of sulfonylureas by halofenate. *N Engl J Med.* 1975;293:1283.

Kudzma DJ, et al. Potentiation of hypoglycemic effect of chlorpropamide and phenformin by halofenate. *Diabetes.* 1977;26:291.

Haloperidol (eg, *Haldol*)

Indomethacin (eg, *Indocin*)

SUMMARY: A preliminary study suggested that the combination of indomethacin and haloperidol resulted in a high incidence of adverse effects such as drowsiness, tiredness, and confusion compared with indomethacin alone, but the role of drug interaction in the reactions was not established.

RISK FACTORS: No specific risk factors are known.

RELATED DRUGS: It is unknown whether other combinations of nonsteroidal anti-inflammatory drugs (NSAIDs) and neuroleptics would result in a higher incidence of adverse effects over either agent alone. Since indomethacin alone has a relatively high incidence of adverse CNS effects compared with most other NSAIDs, it may be that NSAIDs other than indomethacin would be less likely to produce such effects when combined with haloperidol.

MANAGEMENT OPTIONS:

➡ ***Monitor.*** Monistor patients receiving indomethacin and haloperidol for adverse effects such as drowsiness and confusion. If such effects are observed, consider the use of an NSAID other than indomethacin or a neuroleptic other than haloperidol.

REFERENCES:

Bird HA, et al. Drowsiness due to haloperidol/indomethacin in combination. *Lancet.* 1983;1:830.

Haloperidol (eg, *Haldol*)

Lithium (eg, *Eskalith*)

SUMMARY: A number of patients have developed severe neurotoxic extrapyramidal symptoms while receiving lithium and haloperidol, but many other patients have received the combination without such adverse effects.

RISK FACTORS:

➡ *Other Drugs.* Concurrent use of anticholinergic antiparkinsonian drugs can increase the risk.

➡ *Concurrent Diseases.* Presence of acute mania; pre-existing brain damage; the presence of other physiologic disturbances such as infection, fever, or dehydration; or a history of extrapyramidal symptoms with neuroleptic therapy alone can increase the risk of an interaction occurring.

➡ *Dosage Regimen.* Large doses of one or both drugs and failure to discontinue drugs when adverse effects occur can increase the risk of an interaction.

RELATED DRUGS: No information available.

MANAGEMENT OPTIONS:

➡ *Circumvent/Minimize.* It has been recommended that neuroleptics such as haloperidol be used alone for initial control of acute mania symptoms and that lithium be added as the neuroleptic dosage is reduced. Avoid excessive doses of either agent.

➡ *Monitor.* If haloperidol and lithium are used concomitantly, monitor carefully for signs of neurotoxicity, particularly in the presence of one or more of the risk factors described above.

REFERENCES:

Geisler A, et al. Combined effect of lithium and flupenthixol on striatal adenylate cyclase. *Lancet.* 1977;1:430.

Cohen WF, et al. Lithium carbonate, haloperidol and irreversible brain damage. *JAMA.* 1974;230:1283.

Spring G, Frankel M. New data on lithium and haloperidol incompatibility. *Am J Psychiatry.* 1981;138:818.

Kamlana SH, et al. Lithium: some drug interactions. *Practitioner.* 1980;224:1291.

Louden JB, et al. Toxic reactions to lithium and haloperidol. *Lancet.* 1976;2:1088.

Strayhorn JM, et al. Severe neurotoxicity despite "therapeutic" serum lithium levels. *Dis Nerv Syst.* 1977;38:107.

Fetzer J, et al. Lithium encephalopathy: a clinical, psychiatric, and EEG evaluation. *Am J Psychiatry.* 1981;138:1622.

Thomas CJ. Brain damage with lithium/haloperidol. *Br J Psychiatry.* 1979;134:552.

Thornton WE, et al. Lithium intoxication: a report of two cases. *Can Psychiatr Assoc J.* 1975;20:281.

Thomas C, et al. Lithium/haloperidol combinations and brain damage. *Lancet.* 1982;1:626.

Baastrup P, et al. Adverse reactions in treatment with lithium carbonate and haloperidol. *JAMA.* 1976;236:2645.

Juhl RP, et al. Concomitant administration of haloperidol and lithium carbonate in acute mania. *Dis Nerv Syst.* 1977;38:675.

Carman JS, et al. Lithium combined with neuroleptics in chronic schizophrenic and schizoaffective patients. *J Clin Psychiatry.* 1981;42:124.

Biederman J, et al. Combination of lithium carbonate and haloperidol in schizo-affective disorder. *Arch Gen Psychiatry.* 1979;36:327.

Tupin JP, et al. Lithium and haloperidol incompatibility reviewed. *Psychiat J Univ Ottawa.* 1978;3:245.

Haloperidol (eg, *Haldol*)

Quinidine (eg, *Quinora*)

SUMMARY: Quinidine administration increases haloperidol concentrations, potentially increasing the risk of haloperidol toxicity.

RISK FACTORS: No specific risk factors are known.

RELATED DRUGS: No information is available.

MANAGEMENT OPTIONS:

➡ *Monitor.* Until further studies are available, patients taking haloperidol should be monitored for extrapyramidal symptoms, sedation, and hypotension if quinidine is co-administered.

REFERENCES:

Young D, et al. Effect of quinidine on the interconversion kinetics between haloperidol and reduced haloperidol in humans: implications for the involvement of cytochrome P450IID6. *Eur J Clin Pharmacol.* 1993;44:433.

Heparin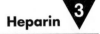

Warfarin (eg, *Coumadin*)

SUMMARY: Warfarin may prolong the activated partial thromboplastin time (aPTT) in patients receiving heparin, and heparin may prolong the prothrombin time (PT) in patients receiving warfarin. These effects should be considered when assessing the anticoagulant effect of each agent.

RISK FACTORS: No specific risk factors known.

RELATED DRUGS: All oral anticoagulants probably interact with heparin in a similar way.

MANAGEMENT OPTIONS:

➡ *Monitor.* In patients receiving both heparin and an oral anticoagulant, monitor for oral anticoagulant-induced increases in aPTT. To minimize the interference of heparin with PT determinations, blood samples for PTs should not be drawn within about 5 or 6 hours of bolus IV heparin administration.

REFERENCES:

Moser KM, et al. Effect of heparin on the one-stage prothrombin time: source of artifactual "resistance" to prothrombinopenic therapy. *Ann Intern Med.* 1967;66:1207.

Mungall D, et al. Bayesian forecasting of APTT response to continuously infused heparin with and without warfarin administration. *J Clin Pharmacol.* 1989;29:1043.

Hauser VM, et al. Effect of warfarin on the activated partial thromboplastin time. *Drug Intell Clin Pharm.* 1986;2:964.

Hexobarbital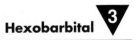

Rifampin (eg, *Rifadin*)

SUMMARY: Hexobarbital serum concentrations are reduced by the administration of rifampin.

RISK FACTORS: No specific risk factors are known.

RELATED DRUGS: The effect of rifampin administration on the disposition of other barbiturates has not been established, but it is possible that they are similarly affected by rifampin.

MANAGEMENT OPTIONS:

➡ **Monitor.** Watch for reduced barbiturate effect. It does not seem necessary to avoid concomitant use of rifampin and barbiturates. However, when patients fail to respond to barbiturates, consider rifampin a potential cause if it is being taken concurrently.

REFERENCES:

Zilly W, et al. Induction of drug metabolism in man after rifampicin treatment measured by increased hexobarbital and tolbutamide clearance. *Eur J Clin Pharmacol.* 1975;9:219-227.

Miguet JP, et al. Induction of hepatic microsomal enzymes after brief administration of rifampicin in man. *Gastroenterology.* 1977;72(5 pt 1):924-926.

Breimer DD, et al. Influence of rifampicin on drug metabolism: differences between hexobarbital and antipyrine. *Clin Pharmacol Ther.* 1977;21:470-481.

Zilly W, et al. Stimulation of drug metabolism by rifampicin in patients with cirrhosis or cholestasis measured by increased hexobarbital and tolbutamide clearance. *Eur J Clin Pharmacol.* 1977;11:287-293.

Smith DA, et al. Age-dependent stereoselective increase in the oral clearance of hexobarbitone isomers caused by rifampicin. *Br J Clin Pharmacol.* 1991;32:735-739.

Hydralazine (eg, *Apresoline*)

Indomethacin (eg, *Indocin*)

SUMMARY: Indomethacin has been shown to inhibit the antihypertensive response to hydralazine in healthy subjects.

RISK FACTORS: No specific risk factors are known.

RELATED DRUGS: Nonsteroidal anti-inflammatory drugs (NSAIDs) other than indomethacin would be expected to produce a similar effect.

MANAGEMENT OPTIONS:

➡ **Monitor.** Monitor for a reduced antihypertensive response when indomethacin or other NSAIDs are given with hydralazine.

REFERENCES:

Cinquegrani MP, et al. Indomethacin attenuates the hypotensive action of hydralazine. *Clin Pharmacol Ther.* 1986;39:564-570.

Jackson SH, et al. Indomethacin does not attenuate the effects of hydralazine in normal subjects. *Eur J Clin Pharmacol.* 1983;25:303-305.

Ibuprofen (eg, *Motrin*)

Lithium (eg, *Eskalith*)

SUMMARY: Ibuprofen increases lithium serum concentrations and may increase the risk of lithium toxicity; the magnitude of the effect appears to vary considerably from patient to patient.

RISK FACTORS:

➡ *Effects of Age.* It has been proposed that older patients may be more susceptible to the interaction; if that is true, it may explain the difference in the magnitude of the interaction noted in the studies.

RELATED DRUGS: Most NSAIDs increase lithium serum concentrations, but sulindac (eg, *Clinoril*) and aspirin appear to have minimal effects.

MANAGEMENT OPTIONS:

➡ *Consider Alternative.* If appropriate for the patient, consider using an anti-inflammatory agent that is less likely to affect lithium, such as sulindac or aspirin.

➡ *Circumvent/Minimize.* Advise patients receiving lithium to avoid ibuprofen-containing products unless approved by the prescriber.

➡ *Monitor.* If ibuprofen therapy is initiated, monitor for lithium toxicity (eg, nausea, vomiting, diarrhea, anorexia, coarse tremor, slurred speech, vertigo, confusion, lethargy; in severe cases, seizures, stupor, coma, cardiovascular collapse) and elevated serum lithium concentrations. In a patient stabilized on lithium and an NSAID, discontinuation of the NSAID may result in inadequate serum lithium concentrations.

REFERENCES:
Ragheb M, et al. Ibuprofen can increase serum lithium level in lithium-treated patients. *J Clin Psychiatry.* 1987;48:161.

Ragheb M, et al. Interaction of indomethacin and ibuprofen with lithium in manic patients under a steady-state lithium level. *J Clin Psychiatry.* 1980;41:397.

Kristoff CA, et al. Effect of ibuprofen on lithium plasma and red blood cell concentrations. *Clin Pharm.* 1986;5:51.

Ibuprofen (eg, *Motrin*)

Methotrexate (eg, *Rheumatrex*)

SUMMARY: Ibuprofen has been reported to increase the serum concentrations of methotrexate, but this has not been a consistent finding. It is not known how often this would result in adverse effects.

RISK FACTORS: No specific risk factors are known.

RELATED DRUGS: Several NSAIDs and aspirin have been shown to increase methotrexate plasma concentrations. Acetaminophen (eg, *Tylenol*) has not been shown to affect methotrexate response.

MANAGEMENT OPTIONS:

➡ *Consider Alternative.* Until more information is available on this interaction, it would be prudent to avoid ibuprofen (as well as other NSAIDs) in patients receiving antineoplastic doses of methotrexate.

➡ *Monitor.* If methotrexate and ibuprofen are used concurrently, observe the patient for signs of methotrexate toxicity including mucosal ulceration, renal dysfunction, and blood dyscrasias. Decreasing the methotrexate dosage may be required.

REFERENCES:

Tracy TS, et al. The effect of NSAIDs on methotrexate disposition in patients with rheumatoid arthritis. *Clin Pharmacol Ther.* 1990;47:138.

Skeith KJ, et al. Lack of significant interaction between low dose methotrexate and ibuprofen or flurbi-profen in patients with arthritis. *J Rheumatol.* 1990;17:1008.

 Ibuprofen (eg, *Motrin*)

Warfarin (eg, *Coumadin*)

SUMMARY: Ibuprofen does not appear to affect the hypoprothrombinemic response to warfarin or phenprocoumon, but cotherapy requires caution because of possible detrimental effects of ibuprofen on the gastric mucosa and platelet function.

RISK FACTORS:

➡ *Concurrent Diseases.* Patients with peptic ulcer disease (PUD) or a history of gastro-intestinal (GI) bleeding are probably at greater risk for this interaction.

RELATED DRUGS: Phenprocoumon interacts similarly. All NSAIDs inhibit platelet func-tion, cause gastric erosions, and probably increase the risk of GI bleeding.

MANAGEMENT OPTIONS:

➡ *Avoid Unless Benefit Outweighs Risk.* Since all NSAIDs probably increase the risk of GI bleeding in patients on oral anticoagulants, use the combination only after careful consideration of the benefit versus risk. If the NSAID is being used as an analge-sic or antipyretic, acetaminophen is probably safer to use with oral anticoagulants. Nonacetylated salicylates (eg, choline salicylate, magnesium salicylate, salsalate, sodium salicylate) also are probably safer with oral anticoagulants than NSAIDs since they have minimal effects on platelet function and the gastric mucosa.

➡ *Monitor.* If any NSAID is used with an oral anticoagulant, one should monitor the prothrombin time carefully and watch for evidence of bleeding, especially from the GI tract.

REFERENCES:

Boekhout-Mussert MJ, et al. Influence of ibuprofen on oral anticoagulation with phenprocoumon. *J Int Med Res.* 1974;2:279.

Thilo D, et al. A study of the effects of the anti-rheumatic drug ibuprofen (*Rufen*) on patients being treated with the oral anticoagulant phenprocoumon (*Marcoumar*). *J Int Med Res.* 1974;2:276.

Penner JA, et al. Lack of interaction between ibuprofen and warfarin. *Curr Ther Res.* 1975;18:862.

McQueen EG. New Zealand committee on adverse drug reactions: tenth annual report, 1975. *N Z Med J.* 1975;82:308.

Shorr RI, et al. Concurrent use of nonsteroidal anti-inflammatory drugs and oral anticoagulants places elderly persons at high risk for hemorrhagic peptic ulcer disease. *Arch Intern Med.* 1993;153:1665.

Imipenem (*Primaxin*)

Theophylline (eg, *Theo-Dur*)

SUMMARY: Several patients receiving theophylline developed generalized seizures following the addition of imipenem, but more study is needed to establish a causal relationship.

RISK FACTORS: No specific risk factors are known.

RELATED DRUGS: No information is available.

MANAGEMENT OPTIONS:

➡ ***Circumvent/Minimize.*** Patients with reduced renal function should have appropriate imipenem dosage adjustments to avoid potentially toxic concentrations.

➡ ***Monitor.*** Until more information is known about this interaction, practitioners should monitor patients for appropriate theophylline and imipenem dosage. Be alert for signs of CNS stimulation or seizures.

REFERENCES:

Semel JD, et al. Seizures in patients simultaneously receiving theophylline and imipenem or ciprofloxacin or metronidazole. *South Med J*. 1991;84:465.

Imipramine (eg, *Tofranil*)

Norepinephrine (eg, *Levophed*)

SUMMARY: Imipramine and other tricyclic antidepressants can markedly enhance the pressor response to norepinephrine.

RISK FACTORS: No specific risk factors are known.

RELATED DRUGS: Desipramine, amitriptyline, and protriptyline interact similarly. Assume that all TCAs will interact with norepinephrine until proven otherwise.

MANAGEMENT OPTIONS:

➡ ***Avoid Unless Benefit Outweighs Risk.*** If IV norepinephrine is used, begin with conservative doses.

➡ ***Monitor.*** Monitor blood pressure carefully if the combination is used.

REFERENCES:

Boakes AJ, et al. Interactions between sympathomimetic amines and antidepressant agents in man. *Br Med J*. 1973;1:311.

Mitchell JR, et al. Guanethidine and related agents. III. Antagonism by drugs which inhibit the norepinephrine pump in man. *J Clin Invest*. 1970;49:1596.

Svedmyr N. The influence of a tricyclic antidepressant agent (protriptyline) on some of the circulatory effects of noradrenaline and adrenaline in man. *Life Sci*. 1968;7:77.

Boakes AJ. Sympathomimetic amines and antidepressant agents. *Br Med J*. 1973;2:114. Letter.

Ghose K. Sympathomimetic amines and tricyclic antidepressant drugs. *Neuropharmacology*. 1980;19:1251.

2 Imipramine (eg, *Tofranil*)

Phenelzine (*Nardil*)

SUMMARY: Severe reactions have occurred in patients receiving combined therapy with tricyclic antidepressants (TCAs) and phenelzine or other nonselective monoamine oxidase inhibitors (MAOIs), but some combinations can be used safely with appropriate precautions.

RISK FACTORS:

➥ *Dosage Regimen.* Large doses of one or both drugs appear to increase the risk.

➥ *Order of Drug Administration.* Most reactions occurred when the cyclic agent was added to established MAOI therapy.

RELATED DRUGS: Antidepressants that inhibit serotonin reuptake such as clomipramine (eg, *Anafranil*), amitriptyline (eg, *Elavil*), desipramine (eg, *Norpramin*), and trazodone (eg, *Desyrel*) may be more likely to result in serotonin syndrome than other tricyclic antidepressants.

MANAGEMENT OPTIONS:

➥ *Avoid Unless Benefit Outweighs Risk.* Some MAOIs and some tricyclics can be used together; however, when cotherapy is contemplated, any possible benefit of the combination should be weighed against the potential hazards. Moreover, it should be noted that the product information for both MAOIs and TCAs states that concurrent use is contraindicated, which may have medicolegal implications. Finally, be aware that a potentially lethal combination (in overdose) will be at the disposal of suicide-prone patients.

➥ *Monitor.* If the combination is used, monitor for evidence of excitation, fever, mania, seizures, or other unexpected adverse effects.

REFERENCES:

Kline NS. Experimental use of monoamine oxidase inhibitors with tricyclic antidepressants (Questions and Answers). *JAMA.* 1974;227:807.

De La Fuente RJ, et al. Mania induced by tricyclic-MAOI combination therapy in bipolar treatment-resistant disorder: case reports. *J Clin Psychiatry.* 1986;47:40.

Beaumont G. Drug interactions with clomipramine (Anafranil). *J Int Med Res.* 1973;1:480.

White K, et al. The combined use of MAOIs and tricyclics. *J Clin Psychiatry.* 1984;45:67.

Winston F. Combined antidepressant therapy. *Br J Psychiatry.* 1971;118:301.

Schuckit U et al. Tricyclic antidepressants and monoamine oxidase inhibitors. Combination therapy in the treatment of depression. *Arch Gen Psychiatry.* 1971;24:509.

Spiker DG, et al. Combining tricyclic and monoamine oxidase inhibitor antidepressants. *Arch Gen Psychiatry.* 1976;33:828.

Ananth J, et al. A review of combined tricyclic and MAOI therapy. *Compr Psychiatry.* 1977;18:221.

White K. Tricyclic overdose in a patient given combined tricyclic MAOI treatment. *Am J Psychiatry.* 1978;135:1411.

Young JPR, et al. Controlled trial of trimipramine, monoamine oxidase inhibitors, and combined treatment in depressed outpatients. *Br Med J.* 1979;2:1315.

White K. Combined tricyclic and monoamine-oxidase inhibitor antidepressant treatment. *West J Med.* 1983;138:406.

Tackley RM, et al. Fatal disseminated intravascular coagulation following a monoamine oxidase inhibitor/tricyclic interaction. *Anaesthesia.* 1987;42:760.

Imipramine (eg, *Tofranil*)

Phenylephrine (eg, *Neo-Synephrine*)

SUMMARY: Imipramine and possibly other tricyclic antidepressants (TCAs) may enhance the pressor response to IV phenylephrine; the effect on oral or nasal phenylephrine is not established.

RISK FACTORS: No specific risk factors are known.

RELATED DRUGS: Until additional information is available, assume that other TCAs would produce a similar effect if combined with IV phenylephrine.

MANAGEMENT OPTIONS:

➡ *Monitor.* Patients receiving TCAs should be given parenteral phenylephrine only with caution and careful monitoring of the blood pressure. Until additional information is available, be alert for enhanced pressor responses to oral phenylephrine.

REFERENCES:

Boakes AJ, et al. Interactions between sympathomimetic amines and antidepressant agents in man. *BMJ.* 1973;1:311-315.

Boakes AJ. Sympathomimetic amines and antidepressant agents. *BMJ.* 1973;2:114. Letter.

Imipramine (eg, *Tofranil*)

Quinidine (eg, *Quinora*)

SUMMARY: Quinidine markedly increases imipramine and desipramine serum concentrations; toxicity may result.

RISK FACTORS:

➡ *Pharmacogenetics.* Extensive metabolizers of the antidepressants are at greater risk.

RELATED DRUGS: Desipramine and nortriptyline concentrations are increased by quinidine. Other cyclic antidepressants may be affected by this interaction but little clinical information is available.

MANAGEMENT OPTIONS:

➡ *Monitor.* Monitor patients maintained on cyclic antidepressants for increased side effects (eg, sedation, arrhythmia, confusion) if quinidine is added to their drug therapy.

REFERENCES:

Steiner E, et al. Inhibition of desipramine 2-hydroxylation by quinidine and quinine. *Clin Pharmacol Ther.* 1988;43:577.

Brosen K, et al. Quinidine inhibits the 2-hydroxylation of imipramine and desipramine but not the demethylation of imipramine. *Eur J Clin Pharmacol.* 1989;37:155.

Pfandl B, et al. Stereoselective inhibition of nortriptyline hydroxylation in man by quinidine. *Xenobiotica.* 1992;22:721.

Imipramine (*Tofranil*)

Venlafaxine (eg, *Effexor*)

SUMMARY: Study in healthy subjects suggests that venlafaxine increases imipramine serum concentrations, but the extent to which this increases the risk of imipramine toxicity is not established.

RISK FACTORS:

➡ *Pharmacogenetics.* Only patients who have CYP2D6 would be expected to experience this interaction.

RELATED DRUGS: Theoretically, other TCAs that are metabolized by CYP2D6, such as amitriptyline (*Elavil*), would be similarly affected.

MANAGEMENT OPTIONS:

➡ *Monitor.* Monitor for altered imipramine effect if venlafaxine is initiated, discontinued, or changed in dosage.

REFERENCES:

Albers LJ, et al. Effect of venlafaxine on imipramine metabolism. *Psychiatry Res.* 2000;96:235-243.

Imipramine (eg, *Tofranil*)

Verapamil (eg, *Calan*)

SUMMARY: Verapamil and diltiazem appear to increase imipramine serum concentrations; the clinical significance is unknown.

RISK FACTORS: No specific risk factors are known.

RELATED DRUGS: Verapamil and diltiazem likely would affect other cyclic antidepressants in a similar manner. The effects of other calcium channel blockers on cyclic antidepressants are unknown.

MANAGEMENT OPTIONS:

➡ *Monitor.* Monitor patients maintained on imipramine for increased serum imipramine concentrations (eg, sedation, dry mouth, tachycardia) if verapamil or diltiazem is initiated concurrently.

REFERENCES:

Hermann DJ, et al. Comparison of verapamil, diltiazem, and labetalol on the bioavailability and metabolism of imipramine. *J Clin Pharmacol.* 1992;32:176-183.

Indinavir (*Crixivan*)

Ketoconazole (eg, *Nizoral*)

SUMMARY: Ketoconazole increases the serum concentration of indinavir; increased toxicity may result.

RISK FACTORS: No specific risk factors are known.

RELATED DRUGS: Other protease inhibitors including ritonavir (*Norvir*), saquinavir (eg, *Fortovase*), and nelfinavir (*Viracept*) may be affected by ketoconazole in a similar manner. Itraconazole (*Sporanox*), miconazole (eg, *Monistat*), and fluconazole (*Diflu-*

can) also are likely to inhibit the metabolism of indinavir. Terbinafine (*Lamisil*) does not appear to affect CYP3A4 activity and may be less likely to affect indinavir metabolism.

MANAGEMENT OPTIONS:

➡ *Circumvent/Minimize.* Pending further clinical studies, the dose or dosing interval of indinavir may need to be altered. The manufacturer has suggested a regimen of 600 mg every 8 hours during concomitant ketoconazole administration.

➡ *Monitor.* Watch for indinavir toxicity (eg, nephrolithiasis, hyperbilirubinemia, nausea).

REFERENCES:

Product information. Indinavir (*Crixivan*). Merck & Company Inc., 1996.

Indinavir (*Crixivan*)

Omeprazole (eg, *Prilosec*)

SUMMARY: Omeprazole reduces the absorption of indinavir; loss of antiviral efficacy may result.

RISK FACTORS: No specific risk factors are known.

RELATED DRUGS: Other proton pump inhibitors (eg, lansoprazole [*Prevacid*], rabeprazole [*Aciphex*], pantoprazole [*Protonix*]) would be expected to produce similar effects on indinavir plasma concentrations. The effect of omeprazole on other protease inhibitors (eg, saquinavir [eg, *Fortovase*], ritonavir [*Norvir*], nelfinavir [*Viracept*]) is unknown.

MANAGEMENT OPTIONS:

➡ *Monitor.* Monitor patients treated with indinavir for reduced antiviral efficacy if omeprazole or other proton pump inhibitors are coadministered.

REFERENCES:

Burger DM, et al. Pharmacokinetic interaction between the proton pump inhibitor omeprazole and the HIV protease inhibitor indinavir. *AIDS.* 1998;12:2080-2082.

Indinavir (*Crixivan*)

Rifabutin (*Mycobutin*)

SUMMARY: Indinavir markedly increases rifabutin serum concentrations while rifabutin lowers indinavir serum concentrations. Rifabutin toxicity and reduction of indinavir efficacy may result.

RISK FACTORS: No specific risk factors are known.

RELATED DRUGS: Rifabutin decreases the AUC of saquinavir (eg, *Invirase*) and would be expected to affect ritonavir (*Norvir*) similarly. Ritonavir increases rifabutin concentrations. Rifampin (eg, *Rifadin*) may affect saquinavir in a similar manner.

MANAGEMENT OPTIONS:

➡ *Circumvent/Minimize.* The dose of rifabutin may require reduction to avoid toxicity; the dose of indinavir may require an increase to maintain efficacy.

➡ *Monitor.* Monitor for rifabutin toxicity (ie, gastrointestinal upset, skin rash) and loss of indinavir efficacy.

REFERENCES:

Product information. Indinavir (*Crixivan*). Merck & Company Inc., 1996.

 Indinavir (*Crixivan*)

Ritonavir (*Norvir*)

SUMMARY: Indinavir plasma concentrations are increased during ritonavir coadministration; less frequent dosage administration may be possible.

RISK FACTORS: No specific risk factors are known.

RELATED DRUGS: Ritonavir had been reported to increase saquinavir (eg, *Fortovase*) concentrations greater than 50-fold. The effect of ritonavir on other protease inhibitors is not established.

MANAGEMENT OPTIONS:

➡ *Circumvent/Minimize.* Because it is likely that ritonavir and indinavir will be used together in some patients, a reduction in the dose or frequency of indinavir administration would be advisable. Guide dosage by monitoring indinavir plasma concentrations if possible.

➡ *Monitor.* Monitor patients for signs of possible indinavir toxicity (eg, neurological or hematological impairment) during combined indinavir/ritonavir therapy.

REFERENCES:

Hsu A, et al. Pharmacokinetic interaction between ritonavir and indinavir in healthy volunteers. *Antimicrob Agents Chemother.* 1998;42:2784-2791.

 Indinavir (*Crixivan*)

Sildenafil (*Viagra*)

SUMMARY: Indinavir increases sildenafil plasma concentrations; increased toxic effects may occur.

RISK FACTORS: No specific risk factors are known.

RELATED DRUGS: Other protease inhibitors such as ritonavir (*Norvir*), saquinavir (*Fortovase*), amprenavir (*Agenerase*), and nelfinavir (*Viracept*) are known to inhibit CYP3A4 activity and would be expected to interact with sildenafil.

MANAGEMENT OPTIONS:

➡ *Circumvent/Minimize.* Because of the potential for serious side effects, counsel patients taking protease inhibitors that are CYP3A4 inhibitors to avoid concurrent sildenafil administration.

➡ *Monitor.* Carefully monitor patients treated with indinavir for side effects if sildenafil is prescribed.

REFERENCES:

Merry C, et al. Interaction of sildenafil and indinavir when coadministered to HIV-positive patients *AIDS.* 1999;13:F101–7.

Indinavir (*Crixivan*)

St. John's Wort AVOID

SUMMARY: The main component of St. John's wort, hypericum extract, significantly reduced the plasma concentration of indinavir; reduction of antiviral efficacy may occur in some patients. Avoid this combination.

RISK FACTORS: No specific risk factors are known.

RELATED DRUGS: Other protease inhibitors (eg, ritonavir [*Norvir*], saquinavir [*Fortovase*], nelfinavir [*Viracept*]) would probably be affected in a similar manner by hypericum extract.

MANAGEMENT OPTIONS:

➡ ***AVOID COMBINATION.*** Patients taking indinavir or other antiviral agents that are metabolized by CYP3A4 should avoid taking St. John's wort.

REFERENCES:

Piscitelli SC, et al. Indinavir concentrations and St. John's wort. *Lancet.* 2000;355(9203):547–48.

Indomethacin (eg, *Indocin*)

Lithium (eg, *Eskalith*)

SUMMARY: Indomethacin may increase plasma lithium concentrations.

RISK FACTORS: No specific risk factors are known.

RELATED DRUGS: Most NSAIDs increase lithium serum concentrations, but sulindac (eg, *Clinoril*) and aspirin appear to have minimal effects.

MANAGEMENT OPTIONS:

➡ ***Consider Alternative.*** If appropriate for the patient, consider using an anti-inflammatory agent that is less likely to affect lithium, such as sulindac or aspirin.

➡ ***Monitor.*** plasma lithium concentrations carefully if indomethacin (or another NSAID) is initiated or discontinued in patients on lithium therapy. Monitor also for lithium toxicity (eg, nausea, vomiting, diarrhea, anorexia, coarse tremor, slurred speech, vertigo, confusion, lethargy; in severe cases, seizures, stupor, coma, cardiovascular collapse).

REFERENCES:

Frolich JC, et al. Indomethacin increases plasma lithium. *Br Med J.* 1978;1:1115.

Ragheb M, et al. Interaction of indomethacin and ibuprofen with lithium in manic patients under a steady-state lithium level. *J Clin Psychiatry.* 1980;41:397.

❷ Indomethacin (eg, *Indocin*)

Methotrexate (eg, *Rheumatrex*)

SUMMARY: Isolated cases indicate that indomethacin may increase the toxicity of antineoplastic doses of methotrexate.

RISK FACTORS:

➡ **Concurrent Diseases.** Particular caution is suggested in patients with pre-existing renal impairment (who may be more susceptible to nonsteroidal anti-inflammatory drug [NSAID]-induced renal failure).

➡ **Dosage Regimen.** The risk of adverse effects from this interaction is primarily in patients receiving antineoplastic doses of methotrexate rather than the lower doses used to treat rheumatoid arthritis, psoriasis, and related diseases.

MANAGEMENT OPTIONS:

➡ **Avoid Unless Benefit Outweighs Risk.** Until more information is available on this interaction, it would be prudent to avoid indomethacin (as well as other NSAIDs) in patients receiving antineoplastic doses of methotrexate. Particular caution is suggested in patients with pre-existing renal impairment who may be more susceptible to NSAID-induced renal failure.

➡ **Monitor.** If the combination is used, monitor for methotrexate toxicity. Findings in methotrexate toxicity can include stomatitis, severe gastrointestinal symptoms (eg, nausea, diarrhea, vomiting), bone marrow suppression, fever, bleeding, skin rashes, nephrotoxicity, and hepatotoxicity. Although decreasing the methotrexate dosage would be expected to reduce the likelihood of toxicity, the magnitude of the required reduction in methotrexate dosage has not been established.

REFERENCES:

Aherne A, et al. Methotrexate kinetics in rheumatoid arthritis: is there an interaction with nonsteroidal antiinflammatory drugs? *J Rheumatol.* 1988;15:1356.

Furst DE, et al. Effect of aspirin and sulindac on methotrexate clearance. *J Pharm Sci.* 1990;79:782.

Dupuis LL, et al. Methotrexate-nonsteroidal antiinflammatory drug interaction in children with arthritis. *J Rheumatol.* 1990;17:1469.

Leigler DG, et al. The effect of organic acids on renal clearance of methotrexate in man. *Clin Pharmacol Ther.* 1969;10:849.

Skeith KJ, et al. Lack of significant interaction between low dose methotrexate and ibuprofen or flurbiprofen in patients with arthritis. *J Rheumatol.* 1990;17:1008.

Stewart CF et al. Effect of aspirin (ASA) on disposition of methotrexate (MTX) in patients with rheumatoid arthritis (RA). *Clin Pharmacol Ther.* 1990;47:139. Abstract PP-56.

Taylor JR et al. Effect of sodium salicylate and indomethacin on methotrexate-serum albumin binding. *Arch Dermatol.* 1977;113:588.

Tracy FS et al. The effect of NSAIDs on methotrexate disposition in patients with rheumatoid arthritis. *Clin Pharmacol Ther.* 1990;47:138. Abstract PP-54.

Daly HM et al. Methotrexate toxicity precipitated by azapropazone. *Br J Dermatol.* 1986;114:733.

Boh LE et al. Low-dose weekly oral methotrexate therapy for inflammatory arthritis. *Clin Pharm.* 1986;5:503.

Anderson PA et al. Weekly pulse methotrexate in rheumatoid arthritis: clinical and immunologic effects in a randomized, double-blind study. *Ann Intern Med.* 1985;103:489.

Tugwell P et al. Methotrexate in rheumatoid arthritis: indications, contraindications, efficacy, and safety. *Ann Intern Med.* 1987;107:358.

Adams JD et al. Drug interactions in psoriasis. *Aust J Dermatol.* 1976;17:39.

Ellison NM et al. Acute renal failure and death following sequential intermediate-dose methotrexate and 5-FU: a possible adverse effect due to concomitant indomethacin administration. *Cancer Treat Rep.* 1985;69:342.

Maiche AG. Acute renal failure due to concomitant action of methotrexate and indomethacin. *Lancet.* 1986;1:1390.

Indomethacin (eg, *Indocin*)

Prazosin (eg, *Minipress*)

SUMMARY: In some patients indomethacin may inhibit the antihypertensive response to prazosin; the effect of other nonsteroidal anti-inflammatory drugs (NSAIDs) is not known, but they may produce a similar effect.

RISK FACTORS: No specific risk factors are known.

RELATED DRUGS: The effect of other NSAIDs on prazosin has not been studied, but they probably produce a similar response. Ibuprofen (eg, *Motrin*) in a dose of 400 mg 3 times/day for 3 weeks has been shown to increase the mean blood pressure by approximately 5 to 7 mm Hg in a parallel trial of 45 hypertensive patients receiving a variety of antihypertensive drugs. Doxazosin (eg, *Cardura*) and terazosin (eg, *Hytrin*) probably interact with NSAIDs in a similar manner.

MANAGEMENT OPTIONS:

➡ **Consider Alternative.** Sulindac (eg, *Clinoril*) appears less likely than other NSAIDs to inhibit the antihypertensive response to beta-blockers, captopril (eg, *Capoten*), and thiazides. It is possible that sulindac also would have less effect on prazosin.

➡ **Monitor.** Monitor for reduced hypotensive response to prazosin (or other antihypertensive agents) when NSAIDs are given concurrently. If blood pressure increases, alteration in antihypertensive drug dosage or the use of alternative antihypertensive agents may be required.

REFERENCES:
Rubin P, et al. Studies on the clinical pharmacology of prazosin. II: The influence of indomethacin and of propranolol on the action and disposition of prazosin. *Br J Clin Pharmacol.* 1980;10:33-39.

Radack KL, et al. Ibuprofen interferes with the efficacy of antihypertensive drugs: a randomized, double-blind, placebo-controlled trial of ibuprofen compared with acetaminophen. *Ann Intern Med.* 1987;107:628-635.

Indomethacin (eg, *Indocin*)

Prednisone (eg, *Deltasone*)

SUMMARY: The combined effects of prednisone and indomethacin may result in an increased incidence or severity of GI ulceration; other combinations of nonsteroidal anti-inflammatory drugs (NSAIDs) and corticosteroids probably produce a similar effect.

RISK FACTORS: No specific risk factors are known.

RELATED DRUGS: If indomethacin does increase GI toxicity of corticosteroids, other NSAIDs would be expected to act similarly.

MANAGEMENT OPTIONS:

➡ **Circumvent/Minimize.** Consider the concurrent use of misoprostol (*Cytotec*).

➡ **Monitor.** Be particularly alert for evidence of GI ulceration and bleeding in patients receiving combinations of NSAIDs and corticosteroids.

REFERENCES:

Hvidberg E, et al. Influence of indomethacin on the distribution of cortisol in man. *Eur J Clin Pharmacol.* 1971;3:102.

Emmanuel JH, et al. Gastric ulcer and the anti-arthritic drugs. *Postgrad Med J.* 1971;47:227-232.

Indomethacin (eg, *Indocin*)

Propranolol (eg, *Inderal*)

SUMMARY: Indomethacin and many other nonsteroidal anti-inflammatory drugs (NSAIDs) can reduce the hypotensive effect of propranolol and other beta blockers.

RISK FACTORS:

➡ **Dosage Regimen.** Chronic administration of an NSAID may inhibit antihypertensive response.

RELATED DRUGS: Other beta blockers may be affected similarly. Other NSAIDs probably produce a similar effect, but there may be differences in the magnitude of the interaction with different NSAIDs.

MANAGEMENT OPTIONS:

➡ **Circumvent/Minimize.** Using the shortest duration of NSAID therapy will minimize the magnitude of the interaction. Using an antihypertensive other than a beta blocker may not circumvent the interaction because NSAIDs generally tend to inhibit the effect of antihypertensives.

➡ **Monitor.** Patients should be monitored for altered antihypertensive or antianginal response to beta blockers when indomethacin is initiated or discontinued. Short-term NSAID use requires no special precautions.

REFERENCES:

Ylitalo P, et al. Inhibition of prostaglandin synthesis by indomethacin interacts with the antihypertensive effect of atenolol. *Clin Pharmacol Ther.* 1985;38:443.

Salvetti A, et al. The influence of indomethacin and sulindac on some pharmacological actions of atenolol in hypertensive patients. *Br J Clin Pharmacol.* 1984;17:108S.

Ebel DL, et al. Effect of sulindac, piroxicam and placebo on the hypotensive effect of propranolol in patients with mild to moderate essential hypertension. *Scand J Rheumatol.* 1986;62:41.

Chalmers JP, et al. Effects of indomethacin, sulindac, naproxen, aspirin, and paracetamol in treated hypertensive patients. *Clin Exp Hypertens.* 1984;6:1077.

Wong DG, et al. Nonsteroidal antiinflammatory drugs (NSAIDs) vs. placebo in hypertension treated with diuretic and beta blocker. *Clin Pharmacol Ther.* 1984;35:284.

Sugimoto K, et al. Influence of indomethacin on a reduction in forearm blood flow induced by propranolol in healthy subjects. *J Clin Pharmacol.* 1989;29:307.

Watkins J, et al. Attenuation of hypotensive effect of propranolol and thiazide diuretics by indomethacin. *Br J Med.* 1980;218:702.

Salvetti A, et al. Interaction between oxprenolol and indomethacin on blood pressure in essential hypertensive patients. *Eur J Clin Pharmacol.* 1982;22:197.

Friedman PL, et al. Coronary vasoconstrictor effect of indomethacin in patients with coronary-artery disease. *N Engl J Med.* 1981;305:1171.

Wong DG, et al. Effect of non-steroidal anti-inflammatory drugs on control of hypertension by beta-blockers and diuretics. *Lancet.* 1986;1:997.

Ferrara LA, et al. Interference by sulphinpyrazone with the antihypertensive effects of oxprenolol. *Eur J Clin Pharmacol.* 1986;29:717.

Abate MA, et al. Interaction of indomethacin and sulindac with labetalol. *Br J Clin Pharmacol.* 1991;31:363.

Schuna AA, et al. Lack of interaction between sulindac or naproxen and propranolol in hypertensive patients. *J Clin Pharmacol.* 1989;29:524.

Forman MB, et al. Effects of indomethacin on systemic coronary hemodynamics in patients with coronary artery disease. *Am Heart J.* 1985;110:311.

Indomethacin (eg, *Indocin*)
Triamterene (*Dyrenium*)

SUMMARY: Some patients develop acute renal failure when indomethacin and triamterene are administered concurrently.

RISK FACTORS: No specific risk factors are known.

RELATED DRUGS: Nephrotoxicity was not seen when indomethacin was combined with furosemide (eg, *Lasix*), hydrochlorothiazide (eg, *Dyazide*), or *spironolactone (eg, Aldactone*) Cases of reduced renal function have been reported with triamterene combined with other nonsteroidal anti-inflammatory drugs (NSAIDs), one involving diclofenac (eg, *Voltaren*) and triamterene and one involving ibuprofen (eg, *Motrin*) and triamterene. Other NSAIDs also may interact, but little information is available.

MANAGEMENT OPTIONS:

➡ *Consider Alternative.* It is possible that spironolactone and amiloride are less likely than triamterene to interact adversely with indomethacin, but this has not been established clinically.

➡ *Monitor.* Carefully monitor renal function in patients on combined therapy with triamterene and indomethacin (or other NSAIDs).

REFERENCES:

Favre L, et al. Reversible acute renal failure from combined triamterene and indomethacin: a study in healthy subjects. *Ann Intern Med.* 1982;96:317.

McCarthy JT, et al. Acute intrinsic renal failure induced by indomethacin. *Mayo Clin Proc.* 1982;57:289.

Weinberg MS, et al. Anuric renal failure precipitated by indomethacin and triamterene. *Nephron.* 1985;40:216.

Harkonen M, et al. Reversible deterioration of renal function after diclofenac in patient receiving triamterene. *Br Med J.* 1986;293:698.

Gehr TWB, et al. Interaction of triamterene-hydrochlorothiazide and ibuprofen. *Clin Pharmacol Ther.* 1990;47:200. Abstract.

Indomethacin (*Indocin*)
Vancomycin (*Vancocin*)

SUMMARY: Indomethacin administration may increase the concentration of vancomycin in neonates; vancomycin toxicity may result.

RISK FACTORS: No specific risk factors known.

RELATED DRUGS: Other nonsteroidal anti-inflammatory drugs may affect vancomycin in a similar manner.

MANAGEMENT OPTIONS:

➥ *Circumvent/Minimize.* Vancomycin dosage may need to be reduced during indomethacin coadministration.

➥ *Monitor.* Vancomycin concentrations should be monitored in neonates receiving indomethacin.

REFERENCES:

Spivey MJ, et al. Vancomycin pharmacokinetics in neonates. *Am J Dis Child.* 1986;149:859. Letter.

  Indomethacin (eg, *Indocin*)

Warfarin (eg, *Coumadin*)

SUMMARY: Although isolated case reports of indomethacin-induced increases in the hypoprothrombinemic response to warfarin have appeared, most patients do not manifest an enhanced anticoagulant effect. Nonetheless, caution is indicated during cotherapy with these drugs because of possible detrimental effects of indomethacin on the gastric mucosa and platelet function.

RISK FACTORS:

➥ *Concurrent Diseases.* Patients with peptic ulcer disease (PUD) or a history of gastrointestinal (GI) bleeding are probably at greater risk.

RELATED DRUGS: All NSAIDs inhibit platelet function, cause gastric erosions, and probably increase the risk of GI bleeding. Some NSAIDs, however, such as ibuprofen (eg, *Motrin*), naproxen (eg, *Naprosyn*), or diclofenac (eg, *Voltaren*) may be less likely to increase oral anticoagulant-induced hypoprothrombinemia than other NSAIDs.

MANAGEMENT OPTIONS:

➥ *Avoid Unless Benefit Outweighs Risk.* Since all NSAIDs probably increase the risk of GI bleeding in patients on oral anticoagulants, use the combination only after careful consideration of the benefit versus risk. If an NSAID must be used with an oral anticoagulant, it would be prudent to use NSAIDs that are unlikely to affect the hypoprothrombinemic response to oral anticoagulants. If the NSAID is being used as an analgesic or antipyretic, acetaminophen is probably safer to use with oral anticoagulants. Non-acetylated salicylates (eg, choline salicylate, magnesium salicylate, salsalate, sodium salicylate) also are probably safer with oral anticoagulants than NSAIDs since such salicylates have minimal effects on platelet function and the gastric mucosa.

➥ *Monitor.* If any NSAID is used with an oral anticoagulant, one should carefully monitor the prothrombin time and watch for evidence of bleeding, especially from the GI tract.

REFERENCES:

Zucker MB, et al. Effect of acetylsalicylic acid, other nonsteroidal antiinflammatory agents, and dipyridamole on human blood platelets. *J Lab Clin Med.* 1970;76:66.

Hoffbrand BI, et al. Potentiation of anticoagulants. *Br Med J.* 1967;2:838. Letter.

Frost H, et al. Concomitant administration of indomethacin and anticoagulants. International Symposium on Inflammation, Freiburg Im Breisgau. Germany. 1966, May.

Vesell ES, et al. Failure of indomethacin and warfarin to interact in normal human volunteers. *J Clin Pharmacol.* 1975;15:486.

Koch-Weser J. Hemorrhagic reactions and drug interactions in 500 warfarin-treated patients. *Clin Pharmacol Ther.* 1973;14:139. Abstract.

Self TH, et al. Drug-enhancement of warfarin activity. *Lancet.* 1975;2:557. Letter.

McQueen EG. New Zealand committee on adverse drug reactions; tenth annual report, 1975. *N Z Med J.* 1975;82:308.

Self TH, et al. Possible interaction of indomethacin and warfarin. *DICP.* 1978;12:580.

Shorr RI, et al. Concurrent use of nonsteroidal anti-inflammatory drugs and oral anticoagulants places elderly persons at high risk hemorrhagic peptic ulcer disease. *Arch Intern Med.* 1993;153:1665.

Chan TYK, et al. Adverse interaction between warfarin and indomethacin. *Drug Safety.* 1994;10:267.

Day R, et al. Adverse interaction between warfarin and indomethacin. *Drug Safety.* 1994;1:213.

Influenza Vaccine

Phenytoin (eg, *Dilantin*)

SUMMARY: Some patients appear to develop an increase in total serum phenytoin concentrations following vaccination, but reductions in free serum phenytoin concentrations also have been reported. The clinical importance of these findings is not established.

RISK FACTORS: No specific risk factors are known.

RELATED DRUGS: No information is available.

MANAGEMENT OPTIONS:

➡ *Monitor.* Although patients should be monitored for evidence of phenytoin toxicity following influenza vaccination, an adjustment in phenytoin dosage rarely is needed. If the phenytoin dose is changed, additional adjustments should be anticipated as the effect of the vaccine dissipates (this has taken as little as 2 weeks but may take much longer).

REFERENCES:

Sawchuk RJ, et al. Effect of influenza vaccination on plasma phenytoin concentration. *Ther Drug Monit.* 1979;1:285.

Levine M, et al. Increased serum phenytoin concentration following influenza vaccination. *Clin Pharm.* 1984;3:505.

Levine M, et al. Phenytoin therapy and immune response to influenza vaccine. *Clin Pharm.* 1985;4:191.

Jann MW, et al. Effect of influenza vaccine on serum anticonvulsant concentrations. *Clin Pharm.* 1986;5:817.

Smith CD, et al. Effect of influenza vaccine on serum concentrations of total and free phenytoin. *Clin Pharm.* 1988;7:828.

Insulin

Marijuana

SUMMARY: Marijuana use may increase serum glucose concentrations.

RISK FACTORS: No specific risk factors are known.

RELATED DRUGS: Marijuana may affect glucose tolerance in patients taking oral hypoglycemic agents.

MANAGEMENT OPTIONS:

➡ *Monitor.* Diabetic patients should be aware that marijuana use might affect glucose tolerance.

REFERENCES:

Lockhart JG. Effects of "speed" and "pot" on the juvenile diabetic (Questions and Answers). *JAMA.* 1970;214:2065.

Pololsky S, et al. Effect of marijuana on the glucose-tolerance test. *Ann NY Acad Sci.* 1971;191:54.

Hughes JE, et al. Marijuana and the diabetic coma. *JAMA.* 1970;214:1113.

Hollister LE, et al. Delta-9-tetrahydrocannabinol and glucose tolerance. *Clin Pharmacol Ther.* 1974;16:297.

Insulin

Prednisone (eg, *Deltasone*)

SUMMARY: Corticosteroids like prednisone may increase blood glucose in patients with diabetes.

RISK FACTORS:

➡ ***Dosage Regimen.*** Chronic administration of corticosteroids can increase glucose concentrations.

RELATED DRUGS: All corticosteroids can increase glucose concentrations during chronic dosing.

MANAGEMENT OPTIONS:

➡ ***Monitor.*** Patients should be observed for evidence of altered diabetic control when corticosteroids are initiated, discontinued or changed in dosage.

REFERENCES:

Gomez EC, et al. Induction of glycosuria and hyperglycemia by topical corticosteroid therapy. *Arch Dermatol.* 1976;112:1559.

Hunder GG, et al. Daily and alternate-day corticosteroid regimens in treatment of giant cell arteritis. Comparison in a prospective study. *Ann Intern Med.* 1975;82:613.

McMahon M, et al. Effects of glucocorticoids on carbohydrate metabolism. *Diabetes Metab Rev.* 1988;4:17.

Insulin

Propranolol (eg, *Inderal*)

SUMMARY: Propranolol and other beta blockers may alter the response to hypoglycemia by prolonging the recovery of normoglycemia, causing hypertension and blocking tachycardia. They also may increase blood glucose concentrations and impair peripheral circulation.

RISK FACTORS: No specific risk factors are known.

RELATED DRUGS: Nonselective beta blockers would be expected to produce results similar to propranolol when administered to patients taking insulin. Oral hypoglycemic agents may interact with the nonselective beta blockers but, since they are less likely to produce hypoglycemia than insulin, the incidence and magnitude of reactions associated with hypoglycemic episodes will be reduced.

MANAGEMENT OPTIONS:

➡ ***Consider Alternative.*** Cardioselective beta blockers (eg, metoprolol, acebutolol, atenolol) are preferable in diabetic patients, especially if the patient is prone to hypoglycemic episodes. The increased safety of cardioselective agents is only relative, as they may exhibit nonselective beta blockade at higher doses.

➡ *Monitor.* Diabetic patients receiving beta blockers should be aware that hypoglycemic episodes may not result in the expected tachycardia, but hypoglycemic-induced sweating will occur or even may be increased.

REFERENCES:

Mills GA, et al. Beta-blockers and glucose control. *DICP.* 1985;19:246.

Hansten PD. Beta-blocking agents and antidiabetic drugs. *DICP.* 1980;14:46.

Molnar GW, et al. Propranolol enhancement of hypoglycemic sweating. *Clin Pharmacol Ther.* 1974;15:490.

Newman RJ. Comparison of propranolol, metoprolol, and acebutolol on insulin-induced hypoglycaemia. *Br Med J.* 1976;2:447.

Deacon SP, et al. Acebutolol, atenolol, and propranolol and metabolic responses to acute hypoglycaemia in diabetics. *Br Med J.* 1977;2:1255.

Deacon SP, et al. Comparison of atenolol and propranolol during insulin-induced hypoglycaemia. *Br Med J.* 1976;2:272.

Sharma SD, et al. Comparison of penbutolol and propranolol during insulin-induced hypoglycaemia. *Curr Ther Res.* 1979;26:252.

Ostman J, et al. Effect of metoprolol and alprenolol on the metabolic, hormonal, and haemodynamic response to insulin-induced hypoglycaemia in hypertensive, insulin-dependent diabetics. *Acta Med Scand.* 1982;211:381.

Shepherd AMM, et al. Hypoglycemia-induced hypertension in a diabetic patient on metoprolol. *Ann Intern Med.* 1981;94:357.

Meyers MG, et al. Effect of d-and dl-propranolol on glucose-stimulated insulin release. *Clin Pharmacol Ther.* 1979;25:303.

Pollare T, et al. Sensitivity to insulin during treatment with atenolol and metoprolol; a randomized, double blind study of effects of carbohydrate and lipoprotein metabolism in hypertensive patients. *Br Med J.* 1989;298:1152.

Mohler H, et al. Glucose intolerance during chronic beta-adrenergic blockade in man. *Clin Pharmacol Ther.* 1979;25:237.

Nardone DA, et al. Hyperglycemia and diabetic coma; possible relationship to diuretic-propranolol therapy. *South Med J.* 1979;72:1607.

Groop L, et al. Influence of beta-blocking drugs on glucose metabolism in patients with non-insulin dependent diabetes mellitus. *Acta Med Scand.* 1982;211:7.

Reeves RL, et al. The effect of metoprolol and propranolol on pancreatic insulin release. *Clin Pharmacol Ther.* 1982;31:262.

Angelo-Nelsen K, et al. Timolol topically and diabetes mellitus. *JAMA.* 1980;244:2263.

Insulin

Thiazides (eg, chlorothiazide)

SUMMARY: Thiazides tend to increase blood glucose and may increase the dosage requirements of antidiabetic drugs.

RISK FACTORS:

➡ *Dosage.* Thiazide dosage greater than 50 mg/day may increase blood glucose.

RELATED DRUGS: Thiazides may inhibit the hypoglycemic effect of chlorpropamide (eg, *Diabinese*) and other oral hypoglycemic agents.

MANAGEMENT OPTIONS:

➡ *Monitor.* Watch for decreased diabetic control when thiazide therapy is started in a patient receiving any antidiabetic drug.

REFERENCES:

Levine R. Mechanisms of insulin secretion. *N Engl J Med.* 1970;283:522.

Grunfeld C, et al. Hypokalemia and diabetes mellitus. *Am J Med.* 1983;75:553.

Helderman JH, et al. Prevention of the glucose intolerance of thiazide diuretics by maintenance of body potassium. *Diabetes*. 1983;32:106.

Fichman MP, et al. Diuretic-induced hyponatremia. *Ann Intern Med*. 1971;75:853.

Amery A, et al. Glucose tolerance during diuretic therapy. Results of trial by the European Working Party on Hypertension in the Elderly. *Lancet*. 1978;1:681.

Murphy MB, et al. Glucose intolerance in hypertensive patients treated with diuretics: a fourteen-year follow-up. *Lancet*. 1982;2:1293.

Lowder NK, et al. Clinically significant diuretic-induced glucose intolerance. *DICP*. 1988;22:969.

 Insulin
Tranylcypromine (*Parnate*)

SUMMARY: Excessive hypoglycemia may occur when tranylcypromine, and other monoamine oxidase inhibitors (MAOIs), are administered to patients with diabetes.

RISK FACTORS: No specific risk factors are known.

RELATED DRUGS: Sulfonylureas such as chlorpropamide and tolbutamide interact with type A MAOIs like tranylcypromine similarly. While it is likely that all type A MAOIs will interact in a similar manner, the effect of type B MAOIs (eg, selegiline [eg, *Eldepryl*]) on glucose tolerance is not established.

MANAGEMENT OPTIONS:

➡ *Monitor.* Until further information on this interaction is available, diabetic patients should be warned about possible hypoglycemic reactions when MAOI therapy is started. Be alert for deterioration of glycemic control when MAOI therapy is discontinued.

REFERENCES:

Cooper AJ, et al. Modification of insulin and sulfonylurea hypoglycemia by monoamine-oxidase inhibitor drugs. *Diabetes*. 1967;16:272.

Adnitt PI. Hypoglycemic action of monoamine oxidase inhibitors (MAOI's). *Diabetes*. 1968;17:628.

Bressler R, et al. Tranylcypromine: a potent insulin secretagogue and hypoglycemic agent. *Diabetes*. 1968;17:617.

Cooper AJ, et al. Potentiation of insulin hypoglycaemia by MAOI antidepressant drugs. *Lancet*. 1966;1:407.

Barrett AM. Modification of the hypoglycaemic response to tolbutamide and insulin by mebanazine, an inhibitor of monoamine oxidase. *J Pharm Pharmacol*. 1965;17:19.

Whickstrom L, et al. Treatment of diabetics with monoamine-oxidase inhibitors. *Lancet*. 1964;2:995.

 Interferon (eg, *Roferon-A*)
Theophylline (eg, *Theo-Dur*)

SUMMARY: Interferon alpha may increase theophylline plasma concentrations, especially in patients with high pre-existing theophylline clearance (ie, those who smoke); the degree to which this increases the risk of theophylline toxicity is not known.

RISK FACTORS:

➡ *Habits.* Limited evidence suggests that the reduction in theophylline clearance by interferon is greater in patients who have high pre-existing theophylline clearance due to smoking.

MANAGEMENT OPTIONS:

➡ *Monitor.* Monitor for excessive theophylline response if interferon is given, especially in theophylline-treated patients who smoke or other patients in whom theophylline clearance may be high (eg, those on enzyme inducers such as barbiturates, carbamazepine [eg, *Tegretol*], phenytoin [eg, *Dilantin*], primidone [eg, *Mysoline*], and rifampin [eg, *Rifadin*]). The effect of interferon on theophylline elimination appears to occur rapidly; expect to see increased plasma theophylline concentrations within 1 to 2 days of interferon administration.

REFERENCES:

Williams SJ, et al. Inhibition of theophylline metabolism by interferon. *Lancet.* 1987;2:939-941.

Okuno H, et al. Depression of drug metabolizing activity in the human liver by interferon-alpha. *Eur J Clin Pharmacol.* 1990;39:365-367.

Jonkman JH, et al. Effects of alpha-interferon on theophylline pharmacokinetics and metabolism. *Br J Clin Pharmacol.* 1989;27:795-802.

Interferon (eg, *Betaseron*)
Zidovudine (eg, *Retrovir*)

SUMMARY: Beta interferon markedly increases the plasma concentrations of zidovudine.

RISK FACTORS: No specific risk factors are known.

RELATED DRUGS: Interleukin-2 interacts similarly.

MANAGEMENT OPTIONS:

➡ *Circumvent/Minimize.* Patients taking zidovudine who are given beta interferon should be given reduced doses of zidovudine. If additional studies substantiate the large degree of metabolic inhibition, zidovudine doses could be reduced 75% or more.

➡ *Monitor.* Monitor for altered zidovudine effect if beta interferon is initiated, discontinued, or changed in dosage; adjust zidovudine dose as needed.

REFERENCES:

Nolta M, et al. Molecular interaction of recombinant beta interferon and zidovudine (AZT): alternations of AZT pharmacokinetics in HIV-infected patients. Fifth International Conference on AIDS. Quebec; 1989:278.

Skinner MH, et al. IL-2 does not alter zidovudine kinetics. *Clin Pharmacol Ther.* 1989;45:128.

Intrauterine Progesterone System (IUDs) (*Progestasert*)
Prednisone (eg, *Deltasone*)

SUMMARY: Corticosteroids like prednisone have been reported to decrease the efficacy of IUDs, but a causal relationship has not been established.

RISK FACTORS: No specific risk factors are known.

RELATED DRUGS: If this interaction is real, it would be expected to occur with other corticosteroids as well.

MANAGEMENT OPTIONS:

➡ *Circumvent/Minimize.* Until more information is available, women using IUDs should consider using another form of contraception during short-term therapy with corticosteroids or other anti-inflammatory drugs. If the anti-inflammatory drug is used chronically, the possibility that the IUD failure rate may be increased somewhat should be considered when selecting a contraceptive method.

➡ *Monitor.* Because pregnancy is the potential outcome, monitoring guidelines are not applicable.

REFERENCES:

Inkeles DM, et al. Unexpected pregnancy in a woman using an intrauterine device and receiving steroid therapy. *Ann Ophthalmol.* 1982;14:975.

Zerner J, et al. Failure of an intrauterine device concurrent with administration of corticosteroids. *Fertil Steril.* 1976;27:1467-1468.

 Irinotecan (*Camptosar*)

AVOID **St. John's wort**

SUMMARY: St. John's wort may reduce irinotecan effect, and the combination should probably be avoided.

RISK FACTORS: No specific risk factors are known.

RELATED DRUGS: Theoretically, topotecan may interact in the same way with St. John's wort.

MANAGEMENT OPTIONS:

➡ *AVOID COMBINATION.* Given the potential risk of reduced irinotecan and the questionable efficacy of St. John's wort, it seems prudent to avoid the combination at this time.

REFERENCES:

Mathijssen RHJ, et al. Effects of St. John's wort on irinotecan metabolism. *J Natl Cancer Inst.* 2002;94:1247-1249.

 Iron

Levodopa (eg, *Larodopa*)

SUMMARY: Oral iron reduced levodopa bioavailability by 50% in a single-dose study of normal subjects; the importance of this interaction in parkinsonian patients on chronic levodopa therapy is not established.

RISK FACTORS: No specific risk factors are known.

RELATED DRUGS: Theoretically, other oral iron preparations would be expected to reduce levodopa absorption; however, the small amounts of iron found in most vitamin-mineral products probably are insufficient to produce much interaction.

MANAGEMENT OPTIONS:

➡ *Circumvent/Minimize.* Until more information is available, separate the doses of iron and levodopa as much as possible, and monitor the patient for inadequate levodopa response.

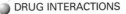

➡ **Monitor.** Monitor for reduced levodopa response if the combination is used.

REFERENCES:
 Campbell NR, et al. Ferrous sulfate reduces levodopa bioavailability: chelation as a possible mechanism. *Clin Pharmacol Ther.* 1989;45:220-225.

Iron

Methyldopa (eg, *Aldomet*)

SUMMARY: Pharmacokinetic studies in healthy subjects and blood pressure measurements in hypertensive patients both indicate that oral iron may inhibit the antihypertensive response to methyldopa.

RISK FACTORS: No specific risk factors are known.

RELATED DRUGS: Although the effect of oral iron salts other than ferrous sulfate and ferrous gluconate on methyldopa is not known, assume that they interact until proven otherwise. The amount of iron in most multivitamins may not be sufficient to inhibit methyldopa absorption, but clinical studies are needed to confirm this. Parenteral iron would not be expected to interact, but this has not been studied. Little is known regarding the effect of iron on antihypertensives other than methyldopa.

MANAGEMENT OPTIONS:

➡ **Consider Alternative.** Methyldopa has disadvantages compared with many other antihypertensives; consider alternative therapy.

➡ **Circumvent/Minimize.** Give methyldopa 2 hours before or 6 hours after oral iron.

➡ **Monitor.** Monitor for reduced antihypertensive response when oral iron and methyldopa are used concurrently.

REFERENCES:
 Campbell N, et al. Alteration of methyldopa absorption, metabolism, and blood pressure control caused by ferrous sulfate and ferrous gluconate. *Clin Pharmacol Ther.* 1988;43:381.

Iron

Moxifloxacin (*Avelox*)

SUMMARY: Iron administration reduces moxifloxacin plasma concentrations; a reduction in antibiotic activity may occur.

RISK FACTORS: No specific risk factors are known.

RELATED DRUGS: Other quinolone antibiotics such as ciprofloxacin (*Cipro*) and norfloxacin (*Noroxin*) are affected in a similar manner by iron.

MANAGEMENT OPTIONS:

➡ **Consider Alternative.** Patients taking moxifloxacin should not take oral iron salts concurrently because of the risk of subtherapeutic moxifloxacin concentrations.

➡ **Circumvent/Minimize.** IV iron could be considered to avoid the interaction. If moxifloxacin is administered to patients taking oral iron, give the antibiotic at least 2 hours before the iron.

➡ *Monitor.* Watch for reduced antibiotic efficacy if moxifloxacin and iron salts are coadministered.

REFERENCES:

Stass H, et al. Effects of iron supplements on the oral bioavailability of moxifloxacin, a novel 8-methoxyfluoroquinolone, in humans. *Clin Pharmacokinet.* 2001;40(suppl 1):57.

② Iron

Mycophenolate Mofetil (*CellCept*)

SUMMARY: Oral iron appears to markedly reduce the bioavailability of mycophenolate mofetil; avoid concurrent use or carefully separate doses.

RISK FACTORS:

➡ *Route of Administration.* The interaction is likely to occur only with oral administration of iron.

RELATED DRUGS: All oral iron preparations would be expected to interact with mycophenolate mofetil.

MANAGEMENT OPTIONS:

➡ *Circumvent/Minimize.* Until more information is available, it would be prudent to give oral iron 4 to 6 hours before or 2 hours after mycophenolate mofetil. Also, warn patients on mycophenolate to avoid taking *otc* iron preparations.

➡ *Monitor.* If oral iron must be used with mycophenolate mofetil, monitor for altered mycophenolate mofetil effect if oral iron is initiated, discontinued, changed in dosage, or if the interval between doses of the 2 drugs is changed.

REFERENCES:

Morii M, et al. Impairment of mycophenolate mofetil absorption by iron ion. *Clin Pharmacol Ther.* 2000;68:613.

③ Iron

Norfloxacin (*Noroxin*)

SUMMARY: The administration of iron salts with norfloxacin lowers the antibiotic serum concentration and may lead to therapeutic failure.

RISK FACTORS: No specific risk factors are known.

RELATED DRUGS: Other quinolones (eg, ciprofloxacin [*Cipro*]) have been reported to be affected similarly by iron. Ofloxacin (*Floxin*) absorption may be less affected by iron.,

MANAGEMENT OPTIONS:

➡ *Consider Alternative.* Patients taking norfloxacin should not take oral iron concurrently because serum norfloxacin concentrations may be subtherapeutic.

➡ *Circumvent/Minimize.* The administration of norfloxacin at least 2 hours before oral iron would theoretically reduce the magnitude of the interaction. IV iron could be used to avoid the interaction.

➥ *Monitor.* If the drugs are used together, watch for lessened antibiotic effect.

REFERENCES:

Campbell NR, et al. Norfloxacin interaction with antacids and minerals. *Br J Clin Pharmacol*. 1992;33:115.

Lehto P, et al. The effect of ferrous sulphate on the absorption of norfloxacin, ciprofloxacin and ofloxacin. *Br J Clin Pharmacol*. 1994;37:82.

Okhamafe AO, et al. Pharmacokinetic interactions of norfloxacin with some metallic medicinal agents. *Int J Pharmacol*. 1991;68:11.

Polk RE, et al. Effect of ferrous sulfate and multivitamins with zinc on absorption of ciprofloxacin in normal volunteers. *Antimicrob Agents Chemother*. 1989;33:1841.

Akerele JO, et al. Influence of oral co-administered metallic drugs on ofloxacin pharmacokinetics. *J Antimicrob Chemother*. 1991;28:87.

Kara M, et al. Clinical and chemical interactions between iron preparations and ciprofloxacin. *Br J Clin Pharmacol*. 1991;31:257.

Iron

Penicillamine (eg, *Cuprimine*)

SUMMARY: Oral iron may reduce plasma penicillamine concentrations substantially; reduced therapeutic response to penicillamine may occur in some patients.

RISK FACTORS: No specific risk factors are known.

RELATED DRUGS: No information is available.

MANAGEMENT OPTIONS:

➥ *Circumvent/Minimize.* Patients receiving penicillamine (eg, for rheumatoid arthritis) should separate penicillamine ingestion from oral iron to minimize mixing in the GI tract. Theoretically, giving the penicillamine a few hours before the iron would minimize the interaction.

➥ *Monitor.* Be alert for evidence of reduced penicillamine response, and adjust the penicillamine dosage as needed.

REFERENCES:

Lyle WH. Penicillamine and iron. *Lancet*. 1976;2:420. Letter.

Osman MA, et al. Reduction in oral penicillamine absorption by food, antacid, and ferrous sulfate. *Clin Pharmacol Ther*. 1983;33:465.

Iron

Tetracycline (eg, *Achromycin V*)

SUMMARY: Oral iron products may reduce the serum concentrations and, possibly, the antibacterial efficacy of tetracycline.

RISK FACTORS: No specific risk factors are known.

RELATED DRUGS: Oxytetracycline, methacycline, and doxycycline interact similarly with oral iron products.

MANAGEMENT OPTIONS:

➥ *Consider Alternative.* On the basis of current evidence, iron preparations should not be administered simultaneously with oral tetracyclines. When possible, a different antibiotic should be chosen if iron is administered.

➡ *Circumvent/Minimize.* If both need to be given to a patient, ferrous sulfate should be administered 3 hours before or 2 hours after tetracycline to minimize the interaction between them. However, the separation of doses may not circumvent interactions between doxycycline and iron preparations.

➡ *Monitor.* If tetracycline and iron are coadministered, be alert for reduced antibiotic effects.

REFERENCES:

Mattila MJ, et al. Interference of iron preparations and milk with the absorption of tetracyclines. In: Exerpta Medica International Congress Series No. 254. Amsterdam: Exerpta Medica; 1972:128–33.

Bateman FJA. Effects of tetracyclines. *Br Med J.* 1970;4:802. Letter.

Neuvonen P, et al. Interference of iron with the absorption of tetracyclines in man. *Br Med J.* 1970;4:532.

Neuvonen PJ, et al. Effect of oral ferrous sulphate on the half-life of doxycycline in man. *Eur J Clin Pharmacol.* 1974;7:361.

 Iron

Vitamin E

SUMMARY: Vitamin E may impair the hematologic response to iron therapy in children with iron-deficiency anemia.

RISK FACTORS: No specific risk factors are known.

RELATED DRUGS: No information is available.

MANAGEMENT OPTIONS:

➡ *Monitor.* Patients with iron-deficiency anemia who are receiving iron therapy should be observed for impaired hematologic response if vitamin E is given concomitantly.

REFERENCES:

Melhorn DK, et al. Relationships between iron-dextran and vitamin E in an iron deficiency anemia in children. *J Lab Clin Med.* 1969;74:789.

 Isocarboxazid (*Marplan*)

AVOID **Venlafaxine (*Effexor*)**

SUMMARY: Severe serotonin syndrome can occur when venlafaxine is used with or within 2 weeks of discontinuation of isocarboxazid or other nonselective monoamine oxidase inhibitor (MAOI). The combination should be strictly avoided.

RISK FACTORS: No specific risk factors are known.

RELATED DRUGS: All nonselective MAOIs should be expected to result in serotonin syndrome if combined with venlafaxine. This would include phenelzine (*Nardil*) and tranylcypromine (*Parnate*); selegiline (eg, *Eldepryl*) can act as a nonselective MAOI in some patients, especially if large doses are used.

MANAGEMENT OPTIONS:

➡ *AVOID COMBINATION.* Combined use of venlafaxine with isocarboxazid (or any other nonselective MAOI) should be avoided. This would include the use of venlafaxine within 2 weeks of discontinuation of a monoamine oxidase inhibitor.

REFERENCES:

Klysner R, et al. Toxic interaction of venlafaxine and isocarboxazide. *Lancet.* 1995;346:1298. Letter.

Isoniazid (INH) (eg, *Laniazid*)
Phenytoin (eg, *Dilantin*)

SUMMARY: INH predictably increases serum phenytoin concentrations; phenytoin intoxication is possible in patients who receive the combination.

RISK FACTORS:

➡ *Pharmacogenetics.* Patients who are slow metabolizers of INH are at increased risk for the interaction.

RELATED DRUGS: No information available.

MANAGEMENT OPTIONS:

➡ *Monitor.* Patients receiving both INH and phenytoin should be watched closely for signs of phenytoin toxicity (eg, ataxia, nystagmus, mental impairment, involuntary muscular movements, seizures); the phenytoin dose should be decreased if necessary. If INH is discontinued, monitor the patient for a decreased therapeutic response to phenytoin and increase the dose as needed.

REFERENCES:

Kutt H, et al. Diphenylhydantoin intoxication. A complication of isoniazid therapy. *Am Rev Respir Dis.* 1970;101:377.

Brennan RW, et al. Diphenylhydantoin intoxication attendant to slow inactivation of isoniazid. *Neurology.* 1970;20:687.

Miller RR, et al. Clinical importance of the interaction of phenytoin and isoniazid. *Chest.* 1979;75:356.

Isoniazid (INH) (eg, *Laniazid*)
Prednisolone (eg, *Prelone*)

SUMMARY: Prednisolone may reduce the plasma concentrations of INH.

RISK FACTORS:

➡ *Pharmacogenetics.* Patients who are rapid INH acetylators are at increased risk for the interaction.

RELATED DRUGS: Other corticosteroids might be similarly affected.

MANAGEMENT OPTIONS:

➡ *Monitor.* In patients receiving concurrent INH and corticosteroids, watch for evidence of reduced INH effect and enhanced corticosteroid effect.

REFERENCES:

Sarma GR, et al. Effect of prednisone and rifampin on isoniazid metabolism in slow and rapid inactivators of isoniazid. *Antimicrob Agents Chemother.* 1980;18:661.

Brodie MJ, et al. Effect of isoniazid on vitamin D metabolism and hepatic monooxygenase activity. *Clin Pharmacol Ther*. 1981;30:363.

Isoniazid (INH) (eg, *Laniazid*)

Rifampin (eg, *Rifadin*)

SUMMARY: Although rifampin may increase the hepatic toxicity of INH in certain predisposed patients, the combination does not cause hepatotoxicity in the vast majority of patients.

RISK FACTORS:

➡ **Concurrent Diseases.** Patients with pre-existing liver disease and those having recently undergone general anesthesia are at increased risk of the interaction.

➡ **Pharmacogenetics.** Patients who are slow INH acetylators are at increased risk for the interaction.

RELATED DRUGS: No information is available.

MANAGEMENT OPTIONS:

➡ **Monitor.** Patients receiving INH and rifampin should be monitored for evidence of hepatotoxicity, especially if they are known to be slow acetylators of INH or have pre-existing liver disease.

REFERENCES:

Lal S, et al. Effect of rifampicin and isoniazid on liver function. *Br Med J*. 1972;1:148.

Beever IW, et al. Circulating hydrazine during treatment with isoniazid and rifampicin in man. *Br J Clin Pharmacol*. 1982;13:599.

Pessayre D, et al. Isoniazid-rifampin fulminant hepatitis. A possible consequence of the enhancement of isoniazid hepatotoxicity by enzyme induction. *Gastroenterology*. 1977;72:284.

Sarma GR, et al. Rifampin-induced release of hydrazine from isoniazid. *Am Rev Resp Dis*. 1986;133:1072.

Bistritzer T, et al. Isoniazid-rifampin-induced fulminant liver disease in an infant. *J Pediatr*. 1980;97:480.

Llorens J, et al. Pharmacodynamic interference between rifampicin and isoniazid. *Chemotherapy*. 1978;24:97.

Steele MA, et al. Toxic hepatitis with isoniazid and rifampin. A metaanalysis. *Chest*. 1991;99:465.

Isoniazid (INH) (eg, *Laniazid*)

Theophylline (eg, *Theo-Dur*)

SUMMARY: Theophylline plasma concentrations increased following several weeks of INH administration; some patients may develop theophylline toxicity.

RISK FACTORS: No specific risk factors are known.

RELATED DRUGS: No information is available.

MANAGEMENT OPTIONS:

➡ **Monitor.** Patients stabilized on theophylline should be monitored for increased theophylline concentrations when INH is administered. The interaction may require several weeks to reach its full potential.

REFERENCES:

Thompson JR, et al. Isoniazid-induced alternations in theophylline pharmacokinetics. *Curr Ther Res*. 1982;32:921.

Hoglund P, et al. Interaction between isoniazid and theophylline. *Eur J Respir Dis*. 1987;70:110.

Torrent J, et al. Theophylline-isoniazid interaction. *DICP*. 1989;23:143.

Dal Nergo R, et al. Rifampicin-isoniazid and delayed elimination of theophylline: a case report. *Int J Clin Pharm Res*. 1988;8:275.

Samigun M, et al. Lowering of theophylline clearance by isoniazid in slow and rapid acetylators. *Br J Clin Pharmacol.*. 1990;29:570.

Isoniazid (INH) (eg, *Laniazid*)
Triazolam (eg, *Halcion*)

SUMMARY: INH may increase triazolam serum concentrations; the clinical significance is unknown.

RISK FACTORS: No specific risk factors are known.

RELATED DRUGS: INH inhibits the metabolism of diazepam (eg, *Valium*).

MANAGEMENT OPTIONS:

➡ *Monitor.* Watch for evidence of increased sedation when triazolam is administered with INH.

REFERENCES:
Ochs HR, et al. Interaction of triazolam with ethanol and isoniazid. *Clin Pharmacol Ther*. 1983;33:241.

Isoniazid (INH) (eg, *Laniazid*)
Valproic Acid (eg, *Depakene*)

SUMMARY: In 1 patient, valproic acid plasma concentrations increased after the addition of INH resulting in symptoms of valproic acid toxicity.

RISK FACTORS:

➡ *Pharmacogenetics.* Patients who are slow acetylators of INH are at increased risk for the interaction.

RELATED DRUGS: No information is available.

MANAGEMENT OPTIONS:

➡ *Monitor.* Patients should be monitored for changes in response to valproic acid when INH is started (ie, nausea, sedation) or stopped (ie, reduced seizure control).

REFERENCES:
Jonville AP, et al. Interaction between isoniazid and valproate: a case of valproate overdosage. *Eur J Clin Pharmacol*. 1991;40:197.

Isoniazid (INH) (eg, *Laniazid*)
Warfarin (eg, *Coumadin*)

SUMMARY: Isolated case reports and theoretical considerations indicate that INH may enhance the effect of oral anticoagulants such as warfarin, but the incidence and clinical significance of this interaction are unknown.

RISK FACTORS: No specific risk factors are known.

RELATED DRUGS: Other oral anticoagulants may be similarly affected.

MANAGEMENT OPTIONS:

➡ **Monitor.** Patients stabilized on oral anticoagulants should be monitored for increased hypoprothrombinemic response when INH therapy is initiated and decreased response when it is discontinued. Initiation of oral anticoagulant therapy in a patient already on chronic INH should not pose difficulties because the patient can be titrated to the proper dose of anticoagulant.

REFERENCES:

Rosenthal AR, et al. Interaction of isoniazid and warfarin. *JAMA*. 1977;238:2177.

Otis PT, et al. An acquired inhibitor of fibrin stabilization associated with isoniazid therapy: clinical and biochemical observations. *Blood*. 1974;44:771.

Isoproterenol (eg, *Isuprel*)

Propranolol (eg, *Inderal*)

SUMMARY: Propranolol and other beta blockers, particularly nonselective agents, may reduce the effectiveness of isoproterenol and other beta agonists in the treatment of asthma.

RISK FACTORS:

➡ **Concurrent Diseases.** Patients with asthma are at increased risk for the interaction.

RELATED DRUGS: Beta blockers, such as metoprolol and practolol, would be expected to inhibit the bronchodilating activity of all beta agonists. Labetalol appears to have a lesser effect on isoproterenol response.

MANAGEMENT OPTIONS:

➡ **Consider Alternative.** The mutually antagonistic effects of propranolol and isoproterenol indicate that their concomitant use would seldom be justified. If beta agonists such as isoproterenol are being used to treat asthma, propranolol and other nonselective beta blockers probably should be avoided. No beta blocker should be considered absolutely safe in patients with asthma.

➡ **Monitor.** If a beta blocker is used in a patient with asthma, carefully monitor for adverse pulmonary effects.

REFERENCES:

Falliers CJ, et al. Effect of single doses of labetalol, metoprolol, and placebo on ventilatory function in patients with bronchial asthma: interaction with isoproterenol. *J Asthma*. 1986;23:251.

Johnson G, et al. Effects of intravenous propranolol and metoprolol and their interaction with isoprenaline on pulmonary function, heart rate, and blood pressure in asthmatics. *Eur J Clin Pharmacol*. 1975;8:175.

Messerli FH, et al. Effects of beta-adrenergic blockade on plasma cyclic AMP and blood sugar responses to glucagon and isoproterenol in man. *Int J Clin Pharmacol*. 1976;14:189.

Thiringer G, et al. Interaction of orally administered metoprolol, practolol and propranolol in asthmatics. *Eur J Clin Pharmacol*. 1976;10:163.

Perruca E, et al. Effect of atenolol, metoprolol, and propranolol on isoproterenol-induced tremor and tachycardia in normal subjects. *Clin Pharmacol Ther*. 1981;29:425.

Isosorbide Mononitrate (ISMO)

Sildenafil (*Viagra*) `AVOID`

SUMMARY: Systolic and diastolic blood pressure may be markedly reduced by the coadministration of sildenafil and isosorbide mononitrate.

RISK FACTORS: No specific risk factors are known.

RELATED DRUGS: It is expected that a similar result would occur with other forms of nitrates including nitroglycerin (eg, *Nitro Dur*) and isosorbide dinitrate (eg, *Isordil*).

MANAGEMENT OPTIONS:

➡ ***AVOID COMBINATION.*** Sildenafil should not be used by patients taking nitrates due to the risk of hypotension.

REFERENCES:

Pfizer Pharmaceuticals. Sildenafil (*Viagra*) product information. 1998.

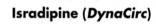

Isradipine (*DynaCirc*)

Lovastatin (*Mevacor*)

SUMMARY: Isradipine decreases lovastatin plasma concentrations; the clinical significance of this reduction is unknown but reduction of efficacy is possible.

RISK FACTORS: No specific risk factors are known.

RELATED DRUGS: The effect of isradipine on other HMG-CoA inhibitors is unknown, but they may be similarly affected.

MANAGEMENT OPTIONS:

➡ ***Monitor.*** Until more information is available, patients taking lovastatin should be monitored for reduced effects during isradipine coadministration.

REFERENCES:

Holtzman JL, et al. Interaction between isradipine and lovastatin in normal male volunteers. *Clin Pharmacol Ther*. 1993;53:164. Abstract.

Zhou L-X, et al. Pharmacokinetic interaction between isradipine and lovastatin in normal, female and male volunteers. *J Pharmacol Exper Ther*. 1995;273:121.

Itraconazole (*Sporanox*)

Lovastatin (*Mevacor*)

SUMMARY: Itraconazole administration produces a very large increase in lovastatin concentrations; toxicity including rhabdomyolysis may occur. Avoid concurrent use.

RISK FACTORS: No specific risk factors are known.

RELATED DRUGS: Simvastatin (*Zocor*) and atorvastatin (*Lipitor*) are metabolized in a similar manner to lovastatin and their metabolism probably would be inhibited by itraconazole. Pravastatin (*Pravachol*) may not be as dependent on CYP3A4 metabolism and therefore may not be inhibited to the same extent by itraconazole. The safety of fluvastatin (*Lescol*) has not been established. Ketoconazole (eg, *Nizoral*), miconazole (eg, *Monistat*), and fluconazole (*Diflucan*) would be expected to inhibit the metabolism of some HMG-CoA reductase inhibitors. Terbinafine (*Lamisil*) may have minimal effect on the metabolism of HMG CoA reductase inhibitors.

MANAGEMENT OPTIONS:

➡ *Use Alternative.* Pending further studies on other HMG-CoA reductase inhibitors, lovastatin and probably simvastatin should not be administered with itraconazole or other inhibitors of CYP3A4. The safety of pravastatin or fluvastatin when combined with itraconazole has not been established. Terbinafine may have minimal effect on the metabolism of the HMG-CoA reductase inhibitors since it does not appear to inhibit CYP3A4 activity. Patients receiving HMG-CoA reductase inhibitors, especially lovastatin or simvastatin, should be monitored carefully for muscle pain or weakness when any drug known to inhibit the activity of CYP3A4 is administered.

REFERENCES:

Lees RS et al. Rhabdomyolysis from the coadministration of lovastatin and the antifungal agent itraconazole. *N Engl J Med.* 1995;333:664.

Neuvonen PJ et al. Itraconazole drastically increases plasma concentrations of lovastatin and lovastatin acid. *Clin Pharmacol Ther.* 1996;60:54.

Itraconazole (*Sporanox*)

Methylprednisolone (eg, *Medrol*)

SUMMARY: Itraconazole increases the plasma concentrations of methylprednisolone; increased side effects associated with corticosteroid use may occur.

RISK FACTORS: No specific risk factors are known.

RELATED DRUGS: The effect of other azole antifungals that inhibit CYP3A4 would likely be similar. Ketoconazole (eg, *Nizoral*) has been noted to increase the concentration of IV methylprednisolone 135%. Fluconazole (*Diflucan*) is a weak CYP3A4 inhibitor, except in high doses. Terbinafine (*Lamisil*) is not known to inhibit CYP3A4 activity. The effect of itraconazole on other corticosteroids has not been established, but the metabolism of prednisone (*Deltasone*) and prednisolone (*Delta-Cortef*) is likely to be reduced by CYP3A4 inhibition.

MANAGEMENT OPTIONS:

➡ *Circumvent/Minimize.* Patients receiving concurrent itraconazole may require reduced doses of methylprednisolone.

➡ *Monitor.* Monitor patients for steroid-induced side effects including myopathy, weakness, and glucose intolerance.

REFERENCES:

Varis T, et al. Plasma concentrations and effects of oral methylprednisolone are considerably increased by itraconazole. *Clin Pharmacol Ther.* 1998;64:363-368.

Linthoudt H, et al. The association of itraconazole and methylprednisolone may give rise to important steroid-related side effects. *J Heart Lung Transplant.* 1996;15:1165.

Itraconazole (*Sporanox*)

Midazolam (*Versed*)

SUMMARY: Itraconazole administration causes a large increase in oral midazolam plasma concentrations and pharmacodynamic effects; increased side effects are likely.

RISK FACTORS:

➡ ***Route of Administration.*** Plasma midazolam concentrations will increase to a greater extent following oral administration than after IV midazolam dosing.

RELATED DRUGS: Ketoconazole (eg, *Nizoral*) and fluconazole (*Diflucan*) also reduce the metabolism of midazolam. Terbinafine (*Lamisil*) does not affect midazolam pharmacokinetics. Other benzodiazepines metabolized by CYP3A4 also will be affected by itraconazole, including alprazolam (eg, *Xanax*) and triazolam (eg, *Halcion*). Benzodiazepines that are metabolized by glucuronidation (eg, oxazepam [eg, *Serax*], lorazepam [eg, *Ativan*], temazepam [eg, *Restoril*]) will likely be minimally affected by itraconazole.

MANAGEMENT OPTIONS:

➡ ***Consider Alternative.*** Prescribe an oral benzodiazepine that is not metabolized via the CYP3A4 enzyme for patients maintained on itraconazole (see Related Drugs). Patients stabilized on midazolam requiring antifungal therapy might be candidates for terbinafine.

➡ ***Monitor.*** Carefully monitor patients receiving oral midazolam and itraconazole for increased sedation and reduced psychomotor performance.

REFERENCES:

Ahonen J, et al. Effect of itraconazole and terbinafine on the pharmacokinetics and pharmacodynamics of midazolam in healthy volunteers. *Br J Clin Pharmacol.* 1995;40:270-272.

Olkkola KT, et al. Midazolam should be avoided in patients receiving the systemic antimycotics ketoconazole and itraconazole. *Clin Pharmacol Ther.* 1994;55:481-485.

Olkkola KT, et al. The effects of the systemic antimycotics, itraconazole and fluconazole, on the pharmacokinetics and pharmacodynamics of intravenous and oral midazolam. *Anesth Analg.* 1996;82:511-516.

Itraconazole (*Sporanox*)

Nifedipine (eg, *Procardia*)

SUMMARY: Itraconazole administration produced increased nifedipine concentrations and enhanced the hypotensive effects of the calcium channel blocker.

RISK FACTORS: No specific risk factors are known.

RELATED DRUGS: It is likely that ketoconazole (eg, *Nizoral*) would inhibit the metabolism of nifedipine in a similar manner. Fluconazole (*Diflucan*) is a weak CYP3A4 inhibitor except in high doses. Terbinafine (*Lamisil*) is not known to inhibit CYP3A4 activity. Other calcium channel blockers would likely be affected by azole antifungals that inhibit CYP3A4.

MANAGEMENT OPTIONS:

➡ ***Consider Alternative.*** If excessive calcium channel blocker effect is observed with concomitant itraconazole therapy, a non-calcium channel blocker antihypertensive agent could be substituted for nifedipine. Consider terbinafine in place of itraconazole if appropriate.

➡ **Monitor.** Monitor patients receiving nifedipine or other calcium channel blockers for exaggerated effect (eg, hypotension, peripheral edema) during the coadministration of itraconazole.

REFERENCES:

Tailor SA, et al. Peripheral edema due to nifedipine-itraconazole interaction: a case report. *Arch Dermatol.* 1996;132:350-352.

Itraconazole (*Sporanox*)

Omeprazole (*Prilosec*)

SUMMARY: Omeprazole administration markedly reduces the plasma concentration of itraconazole; loss of antifungal effect may occur.

RISK FACTORS:

➡ **Pharmacogenetics.** Patients who are slow CYP2C19 metabolizers of omeprazole will likely be affected to a greater degree.

RELATED DRUGS: Ketoconazole is also dependent on an acidic gastric pH for complete absorption. All proton pump inhibitors (eg, esomeprazole [*Nexium*], lansoprazole [*Prevacid*], pantoprazole [*Protonix*], and rabeprazole [*Aciphex*]) will reduce the absorption of itraconazole and ketoconazole. Fluconazole (*Diflucan*) and voriconazole (*Vfend*) absorption does not appear to be affected by alkalinization of the stomach.

MANAGEMENT OPTIONS:

➡ **Circumvent/Minimize.** The administration of acidic drinks such as *Coca-Cola* or *Pepsi* (both have a pH of 2.5) will increase the absorption of itraconazole and ketoconazole in patients who have an elevated gastric pH., Theoretically, a solution of itraconazole (eg, *Sporanox* oral solution) would not be affected by changes in gastric pH, although no data are available. Consider using an alternative antifungal such as fluconazole or voriconazole.

➡ **Monitor.** Monitor patients taking itraconazole for possible loss of antifungal efficacy if drugs are coadministered that can increase gastric pH.

REFERENCES:

Jaruratanasirikul S, et al. Effect of omeprazole on the pharmacokinetics of itraconazole. *Eur J Clin Pharmacol.* 1998;54:159-161.

Lange D, et al. The effect of coadministration of a cola beverage on the bioavailability of itraconazole in patients with acquired immunodeficiency syndrome. *Curr Ther Res Clin Exp.* 1997;8:202-212.

Jaruratanasirikul S, et al. Influence of an acidic beverage (*Coca-Cola*) on the absorption of itraconazole. *Eur J Clin Pharmacol.* 1997;52:235-237.

Itraconazole (*Sporanox*)

Phenytoin (eg, *Dilantin*)

SUMMARY: Phenytoin dramatically reduces itraconazole serum concentrations and is likely to reduce its therapeutic response.

RISK FACTORS: No specific risk factors are known.

RELATED DRUGS: Enzyme inducers other than phenytoin also have been shown to reduce itraconazole serum concentrations.

MANAGEMENT OPTIONS:

➡ *Use Alternative.* Given the marked reduction in itraconazole serum concentrations, it would be prudent to use an alternative antifungal agent in patients receiving phenytoin. Ketoconazole (eg, *Nizoral*) metabolism also is increased by enzyme inducers and probably would not be a suitable alternative. Phenytoin is not likely to substantially affect fluconazole (*Diflucan*) (eliminated primarily unchanged by the kidneys), but fluconazole can inhibit phenytoin metabolism (via inhibition of CYP2C9). Thus, if fluconazole is used, monitor for increased phenytoin effect.

REFERENCES:

Ducharme MP, et al. Itraconazole and hydroxyitraconazole serum concentrations are reduced more than tenfold by phenytoin. *Clin Pharmacol Ther*. 1995;58:617-624.

Itraconazole (*Sporanox*) ▼

Quinidine

SUMMARY: Itraconazole administration increases quinidine plasma concentrations; cardiac toxicity could result.

RISK FACTORS: No specific risk factors are known.

RELATED DRUGS: Ketoconazole (eg, *Nizoral*) is known to reduce quinidine clearance; fluconazole (*Diflucan*) is also likely to increase quinidine concentrations. Terbinafine (*Lamisil*) does not affect CYP3A4 and would not be expected to alter quinidine concentrations.

MANAGEMENT OPTIONS:

➡ *Consider Alternative.* Consider the use of an antifungal agent that does not reduce CYP3A4 activity, such as terbinafine, for patients taking quinidine.

➡ *Monitor.* Observe patients taking quinidine for increased plasma concentrations and electrocardiographic changes, including increased QTc intervals.

REFERENCES:

Kaukonen KM, et al. Itraconazole increases plasma concentrations of quinidine. *Clin Pharmacol Ther*. 1997;62:510.

Itraconazole (*Sporanox*)

Repaglinide (*Prandin*)

SUMMARY: Itraconazole increases the serum concentration of repaglinide; enhanced hypoglycemic effects may result.

RISK FACTORS: No specific risk factors are known.

RELATED DRUGS: The elimination of other oral hypoglycemic agents (eg, pioglitazone [*Actos*]) metabolized by CYP3A4 may be reduced by itraconazole coadministration. Ketoconazole (eg, *Nizoral*), fluconazole (*Diflucan*), and voriconazole (*Vfend*) also inhibit CYP3A4 activity and may increase repaglinide serum concentrations.

MANAGEMENT OPTIONS:

➡ ***Consider Alternative.*** Consider using alternative lipid-lowering drugs not metabolized by CYP3A4 (eg, fluvastatin [*Lescol*] or pravastatin [*Pravachol*]) in patients receiving itraconazole. Terbinafine (*Lamisil*) does not inhibit CYP3A4 and could be considered as an alternative antifungal agent.

➡ ***Monitor.*** Monitor patients taking repaglinide for changes in blood glucose concentrations if itraconazole is added to or discontinued from the drug regimen.

REFERENCES:

Niemi M, et al. Effects of gemfibrozil, itraconazole, and their combination on the pharmacokinetics and pharmacodynamics of repaglinide: potentially hazardous interaction between gemfibrozil and repaglinide. *Diabetologia*. 2003;46:347-351.

Itraconazole (*Sporanox*)

Rifampin (eg, *Rifadin*)

SUMMARY: Rifampin appears to reduce itraconazole plasma concentrations; the interaction may reduce the efficacy of itraconazole.

RISK FACTORS: No specific risk factors are known.

RELATED DRUGS: Rifampin also reduces the concentration of fluconazole (*Diflucan*) and ketoconazole (eg, *Nizoral*).

MANAGEMENT OPTIONS:

➡ ***Monitor.*** Until further information is available, patients should be observed for reduced itraconazole concentrations and response when receiving rifampin.

REFERENCES:

Blomley M, et al. Itraconazole and anti-tuberculosis drugs. *Lancet*. 1990;336:1255.

Tucker RM, et al. Interaction of azoles with rifampin, phenytoin, and carbamazepine: in vitro and clinical observations. *Clin Infect Dis*. 1992;14:165-174.

Drayton J, et al. Coadministration of rifampin and itraconazole leads to undetectable levels of serum itraconazole. *Clin Infect Dis*. 1994;18:266.

Itraconazole (*Sporanox*)

Simvastatin (*Zocor*)

SUMMARY: Itraconazole increases the plasma concentrations of simvastatin and simvastatin acid; skeletal muscle toxicity could result.

RISK FACTORS: No specific risk factors are known.

RELATED DRUGS: Lovastatin (eg, *Mevacor*) undergoes metabolism similar to simvastatin and would likely be affected in a similar manner. Other antifungal agents (eg, ketoconazole [eg, *Nizoral*], fluconazole [*Diflucan*]) are likely to increase simvastatin concentrations. Pravastatin (*Pravachol*) and fluvastatin (*Lescol*) are not metabolized by CYP3A4 and would not be expected to interact with itraconazole.

MANAGEMENT OPTIONS:

➡ *Use Alternative.* Give fluvastatin or pravastatin to patients taking itraconazole who require an HMG-CoA reductase inhibitor.

REFERENCES:

Neuvonen PJ, et al. Simvastatin but not pravastatin is very susceptible to interaction with the CYP3A4 inhibitor itraconazole. *Clin Pharmacol Ther.* 1998;63:332-341.

Itraconazole (*Sporanox*)

Tacrolimus (*Prograf*)

SUMMARY: Itraconazole administration appears to increase tacrolimus concentrations; adjust tacrolimus dosage as required.

RISK FACTORS: No specific risk factors are known.

RELATED DRUGS: Other antifungal agents (eg, ketoconazole [eg, *Nizoral*], fluconazole [*Diflucan*]) are likely to increase tacrolimus concentrations. Cyclosporine (eg, *Neoral*) concentrations have been noted to increase when it is administered with itraconazole.

MANAGEMENT OPTIONS:

➡ *Consider Alternative.* Consider the use of an antifungal agent that does not inhibit CYP3A4 (eg, terbinafine [*Lamisil*]).

➡ *Monitor.* The concentration of tacrolimus should be monitored during coadministration of itraconazole. Be alert for evidence of tacrolimus toxicity including nephrotoxicity, hypertension, or hyperkalemia.

REFERENCES:

Billaud EM, et al. Evidence for a pharmacokinetic interaction between itraconazole and tacrolimus in organ transplant patients. *Br J Clin Pharmacol.*1998;46:271–74.

Itraconazole (*Sporanox*)

AVOID **Terfenadine†**

SUMMARY: Itraconazole administration produces elevated plasma concentrations of terfenadine that can lead to prolonged QTc intervals and ventricular arrhythmias. Terfenadine should not be taken by patients requiring itraconazole for antifungal therapy.

RISK FACTORS: No specific risk factors are known.

RELATED DRUGS: Other antifungal agents, including ketoconazole (*Nizoral*) and fluconazole (*Diflucan*), have been noted to increase terfenadine concentrations. Astemizole† concentrations have been noted to increase when it is administered with antifungal agents. Cetirizine (*Zyrtec*) and loratadine (*Claritin*) appear to be less likely to interact with itraconazole and produce cardiotoxicity.

MANAGEMENT OPTIONS:

➡ *AVOID COMBINATION.* Until more information on the interaction between itraconazole and terfenadine is available, it would be prudent to avoid giving the 2 drugs together. The use of sedating antihistamines or perhaps loratadine instead of terfenadine would seem to be preferred in patients taking itraconazole or other oral antifungal agents.

REFERENCES:

Honig PK, et al. Itraconazole affects single-dose terfenadine pharmacokinetics and cardiac repolarization pharmacodynamics. *J Clin Pharmacol*. 1993;33:1201.

Crane JK, et al. Syncope and cardiac arrhythmia due to an interaction between itraconazole and terfenadine. *Am J Med*. 1993;95:445.

Pohjola-Sintonen S et al. Itraconazole prevents terfenadine metabolism and increases risk of torsades de pointes ventricular tachycardia. *Eur J Clin Pharmacol*. 1993;45:191.

† Not available in the US.

2 **Itraconazole (*Sporanox*)**

Triazolam (eg, *Halcion*)

SUMMARY: Itraconazole administration produces large increases in triazolam concentrations and pharmacologic effects.

RISK FACTORS:

➡ *Route of Administration.* Oral administration of triazolam increases the risk for the interaction.

RELATED DRUGS: Midazolam (*Versed*) and diazepam (eg, *Valium*) concentrations are likely to be increased by itraconazole. Ketoconazole (*Nizoral*) or fluconazole (*Diflucan*) administration may result in increased triazolam concentrations.

MANAGEMENT OPTIONS:

➡ *Avoid Unless Benefit Outweighs Risk.* The concomitant administration of triazolam and itraconazole should be avoided.

➡ *Monitor.* Patients receiving triazolam and itraconazole should be monitored for increased triazolam effects including drowsiness and prolonged amnesia. Reduced doses of triazolam should be considered in patients taking itraconazole.

REFERENCES:
Varhe A, et al. Oral triazolam is potentially hazardous to patients receiving systemic antimycotics ketoconazole or itraconazole. *Clin Pharmacol Ther.* 1994;56:601.

Itraconazole (*Sporanox*)

Vincristine (*Oncovin*)

SUMMARY: Itraconazole may increase the risk of neurotoxicity in patients receiving vincristine.

RISK FACTORS: No specific risk factors are known.

RELATED DRUGS: Vinblastine (*Velban*) is metabolized by CYP3A4 and may be affected by itraconazole in a similar manner. Ketoconazole (*Nizoral*) is an inhibitor of CYP3A4 and P-glycoprotein and may interact in a similar manner with vincristine.

MANAGEMENT OPTIONS:

➡ *Monitor.* Carefully monitor patients receiving vincristine and itraconazole for evidence of neurotoxicity.

REFERENCES:
Bohme A, et al. Aggravation of vincristine-induced neurotoxicty by itraconazole in the treatment of adult ALL. *Ann Hematol.* 1995;71:311-312.

Itraconazole (*Sporanox*)

Warfarin (eg, *Coumadin*)

SUMMARY: A patient stabilized on warfarin developed excessive hypoprothrombinemia and severe bleeding after itraconazole was added to her regimen.

RISK FACTORS: No specific risk factors are known.

RELATED DRUGS: Other azole antifungal agents such as fluconazole (*Diflucan*), ketoconazole (*Nizoral*), and miconazole (eg, *Monistat*) also have been reported to increase the hypoprothrombinemic response to warfarin. The effect of itraconazole on oral anticoagulants other than warfarin is unknown, but theoretically phenprocoumon would be less likely to interact.

MANAGEMENT OPTIONS:

➡ *Monitor.* Monitor for altered oral anticoagulant effect if itraconazole is initiated, discontinued, or changed in dosage. Adjust the anticoagulant dose as needed.

REFERENCES:
Yeh J, et al. Potentiation of action of warfarin by itraconazole. *Br Med J.* 1990;301:669.

Kaolin-Pectin (eg, *Kao-Spen*)

Lincomycin (eg, *Lincocin*)

SUMMARY: Kaolin-pectin mixtures may reduce the antibacterial efficacy of lincomycin.

RISK FACTORS: No specific risk factors are known.

RELATED DRUGS: Clindamycin (eg, *Cleocin*) may be similarly affected by kaolin-pectin.

MANAGEMENT OPTIONS:

➡ ***Avoid Unless Benefit Outweighs Risk.*** Do not generally administer kaolin-pectin to patients taking lincomycin.

➡ ***Monitor.*** Monitor for reduced lincomycin efficacy if administered with kaolin-pectin.

REFERENCES:

Wagner JG. Pharmacokinetics. 1. Definitions, modeling and reasons for measuring blood levels and urinary excretion. *Drug Intell.* 1968;2:38.

McCall CE, et al. Lincomycin: activity in vitro and absorption and excretion in normal young men. *Am J Med Sci.* 1967;254:144-155.

McGehee RF Jr, et al. Comparative studies of antibacterial activity in vitro and absorption and excretion of lincomycin and clindamycin. *Am J Med Sci.* 1968;256:279-292.

Kaolin-Pectin (eg, *Kao-Spen*)

Quinidine (eg, *Quinora*)

SUMMARY: Kaolin-pectin reduces quinidine plasma concentrations when the 2 drugs are administered concurrently.

RISK FACTORS: No specific risk factors are known.

RELATED DRUGS: No information is available.

MANAGEMENT OPTIONS:

➡ ***Circumvent/Minimize.*** Although no data are available on the effect of separating the doses of quinidine and kaolin-pectin, it would be prudent to administer kaolin-pectin suspension several hours after quinidine to minimize this interaction.

➡ ***Monitor.*** Monitor quinidine concentrations and diminished antiarrhythmic efficacy if kaolin-pectin is coadministered.

REFERENCES:

Moustafa MA, et al. Decreased bioavailability of quinidine sulphate due to interactions with adsorbent antacids and antidiarrheal mixtures. *Int J Pharm.* 1987;34:207.

Ketoconazole (*Nizoral*)

Loratadine (*Claritin*)

SUMMARY: Ketoconazole administration increases loratadine plasma concentrations; the clinical significance of this effect is unknown.

RISK FACTORS: No specific risk factors are known.

RELATED DRUGS: Other antifungal agents (eg, miconazole [eg, *Monistat*], itraconazole [*Sporanox*], fluconazole [*Diflucan*]) are likely to increase loratadine concentrations.

MANAGEMENT OPTIONS:

➥ *Monitor.* Monitor patients receiving ketoconazole and loratadine for increased loratadine effects.

REFERENCES:

Brannan MD, et al. Effects of various cytochrome P450 inhibitors on the metabolism of loratadine. *Clin Pharmacol Ther.* 1995;57:193.

Ketoconazole (eg, *Nizoral*)

Lovastatin (*Mevacor*)

SUMMARY: Like itraconazole, ketoconazole administration may produce very large increases in lovastatin concentrations; toxicity including rhabdomyolysis may occur. Avoid concurrent use.

RISK FACTORS: No specific risk factors are known.

RELATED DRUGS: Simvastatin (*Zocor*) and atorvastatin (*Lipitor*) are metabolized in a similar manner to lovastatin and their metabolism probably would be inhibited by ketoconazole. Pravastatin (*Pravachol*) may not be as dependent on CYP3A4 metabolism and therefore may not be inhibited to the same extent by itraconazole. The safety of fluvastatin (*Lescol*) has not been established. Itraconazole (*Sporanox*), miconazole (eg, *Monistat*), and fluconazole (*Diflucan*) would be expected to inhibit the metabolism of some HMG-CoA reductase inhibitors. Terbinafine (*Lamisil*) may have minimal effect on the metabolism of HMG-CoA reductase inhibitors.

MANAGEMENT OPTIONS:

➥ *Use Alternative.* Pending studies on other HMG-CoA reductase inhibitors, lovastatin and probably simvastatin should not be administered with ketoconazole or other inhibitors of CYP3A4. The safety of pravastatin or fluvastatin when combined with ketoconazole has not been established. Terbinafine may have minimal effect on the metabolism of the HMG-CoA reductase inhibitors since it does not appear to inhibit CYP3A4 activity. Patients receiving HMG-CoA reductase inhibitors, especially lovastatin or simvastatin, should be monitored carefully for muscle pain or weakness when any drug known to inhibit the activity of CYP3A4 is administered.

REFERENCES:

Neuvonen PJ, et al. Itraconazole drastically increases plasma concentrations of lovastatin and lovastatin acid. *Clin Pharmacol Ther.* 1996;60:54.

Ketoconazole (*Nizoral*)

Methylprednisolone (eg, *Medrol*)

SUMMARY: Ketoconazole increases methylprednisolone concentrations and enhances methylprednisolone-induced suppression of cortisol secretion.

RISK FACTORS: No specific risk factors are known.

RELATED DRUGS: Ketoconazole has been reported to inhibit the metabolism of prednisolone.

MANAGEMENT OPTIONS:

➡ *Monitor.* Patients receiving methylprednisolone may require dosage adjustments when ketoconazole is added to or removed from their drug regimens.

REFERENCES:

Glynn AM, et al. Effects of ketoconazole on methylprednisolone pharmacokinetics and cortisol secretion. *Clin Pharmacol Ther.* 1986;39:654.

Kandrotas RJ, et al. Ketoconazole effects on methylprednisolone disposition and their joint suppression of endogenous cortisol. *Clin Pharmacol Ther.* 1987;42:465.

▼ Ketoconazole (eg, *Nizoral*)

Midazolam (*Versed*)

SUMMARY: Oral midazolam concentrations were markedly increased following ketoconazole administration; increased sedation and psychomotor impairment should be expected.

RISK FACTORS:

➡ *Route of Administration.* Plasma midazolam concentrations will increase to a greater extent following oral administration than after IV midazolam dosing.

RELATED DRUGS: Itraconazole (*Sporanox*), fluconazole (*Diflucan*), and miconazole (eg, *Monistat*) are likely to reduce midazolam's metabolism. Ketoconazole is likely to inhibit other benzodiazepines that are metabolized by CYP3A4 such as alprazolam (eg, *Xanax*) and triazolam (eg, *Halcion*). Benzodiazepines not metabolized via the CYP3A4 enzyme (eg, lorazepam [eg, *Ativan*], oxazepam [eg, *Serax*], temazepam [eg, *Restoril*]) are less likely to be affected.

MANAGEMENT OPTIONS:

➡ *Consider Alternative.* Prescribe patients maintained on ketoconazole a benzodiazepine that is not metabolized via the CYP3A4 enzyme (see Related Drugs). Consider patients stabilized on midazolam requiring antifungal therapy for terbinafine.

➡ *Monitor.* Carefully monitor patients receiving both midazolam and ketoconazole for increased sedation and reduced psychomotor performance.

REFERENCES:

Olkkola KT, et al. Midazolam should be avoided in patients receiving the systemic antimycotics ketoconazole and itraconazole. *Clin Pharmacol Ther.* 1994;55:481.

▼ Ketoconazole (*Nizoral*)

Nisoldipine (*Sular*)

SUMMARY: Ketoconazole markedly increases nisoldipine concentrations; increased hypotensive effects may occur.

RISK FACTORS: No specific risk factors are known.

RELATED DRUGS: Other antifungal drugs (eg, itraconazole [*Sporanox*] or fluconazole [*Diflucan*]) that can inhibit CYP3A4 would be expected to have a similar effect on nisoldipine pharmacokinetics. Several other calcium channel blockers are substrates for CYP3A4 and ketoconazole has been shown to reduce their first-pass metabolism and increase their plasma concentrations.

MANAGEMENT OPTIONS:

➡ *Circumvent/Minimize.* Calcium channel blockers with less first-pass metabolism (eg, amlodipine [*Norvasc*]) would be less affected by ketoconazole; however, one should still be alert for increased hypotensive effects. Terbinafine (*Lamisil*) does not appear to inhibit CYP3A4 activity and could be considered as an alternative antifungal agent in patients taking nisoldipine.

➡ *Monitor.* Monitor patients stabilized on nisoldipine for orthostatic hypotension and tachycardia if ketoconazole is administered.

REFERENCES:

Heinig R, et al. The effect of ketoconazole on the pharmacokinetics, pharmacodynamics and safety of nisoldipine. *Eur J Clin Pharmacol.* 1999;55:57-60.

Ketoconazole (eg, *Nizoral*)

Omeprazole (eg, *Prilosec*)

SUMMARY: Omeprazole markedly reduces the bioavailability of ketoconazole; loss of antifungal effect may occur. Ketoconazole increases omeprazole concentrations; some patients may experience increased side effects.

RISK FACTORS:

➡ *Pharmacogenetics.* Patients who are slow CYP2C19 metabolizers of omeprazole will likely be affected to a greater degree, both for the effect of omeprazole on ketoconazole absorption and the effect of ketoconazole on omeprazole metabolism.

RELATED DRUGS: Itraconazole (*Sporanox*) also is dependent on an acidic gastric pH for absorption. All proton pump inhibitors (PPIs) will reduce the absorption of ketoconazole and itraconazole. Lansoprazole (*Prevacid*), esomeprazole (*Nexium*), and pantoprazole (*Protonix*) are metabolized partially by CYP2C19 and CYP3A4 and would be expected to interact with ketoconazole and other azole antifungal agents that inhibit CYP3A4 (eg, itraconazole, voriconazole [*Vfend*], fluconazole [*Diflucan*]). Rabeprazole (*Aciphex*) has minimal CYP3A4 metabolism and would not likely be affected to a significant degree by azole antifungal agents.

MANAGEMENT OPTIONS:

➡ *Circumvent/Minimize.* The administration of acidic drinks such as *Coca-Cola* or *Pepsi* (both have a pH of 2.5) will increase the absorption of ketoconazole and itraconazole in patients who have elevated gastric pH. Theoretically, a solution formulation of the azole antifungal agent (eg, *Sporanox Oral Solution*) would not be affected by changes in gastric pH, although no data are available.

➡ *Monitor.* Monitor patients taking ketoconazole for possible loss of antifungal efficacy if drugs are coadministered that can increase gastric pH. While the PPIs are generally well tolerated, be alert for increased side effects (eg, headache, diarrhea) if ketoconazole is administered to patients taking PPIs metabolized by CYP3A4.

REFERENCES:

Chin TW, et al. Effects of an acidic beverage (*Coca-Cola*) on absorption of ketoconazole. *Antimicrob Agents Chemother.* 1995;39:1671-1675.

Bottiger Y, et al. Inhibition of the sulfoxidation of omeprazole by ketoconazole in poor and extensive metabolizers of S-mephenytoin. *Clin Pharmacol Ther.* 1997;62:384-391.

Lange D, et al. The effect of coadministration of a cola beverage on the bioavailability of itraconazole in patients with acquired immunodeficiency syndrome. *Curr Ther Res.* 1997;8:202-212.

Ketoconazole (eg, *Nizoral*)

Pimozide (*Orap*)

SUMMARY: Elevated pimozide concentrations and cardiac arrhythmias may occur if pimozide and ketoconazole are coadministered.

RISK FACTORS: No specific risk factors are known.

RELATED DRUGS: Itraconazole (*Sporanox*) would also be likely to produce increased pimozide plasma concentrations. Fluconazole (*Diflucan*) and voriconazole (*Vfend*) are less potent CYP3A4 inhibitors but may result in increased pimozide plasma concentrations and thus increase the risk of QTc prolongation.

MANAGEMENT OPTIONS:

➡ ***Use Alternative.*** Do not administer ketoconazole or any antifungal agent that is known to inhibit CYP3A4 to patients receiving pimozide. Consider terbinafine (*Lamisil*) as an alternative because it does not affect CYP3A4 activity.

➡ ***Monitor.*** If ketoconazole is coadministered with pimozide, monitor the ECG for evidence of QTc prolongation.

REFERENCES:
Product Information. Pimozide (*Orap*). Gate Pharmaceuticals. 1999.

 Ketoconazole (eg, *Nizoral*)

Quinidine (eg, *Quinora*)

SUMMARY: In a patient stabilized on quinidine, ketoconazole was associated with a marked increase in quinidine plasma concentrations.

RISK FACTORS: No specific risk factors are known.

RELATED DRUGS: Other azole CYP3A4-inhibiting antifungals (eg, fluconazole [*Diflucan*], miconazole [eg, *Monistat*], itraconazole [*Sporanox*]) would be expected to have similar effects on quinidine metabolism.

MANAGEMENT OPTIONS:

➡ ***Monitor.*** Until more definitive studies are available, patients stabilized on quinidine should be observed for increased plasma concentrations and electrocardiographic changes (prolonged QRS) when ketoconazole is added to their regimen.

REFERENCES:
McNulty RM, et al. Transient increase in plasma quinidine concentrations during ketoconazole-quinidine therapy. *Clin Pharm.* 1989;8:222.

Ketoconazole (eg, *Nizoral*)

Ranitidine (eg, *Zantac*)

SUMMARY: Ranitidine administration reduces the plasma concentrations of ketoconazole, potentially resulting in loss of antifungal effect.

RISK FACTORS: No specific risk factors are known.

RELATED DRUGS: Other oral antifungal agents may be similarly affected by ranitidine administration. Other H_2-receptor antagonists (eg, cimetidine [eg, *Tagamet*], nizatidine [*Axid*], famotidine [eg, *Pepcid*]) and proton pump inhibitors (eg, omeprazole [*Prilosec*], lansoprazole [*Prevacid*]) would be expected to produce similar reactions with ketoconazole.

MANAGEMENT OPTIONS:

➡ *Circumvent/Minimize.* Several recommendations have been made to avoid this interaction in patients with elevated gastric pH. The product information for ketoconazole suggests that each ketoconazole tablet should be dissolved in 4 mL of an aqueous solution of 0.2 N hydrochloric acid with the resulting mixture ingested with a straw (to avoid contact with teeth) and followed by a glass of water. Others suggest that an easier and equally effective method is to give 2 capsules of glutamic acid hydrochloride 15 minutes before the ketoconazole.

➡ *Monitor.* Until more is known about this interaction, be alert for evidence of reduced ketoconazole effect when ranitidine or other agents that increase gastric pH are coadministered.

REFERENCES:

Piscitelli SC, et al. Effects of ranitidine and sucralfate on ketoconazole bioavailability. *Antimicrob Agents Chemother*. 1991;35:1795.

Product information. Ketoconazole (*Nizoral*). Janssen Pharmaceutica. 1993.

Lelawongs P, et al. Effect of food and gastric acidity on absorption of orally administered ketoconazole. *Clin Pharm*. 1988;7:228.

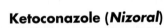

Ketoconazole (*Nizoral*)

Rifampin (eg, *Rifadin*)

SUMMARY: Rifampin and isoniazid (INH) decrease the plasma concentration of ketoconazole, and ketoconazole appears to decrease the peak plasma concentration of rifampin.

RISK FACTORS: No specific risk factors are known.

RELATED DRUGS: Rifampin reduces the concentration of fluconazole (*Diflucan*) and itraconazole (*Sporanox*).

MANAGEMENT OPTIONS:

➡ *Circumvent/Minimize.* Separation of the rifampin and ketoconazole doses by 12 hours may prevent depression of rifampin concentrations.

➡ *Monitor.* Patients should be observed for therapeutic failure when rifampin or INH are administered with ketoconazole. Likewise, the response to rifampin should be checked when ketoconazole is coadministered.

REFERENCES:

Engelhard D, et al. Interaction of ketoconazole with rifampin and isoniazid. *N Engl J Med*. 1984;311:1681.

Meunier F. Serum fungistatic and fungicidal activity in volunteers receiving antifungal agents. *Eur J Clin Microbiol*. 1986;5:103.

Drouhet E, et al. Laboratory and clinical assessment of ketoconazole in deep-seated mycoses. *Am J Med*. 1983;74(1B):30.

Brass C, et al. Disposition of ketoconazole, an oral antifungal, in humans. *Antimicrob Agents Chemother*. 1982;21:151.

Doble N, et al. Pharmacokinetic study of the interaction between rifampicin and ketoconazole. *J Antimicrob Chemother*. 1988;21:633.

Ketoconazole (eg, *Nizoral*)

Ritonavir (*Norvir*)

SUMMARY: Ketoconazole administration increases the plasma concentration of ritonavir; increased side effects could occur in some patients.

RISK FACTORS: No specific risk factors are known.

RELATED DRUGS: Ketoconazole has been reported to increase the concentrations of nelfinavir (*Viracept*) and saquinavir (*Fortovase*). Other protease inhibitors such as indinavir (*Crixivan*) may be affected in a similar manner. Itraconazole (*Sporanox*) and fluconazole (*Diflucan*) are inhibitors of CYP3A4 and may reduce the metabolism of ritonavir. Terbinafine (*Lamisil*) does not appear to inhibit CYP3A4 activity and may not increase ritonavir concentrations.

MANAGEMENT OPTIONS:

➡ **Consider Alternative.** Although no data are available, consider terbinafine as an alternative antifungal agent in patients receiving protease inhibitors.

➡ **Monitor.** Monitor patients taking protease inhibitors for increased concentrations and symptoms of toxicity (eg, nausea, vomiting, diarrhea) when ketoconazole is administered.

REFERENCES:

Khaliq Y, et al. Effect of ketoconazole on ritonavir and saquinavir concentrations in plasma and cerebrospinal fluid from patients infected with human immunodeficiency virus. *Clin Pharmacol Ther.* 2000;68:637-646.

Bertz R, et al. Evaluation of the pharmacokinetics of multiple dose ritonavir and ketoconazole in combination. *Clin Pharmacol Ther.* 1998;63:228.

Ketoconazole (eg, *Nizoral*)

Saquinavir (eg, *Invirase*)

SUMMARY: Ketoconazole administration can result in a large increase in saquinavir serum concentrations; toxicity may result in some patients.

RISK FACTORS: No specific risk factors are known.

RELATED DRUGS: Ketoconazole is known to increase the serum concentration of indinavir (*Crixivan*). The effects of other azole antifungal agents (eg, itraconazole [*Sporanox*], fluconazole [*Diflucan*]) that inhibit CYP3A4 metabolism on saquinavir is unknown, but some increase in saquinavir serum concentration would be expected. Terbinafine (*Lamisil*) does not appear to inhibit CYP3A4 activity and may not increase saquinavir concentrations.

MANAGEMENT OPTIONS:

➡ **Consider Alternative.** Although no specific data are available, terbinafine does not appear to inhibit CYP3A4 activity and might provide an alternative antifungal agent that may not increase saquinavir concentrations.

➡ **Circumvent/Minimize.** It may be necessary to reduce the dose of saquinavir when ketoconazole is coadministered.

➡ *Monitor.* Pending further information on this interaction, monitor patients for increased saquinavir serum concentrations and abdominal discomfort or diarrhea.

REFERENCES:
Product information. Saquinavir (*Invirase*). Hoffman-La Roche, Inc. 1995.

Ketoconazole (*Sporanox*)

Simvastatin (*Zocor*)

SUMMARY: Ketoconazole can cause elevated simvastatin concentrations leading to myopathy and, potentially, rhabdomyolysis.

RISK FACTORS: No specific risk factors are known.

RELATED DRUGS: Itraconazole (*Nizoral*), and to a lesser extent, fluconazole (*Diflucan*) and voriconazole (*Vfend*) will reduce the metabolism of simvastatin. The metabolism of lovastatin (*Mevacor*) is markedly reduced by coadministration of ketoconazole. Ketoconazole also reduces the clearance of atorvastatin (*Lipitor*) but to a lesser degree than observed with lovastatin.

MANAGEMENT OPTIONS:

➡ *Use Alternative.* Avoid coadministration of ketoconazole or itraconazole with simvastatin. Use a statin not dependent on CYP3A4 metabolism (eg, fluvastatin [*Luvox*], pravastatin [*Pravachol*]) with ketoconazole. If possible, use an antifungal without CYP3A4 inhibition (eg, Terbinafine [*Lamisil*]). If a suitable alternative antifungal is not available, withhold statin administration during antifungal therapy. Monitor for evidence of muscle pain or weakness.

REFERENCES:
Gilad R, et al. Rhabdomyolysis induced by simvastatin and ketoconazole treatment. *Clin Neuropharmacol.* 1999;22:295-297.

Ketoconazole (eg, *Nizoral*)

Sirolimus (*Rapamune*)

SUMMARY: Ketoconazole produced a marked increase in the plasma concentration of sirolimus. Sirolimus-induced toxicity may result.

RISK FACTORS: No specific risk factors are known.

RELATED DRUGS: Itraconazole (*Sporanox*) and fluconazole (*Diflucan*) may also increase the bioavailability of orally administered sirolimus. Tacrolimus (*Prograf*) plasma concentrations are also increased by ketoconazole.

MANAGEMENT OPTIONS:

➡ *Consider Alternative.* Consider the use of an antifungal agent that does not inhibit CYP3A4 (eg, terbinafine [*Lamisil*]) in patients stabilized on sirolimus who require antifungal therapy.

➡ *Monitor.* Monitor sirolimus concentrations and adjust the dose as necessary if ketoconazole is added to or discontinued from a patient's regimen. Be alert for signs of sirolimus toxicity, including hyperlipidemia and bone marrow depression.

REFERENCES:

Foren LC, et al. Sirolimus oral bioavailability increases ten-fold with concomitant ketoconazole. *Clin Pharmacol Ther.* 1999;65:159.

Ketoconazole (eg, *Nizoral*)

Sucralfate (eg, *Carafate*)

SUMMARY: The coadministration of sucralfate and ketoconazole reduces the plasma concentration of the antifungal agent; the clinical importance of the reduction is unknown.

RISK FACTORS: No specific risk factors are known.

RELATED DRUGS: No information is available.

MANAGEMENT OPTIONS:

➡ *Circumvent/Minimize.* Administer ketoconazole at least 2 hours before sucralfate to minimize any interaction.

➡ *Monitor.* If ketoconazole and sucralfate are coadministered, monitor for reduced antifungal effects.

REFERENCES:

Piscitelli SC, et al. Effects of ranitidine and sucralfate on ketoconazole bioavailability. *Antimicrob Agents Chemother.* 1991;35:1765-1771.

Carver PL, et al. In vivo interaction of ketoconazole and sucralfate in healthy volunteers. *Antimicrob Agents Chemother.* 1994;38:326-329.

Ketoconazole (eg, *Nizoral*)

Tacrolimus (*Prograf*)

SUMMARY: Ketoconazole increases the concentration of orally administered tacrolimus; toxicity may result.

RISK FACTORS:

➡ *Route of Administration.* The oral administration of tacrolimus will produce an interaction of greater magnitude with ketoconazole than that following the intravenous (IV) administration of tacrolimus.

RELATED DRUGS: Cyclosporine (eg, *Neoral*) is similarly affected by ketoconazole administration. Other azole antifungal agents (eg, itraconazole [*Sporanox*], fluconazole [*Diflucan*]) are likely to affect orally administered tacrolimus in a similar manner.

MANAGEMENT OPTIONS:

➡ *Consider Alternative.* Consider patients stabilized on tacrolimus who require antifungal therapy for an alternative antifungal agent. Since itraconazole and fluconazole may produce similar effects on the bioavailability of tacrolimus, consider terbinafine (*Lamisil*), which does not appear to reduce CYP3A4 or P-glycoprotein activity.

➡ *Circumvent/Minimize.* Reduce the dose of tacrolimus, based upon blood concentrations, if it is administered with ketoconazole.

➡ *Monitor.* Check tacrolimus blood concentrations during coadministration with ketoconazole.

REFERENCES:

Floren LC, et al. Tacrolimus oral bioavailability doubles with coadministration of ketoconazole. *Clin Pharmacol Ther.* 1997;62:41-49.

Ketoconazole (*Nizoral*)

Terfenadine† AVOID

SUMMARY: Excessive terfenadine concentrations following concomitant ketoconazole administration may increase the risk of cardiac arrhythmias.

RISK FACTORS:

➡ *Concurrent Diseases.* Pre-existing cardiac conduction problems increase the risk for the interaction.

RELATED DRUGS: Other oral antifungal agents (eg, itraconazole [*Sporanox*], fluconazole [*Diflucan*]) have been reported to inhibit the metabolism of terfenadine. Astemizole† metabolism also has been noted to be reduced during oral antifungal therapy.

MANAGEMENT OPTIONS:

➡ *AVOID COMBINATION.* Until more information on the interaction between ketoconazole and terfenadine is available, it would be prudent to avoid giving the 2 drugs together. The use of sedating antihistamines or perhaps cetirizine (*Zyrtec*) or loratadine (*Claritin*) instead of terfenadine would seem to be preferred in patients taking ketoconazole or other oral antifungal agents.

REFERENCES:

Monahan BP, et al. Torsades de pointes occurring in association with terfenadine use. *JAMA.* 1990;264:2788.

Zimmermann M, et al. Torsades de pointes after treatment with terfenadine and ketoconazole. *Eur Heart J.* 1992;13:1002.

Eller MG, et al. Pharmacokinetic interaction between terfenadine and ketoconazole. *Clin Pharmacol Ther.* 1991;49:130. Abstract.

Honig P, et al. The pharmacokinetics and cardiac consequences of the terfenadine-ketoconazole interaction. *Clin Pharmacol Ther.* 1993;53:206. Abstract.

† Not available in the US.

Ketoconazole (eg, *Nizoral*)

Tolterodine (*Detrol*)

SUMMARY: Ketoconazole moderately increased tolterodine serum concentrations, but it is not known how often this effect would result in adverse outcomes.

RISK FACTORS:

➡ *Pharmacogenetics.* This interaction is likely to be significant only in patients who are deficient in CYP2D6.

RELATED DRUGS: Itraconazole (*Sporanox*) is also a potent inhibitor of CYP3A4; fluconazole (*Diflucan*) is somewhat weaker, but in larger doses it also inhibits CYP3A4.

MANAGEMENT OPTIONS:

➥ *Circumvent/Minimize.* The manufacturer recommends that patients receiving CYP3A4 inhibitors such as ketoconazole and itraconazole, should not take tolterodine in doses greater than 1 mg twice daily.

➥ *Monitor.* In patients receiving tolterodine with ketoconazole or other CYP3A4 inhibitors, monitor for excessive antimuscarinic effects (eg, dry mouth, constipation, blurred vision, dry eyes).

REFERENCES:

Brynne N, et al. Ketoconazole inhibits the metabolism of tolterodine in subjects with deficient CYP2D6 activity. *Br J Clin Pharmacol.* 1999;48:564–72.

Short DD. Tolterodine, a new antimuscarinic drug for treatment of bladder overactivity—a comment. *Pharmacotherapy.* 1999;19:1188.

Ketoconazole (eg, *Nizoral*)

Triazolam (eg, *Halcion*)

SUMMARY: Triazolam plasma concentrations are markedly elevated by the coadministration of ketoconazole; increased toxicity is likely to result.

RISK FACTORS: No specific risk factors are known.

RELATED DRUGS: Itraconazole (*Sporanox*), fluconazole (*Diflucan*), and miconazole (eg, *Monistat*) are likely to reduce triazolam's metabolism. Ketoconazole is likely to inhibit other benzodiazepines that are metabolized by CYP3A4 such as alprazolam (eg, *Xanax*) and oral midazolam (*Versed*). Benzodiazepines not metabolized via the CYP3A4 enzyme (eg, lorazepam [eg, *Ativan*], oxazepam [eg, *Serax*]) are less likely to be affected.

MANAGEMENT OPTIONS:

➥ *Consider Alternative.* Patients maintained on ketoconazole should be prescribed a benzodiazepine that is not metabolized via the CYP3A4 enzyme (see Related Drugs). Patients stabilized on triazolam requiring antifungal therapy should be considered for terbinafine.

➥ *Monitor.* Patients receiving both triazolam and ketoconazole should be carefully monitored for increased sedation and reduced psychomotor performance.

REFERENCES:

Von Moltke LL, et al. Triazolam biotransformation by human liver microsomes *in vitro*: effects of metabolic inhibitors and clinical confirmation of a predicted interaction with ketoconazole. *J Pharmacol Exper Ther.* 1996;276:370.

Wright CE, et al. Ketoconazole inhibition of triazolam and alprazolam clearance: differential kinetic and dynamic consequences. *Clin Pharmacol Ther.* 1997;61:183. Abstract.

Ketoconazole (*Nizoral*)

Warfarin (eg, *Coumadin*)

SUMMARY: Isolated case reports, as well as the known interactive properties of the 2 drugs, suggest that ketoconazole increases the hypoprothrombinemic response of warfarin.

RISK FACTORS: No specific risk factors are known.

RELATED DRUGS: Other azole antifungal agents such as fluconazole (*Diflucan*), itraconazole (*Sporanox*), and miconazole (eg, *Monistat*) also have been reported to increase the hypoprothrombinemic response to warfarin. The effect of ketoconazole on oral anticoagulants other than warfarin is not established, but an interaction may occur (with the possible exception of phenprocoumon, which is metabolized primarily by glucuronidation).

MANAGEMENT OPTIONS:

➡ *Monitor.* Monitor for altered oral anticoagulant effect if ketoconazole is initiated, discontinued, or changed in dosage. Adjust the anticoagulant dose as needed.

REFERENCES:
Smith AG. Potentiation of oral anticoagulants by ketoconazole. *Br Med J*. 1984;288:188-189.

Ketoconazole (*Nizoral*)

Ziprasidone (*Geodon*)

SUMMARY: Ketoconazole administration resulted in a modest increase in ziprasidone plasma concentrations; some increase in side effects might occur.

RISK FACTORS: No specific risk factors are known.

RELATED DRUGS: Itraconazole (*Sporanox*) and fluconazole (*Diflucan*) can inhibit CYP3A4 activity and may reduce the metabolism of ziprasidone.

MANAGEMENT OPTIONS:

➡ *Circumvent/Minimize.* Terbinafine (*Lamisil*) does not appear to inhibit CYP3A4 activity and could be considered as an alternative antifungal agent in patients taking ziprasidone.

➡ *Monitor.* Be alert for some increase in side effects including dizziness, asthenia, and somnolence if ketoconazole and ziprasidone are administered concomitantly.

REFERENCES:
Miceli JJ, et al. The effects of ketoconazole on ziprasidone pharmacokinetics–a placebo-controlled crossover study in healthy volunteers. *Br J Clin Pharmacol*. 2000;49(suppl 1):71S-76S.

Ketoconazole (eg, *Nizoral*)

Zolpidem (*Ambien*)

SUMMARY: Ketoconazole produces an increase in zolpidem concentrations; increased sedation may occur.

RISK FACTORS: No specific risk factors are known.

RELATED DRUGS: Itraconazole (*Sporanox*) and fluconazole (*Diflucan*) have been reported to produce a minimal increase in zolpidem plasma concentrations.

MANAGEMENT OPTIONS:

➡ *Consider Alternative.* Because itraconazole and fluconazole produce minimal changes in zolpidem concentrations, they may be safer alternatives to ketoconazole. Terbinafine (*Lamisil*) is not an inhibitor of CYP3A4 and would not be expected to affect zolpidem metabolism. A benzodiazepine that is not a substrate for CYP3A4 (eg, lorazepam [eg, *Ativan*], oxazepam [eg, *Serax*]), could be substituted for zolpidem to avoid an interaction with ketoconazole.

➡ *Monitor.* Observe patients taking ketoconazole and zolpidem for enhanced sedation.

REFERENCES:

Greenblatt DJ, et al. Kinetic and dynamic interaction study of zolpidem with ketoconazole, itraconazole, and fluconazole. *Clin Pharmacol Ther.* 1998;64:661–671.

 Ketoprofen (eg, *Orudis*)

Methotrexate (eg, *Rheumatrex*)

SUMMARY: Isolated cases indicate that ketoprofen may increase the toxicity of antineoplastic doses of methotrexate.

RISK FACTORS:

➡ *Concurrent Diseases.* Particular caution is suggested in patients with preexisting renal impairment (who may be more susceptible to nonsteroidal anti-inflammatory drug [NSAID]-induced renal failure).

➡ *Dosage Regimen.* The risk of adverse effects from this interaction is primarily in patients receiving antineoplastic doses of methotrexate, rather than the lower doses used to treat rheumatoid arthritis, psoriasis, and related diseases.

RELATED DRUGS: Other NSAIDs may interact similarly; however, more information is needed.

MANAGEMENT OPTIONS:

➡ *Avoid Unless Benefit Outweighs Risk.* Until more information is available on this interaction, it would be prudent to avoid ketoprofen (as well as other NSAIDs) in patients receiving antineoplastic doses of methotrexate. Particular caution is suggested in patients with preexisting renal impairment, who may be more susceptible to NSAID-induced renal failure.

➡ *Monitor.* If the combination is used, monitor for methotrexate toxicity. Findings in methotrexate toxicity can include stomatitis, severe GI symptoms (eg, nausea, diarrhea, vomiting), bone marrow suppression, fever, bleeding, skin rashes, nephrotoxicity, and hepatotoxicity. Although decreasing the methotrexate dosage would be expected to reduce the likelihood of toxicity, the magnitude of the required reduction in methotrexate dosage has not been established.

REFERENCES:

Ahern AM, et al. Methotrexate kinetics in rheumatoid arthritis: is there an interaction with nonsteroidal antiinflammatory drugs? *J Rheumatol.* 1988;15:1356-1360.

Furst DE, et al. Effect of aspirin and sulindac on methotrexate clearance. *J Pharm Sci.* 1990;79:782-786.

Dupuis LL, et al. Methotrexate-nonsteroidal antiinflammatory drug interaction in children with arthritis. *J Rheumatol.* 1990;17:1469-1473.

Liegler DG, et al. The effect of organic acids on renal clearance of methotrexate in man. *Clin Pharmacol Ther.* 1969;10:849-857.

Skeith KJ, et al. Lack of significant interaction between low dose methotrexate and ibuprofen or flurbiprofen in patients with arthritis. *J Rheumatol.* 1990;17:1008-1010.

Stewart CF, et al. Effect of aspirin (ASA) on the disposition of methotrexate (MTX) in patients with rheumatoid arthritis (RA). *Clin Pharmacol Ther.* 1990;47:139.

Taylor JR, et al. Effect of sodium salicylate and indomethacin on methotrexate-serum albumin binding. *Arch Dermatol.* 1977;113:588-591.

Tracy FS, et al. The effect of NSAIDS on methotrexate disposition in patients with rheumatoid arthritis. *Clin Pharmacol Ther.* 1990;47:138.

Thyss A, et al. Clinical and pharmacokinetic evidence of a life-threatening interaction between methotrexate and ketoprofen. *Lancet.* 1986;1:256-258.

Boh LE, et al. Low-dose weekly oral methotrexate therapy for inflammatory arthritis. *Clin Pharm.* 1986;5:503.

Andersen PA, et al. Weekly pulse methotrexate in rheumatoid arthritis: clinical and immunologic effects in a randomized, double-blind study. *Ann Intern Med.* 1985;103:489-496.

Tugwell P, et al. Methotrexate in rheumatoid arthritis: indications, contraindications, efficacy, and safety. *Ann Intern Med.* 1987;107:358-366.

Daly HM, et al. Methotrexate toxicity precipitated by azapropazone. *Br J Dermatol.* 1986;114:733.

Adams JD, et al. Drug interactions in psoriasis. *Australas J Dermatol.* 1976;17:39-40.

Ketoprofen (eg, *Orudis*)

Warfarin (eg, *Coumadin*)

SUMMARY: A patient well controlled on chronic warfarin therapy developed excessive hypoprothrombinemia and bleeding after starting ketoprofen therapy. However, this patient may have been particularly predisposed to the interaction, and more study will be needed to determine the incidence and magnitude of the effect.

RISK FACTORS:

➡ ***Concurrent Diseases.*** Patients with peptic ulcer disease or a history of gastrointestinal (GI) bleeding are probably at greater risk for the interaction.

RELATED DRUGS: All NSAIDs inhibit platelet function, cause gastric erosions, and probably increase the risk of GI bleeding. Some NSAIDs, however, such as ibuprofen (eg, *Advil*), naproxen (eg, *Naprosyn*), or diclofenac (eg, *Voltaren*), may be less likely to increase oral anticoagulant-induced hypoprothrombinemia than other NSAIDs.

MANAGEMENT OPTIONS:

➡ ***Avoid Unless Benefit Outweighs Risk.*** Since all NSAIDs probably increase the risk of GI bleeding in patients on oral anticoagulants, use the combination only after careful consideration of the benefit versus risk. If an NSAID must be used with an oral anticoagulant, it would be prudent to use NSAIDs that are unlikely to affect the hypoprothrombinemic response to oral anticoagulants. If the NSAID is being used as an analgesic or antipyretic, acetaminophen (eg, *Tylenol*) probably is safer to use with oral anticoagulants. Nonacetylated salicylates (eg, choline salicylate, magnesium salicylate, salsalate, sodium salicylate) also probably are safer with oral anticoagulants than NSAIDs, since such salicylates have minimal effects on platelet function and the gastric mucosa.

➡ **Monitor.** If any NSAID is used with an oral anticoagulant, one should carefully monitor the prothrombin time and watch for evidence of bleeding, especially from the GI tract.

REFERENCES:

Flessner MF, et al. Prolongation of prothrombin time and severe gastrointestinal bleeding associated with combined use of warfarin and ketoprofen. *JAMA.* 1988;259:353.

Jahnchen E, et al. Interaction of allopurinol with phenprocoumon in man. *Klin Wschr.* 1977;55:759.

McInnes GT, et al. Acute adverse reactions attributed to allopurinol in hospitalized patients. *Ann Rheum Dis.* 1981;40:245.

Bach D, et al. The effect of verapamil on antipyrine pharmacokinetics and metabolism in man. *Br J Clin Pharmacol.* 1986;21:655.

Shorr RI, et al. Concurrent use of nonsteroidal anti-inflammatory drugs and oral anticoagulants places elderly persons at high risk for hemorrhagic peptic ulcer disease. *Arch Intern Med.* 1993;153:1665.

Mieszczak C, et al. Lack of interaction of ketoprofen with warfarin. *Eur J Clin Pharmacol.* 1993;44:205.

Ketorolac (eg, *Toradol*)

Lithium (eg, *Eskalith*)

SUMMARY: A patient receiving lithium developed about a doubling of his lithium serum concentrations after starting ketorolac, but the incidence and magnitude of this interaction is not established.

RISK FACTORS: No specific risk factors are known.

RELATED DRUGS: Most NSAIDs increase lithium serum concentrations, but sulindac (eg, *Clinoril*) and aspirin appear to have minimal effects.

MANAGEMENT OPTIONS:

➡ **Consider Alternative.** If appropriate for the patient, consider using an anti-inflammatory agent that is less likely to affect lithium, such as sulindac or aspirin.

➡ **Monitor.** If ketorolac therapy is initiated in a patient taking lithium, monitor serum lithium concentrations and look for evidence of lithium toxicity (eg, nausea, vomiting, diarrhea, anorexia, coarse tremor, slurred speech, vertigo, confusion, lethargy; in severe cases, seizures, stupor, coma, cardiovascular collapse). In a patient stabilized on lithium and an NSAID, discontinuation of the NSAID may result in inadequate lithium serum concentrations.

REFERENCES:

Langlois R, et al. Increased serum lithium levels due to ketorolac therapy. *CMAJ.* 1994;150:1455-1456.

Lamotrigine (*Lamictal*)

Phenytoin (eg, *Dilantin*)

SUMMARY: Phenytoin stimulates the metabolism of lamotrigine, resulting in lower plasma concentrations and decreased elimination half-life.

RISK FACTORS: No specific risk factors are known.

RELATED DRUGS: The effect of phenobarbital (eg, *Solfoton*) on lamotrigine has not been studied directly. However, the known inducing properties of phenobarbital and carbamazepine would be consistent with decreasing lamotrigine concentrations.

MANAGEMENT OPTIONS:

➡ *Monitor.* In patients stabilized on enzyme-inducing drugs, monitor for the need to use larger than expected doses of lamotrigine. Also be aware that discontinuing phenytoin may affect lamotrigine dosage requirements.

REFERENCES:

Binnie CD, et al. Double blind crossover trial of lamotrigine (*Lamictal*) as add-on therapy in intractable epilepsy. *Epilepsy Res.* 1986;4:222.

Jawad S, et al. Lamotrigine: single dose pharmacokinetics and initial 1 week experience in refractory epilepsy. *Epilepsy Res.* 1987;1:194.

Cohen AF, et al. Lamotrigine, a new anticonvulsant: pharmacokinetics in normal humans. *Clin Pharmacol Ther.* 1987;41:535-541.

Wolf P, et al. Lamotrigine: preliminary clinical observations on pharmacokinetics and interactions with traditional antiepileptic drugs. *J Epilepsy.* 1992;5:73.

Lamotrigine (*Lamictal*)

Rifampin (eg, *Rifadin*)

SUMMARY: Rifampin reduces the plasma concentration of lamotrigine; reduced antiepileptic efficacy may result.

RISK FACTORS: No specific risk factors are known.

RELATED DRUGS: Rifampin is known to induce the metabolism of several other antiepileptic agents. While no data are available, rifabutin (*Mycobutin*) also may increase lamotrigine metabolism.

MANAGEMENT OPTIONS:

➡ *Monitor.* Monitor patients receiving lamotrigine and rifampin for reduced lamotrigine plasma concentrations and reduced antiepileptic effect.

REFERENCES:

Ebert U, et al. Effects of rifampicin and cimetidine on pharmacokinetics and pharmacodynamics of lamotrigine in healthy subjects. *Eur J Clin Pharmacol.* 2000;56:299-304.

Lamotrigine (*Lamictal*)

Valproic Acid (eg, *Depakene*)

SUMMARY: Clinical evidence suggests that combined therapy with lamotrigine and valproic acid may increase the risk of toxic epidermal necrolysis, but a causal relationship has not been proved.

RISK FACTORS: No specific risk factors are known.

RELATED DRUGS: No information is available.

MANAGEMENT OPTIONS:

➥ *Circumvent/Minimize.* In patients receiving lamotrigine and valproic acid, it would be prudent to discontinue lamotrigine immediately if any rash appears.

➥ *Monitor.* The health care practitioner and patient should be alert for any evidence of rash.

REFERENCES:

Page RL II, et al. Fatal toxic epidermal necrolysis related to lamotrigine administration. *Pharmacotherapy.* 1998;18:392-398.

 Levodopa (eg, *Larodopa*)

Methionine

SUMMARY: L-methionine may inhibit the clinical response to levodopa in parkinsonian patients.

RISK FACTORS: No specific risk factors are known.

RELATED DRUGS: No information is available.

MANAGEMENT OPTIONS:

➥ *Circumvent/Minimize.* Large doses of methionine probably should be avoided in parkinsonian patients receiving levodopa.

➥ *Monitor.* Monitor for reduced levodopa effect if the combination is used.

REFERENCES:

Pearce LA, et al. L-methionine: a possible levodopa antagonist. *Neurology.* 1974;24:640.

Levodopa (eg, *Larodopa*)

Moclobemide

SUMMARY: Moclobemide appeared to increase the risk of adverse effects (eg, headache, nausea) in healthy subjects receiving levodopa; but more study is needed.

RISK FACTORS: No specific risk factors are known.

RELATED DRUGS: The effect of other MAO-A inhibitors on levodopa is not established.

MANAGEMENT OPTIONS:

➥ *Monitor.* If moclobemide is used in a patient receiving levodopa, one should monitor for the need to adjust the levodopa dosage.

REFERENCES:

Dingemanse J. An update of recent moclobemide interaction data. *Int Clin Psychopharmacol.* 1993;7:167.

Levodopa (eg, *Larodopa*)
Phenelzine (*Nardil*)

SUMMARY: The administration of levodopa with nonselective monoamine oxidase inhibitors (MAOIs) may result in a hypertensive response.

RISK FACTORS:

➥ *Other Drugs.* Concurrent use of carbidopa with levodopa appears to minimize the interaction with nonselective MAOIs.

➥ *Dosage Regimen.* One patient receiving phenelzine became hypertensive with a 50 mg dose of levodopa but not with a 25 mg dose.

RELATED DRUGS: All nonselective MAOIs including isocarboxazid (*Marplan*) and tranylcypromine would be expected to interact with levodopa in the absence of a decarboxylase inhibitor.

MANAGEMENT OPTIONS:

➥ *Circumvent/Minimize.* The use of a decarboxylase inhibitor (eg, carbidopa) with levodopa apparently prevents the hypertensive reactions.

➥ *Monitor.* The use of nonselective MAOIs with levodopa (in the absence of a decarboxylase inhibitor) generally should be avoided. Remember that the effects of nonselective MAOIs should be assumed to persist for 2 weeks after they are discontinued. If they are given concomitantly, blood pressure must be monitored very carefully. If hypertension ensues, the results of 1 case indicate that phentolamine (eg, *Regitine*) may reverse the hypertension.

REFERENCES:

Sharpe J, et al. Idiopathic orthostatic hypotension treated with levodopa and MAO inhibitor: a preliminary report. *Can Med Assoc J.* 1972;107:296.

Friend DG, et al. The action of 1-dihydroxyphenylalanine in patients receiving nialamide. *Clin Pharmacol Ther.* 1965;6:362.

Cotzias GC, et al. L-dopa in Parkinson's syndrome. *N Engl J Med.* 1969;281:272.

Cotzias GC. Metabolic modification of some neurologic disorders. *JAMA.* 1969;210:1255.

Hunter KR, et al. Monoamine oxidase inhibitors and L-dopa. *Br Med J.* 1970;3:388.

Kott E, et al. Excretion of dopa metabolites. *N Engl J Med.* 1971;284:395. Letter.

Goldberg LI, et al. Cardiovascular effects of levodopa. *Clin Pharmacol Ther.* 1971;12:376.

Teychenne PF, et al. Interactions of levodopa with inhibitors of monoamine oxidase and L-aromatic amino acid decarboxylase. *Clin Pharmacol Ther.* 1975;18:273.

Birkmayer W et al. Implications of combined treatment with "madopar" and L-Deprenil in Parkinson's disease. *Lancet.* 1977;1:439.

Corder CN, et al. Postural hypotension:adrenergic responsivity and levodopa therapy. *Neurology.* 1977;27:921.

Collier DS, et al. Parkinsonism treatment: Part III—update. *Ann Pharmacother.* 1992;26:227.

Levodopa (eg, *Larodopa*)

Phenytoin (eg, *Dilantin*)

SUMMARY: Preliminary patient data indicate that phenytoin may inhibit the antiparkinsonian effect of levodopa.

RISK FACTORS: No specific risk factors are known.

RELATED DRUGS: No information is available.

MANAGEMENT OPTIONS:

➥ *Consider Alternative.* Although this interaction is based on limited evidence, consider alternatives to phenytoin in parkinsonian patients receiving levodopa.

➥ *Circumvent/Minimize.* If the combination is used, a larger dose of levodopa may be required.

➥ *Monitor.* Be alert for evidence of levodopa's reduced antiparkinson effect if phenytoin is taken concurrently.

REFERENCES:

Mendez JS, et al. Diphenylhydantoin blocking of levodopa effects. *Arch Neurol.* 1975;32:44.

Levodopa (eg, *Larodopa*)

Pyridoxine (Vitamin B$_6$)

SUMMARY: Pyridoxine inhibits the antiparkinsonian effect of levodopa, but few patients are affected since concurrent use of carbidopa negates the interaction.

RISK FACTORS:

➥ *Other Drugs.* The interaction occurs only in the absence of concurrent therapy with a peripheral decarboxylase inhibitor (eg, carbidopa [*Lodosyn*]).

RELATED DRUGS: No information is available.

MANAGEMENT OPTIONS:

➥ *Circumvent/Minimize.* Pyridoxine and vitamin preparations containing pyridoxine should be avoided in patients receiving levodopa unless a peripheral decarboxylase inhibitor (eg, carbidopa) is also being given.

➥ *Monitor.* Monitor for reduced levodopa response if pyridoxine is used in the absence of a decarboxylase inhibitor.

REFERENCES:

Fahn S. "On-off" phenomenon with levodopa therapy in parkinsonism. *Neurology.* 1974;24:431.

Bianchine JR, et al. Levodopa and pyridoxine co-administration:differential metabolic effect in parkinsonian and normal subjects. *Ann Intern Med.* 1973;78:830. Abstract.

Carter AB. Pyridoxine and parkinsonism. *Br Med J.* 1973;4:236. Letter.

Mars H. Levodopa, carbidopa, and pyridoxine in Parkinson disease. Metabolic interactions. *Arch Neurol.* 1974;30:444.

Duvoisin RC, et al. Pyridoxine reversal of L-DOPA effects in parkinsonism. *Trans Am Neurol Assoc.* 1969;94:81.

Cotzias GC. Metabolic modification of some neurologic disorders. *JAMA.* 1969;210:1255.

Leon AS. Pyridoxine antagonism of levodopa in parkinsonism. *JAMA.* 1971;218:1924.

Papavasiliou PS, et al. Levodopa in parkinsonism: potentiation of central effects with a peripheral inhibitor. *N Engl J Med*. 1972;286:8.

Cotzias GC, et al. Blocking the negative effects of pyridoxine on patients receiving levodopa. *JAMA*. 1971;215:1504. Letter.

Mims RB et al. Inhibition of L-dopa-induced growth hormone stimulation of pyridoxine and chlorpromazine. *J Clin Endocrinol Metab*. 1975;40:256.

Hildick-Smith M. Pyridoxine in parkinsonism. *Lancet*. 1973;2:1029. Letter.

Jones CJ. Pyridoxine in parkinsonism. *Lancet*. 1973;2:1030. Letter.

Yahr MD, et al. Pyridoxine and levodopa in the treatment of parkinsonism. *JAMA*. 1972;220:861. Letter.

Levodopa (eg, *Larodopa*)
Spiramycin[†]

SUMMARY: Spiramycin reduces the plasma concentration of levodopa: antiparkinson efficacy may be reduced.

RISK FACTORS: No specific risk factors are known.

RELATED DRUGS: It is not known whether other macrolide antibiotics (eg, erythromycin [eg, *E-Mycin*]) that stimulate gastric motility would produce a similar effect.

MANAGEMENT OPTIONS:

➡ ***Monitor.*** Until studies in patients with Parkinson disease are available, administer spiramycin and other macrolide antibiotics that increase GI transit to patients taking levodopa-carbidopa combinations only with close observation for increased symptoms of Parkinson disease.

REFERENCES:
Brion N, et al. Effect of a macrolide (spiramycin) on the pharmacokinetics of L-dopa and carbidopa in healthy volunteers. *Clin Neuropharmacol*. 1992;15:229-235.

† Not available in the US.

Levodopa (eg, *Larodopa*)
Tacrine (*Cognex*)

SUMMARY: Tacrine may inhibit the effect of levodopa in patients with parkinsonism; dosage adjustments of one or both drugs may be required.

RISK FACTORS: No specific risk factors are known.

RELATED DRUGS: No information is available.

MANAGEMENT OPTIONS:

➡ ***Consider Alternative.*** Before giving tacrine to a patient with parkinsonism (whether on levodopa or not) consider the risk of worsening the parkinsonism.

➡ ***Monitor.*** If tacrine is used in a patient with parkinsonism, the doses of the tacrine or the antiparkinson drugs may need to be adjusted.

REFERENCES:
Ott BR, et al. Exacerbation of parkinsonism by tacrine. *Clin Neuropharmacol*. 1992;15:322-325.

Lidocaine (eg, *Xylocaine*)

Morphine (eg, *Duramorph*)

SUMMARY: A patient who had received morphine and fentanyl (eg, *Sublimaze*) during anesthetic induction developed respiratory depression and lost consciousness after receiving IV lidocaine; carefully monitor patients receiving opioids and lidocaine for excessive opioid effects.

RISK FACTORS:

➡ ***Route of Administration.*** The observed reaction occurred following IV use of lidocaine. Theoretically, an interaction with opioids would be unlikely to occur with routes of lidocaine administration that do not result in lidocaine reaching the CNS.

RELATED DRUGS: Theoretically, lidocaine would enhance the effect of any opioid.

MANAGEMENT OPTIONS:

➡ ***Monitor.*** If lidocaine is used concurrently with opioids, monitor for excessive opioid effects (eg, respiratory depression, CNS depression). Based on the case reported, administration of an opioid antagonist such as naloxone may be effective in reversing the reaction.

REFERENCES:

Jensen E, et al. Potentiation of narcosis after intravenous lidocaine in a patient given spinal opioids. *Anesth Analg.* 1999;89:758–59.

Lidocaine (eg, *Xylocaine*)

Propranolol (eg, *Inderal*)

SUMMARY: Lidocaine concentrations may become excessive during concomitant propranolol administration.

RISK FACTORS: No specific risk factors are known.

RELATED DRUGS: Metoprolol and nadolol interact similarly with lidocaine. Other beta blockers also may enhance the negative inotropic effects of lidocaine. Pindolol (eg, *Visken*) reportedly has no effect on lidocaine clearance.

MANAGEMENT OPTIONS:

➡ ***Monitor.*** Patients who receive concurrent therapy with beta blockers and lidocaine should be monitored carefully for increased lidocaine effects. The magnitude of the reduction in lidocaine clearance probably varies with different beta blockers, but no generalizations are possible at this time.

REFERENCES:

Bax NDS, et al. The impairment of lidocaine clearance by propranolol—major contribution from enzyme inhibition. *Br J Clin Pharmacol.* 1985;19:597.

Svendsen TL, et al. Effects of propranolol and pindolol on plasma lignocaine clearance in man. *Br J Clin Pharmacol.* 1982;13:223S.

Schneck DW, et al. Effects of nadolol and propranolol on plasma lidocaine clearance. *Clin Pharmacol Ther.* 1984;36:584.

Greenblatt DJ. Impairment of antipyrine clearance in humans by propranolol. *Circulation.* 1978;57:1161.

Branch RA, et al. The reduction of lidocaine clearance by dl-propranolol: an example of hemodynamic drug interaction. *J Pharmacol Exp Ther.* 1973;184:515.

Ochs HR, et al. Reduction in lidocaine clearance during continuous infusion and by coadministration of propranolol. *N Engl J Med.* 1980;303:373.

Graham CF, et al. Lidocaine-propranolol interactions. *N Engl J Med.* 1981;304:1301.

Conrad KA, et al. Lidocaine elimination: effects of metoprolol and of propranolol. *Clin Pharmacol Ther.* 1983;33:133.

Deacon CS, et al. Inhibition of oxidative drug metabolism by betaadrenoreceptor antagonist is related to their lipid solubility. *Br J Clin Pharmacol.* 1981;12:429.

Boudoulas H, et al. Negative inotropic effect of lidocaine in patients with coronary arterial disease and normal subjects. *Chest.* 1977;71:170.

Greenblatt DJ, et al. Impairment of antipyrine clearance in humans by propranolol. *Circulation.* 1978;57:1161.

Lisinopril (eg, *Prinivil*)

Lithium (eg, *Eskalith*)

SUMMARY: Several case reports suggest that lisinopril and other angiotensin-converting enzyme (ACE) inhibitors may increase the risk of serious lithium toxicity, but the incidence of this effect is unknown.

RISK FACTORS: No specific risk factors are known.

RELATED DRUGS: Given the proposed mechanism, it appears likely that all ACE inhibitors (eg, enalapril [eg, *Vasotec*]) have the potential to produce lithium toxicity.

MANAGEMENT OPTIONS:

➡ *Consider Alternative.* If possible, avoid the concurrent use of an ACE inhibitor and lithium. Although it appears that patients can be stabilized on the 2 drugs, it is possible that other factors (eg, diarrhea) may unmask the interaction, resulting in lithium toxicity. If an alternative to an ACE inhibitor is used, remember that other antihypertensives such as thiazides, calcium channel blockers, methyldopa, and possibly propranolol (eg, *Inderal*) and spironolactone (eg, *Aldactone*), also may affect lithium response.

➡ *Monitor.* If the combination of an ACE inhibitor and lithium is used, monitor the serum lithium concentration if the ACE inhibitor is initiated, discontinued, or changed in dosage. Monitor the patient for clinical evidence of lithium toxicity (eg, nausea, vomiting, diarrhea, anorexia, coarse tremor, slurred speech, vertigo, confusion, lethargy; in severe cases, seizures, stupor, coma, cardiovascular collapse). Adjust lithium dose as needed.

REFERENCES:
Baldwin CM, et al. A case of lisinopril-induced lithium toxicity. *DICP.* 1990;24:946-947.

Navis GJ, et al. Volume homeostasis, angiotensin converting enzyme inhibition, and lithium therapy. *Am J Med.* 1989;86:621.

Douste-Blazy P, et al. Angiotensin converting enzyme inhibitors and lithium treatment. *Lancet.* 1986;1:1448.

Correa FJ, et al. Angiotensin-converting enzyme inhibitors and lithium toxicity. *Am J Med.* 1992;93:108-109.

Lisinopril (eg, *Prinivil*)

Rofecoxib (*Vioxx*)

SUMMARY: Rofecoxib appears to inhibit the antihypertensive effect of lisinopril; monitor blood pressure and adjust lisinopril dosage as needed.

RISK FACTORS: No specific risk factors are known.

RELATED DRUGS: Theoretically, other COX-2 inhibitors such as celecoxib (*Celebrex*) would interact similarly with lisinopril and other ACE inhibitors, but little information is available. Several NSAIDs have been shown to inhibit the antihypertensive effect of ACE inhibitors.

MANAGEMENT OPTIONS:

➡ ***Consider Alternative.*** Antihypertensive agents other than ACE inhibitors (eg, calcium-channel blockers) may be less affected by COX-2 inhibitors.

➡ ***Monitor.*** If rofecoxib or other COX-2 inhibitors are used with lisinopril or other ACE inhibitors, monitor the blood pressure carefully. Based on limited evidence, increasing the ACE inhibitor dose may circumvent the interaction in patients with mild hypertension.

REFERENCES:

Brown CH. Effect of rofecoxib on the antihypertensive activity of lisinopril. *Ann Pharmacother.* 2000;34:1486. Letter.

Lithium (eg, *Eskalith*)

Losartan (eg, *Cozaar*)

SUMMARY: An elderly patient developed lithium toxicity after starting losartan, but more study is needed to establish the clinical importance of this effect.

RISK FACTORS: No specific risk factors are known.

RELATED DRUGS: The effect of angiotensin-2 receptor antagonists other than losartan on lithium is not established; theoretically they should interact similarly.

MANAGEMENT OPTIONS:

➡ ***Monitor.*** Be alert for evidence of lithium toxicity (eg, nausea, vomiting, diarrhea, anorexia, coarse tremor, slurred speech, vertigo, confusion, lethargy; in severe cases, seizures, stupor, coma, cardiovascular collapse). Adjust lithium dose as needed.

REFERENCES:

Blanche P, et al. Lithium intoxication in an elderly patient after combined treatment with losartan. *Eur J Clin Pharmacol.* 1997;52:501.

Lithium (eg, *Eskalith*)

Mefenamic Acid (*Ponstel*)

SUMMARY: Isolated cases of lithium toxicity have been associated with mefenamic acid therapy.

RISK FACTORS: No specific risk factors are known.

RELATED DRUGS: Most NSAIDs increase lithium serum concentrations, but sulindac (eg, *Clinoril*) and aspirin appear to have minimal effects.

MANAGEMENT OPTIONS:

➡ ***Consider Alternative.*** If appropriate for the patient, consider using an anti-inflammatory agent that is less likely to affect lithium, such as sulindac or aspirin.

➡️ *Monitor.* If mefenamic acid therapy is initiated in the presence of lithium therapy, monitor serum lithium concentrations and for symptoms consistent with lithium toxicity (eg, nausea, vomiting, diarrhea, anorexia, coarse tremor, slurred speech, vertigo, confusion, lethargy; in severe cases, seizures, stupor, coma, and cardiovascular collapse). In a patient stabilized on lithium and an NSAID, discontinuation of the NSAID may result in inadequate serum lithium concentrations.

REFERENCES:

MacDonald J, et al. Toxic interaction of lithium carbonate and mefenamic acid. *BMJ.* 1988;297:1339.

Shelly RK. Lithium toxicity and mefenamic acid: a possible interaction and the role of prostaglandin inhibition. *Br J Psychiatry.* 1987;151:847.

Lithium (eg, *Eskalith*)
Meloxicam (*Mobic*)

SUMMARY: Meloxicam increases lithium plasma concentrations and may produce lithium toxicity; the magnitude of the effect varies considerably among patients.

RISK FACTORS: No specific risk factors are known.

RELATED DRUGS: Most NSAIDs appear to increase lithium plasma concentrations, and available evidence suggests that COX-2 inhibitors such as celecoxib (*Celebrex*) and rofecoxib (*Vioxx*) do as well. Some evidence suggests that sulindac (eg, *Clinoril*) does not interact with lithium, but isolated cases of increased lithium levels have been reported. Available evidence suggests that aspirin (even large doses) has little effect on lithium.

MANAGEMENT OPTIONS:

➡️ *Monitor.* If meloxicam or another NSAID is used with lithium, monitor plasma lithium concentrations for symptoms consistent with lithium toxicity (eg, nausea, vomiting, diarrhea, anorexia, coarse tremor, slurred speech, vertigo, confusion, lethargy; in severe cases, seizures, stupor, coma, and cardiovascular collapse).

REFERENCES:

Turck D, et al. Steady-state pharmacokinetics of lithium in healthy volunteers receiving concomitant meloxicam. *Br J Clin Pharmacol.* 2000;50:197-204.

Lithium (eg, *Eskalith*)
Methyldopa (eg, *Aldomet*)

SUMMARY: Methyldopa was associated with evidence of lithium toxicity in several patients, but a causal relationship was not firmly established.

RISK FACTORS: No specific risk factors are known.

RELATED DRUGS: No information is available.

MANAGEMENT OPTIONS:

➡️ *Consider Alternative.* In patients who need lithium therapy, consider using antihypertensive therapy other than methyldopa.

➡️ *Monitor.* If the combination is used, monitor for evidence of lithium intoxication (eg, nausea, vomiting, tremor, confusion, weakness, dizziness, slurred speech).

Plasma lithium concentrations may not be useful in detecting this interaction because they may be in the therapeutic range.

REFERENCES:

O'Regan JB. Adverse interactions of lithium carbonate and methyldopa. *Can Med Assoc J.* 1976;115:385. Letter.

Byrd GJ. Methyldopa and lithium carbonate: suspected interaction. *JAMA.* 1975;233:320. Letter.

Osanloo E, et al. Interaction of lithium and methyldopa. *Ann Intern Med.* 1980;92:433.

Walker N, et al. Lithium-methyldopa interactions in normal subjects. *DICP.* 1980;14:638.

Yassa R. Lithium-methyldopa interaction. *Can Med Assoc J.* 1986;134:141.

Lithium (eg, *Eskalith*)

Naproxen (eg, *Naprosyn*)

SUMMARY: Naproxen increases lithium serum concentrations and may increase the risk of lithium toxicity; the magnitude of the effect appears to vary considerably from patient to patient.

RISK FACTORS: No specific risk factors are known.

RELATED DRUGS: Most NSAIDs increase lithium serum concentrations, but sulindac (eg, *Clinoril*) and aspirin appear to have minimal effects.

MANAGEMENT OPTIONS:

➡ *Consider Alternative.* If appropriate for the patient, consider using an anti-inflammatory agent that is less likely to affect lithium, such as sulindac or aspirin.

➡ *Monitor.* If naproxen therapy is initiated in the presence of lithium therapy, monitor serum lithium concentrations and for symptoms consistent with lithium toxicity (eg, nausea, vomiting, diarrhea, anorexia, coarse tremor, slurred speech, vertigo, confusion, lethargy; in severe cases, seizures, stupor, coma, cardiovascular collapse). In a patient stabilized on lithium and an NSAID, discontinuation of the NSAID may result in inadequate serum lithium concentrations.

REFERENCES:

Ragheb M, et al. Lithium interaction with sulindac and naproxen. *J Clin Psychopharmacol.* 1986;6:150.

Lithium (eg, *Eskalith*)

Phenelzine (*Nardil*)

SUMMARY: Two fatal cases of malignant hyperpyrexia have been reported in patients taking lithium and phenelzine, but a causal relationship was not established.

RISK FACTORS: No specific risk factors are known.

RELATED DRUGS: Until more information is available, one should assume that other nonselective monoamine oxidase inhibitors (MAOIs) such as isocarboxazid (*Marplan*) and tranylcypromine (*Parnate*) also can interact with lithium.

MANAGEMENT OPTIONS:

➡ *Avoid Unless Benefit Outweighs Risk.* Given the severity of the reported interactions, it would be prudent to avoid concurrent use of lithium with nonselective MAOIs until additional information is available. The effects of nonselective MAOIs should be assumed to persist for 2 weeks after they are discontinued.

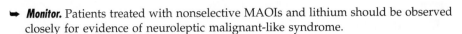
➥ *Monitor.* Patients treated with nonselective MAOIs and lithium should be observed closely for evidence of neuroleptic malignant-like syndrome.

REFERENCES:
Brennan D, et al. Neuroleptic malignant syndrome without neuroleptics. *Br J Psychiatry.* 1988;152:578.
Staufenberg EF, et al. Malignant hyperpyrexia syndrome in combined treatment. *Br J Psychiatry.* 1989;154:577.

Lithium (eg, *Eskalith*)
Phenylbutazone

SUMMARY: Phenylbutazone appears to increase lithium serum concentrations, but the magnitude of the effect appears to vary considerably from patient to patient. Limited evidence suggests that phenylbutazone may result in adverse psychiatric symptoms in patients receiving lithium.

RISK FACTORS: No specific risk factors are known.

RELATED DRUGS: Most NSAIDs increase lithium serum concentrations, but sulindac (eg, *Clinoril*) and aspirin appear to have minimal effects.

MANAGEMENT OPTIONS:

➥ *Consider Alternative.* If appropriate for the patient, consider using an anti-inflammatory agent that is less likely to affect lithium, such as sulindac or aspirin.

➥ *Monitor.* Monitor serum lithium concentrations and for symptoms consistent with lithium toxicity (eg, nausea, vomiting, diarrhea, anorexia, coarse tremor, slurred speech, vertigo, confusion, lethargy; in severe cases, seizures, stupor, coma, cardiovascular collapse) when phenylbutazone therapy is initiated. In a patient stabilized on lithium and an NSAID, discontinuation of the NSAID may result in inadequate serum lithium concentrations.

REFERENCES:
Ragheb M. The interaction of lithium with phenylbutazone in bipolar affective patients. *J Clin Psychopharmacol.* 1990;10:149. Letter.

Lithium (eg, *Eskalith*)
Phenytoin (eg, *Dilantin*)

SUMMARY: Some patients have developed lithium intoxication following phenytoin use, but a causal relationship has not been established.

RISK FACTORS: No specific risk factors are known.

RELATED DRUGS: No information is available.

MANAGEMENT OPTIONS:

➥ *Monitor.* Until more information is available, be alert for evidence of lithium toxicity when phenytoin is given concurrently.

REFERENCES:
Salem RB, et al. Ataxia as the primary symptom of lithium toxicity. *Drug Intell Clin Pharm.* 1980;14:621.
Spiers J et al. Severe lithium toxicity within normal serum concentrations. *Br Med J.* 1978;1:815.
MacCallum WAG. Interaction of lithium and phenytoin. *Br Med J.* 1980;280:610.

Lithium (eg, *Eskalith*)

Piroxicam (eg, *Feldene*)

SUMMARY: Piroxicam was associated with symptoms of lithium toxicity in one well-documented case report, but the incidence of this effect in patients receiving this drug combination is not known.

RISK FACTORS: No specific risk factors are known.

RELATED DRUGS: Most nonsteroidal anti-inflammatory drugs increase lithium serum concentrations, but sulindac (eg, *Clinoril*) and aspirin appear to have minimal effects.

MANAGEMENT OPTIONS:

➡ ***Consider Alternative.*** If appropriate for the patient, consider using an anti-inflammatory agent that is less likely to affect lithium, such as sulindac or aspirin.

➡ ***Monitor.*** Be alert for evidence of increased lithium effect when piroxicam is started or stopped (eg, nausea, vomiting, diarrhea, anorexia, coarse tremor, slurred speech, vertigo, confusion, lethargy; in severe cases, seizures, stupor, coma, cardio-vascular collapse). Serum lithium determinations would be useful in monitoring this interaction.

REFERENCES:

Kerry RJ, et al. Possible toxic interaction between lithium and piroxicam. *Lancet.* 1983;1:418.

 # Lithium (eg, *Eskalith*)

Potassium Iodide

SUMMARY: Hypothyroidism may be more likely in patients receiving both lithium and potassium iodide than in those receiving either drug alone, but the degree of increased risk is not established.

RISK FACTORS: No specific risk factors are known.

RELATED DRUGS: No information is available.

MANAGEMENT OPTIONS:

➡ ***Monitor.*** If it is necessary to use lithium and iodide concomitantly, monitor the patient for signs of hypothyroidism.

REFERENCES:

Shopsin B, et al. Iodine and lithium-induced hypothyroidism: documentation of synergism. *Am J Med.* 1973;55:695.

Swedberg K, et al. Heart failure as complication of lithium treatment. *Acta Med Scand.* 1974;196:279.

Wiener JD. Lithium carbonate-induced myxedema. *JAMA.* 1972;220:587. Letter.

Jorgensen JV, et al. Possible synergism between iodine and lithium carbonate. *JAMA.* 1973;223:192. Letter.

 # Lithium (eg, *Eskalith*)

Sibutramine (*Meridia*)

SUMMARY: The risk of serotonin syndrome would theoretically increase when sibutramine is combined with other sero-tonergic drugs such as lithium.

RISK FACTORS: No specific risk factors are known.

RELATED DRUGS: No information is available.

MANAGEMENT OPTIONS:

➡ *Avoid Unless Benefit Outweighs Risk.* The manufacturer states that sibutramine should not be used with lithium. This is a prudent recommendation until more information is available.

➡ *Monitor.* Serotonin syndrome can result in neurotoxicity (ie, myoclonus, tremors, rigidity, incoordination, restlessness, hyperreflexia, seizures, coma), psychiatric symptoms (ie, agitation, confusion, hypomania), and temperature regulation abnormalities (ie, fever, sweating). Note that mild forms of serotonin syndrome have also been reported, so any combination of the above symptoms should be considered possibly related to excessive serotonin activity.

REFERENCES:

Product information. Sibutramine (*Meridia*). Knoll Pharmaceuticals. 1997.

Mills KC. Serotonin syndrome: a clinical update. *Crit Care Clin.* 1997;13:763.

Lithium (eg, *Eskalith*)

Sodium Bicarbonate

SUMMARY: Sodium bicarbonate may lower plasma lithium concentrations.

RISK FACTORS: No specific risk factors are known.

RELATED DRUGS: No information is available.

MANAGEMENT OPTIONS:

➡ *Monitor.* Patients on combined sodium bicarbonate and lithium therapy should be monitored for decreased lithium effect. Lithium blood levels may be helpful in assessing this interaction.

REFERENCES:

Thomsen K, et al. Renal lithium excretion in man. *Am J Physiol.* 1968;215:823.

Lithium (eg, *Eskalith*)

Sodium Chloride

SUMMARY: High sodium intake may reduce serum lithium concentrations, while restriction of sodium may increase serum lithium.

RISK FACTORS: No specific risk factors are known.

RELATED DRUGS: No information is available.

MANAGEMENT OPTIONS:

➡ *Circumvent/Minimize.* Extremely large or small intakes of sodium chloride should be avoided in patients receiving lithium carbonate. Patients on severe salt-restricted diets probably should not be given lithium carbonate.

➡ *Monitor.* Monitor for increased lithium response if sodium intake is reduced and for decreased lithium response if sodium intake is increased.

REFERENCES:

Hurtig HI, et al. Lithium toxicity enhanced by diuresis. *N Engl J Med.* 1974;290:748.

Platman SR, et al. Lithium retention and excretion. The effect of sodium and fluid intake. *Arch Gen Psychiatry.* 1969;20:285.

Bleiweiss H. Salt supplements with lithium. *Lancet.* 1970;1:416. Letter.

Levy ST, et al. Lithium-induced diabetes insipidus: manic symptoms, brain and electrolyte correlates, and chlorothiazide treatment. *Am J Psychiatry.* 1973;130:1014.

Demers RG, et al. Sodium intake and lithium treatment in mania. *Am J Psychiatry.* 1971;128:1.

Lithium (eg, *Eskalith*)

Theophylline (eg, *Theo-Dur*)

SUMMARY: Theophylline appears to increase renal lithium clearance in most patients; the magnitude of the effect probably is sufficient to reduce lithium efficacy in some patients.

RISK FACTORS: No specific risk factors are known.

RELATED DRUGS: No information is available.

MANAGEMENT OPTIONS:

➡ *Circumvent/Minimize.* Intermittent use of theophylline in a patient on chronic lithium is best avoided, since the patient's response to lithium may fluctuate each time the theophylline is started or stopped.

➡ *Monitor.* When initiating theophylline therapy in a patient on chronic lithium, be alert for evidence of reduced lithium response. Discontinuation of theophylline therapy in a patient receiving lithium may result in excessive lithium response. When initiating lithium therapy in a patient on chronic theophylline, lithium dosage requirements may be higher than anticipated. Measurement of serum lithium concentrations would be useful in monitoring this interaction.

REFERENCES:

Thomsen K, et al. Renal lithium excretion in man. *Am J Physiol.* 1968;215:823.

Sierles FS, et al. Concurrent use of theophylline and lithium in a patient with chronic obstructive lung disease and bipolar disorder. *Am J Psychiatry.* 1982;139:117.

Cook BL, et al. Theophylline-lithium interaction. *J Clin Psychiatry.* 1985;46:278.

Lithium (eg, *Eskalith*)

Verapamil (eg, *Calan*)

SUMMARY: The addition of verapamil or diltiazem (eg, Cardizem) to patients stabilized on lithium therapy may result in neurotoxicity.

RISK FACTORS: No specific risk factors are known.

RELATED DRUGS: If this interaction is due to additive effects on cellular calcium transport, other calcium channel blockers might interact in a similar manner. Other case reports describe the development of stiffness and rigidity or psychosis after diltiazem (eg, *Cardizem*) was added to lithium therapy.

MANAGEMENT OPTIONS:

➡ *Monitor.* The use of calcium blockers in the treatment of patients with bipolar disorders receiving lithium should be commenced carefully with observation for neurotoxic effects. More experience with this interaction is necessary to determine if anticholinergic agents will be useful in controlling some of the symptoms associated with the interaction.

REFERENCES:

Price WA, et al. Neurotoxicity caused by lithium-verapamil synergism. *J Clin Pharmacol.* 1986;26:717.

Price WA, et al. Lithium-verapamil toxicity in the elderly. *J Am Geriatr Soc.* 1987;35:177.

Valdiserri EV. A possible interaction between lithium and diltiazem: case report. *J Clin Psychiatry.* 1985;46:540.

Helmuth D, et al. Choreoathetosis induced by verapamil and lithium treatment. *J Clin Psychopharmacol.* 1989;9:454. Letter.

Binder EF, et al. Diltiazem-induced psychosis and a possible diltiazem-lithium interaction. *Arch Intern Med.* 1991;151:373.

Lopinavir/Ritonavir (*Kaletra*)

Disulfiram (*Antabuse*) `AVOID`

SUMMARY: The oral solution of *Kaletra* contains a considerable amount of alcohol and should not be used by patients taking disulfiram.

RISK FACTORS: No specific risk factors are known.

RELATED DRUGS: All solutions containing alcohol are contraindicated in patients taking disulfiram.

MANAGEMENT OPTIONS:

➡ *AVOID COMBINATION.* Do not use *Kaletra* oral solution in patients taking disulfiram; *Kaletra* capsules can be used.

REFERENCES:

Product information. Lopinavir/Ritonavir (*Kaletra*). Abbott Laboratories. 2000.

Loratadine (eg, *Claritin*)

Nefazodone (*Serzone*)

SUMMARY: Nefazodone increases loratadine serum concentrations resulting in a modest increase in the corrected QT (QTc) interval on the electrocardiogram (ECG), but the clinical importance of this effect is not established.

RISK FACTORS:

➡ *Hypokalemia.* The QTc interval on the ECG may be prolonged in patients with hypokalemia, increasing the risk of this interaction.

➡ *Miscellaneous.* Other factors that may prolong the QTc interval (eg, hypomagnesemia, bradycardia, impaired liver function, hypothyroidism) also may increase the risk of ventricular arrhythmias.

RELATED DRUGS: Sertraline (*Zoloft*), venlafaxine (*Effexor*), and citalopram (*Celexa*) have little effect on CYP3A4 or CYP2D6, and theoretically would be unlikely to interact with loratadine. Cetirizine (*Zyrtec*) and fexofenadine (*Allegra*) do not appear to be metabolized by cytochrome P450 isozymes, and do not appear to affect the QTc interval. Thus, they would theoretically be unlikely to interact with nefazodone.

MANAGEMENT OPTIONS:

➡ **Consider Alternative.** Consider using an alternative antihistamine (eg, fexofenadine, cetirizine) instead of loratadine. Or consider an alternative antidepressant (eg, sertraline, venlafaxine, citalopram) in place of nefazodone (see Related Drugs).

➡ **Monitor.** If loratadine and nefazodone are used concurrently, monitor for evidence of arrhythmias (eg, syncope) and for prolonged QT intervals.

REFERENCES:

De Ponti F, et al. QT-interval prolongation by non-cardiac drugs: lessons to be learned from recent experience. *Eur J Clin Pharmacol.* 2000;56:1-18.

Abernethy DR, et al. Loratadine and terfenadine interaction with nefazodone: both antihistamines are associated with QTc prolongation. *Clin Pharmacol Ther.* 2001;69:96-103.

Lorazepam (*Ativan*)

Loxapine (eg, *Loxitane*)

SUMMARY: Isolated cases of respiratory depression, stupor, and hypotension have been observed in patients receiving loxapine and lorazepam, but the role that a drug interaction played in these cases was not established.

RISK FACTORS: No specific risk factors are known.

RELATED DRUGS: Positive results of combining benzodiazepines and neuroleptics have been reported. Diazepam increased the antipsychotic response to neuroleptic agents in schizophrenic patients, and lorazepam appeared to alleviate auditory hallucinations in a schizophrenic patient receiving 1 g/day of chlorpromazine (eg, *Thorazine*). Other combinations of neuroleptics and benzodiazepines have been used without excessive adverse effects.

MANAGEMENT OPTIONS:

➡ **Monitor.** Until more information is available, carefully monitor patients receiving loxapine and lorazepam for excessive sedation and respiratory depression. With any other combination of a neuroleptic and a benzodiazepine, consider the possibility of additive sedative effects and monitor patients accordingly.

REFERENCES:

Cohen S, et al. Respiratory distress with use of lorazepam in mania. *J Clin Psychopharmacol.* 1987;7:199-200.

Battaglia, et al. Loxapine-lorazepam-induced hypotension and stupor. *J Clin Psychopharmacol.* 1989;9:227-228.

Lingjaerde O, et al. Antipsychotic effect of diazepam when given in addition to neuroleptics in chronic psychotic patients: a double-blind clinical trial. *Curr Ther Res.* 1979;26:505.

Yassa R, et al. Lorazepam as an adjunct in the treatment of auditory hallucinations in a schizophrenic patient. *J Clin Psychopharmacol.* 1989;9:386.

Lorcainide†

Rifampin (eg, *Rifadin*)

SUMMARY: Evidence from 1 patient suggests that rifampin may decrease lorcainide plasma concentrations.

RISK FACTORS: No specific risk factors are known.

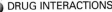

RELATED DRUGS: No information is available.

MANAGEMENT OPTIONS:

➥ *Monitor.* Patients receiving lorcainide may require increased doses while taking rifampin; be alert for loss of efficacy.

REFERENCES:

Mauro VF, et al. Drug interaction between lorcainide and rifampicin. *Eur J Clin Pharmacol.* 1987;31:737-738.

† Not available in the US.

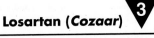

Losartan (*Cozaar*)

Rifampin (eg, *Rifadin*)

SUMMARY: Rifampin administration reduces the plasma concentrations of losartan and its active metabolite. A reduction in hypotensive efficacy may occur.

RISK FACTORS: No specific risk factors are known.

RELATED DRUGS: Eprosartan (*Teveten*), a related angiotensin II receptor inhibitor, is not metabolized by the cytochrome P450 system and would not be expected to interact with rifampin. Rifabutin (*Mycobutin*) would be expected to have a similar effect on eprosartan.

MANAGEMENT OPTIONS:

➥ *Consider Alternative.* Switch patients stabilized on losartan who require rifampin to an alternative hypotensive agent that does not interact with rifampin, such as an angiotensin-converting enzyme inhibitor.

➥ *Monitor.* Observe patients who receive rifampin and losartan for loss of hypotensive effect.

REFERENCES:

Williamson KM, et al. Effects of erythromycin or rifampin on losartan pharmacokinetics in healthy volunteers. *Clin Pharmacol Ther.* 1998;63:316-323.

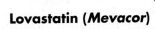

Lovastatin (*Mevacor*)

Nicotinic Acid (Niacin)

SUMMARY: Isolated cases of myopathy and rhabdomyolysis have occurred in patients receiving lovastatin and niacin, but a causal relationship has not been established.

RISK FACTORS: No specific risk factors are known.

RELATED DRUGS: Little is known about whether niacin increases the risk of myopathy when it is combined with simvastatin (*Zocor*). Fluvastatin (*Lescol*) does not appear to result in myopathy when combined with niacin. Theoretically, pravastatin (*Pravachol*) also would be unlikely to interact with niacin.

MANAGEMENT OPTIONS:

➥ *Monitor.* Although the interaction between lovastatin and niacin is not well documented, patients receiving the combination should be alert for muscular symptoms such as pain, tenderness, or weakness; creatine kinase should be measured in patients with such symptoms. Early recognition of this disorder is important as

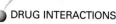

it may progress to acute renal failure in some patients if the drugs are not discontinued promptly.

REFERENCES:

Reaven P, et al. Lovastatin, nicotinic acid, and rhabdomyolysis. *Ann Intern Med.* 1988;109:597.

Tobert JA. Rhabdomyolysis in patients receiving lovastatin after cardiac transplantation. *N Engl J Med.* 1988;318:47.

Malloy MJ, et al. Complementarity of colestipol, niacin, and lovastatin in treatment of severe familial hypercholesterolemia. *Ann Intern Med.* 1987;107:616.

McKenney JM. Lovastatin: a new cholesterol-lowering agent. *Clin Pharm.* 1988;7:21.

Norman DJ, et al. Myolysis and acute renal failure in a heart-transplant recipient receiving lovastatin. *N Engl J Med.* 1988;318:46.

 Lovastatin (*Mevacor*)

Pectin (eg, *Kapectolin*)

SUMMARY: Preliminary results from a few patients suggest that pectin inhibits the cholesterol-lowering effect of lovastatin; more study is needed to assess the clinical importance.

RISK FACTORS: No specific risk factors are known.

RELATED DRUGS: The effect of pectin on HMG-CoA reductase inhibitors other than lovastatin is not established.

MANAGEMENT OPTIONS:

➡ *Circumvent/Minimize.* Although it is unknown whether separating the administration of lovastatin and pectin would avoid the interaction, it would be prudent to give lovastatin 2 hours before or 4 hours after pectin.

➡ *Monitor.* Monitor for reduced lovastatin response if the combination is given.

REFERENCES:

Richter WO, et al. Interaction between fibre and lovastatin. *Lancet.* 1991;338:706.

 Lovastatin (*Mevacor*)

Warfarin (eg, *Coumadin*)

SUMMARY: Lovastatin has been associated with increased hypoprothrombinemic response to warfarin in a number of patients, but the incidence with magnitude of this effect is not established.

RISK FACTORS: No specific risk factors are known.

RELATED DRUGS: The effect of lovastatin on oral anticoagulants other than warfarin is unknown, but assume that an interaction occurs until proven otherwise. Fluvastatin (*Lescol*) appears to inhibit CYP2C9, the primary enzyme in the metabolism of warfarin; thus, one would expect fluvastatin to increase warfarin response. Simvastatin (*Zocor*) appears to produce a small increase in warfarin effect, while available evidence suggests that pravastatin (*Pravachol*) does not affect warfarin. Clofibrate (*Atromid-S*) and gemfibrozil (eg, *Lopid*) may enhance the hypoprothrombinemic response to warfarin, while cholestyramine (eg, *Questran*) and colestipol (*Colestid*) may reduce its effect.

MANAGEMENT OPTIONS:

➡ *Consider Alternative.* Pravastatin appears less likely to interact with warfarin, but one still should monitor for altered hypoprothrombinemic response.

➡ *Monitor.* If lovastatin is used with oral anticoagulants, monitor for altered hypoprothrombinemic response if lovastatin is initiated, discontinued, or changed in dosage. Adjust the anticoagulant dose as needed.

REFERENCES:

Ahmad S. Lovastatin warfarin interaction. *Arch Intern Med.* 1990;150:2407.

Tobert JA, et al. Clinical experience with lovastatin. *Am J Cardiol.* 1990;65:23F.

Product information. Lovastatin (*Mevacor*). Merck Sharp & Dohme. 1993.

Transon C, et al. In vivo inhibition profile of cyctochrome P450TB (CYP2C9) by (±) fluvastatin. *Clin Pharmacol Ther.* 1995;58:412.

O'Rangers EA, et al. The effect of HMG coA reductase inhibitors on the anticoagulant response to warfarin. *Pharmacotherapy.* 1994;14:349. Abstract.

Magnesium (eg, *Mag-200*)

Nifedipine (eg, *Procardia*)

SUMMARY: The addition of nifedipine to methyldopa (eg, *Aldomet*) and magnesium sulfate produced transient hypotensive effects.

RISK FACTORS: No specific risk factors are known.

RELATED DRUGS: Other calcium channel blockers would be expected to enhance the hypotensive actions of magnesium.

MANAGEMENT OPTIONS:

➡ *Monitor.* Carefully monitor patients receiving magnesium for pre-eclampsia for hypotension if calcium channel blockers are given concomitantly.

REFERENCES:

Waisman GD, et al. Magnesium plus nifedipine: potentiation of hypotensive effect in preeclampsia? *Am J Obstet Gynecol.* 1988;159:308.

Magnesium (eg, *Mag-200*)

Succinylcholine (eg, *Anectine*)

SUMMARY: Parenteral magnesium salts may enhance the effect of neuromuscular blockers like succinylcholine.

RISK FACTORS: No specific risk factors are known.

RELATED DRUGS: Tubocurarine does not appear to interact.

MANAGEMENT OPTIONS:

➡ *Monitor.* Monitor for increased effect of succinylcholine (and other neuromuscular blocking agents) if parenteral magnesium is used concurrently. IV administration of calcium may partially ameliorate the excessive neuromuscular blockade that may occur.

REFERENCES:

Giesecke AH Jr, et al. Of magnesium, muscle relaxants, toxemic parturients, and cats. *Anesth Analg.* 1968;47:689.

Ghoneim MM, et al. The interaction between magnesium and other neuromuscular blocking agents. *Anesthesiology.* 1970;32:23.

Morris R, et al. Potentiation of muscle relaxants by magnesium sulfate therapy in toxemia of pregnancy. *South Med J.* 1968;61:25.

Aldrete JA, et al. Prevention of succinylcholine-induced hyperkalaemia by magnesium sulfate. *Can Anaesth Soc J.* 1970;17:477.

Mebendazole (*Vermox*)

Phenytoin (eg, *Dilantin*)

SUMMARY: In patients receiving high oral doses of mebendazole for *Echinococcus multilocularis* or *E. granulosus* (hydatid disease), phenytoin has been shown to lower plasma mebendazole concentrations, possibly impairing its therapeutic effect.

RISK FACTORS:

➡ *Concurrent Diseases.* Patients with tissue-dwelling organisms appear to be at greater risk for the interaction than those with intestinal helminths.

RELATED DRUGS: Other enzyme-inducing agents would be expected to produce a similar effect.

MANAGEMENT OPTIONS:

➡ *Avoid Unless Benefit Outweighs Risk.* In patients receiving mebendazole for tissue-dwelling organisms, try to avoid using enzyme-inducing drugs. No precautions appear necessary during cotherapy with phenytoin in patients receiving mebendazole to treat intestinal helminths. If possible, use valproic acid in place of phenytoin because it does not appear to reduce plasma mebendazole concentrations.

➡ *Monitor.* Be alert for evidence of reduced mebendazole response if phenytoin or other enzyme inducers are used with mebendazole.

REFERENCES:

Witassek F, et al. Chemotherapy of larval echinococcus with mebendazole: microsomal liver function and cholestasis as determinants of plasma drug level. *Eur J Clin Pharmacol.* 1983;25:85.

Bekhti A, et al. A correlation between serum mebendazole concentrations and the aminopyrine breath test. Implications in the treatment of hydatid disease. *Br J Clin Pharmacol.* 1986;21:223.

Luder PJ, et al. Treatment of hydatid disease with high oral doses of mebendazole. Long-term follow-up of plasma mebendazole levels and drug interactions. *Eur J Clin Pharmacol.* 1986;31:443.

Meclofenamate

Warfarin (eg, *Coumadin*)

SUMMARY: Preliminary evidence indicates that meclofenamate may increase the hypoprothrombinemic response to warfarin; presumably, it also might effect the response to other oral anticoagulants. The possible detrimental effects of meclofenamate on the gastric mucosa and platelet function is another reason to undertake cotherapy with caution.

RISK FACTORS:

➡ *Concurrent Diseases.* Patients with peptic ulcer disease (PUD) or a history of GI bleeding probably are at greater risk for the interaction.

RELATED DRUGS: All nonsteroidal anti-inflammatory drugs (NSAIDs) inhibit platelet function, cause gastric erosions, and probably increase the risk of GI bleeding. Some NSAIDs; however, such as ibuprofen (eg, *Advil*), naproxen (eg, *Naprosyn*), or diclofenac (eg, *Voltaren*), may be less likely to increase oral anticoagulant-induced hypoprothrombinemia than other NSAIDs.

MANAGEMENT OPTIONS:

➡ *Avoid Unless Benefit Outweighs Risk.* Because all NSAIDs probably increase the risk of GI bleeding in patients on oral anticoagulants, use the combination only after careful consideration of the benefit versus risk. If an NSAID must be used with an oral anticoagulant, it would be prudent to use NSAIDs that are unlikely to affect the hypoprothrombinemic response to oral anticoagulants as mentioned in Related Drugs. If the NSAID is being used as an analgesic or antipyretic, aceta-minophen (eg, *Tylenol*) probably is safer to use with oral anticoagulants. Nonacety-lated salicylates (eg, choline salicylate, magnesium salicylate, salsalate, sodium salicylate) also probably are safer with oral anticoagulants than NSAIDs, because such salicylates have minimal effects on platelet function and the gastric mucosa.

➡ *Monitor.* If any NSAID is used with an oral anticoagulant, one should carefully monitor the prothrombin time and watch for evidence of bleeding, especially from the GI tract.

REFERENCES:

AMA Drug Evaluation. 6th ed. American Medical Association. Chicago; 1986:1066.

Product information. Meclofenamate (*Meclomen*). Parke-Davis. 1990.

Shorr RI, et al. Concurrent use of nonsteroidal anti-inflammatory drugs and oral anticoagulants places elderly persons at high risk for hemorrhagic peptic ulcer disease. *Arch Intern Med.* 1993;153:1665.

② Mefenamic Acid (*Ponstel*)

Warfarin (eg, *Coumadin*)

SUMMARY: Limited clinical evidence indicates that mefenamic acid may produce a small increase in the hypoprothrombinemic response to warfarin and, presumably, other oral anticoagulants. Another reason for caution during cotherapy with these drugs is the possible detrimental effects of mefenamic acid on the gastric mucosa and platelet function.

RISK FACTORS:

➡ *Concurrent Diseases.* Patients with peptic ulcer disease (PUD) or a history of GI bleeding probably are at greater risk for the interaction.

RELATED DRUGS: All nonsteroidal anti-inflammatory drugs (NSAIDs) inhibit platelet function, cause gastric erosions, and probably increase the risk of GI bleeding. Some NSAIDs; however, such as ibuprofen (eg, *Advil*), naproxen (eg, *Naprosyn*), or diclofenac (eg, *Voltaren*), may be less likely to increase oral anticoagulant-induced hypoprothrombinemia than other NSAIDs.

MANAGEMENT OPTIONS:

➡ *Avoid Unless Benefit Outweighs Risk.* Because all NSAIDs probably increase the risk of GI bleeding in patients on oral anticoagulants, use the combination only after careful consideration of the benefit versus risk. If an NSAID must be used with an oral anticoagulant, it would be prudent to use NSAIDs that are unlikely to affect the hypoprothrombinemic response to oral anticoagulants as mentioned in the Related Drugs. If the NSAID is being used as an analgesic or antipyretic, aceta-minophen (eg, *Tylenol*) probably is safer to use with oral anticoagulants. Nonacety-lated salicylates (eg, choline salicylate, magnesium salicylate, salsalate, sodium salicylate) also probably are safer with oral anticoagulants than NSAIDs, because such salicylates have minimal effects on platelet function and the gastric mucosa.

➡ *Monitor.* If any NSAID is used with an oral anticoagulant, one should carefully monitor the prothrombin time and watch for evidence of bleeding, especially from the GI tract.

REFERENCES:

Anon. Today's drugs. Mefenamic acid. *BMJ.* 1966;2:1506.

Homes EL. Pharmacology of the fenamates. IV. Toleration by normal human subjects. *Ann Phys Med.* 1967;9(Suppl.):36.

Sellers EM, et al. Displacement of warfarin from human albumin by diazoxide and ethacrynic, mefenamic and nalidixic acids. *Clin Pharmacol Ther.* 1970;11:524.

Sellers EM, et al. Kinetics and clinical importance of displacement of warfarin from albumin by acidic drugs. *Ann NY Acad Sci.* 1971;179:213.

Shorr RI, et al. Concurrent use of nonsteroidal anti-inflammatory drugs and oral anticoagulants places elderly persons at high risk for hemorrhagic peptic ulcer disease. *Arch Intern Med.* 1993;153:1665.

Meperidine (eg, *Demerol*)

Phenelzine (*Nardil*) `AVOID`

SUMMARY: Some patients receiving nonselective monoamine oxidase inhibitors (MAOIs) and meperidine have developed life-threatening serotonin syndrome.

RISK FACTORS: No specific risk factors are known.

RELATED DRUGS: Meperidine is contraindicated in patients receiving any nonselective MAOI, including isocarboxazid (*Marplan*) and tranylcypromine (*Parnate*). Morphine (eg, *Roxanol*) does not appear likely to cause such severe reactions; thus, although it cannot be used with impunity with nonselective MAOIs, it is preferable to meperidine. Epidural fentanyl (eg, *Sublimaze*) has been reported to be an acceptable analgesic for postoperative pain in a patient taking tranylcypromine.

MANAGEMENT OPTIONS:

➡ *AVOID COMBINATION.* Meperidine should be avoided in patients receiving nonselective MAOIs. Remember that the effects of nonselective MAOIs should be assumed to persist for 2 weeks after they are discontinued. Available evidence suggests that morphine is safer than meperidine in patients receiving nonselective MAOIs.

REFERENCES:

Evans-Prosser CDG. The use of pethidine and morphine in the presence of monoamine oxidase inhibitors. *Br J Anaesthesiol.* 1968;40:279.

Browne B, et al. Monoamine oxidase inhibitors and narcotic analgesics. A critical review of the implications for treatment. *Br J Psych.* 1987;151:210.

Goldberg LI. Monoamine oxidase inhibitors. Adverse reactions and possible mechanism. *JAMA.* 1964;190:456.

Sjoqvist F. Psychotropic drugs (2). Interaction between monoamine oxidase (MAO) inhibitors and other substances. *Proc R Soc Med.* 1965;58:967.

Vigran IM. Dangerous potentiation of meperidine hydrochloride by pargyline hydrochloride. *JAMA.* 1964;187:953.

Anon. Analgesics and monoamine oxidase inhibitors. *BMJ.* 1967;4:284.

Youssef MS, et al. Epidural fentanyl and monoamine oxidase inhibitors. *Anaesthesia.* 1988;43:210.

Meperidine (eg, *Demerol*)

Phenobarbital (eg, *Solfoton*)

SUMMARY: Phenobarbital and meperidine cotherapy can result in excessive CNS depression.

RISK FACTORS: No specific risk factors are known.

RELATED DRUGS: Most combinations of barbiturates and narcotic analgesics would be expected to exhibit additive CNS depressant effects. Moreover, the metabolism of narcotic analgesics that are converted to inactive products might be enhanced by barbiturates thus reducing their effect.

MANAGEMENT OPTIONS:

➡ **Monitor.** Monitor for excessive CNS depression when barbiturates and narcotic analgesics are given concurrently; adjust dosage of 1 or both drugs as needed.

REFERENCES:

Stambaugh JE, et al. The effect of phenobarbital on the metabolism of meperidine in normal volunteers. *J Clin Pharmacol.* 1978;18:482.

Bellville JW, et al. The hypnotic effects of codeine and secobarbital and their interaction in man. *Clin Pharmacol Ther.* 1971;12:607.

Stambaugh JE, et al. A potentially toxic drug interaction between pethidine (meperidine) and phenobarbitone. *Lancet.* 1977;1:398.

Meperidine (eg, *Demerol*)

Phenytoin (*Dilantin*)

SUMMARY: Phenytoin may reduce meperidine serum concentrations, but the clinical importance of this effect is not established.

RISK FACTORS: No specific risk factors are known.

RELATED DRUGS: No information is available.

MANAGEMENT OPTIONS:

➡ **Monitor.** Until more information is available, be alert for evidence of reduced analgesic efficacy or increased toxicity when meperidine is used in patients receiving phenytoin.

REFERENCES:

Pond SM, et al. Effect of phenytoin on meperidine clearance and normeperidine formation. *Clin Pharmacol Ther.* 1981;30:680.

Meperidine (eg, *Demerol*)

Selegiline (eg, *Eldepryl*)

SUMMARY: A patient on selegiline developed agitation, delirium, rigidity, sweating, and hyperpyrexia after starting meperidine, but it was not established that it resulted from an interaction between selegiline and meperidine.

RISK FACTORS:

➥ *Other Drugs.* The concurrent use of other drugs that inhibit serotonin reuptake may increase the risk.

RELATED DRUGS: Theoretically, morphine (eg, *Roxanol*) would be less likely to interact than meperidine, but little is known about other opiates.

MANAGEMENT OPTIONS:

➥ *Use Alternative.* Although it is not clear that the reported reaction resulted from a selegiline-meperidine interaction, the potential severity of the reaction dictates caution. Until more data are available, it would be prudent to use analgesics other than meperidine in patients on selegiline. Nonetheless, the manufacturer recommends caution.

REFERENCES:

Zornberg GL, et al. Severe adverse interaction between pethidine and selegiline. *Lancet.* 1991;337:246.

Product information. Selegiline (*Eldepryl*). Somerset Pharmaceuticals, Inc. 1996.

Meperidine (eg, *Demerol*)

Sibutramine (*Meridia*)

SUMMARY: The risk of serotonin syndrome would theoretically increase when sibutramine is combined with other serotonergic drugs such as meperidine.

RISK FACTORS: No specific risk factors are known.

RELATED DRUGS: Little is known regarding the serotonergic effects of opioids other than meperidine.

MANAGEMENT OPTIONS:

➥ *Avoid Unless Benefit Outweighs Risk.* The manufacturer states that sibutramine should not be used with meperidine. This is a prudent recommendation until more information is available.

➥ *Monitor.* Serotonin syndrome can result in neurotoxicity (eg, myoclonus, tremors, rigidity, incoordination, restlessness, hyperreflexia, seizures, coma), psychiatric symptoms (eg, agitation, confusion, hypomania), and temperature regulation abnormalities (eg, fever, sweating). Note that mild forms of serotonin syndrome have also been reported, so consider any combination of the above symptoms possibly related to excessive serotonin activity.

REFERENCES:

Product information. Sibutramine (*Meridia*). Knoll Pharmaceuticals. 1997.

Mills KC. Serotonin syndrome. A clinical update. *Crit Care Clin.* 1997;13:763.

Mercaptopurine (6-MP; *Purinethol*)

Warfarin (eg, *Coumadin*)

SUMMARY: Mercaptopurine appeared to inhibit the hypoprothrombinemic response to warfarin in 1 patient, a finding consistent with animal studies. More study is needed to evaluate the incidence and significance of this interaction.

RISK FACTORS: No specific risk factors are known.

RELATED DRUGS: Azathioprine (eg, *Imuran*) is metabolized to mercaptopurine and also has been reported to inhibit the hypoprothrombinemic response to warfarin. The effect of mercaptopurine on oral anticoagulants other than warfarin is unknown, but be alert for a similar effect with all oral anticoagulants until information to the contrary is available.

MANAGEMENT OPTIONS:

➡ ***Monitor.*** Monitor for altered oral anticoagulant effect if mercaptopurine is initiated, discontinued, or changed in dosage. Adjust the anticoagulant dose as needed.

REFERENCES:

Martini A, et al. Studies in rats on the mechanisms by which 6-mercaptopurine inhibits the anticoagulant effect of warfarin. *J Pharmacol Exp Ther.* 1977;201:547.

Spiers ASD, et al. Increased warfarin requirement during mercaptopurine therapy: a new drug interaction. *Lancet.* 1974;2:221.

Mesalamine (eg, *Asacol*)

Warfarin (eg, *Coumadin*)

SUMMARY: Mesalamine appeared to inhibit warfarin effect in 1 patient, but a causal relationship was not established.

RISK FACTORS: No specific risk factors are known.

RELATED DRUGS: No information is available.

MANAGEMENT OPTIONS:

➡ ***Circumvent/Minimize.*** If the mesalamine inhibits warfarin absorption, separating the doses might reduce the magnitude of the interaction. But because the mechanism of this purported interaction is not known, it is premature to make such recommendations. Moreover, because warfarin undergoes enterohepatic circulation, separation of doses of warfarin from binding agents does not completely eliminate such interactions.

➡ ***Monitor.*** Closely monitor the hypoprothrombinemic response to warfarin if mesalamine is initiated, discontinued, or changed in dosage.

REFERENCES:

Marinella MA. Mesalamine and warfarin therapy resulting in decreased warfarin effect. *Ann Pharmacother.* 1998;32:841.

Metaraminol (*Aramine*)

Pargyline AVOID

SUMMARY: Metaraminol administration in patients taking a monoamine oxidase (MAO) inhibitor, such as pargyline, may result in a severe hypertensive response.

RISK FACTORS: No specific risk factors are known.

RELATED DRUGS: Metaraminol is contraindicated in patients receiving any nonselective MAO inhibitor, including isocarboxazid (*Marplan*), phenelzine (*Nardil*), and tranylcypromine (*Parnate*). Levarterenol (*Levophed*) is likely to be a safer pressor agent than metaraminol in such patients.

MANAGEMENT OPTIONS:

➡ *AVOID COMBINATION.* Avoid metaraminol in patients taking a monoamine inhibitor. Remember that the effects of nonselective monoamine inhibitors should be assumed to persist for 2 weeks after they are discontinued.

REFERENCES:

Sjoqvist F. Psychotropic drugs (2). Interaction between monoamine oxidase (MAO) inhibitors and other substances. *Proc R Soc Med.* 1965;58:967-978.

Horler AR, et al. Hypertensive crisis due to pargyline and metaraminol. *BMJ.* 1965;3:460.

Methadone (eg, *Dolophine*)

Nevirapine (*Viramune*)

SUMMARY: Nevirapine reduces methadone concentrations; methadone withdrawal symptoms may result.

RISK FACTORS: No specific risk factors are known.

RELATED DRUGS: Efavirenz (*Sustiva*) has been noted to reduce methadone plasma concentrations.

MANAGEMENT OPTIONS:

➡ *Consider Alternative.* Consider the use of an analgesic (eg, morphine, codeine) not metabolized by CYP3A4 in patients taking methadone for its analgesic activity.

➡ *Monitor.* Observe patients on methadone maintenance therapy for evidence of withdrawal symptoms if nevirapine is instituted. Methadone dosage may require an increase to prevent withdrawal symptoms. Monitor for excess methadone effect if the nevirapine is discontinued in a patient taking methadone.

REFERENCES:

Clarke SM, et al. Pharmacokinetic interactions of nevirapine and methadone and guidelines for use of nevirapine to treat injection drug users. *Clin Infect Dis.* 2001;33:1595-1597.

Otero MJ, et al. Nevirapine-induced withdrawal symptoms in HIV patients on methadone maintenance programme: an alert. *AIDS.* 1999;13:1004-1005.

Altice FL, et al. Nevirapine-induced opiate withdrawal among injection drug users with HIV infection receiving methadone. *AIDS.* 1999;13:957-962.

Heelon MW, et al. Methadone withdrawal when starting an antiretroviral regimen including nevirapine. *Pharmacotherapy.* 1999;19:471-472.

Methadone (eg, *Dolophine*)

Phenobarbital (eg, *Solfoton*)

SUMMARY: Phenobarbital may enhance methadone metabolism, resulting in methadone withdrawal.

RISK FACTORS: No specific risk factors are known.

RELATED DRUGS: All barbiturates would be expected to enhance methadone metabolism.

MANAGEMENT OPTIONS:

➡ *Monitor.* Monitor for methadone withdrawal if barbiturates are given concurrently.

REFERENCES:

Liu SJ, et al. Case report of barbiturate-induced enhancement of methadone metabolism and withdrawal syndrome. *Am J Psychiatry.* 1984;141:1287-1288.

 Methadone (eg, *Dolophine*)

Phenytoin (*Dilantin-125*)

SUMMARY: Phenytoin may reduce serum methadone concentrations, resulting in symptoms of methadone withdrawal.

RISK FACTORS: No specific risk factors are known.

RELATED DRUGS: Other enzyme inducers such as barbiturates, carbamazepine (eg, *Tegretol*), primidone (*Mysoline*), and rifampin probably also enhance methadone metabolism.

MANAGEMENT OPTIONS:

➡ *Avoid Unless Benefit Outweighs Risk.* If possible, avoid using methadone with enzyme inducers such as phenytoin.

➡ *Monitor.* If the combination is necessary, monitor for the need to adjust the methadone dose if phenytoin therapy is initiated, discontinued, or changed in dosage.

REFERENCES:

Finelli PF. Phenytoin and methadone tolerance. *N Engl J Med.* 1976;294:227.

Tong TG, et al. Phenytoin-induced methadone withdrawal. *Ann Intern Med.* 1981;94:349-351.

 Methadone (eg, *Dolophine*)

Rifampin (eg, *Rifadin*)

SUMMARY: Rifampin can decrease methadone serum concentrations, resulting in withdrawal symptoms.

RISK FACTORS: No specific risk factors are known.

RELATED DRUGS: No information is available.

MANAGEMENT OPTIONS:

➡ *Monitor.* Observe methadone-treated patients for evidence of methadone withdrawal when they are started on rifampin. If the methadone dose is increased to offset the effect of rifampin, be alert for excessive methadone effect when the rifampin is discontinued.

REFERENCES:

Kreek MJ, et al. Rifampin-induced methadone withdrawal. *N Engl J Med.* 1976;294:1104-1106.

Bending MR, et al. Rifampicin and methadone withdrawal. *Lancet.* 1977;1:1211.

Holmes VE. Rifampin-induced methadone withdrawal in AIDS. *J Clin Psychopharmacol.* 1990;10:443-444.

Methadone (eg, *Dolophine*)
Ritonavir (*Norvir*)

SUMMARY: Ritonavir appears to reduce methadone activity; loss of analgesia or narcotic withdrawal may result.

RISK FACTORS: No specific risk factors are known.

RELATED DRUGS: While there is no information regarding the potential for other antiviral agents to reduce the concentration of methadone, agents that induce CYP3A4 activity such as nevirapine (*Viramune*) may affect methadone in a similar manner.

MANAGEMENT OPTIONS:

➡ *Monitor.* Observe patients taking methadone for a loss of efficacy during ritonavir administration.

REFERENCES:

Geletko SM, et al. Decreased methadone effect after ritonavir initiation. *Pharmacotherapy.* 2000;20:93-94.

Methadone (eg, *Dolophine*)
Somatostatin (*Zecnil*)

SUMMARY: Somatostatin appeared to inhibit the analgesic effect of methadone in 1 patient; the clinical importance of this effect is not established.

RISK FACTORS: No specific risk factors are known.

RELATED DRUGS: It is not known whether the somatostatin analog octreotide (eg, *Sandostatin*) also inhibits methadone analgesia, but be alert for the possibility. Somatostatin has also been reported to inhibit morphine analgesia (see Morphine/Somatostatin), but its effect on other opioids is not established.

MANAGEMENT OPTIONS:

➡ *Monitor.* Watch for evidence of reduced analgesia if somatostatin is used with methadone or other opioid analgesics. If methadone analgesia appears diminished, it would be prudent to stop somatostatin. If somatostatin cannot be stopped, evidence suggests that it may be difficult to achieve adequate analgesia.

REFERENCES:

Ripamonti C, et al. Can somatostatin be administered in association with morphine in advanced cancer patients with pain? *Ann Oncol.* 1998;9:921-923.

Methadone (eg, *Dolophine*)

St. John's Wort

SUMMARY: St. John's wort appears to reduce methadone plasma concentrations and may lead to symptoms of methadone withdrawal.

RISK FACTORS: No specific risk factors are known.

RELATED DRUGS: No information is available.

MANAGEMENT OPTIONS:

➡ *Monitor.* Observe methadone-treated patients for evidence of methadone withdrawal if they take St. John's wort concurrently. If the methadone dose is increased to offset the effect of St. John's wort, be alert for excessive methadone effect when rifampin is discontinued.

REFERENCES:

Eich-Höchli D, et al. Methadone maintenance treatment and St. John's wort. *Pharmacopsychiatry.* 2003;36:35-37.

Methandrostenolone

Tolbutamide (eg, *Orinase*)

SUMMARY: Anabolic steroids may enhance the hypoglycemic effect of tolbutamide and possibly other antidiabetic agents.

RISK FACTORS: No specific risk factors are known.

RELATED DRUGS: Although some anabolic steroids would be expected to enhance the hypoglycemic response to other antidiabetic drugs, specific data demonstrating this effect on hypoglycemic agents other than tolbutamide are lacking.

MANAGEMENT OPTIONS:

➡ *Consider Alternative.* Nandrolone (eg, *Durabolin*) and methenolone acetate did not appear to affect tolbutamide's hypoglycemic effects.

➡ *Monitor.* If anabolic steroids are added to antidiabetic drug therapy, the patient should be monitored more closely for evidence of hypoglycemia.

REFERENCES:

Sotaniemi EA, et al. Drug metabolism and androgen control therapy in prostatic cancer. *Clin Pharmacol Ther.* 1973;14:413.

Kontturi M, et al. Estrogen-induced metabolic changes during treatment of prostatic cancer. *Scan J Lab Clin Invest.* 1970;25(Suppl. 113):45.

Sachs BA, et al. Effect of oxandrolone on plasma lipids and lipoproteins of patients with disorders of lipid metabolism. *Metabolism.* 1968;17:400.

Landon J, et al. The effect of anabolic steroids on blood sugar and plasma insulin levels in man. *Metabolism.* 1963;12:924.

Methenamine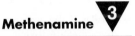

Sodium Bicarbonate

SUMMARY: Sodium bicarbonate administration interferes with the antibacterial activity of methenamine compounds.

RISK FACTORS: No specific risk factors are known.

RELATED DRUGS: Certain antacids (eg, magnesium, aluminum hydroxides) and acetazolamide (eg, *Diamox*) also may alkalinize the urine somewhat, but it is unknown whether this effect would be sufficient to affect methenamine.

MANAGEMENT OPTIONS:

➡ *Monitor.* If the urine cannot be kept at approximately pH 5.5 or lower during the use of sodium bicarbonate, methenamine compounds should not be used.

REFERENCES:

Product information. Mandelamine. Warner-Chilcott. 1993.

Kevorkian CG, et al. Methenamine mandelate with acidification: an effective urinary antiseptic in patients with neurogenic bladder. *Mayo Clin Proc.* 1984;59:523.

Pearman JW, et al. The antimicrobial activity of urine of paraplegic patients receiving methenamine mandelate. *Invest Urol.* 1978;16:91.2.

Methenamine

Sulfadiazine

SUMMARY: The combination of methenamine and sulfadiazine may result in crystalluria.

RISK FACTORS: No specific risk factors are known.

RELATED DRUGS: Sulfamethizole and sulfathiazole interact similarly with methenamine. However, more soluble agents, such as sulfisoxazole, rarely interact.

MANAGEMENT OPTIONS:

➡ *Consider Alternative.* Methenamine compounds should not be used with sulfonamides that may precipitate in an acid urine. The use of sulfathiazole or sulfamethizole with methenamine compounds should be avoided. If a methenamine product and a sulfonamide are to be used together, it would be preferable to use the more soluble sulfonamides, such as sulfisoxazole.

➡ *Monitor.* Patients receiving methenamine and sulfadiazine should be monitored for crystalluria.

REFERENCES:

Mandelamine. Physician's Desk Reference. 47th ed. Oradell: Medical Economics Data; 1993:1780.

② Methotrexate (eg, *Rheumatrex*)

Naproxen (eg, *Naprosyn*)

SUMMARY: A patient on chronic methotrexate for arthritis developed evidence of methotrexate toxicity and died after receiving naproxen.

RISK FACTORS:

➡ **Concurrent Diseases.** Particular caution is suggested in patients with pre-existing renal impairment (who may be more susceptible to nonsteroidal anti-inflammatory drug [NSAID]-induced renal failure).

➡ **Dosage Regimen.** The risk of adverse effects from this interaction is primarily in patients receiving antineoplastic doses of methotrexate, rather than the lower doses used to treat rheumatoid arthritis, psoriasis, and related diseases.

MANAGEMENT OPTIONS:

➡ **Avoid Unless Benefit Outweighs Risk.** Until more information is available on this interaction, it would be prudent to avoid naproxen (as well as other NSAIDs) in patients receiving antineoplastic doses of methotrexate. Particular caution is suggested in patients with pre-existing renal impairment, who may be more susceptible to NSAID-induced renal failure.

➡ **Monitor.** If the combination is used, monitor for methotrexate toxicity. Findings in methotrexate toxicity can include stomatitis, severe GI symptoms (nausea, diarrhea, vomiting), bone marrow suppression, fever, bleeding, skin rashes, nephrotoxicity, and hepatotoxicity. Although decreasing the methotrexate dosage would be expected to reduce the likelihood of toxicity, the magnitude of the required reduction in methotrexate dosage has not been established.

REFERENCES:

Aherene A, et al. Methotrexate kinetics in rheumatoid arthritis: is there an interaction with nonsteroidal antiinflammatory drugs? *J Rheumatol.* 1988;15:1356.

Furst DE, et al. Effect of aspirin and sulindac on methotrexate clearance. *J Pharm Sci.* 1990;79:782.

Dupuis LL, et al. Methotrexate-nonsteroidal antiinflammatory drug interaction in children with arthritis. *J Rheumatol.* 1990;17:469.

Liegler DG, et al. The effect of organic acids on renal clearance of methotrexate in man. *Clin Pharmacol Ther.* 1969;10:849.

Skeith KJ, et al. Lack of significant interaction between low dose methotrexate and ibuprofen or flurbiprofen in patients with arthritis. *J Rheumatol.* 1990;17:1008.

Stewart CF, et al. Effect of aspirin (ASA) on the disposition of methotrexate (MTX) in patients with rheumatoid arthritis (RA). *Clin Pharmacol Ther.* 1990;47:139. Abstract PP-56.

Taylor JR, et al. Effect of sodium salicylate and indomethacin on methotrexate-serum albumin binding. *Arch Dermatol.* 1977;113:588.

Tracy FS, et al. The effect of NSAIDS on methotrexate disposition in patients with rheumatoid arthritis. *Clin Pharmacol Ther.* 1990;47:138. Abstract PP-54.

Daly HM, et al. Methotrexate toxicity precipitated by azapropazone. *Br J Dermatol.* 1986;114:733.

Boh LE, et al. Low-dose weekly oral methotrexate therapy for inflammatory arthritis. *Clin Pharm.* 1986;5:503.

Anderson PA, et al. Weekly pulse methotrexate in rheumatoid arthritis: clinical and immunologic effects in a randomized, double-blind study. *Ann Intern Med.* 1985;103:489.

Tugwell P, et al. Methotrexate in rheumatoid arthritis: indications, contraindications, efficacy, and safety. *Ann Intern Med.* 1987;107:358.

Adams JD, et al. Drug interactions in psoriasis. *Aust J Dermatol.* 1976;17:39.

Singh RR, et al. Fatal interaction between methotrexate and naproxen. *Lancet.* 1986;1:1390.

Methotrexate (eg, *Rheumatrex*)

Neomycin (eg, *Neo-fradin*) AVOID

SUMMARY: Oral absorption of methotrexate is decreased by 30% to 50% in patients receiving oral antibiotic mixtures including paromomycin (*Humatin*), neomycin, nystatin (eg, *Mycostatin*), and vancomycin (eg, *Vancocin*).

RISK FACTORS: No specific risk factors are known.

RELATED DRUGS: No information is available.

MANAGEMENT OPTIONS:

➡ *AVOID COMBINATION.* Patients receiving oral methotrexate should not receive oral nonabsorbable antibiotics. It is not known whether this interaction occurs with parenteral methotrexate; however, the possibility cannot be excluded.

REFERENCES:
Cohen MH, et al. Effect of oral prophylactic broad spectrum nonabsorbable antibiotics on the gastrointestinal absorption of nutrients and methotrexate in small cell bronchogenic carcinoma patients. *Cancer.* 1976;38:1556–1559.

Methotrexate (eg, *Rheumatrex*)

Omeprazole (*Prilosec*)

SUMMARY: A patient with osteosarcoma developed elevated methotrexate serum concentrations while receiving concurrent omeprazole; more study is needed to establish the clinical importance of this purported interaction.

RISK FACTORS: No specific risk factors are known.

RELATED DRUGS: Theoretically, H_2-receptor antagonists such as ranitidine (eg, *Zantac*), cimetidine (eg, *Tagamet*), famotidine (eg, *Pepcid*), and nizatidine (*Axid*) would be less likely than omeprazole to interact with methotrexate, but little clinical information is available.

MANAGEMENT OPTIONS:

➡ *Monitor.* Until more data are available, monitor for excessive methotrexate effect if omeprazole is given concurrently.

REFERENCES:
Reid T, et al. Impact of omeprazole on the plasma clearance of methotrexate. *Cancer Chemother Pharmacol.* 1993;33:82-84.

Methotrexate (eg, *Rheumatrex*)

Oxacillin (*Bactocill*)

SUMMARY: A patient developed severe methotrexate toxicity following 3 doses of oxacillin.

RISK FACTORS: No specific risk factors are known.

RELATED DRUGS: Other penicillins (eg, amoxicillin, piperacillin, mezlocillin) are known to inhibit methotrexate elimination.

MANAGEMENT OPTIONS:

➡ ***Consider Alternative.*** Treat patients receiving methotrexate with alternative antibiotics that do not compete with the renal organic anion transporter.

➡ ***Monitor.*** Watch patients for evidence of enhanced methotrexate effect and possible toxicity when large doses of oxacillin or other penicillins are coadministered.

REFERENCES:

Titier K, et al. Pharmacokinetic interaction between high-dose methotrexate and oxacillin. *Ther Drug Monit.* 2002;24:570-572.

 Methotrexate

Pantoprazole (*Protonix*)

SUMMARY: A patient on pantoprazole developed myopathy following low-dose methotrexate. A causal relationship was strong in this case, but it is not known how often the combination would produce adverse outcomes.

RISK FACTORS: Not established.

RELATED DRUGS: Omeprazole (eg, *Prilosec*) also has been associated with methotrexate toxicity, so it is possible that other proton pump inhibitors also would interact with methotrexate.

MANAGEMENT OPTIONS:

➡ ***Monitor.*** In patients receiving methotrexate, one should be particularly alert for evidence of methotrexate toxicity if pantoprazole, omeprazole, or other proton pump inhibitor is given concurrently.

REFERENCES:

Troger U, et al. Severe myalgia from an interaction between treatments with pantoprazole and methotrexate. *BMJ.* 2002;324:1497.

Beorlegui B, et al. Potential interaction between methotrexate and omeprazole. *Ann Pharmacother.* 2000;34:1024-1027.

Reid T, et al. Impact of omeprazole on the plasma clearance of methotrexate. *Cancer Chemother Pharmacol.* 1993;33:82-84.

 Methotrexate (eg, *Rheumatrex*)

Phenylbutazone

SUMMARY: Two patients on methotrexate developed evidence of severe methotrexate toxicity after starting phenylbutazone; 1 patient died.

RISK FACTORS:

➡ ***Concurrent Diseases.*** Particular caution is suggested in patients with pre-existing renal impairment (who may be more susceptible to nonsteroidal anti-inflammatory drug [NSAID]-induced renal failure).

➡ ***Dosage Regimen.*** The risk of adverse effects from this interaction is primarily in patients receiving antineoplastic doses of methotrexate, rather than the lower doses used to treat rheumatoid arthritis, psoriasis, and related diseases.

RELATED DRUGS: Oxyphenbutazone also would be expected to enhance methotrexate toxicity, but clinical data are lacking.

MANAGEMENT OPTIONS:

➡ *Avoid Unless Benefit Outweighs Risk.* Although only limited clinical evidence exists, it would be prudent to avoid phenylbutazone (as well as other NSAIDs) in patients receiving antineoplastic doses of methotrexate. Particular caution is suggested in patients with pre-existing renal impairment who may be more susceptible to NSAID-induced renal failure.

➡ *Monitor.* If the combination is used, monitor for methotrexate toxicity. Findings in methotrexate toxicity can include stomatitis, severe GI symptoms (eg, nausea, diarrhea, vomiting), bone marrow suppression, fever, bleeding, skin rashes, nephrotoxicity, and hepatotoxicity. Although decreasing the methotrexate dosage would be expected to reduce the likelihood of toxicity, the magnitude of the required reduction in methotrexate dosage has not been established.

REFERENCES:

Ahern M, et al. Methotrexate kinetics in rheumatoid arthritis: is there an interaction with nonsteroidal anti-inflammatory drugs? *J Rheumatol.* 1988;15:1356-1360.

Furst DE, et al. Effect of aspirin and sulindac on methotrexate clearance. *J Pharm Sci.* 1990;79:782-786.

Dupuis LL, et al. Methotrexate-nonsteroidal anti-iflammatory drug interaction in children with arthritis. *J Rheumatol.* 1990;17:1469-1473.

Liegler DG, et al. The effect of organic acids on renal clearance of methotrexate in man. *Clin Pharmacol Ther.* 1969;10:849-857.

Skeith KJ, et al. Lack of significant interaction between low dose methotrexate and ibuprofen or flurbiprofen in patients with arthritis. *J Rheumatol.* 1990;17:1008-1010.

Stewart CF, et al. Effect of aspirin (ASA) on the disposition of methotrexate (MTX) in patients with rheumatoid arthritis (RA). *Clin Pharmacol Ther.* 1990;47:139.

Taylor JR, et al. Effect of sodium salicylate and indomethacin on methotrexate-serum albumin binding. *Arch Dermatol.* 1977;113:588-591.

Tracy FS, et al. The effect of NSAIDs on methotrexate disposition in patients with rheumatoid arthritis. *Clin Pharmacol Ther.* 1990;47:138.

Greenstone M, et al. Acute nephrotic syndrome with reversible renal failure after phenylbutazone. *Br Med J.* 1981;282:950-951.

Adams JD, et al. Drug interaction in psoriasis. *Australas J Dermatol.* 1976;17:39-40.

Methotrexate (eg, *Rheumatrex*)

Polio Vaccine AVOID

SUMMARY: Administration of live-virus vaccines such as oral polio vaccine (OPV) to immunosuppressed patients, including those undergoing cytotoxic chemotherapy, may result in infection by the live virus.

RISK FACTORS: No specific risk factors are known.

RELATED DRUGS: Other vaccines that may result in infections in immunocompromised patients include BCG vaccine, typhoid vaccine, measles vaccine, mumps vaccine, rubella vaccine, or yellow fever vaccine.

MANAGEMENT OPTIONS:

➡ *AVOID COMBINATION.* Current recommendations state that patients with leukemia in remission should not receive live vaccines until at least 3 months have passed since the completion of all chemotherapy., Similar guidelines should be followed for patients receiving chemotherapy for other malignancies.

REFERENCES:

Allison J. Methotrexate and smallpox vaccination. *Lancet.* 1968;2:1250. Letter.

Mitus A, et al. Attenuated measles vaccine in children with acute leukemia. *Am J Dis Child.* 1962;103:243.

Pizzo PA, et al. Infections in the cancer patient. In: DeVita VT et al., eds. Cancer: principles and practice of oncology. 4th ed. Philadelphia: J. B. Lippincott; 1993:2292.

Immunization Practices Advisory Committee. Update on adult immunization. Recommendations of the Immunization practices advisory committee (ACIP). *MMWR.* 1991;40(RR-12):1.

2   Methotrexate (eg, *Rheumatrex*)

Probenecid

SUMMARY: Probenecid markedly increases serum methotrexate concentrations and would be expected to increase both the therapeutic effect and toxicity of methotrexate.

RISK FACTORS: No specific risk factors are known.

RELATED DRUGS: Sulfinpyrazone (eg, *Anturane*) would be expected to produce a similar effect on methotrexate.

MANAGEMENT OPTIONS:

➡ *Avoid Unless Benefit Outweighs Risk.* Probenecid and sulfinpyrazone generally should be avoided in patients receiving methotrexate.

➡ *Monitor.* If the combination is used, one should anticipate that a reduction in methotrexate dosage may be required. Serum methotrexate determinations would be helpful, and one also should monitor for excessive methotrexate effect (eg, gastrointestinal toxicity, stomatitis, bone marrow suppression, hepatotoxicity, infection).

REFERENCES:

Aherne GW, et al. Prolongation and enhancement of serum methotrexate concentrations by probenecid. *BMJ.* 978;1:1097.

Lilly MB, et al. Clinical pharmacology of oral intermediate-dose methotrexate with or without probenecid. *Cancer Chemother Pharmacol.* 1985;15:220.

Ramu A, et al. Probenecid inhibition of methotrexate excretion from cerebrospinal fluid in dogs. *J Pharmacokinet Biopharm.* 1978;6:389.

Howell SB, et al. Effect of probenecid on cerebrospinal fluid methotrexate kinetics. *Clin Pharmacol Ther.* 1979;26:641.

3   Methotrexate (eg, *Rheumatrex*)

Thiazides

SUMMARY: Thiazides may increase bone marrow suppression in patients on chemotherapy, possibly by increasing the effect of methotrexate.

RISK FACTORS: No specific risk factors are known.

RELATED DRUGS: No information is available.

MANAGEMENT OPTIONS:

➥ *Monitor.* Patients should be monitored for enhanced bone marrow suppression when thiazides are used with methotrexate (or other cytotoxic agents). Adjust cytotoxic drug dosage as needed.

REFERENCES:

Orr LE. Potentiation of myelosuppression from cancer chemotherapy and thiazide diuretics. *Drug Intell Clin Pharm.* 1981;15:967.

Methotrexate (eg, *Rheumatrex*)

Trimethoprim (eg, *Bactrim*)

SUMMARY: The administration of trimethoprim and methotrexate has resulted in severe methotrexate toxicity.

RISK FACTORS:

➥ *Concurrent Diseases.* Preexisting renal disease will reduce methotrexate elimination.

RELATED DRUGS: None known.

MANAGEMENT OPTIONS:

➥ *Use Alternative.* Do not administer trimethoprim to patients taking methotrexate. Choose an alternative antibiotic. Avoid penicillins because they can have a similar effect on methotrexate renal elimination.

REFERENCES:

Ferrazzini G, et al. Interaction between trimethoprim-sulfamethoxazole and methotrexate in children with leukemia. *J Pediatr.* 1990;117:823-826.

Govert JA, et al. Pancytopenia from using trimethoprim and methotrexate. *Ann Intern Med.* 1992;117:877-878.

Groenendal H, et al. Methotrexate and trimethoprim-sulphamethoxazole—a potentially hazardous combination. *Clin Exper Derm.* 1990;15:358-360.

Steuer A, et al. Methotrexate and trimethoprim: a fatal interaction. *Br J Rheumatol.* 1998;37:105-106.

Saravana S, et al. Myelotoxicity due to methotrexate - an iatrogenic cause. *Eur J Haematol.* 2003;71:315-316.

Methotrexate (eg, *Rheumatrex*)

Vancomycin (eg, *Vancocin*)

SUMMARY: Methotrexate serum concentrations can be reduced by oral vancomycin and aminoglycosides.

RISK FACTORS: No specific risk factors are known.

RELATED DRUGS: No information is available.

MANAGEMENT OPTIONS:

➥ *Monitor.* Watch for decreased methotrexate response if oral aminoglycosides are administered.

REFERENCES:

Cohen MH, et al. Effect of oral prophylactic broad spectrum nonabsorbable antibiotics on the gastrointestinal absorption of nutrients and methotrexate in small cell bronchogenic carcinoma patients. *Cancer.* 1976;38:1556-1559.

Methotrimeprazine

AVOID **Pargyline**

SUMMARY: Coadministration of pargyline and methotrimeprazine was associated with fatality in 1 reported case.

RISK FACTORS: No specific risk factors are known.

RELATED DRUGS: All nonselective monoamine oxidase (MAO) inhibitors, including iso-carboxazid (*Marplan*), phenelzine (*Nardil*), and tranylcypromine (*Parnate*), should be considered contraindicated with methotrimeprazine.

MANAGEMENT OPTIONS:

➡ *AVOID COMBINATION.* Although the interaction between methotrimeprazine and MAO inhibitors is not well documented, the possibility of a fatal reaction contra-indicates concomitant use of these drugs. Remember that the effects of nonselective MAO inhibitors should be assumed to persist for 2 weeks after they are discontinued.

REFERENCES:

Sjoqvist F. Psychotropic drugs (2). Interaction between monoamine oxidase (MAO) inhibitors and other substances. *Proc R Soc Med.* 1965;58(11 pt 2):967-978.

Barsa JA, et la. A comparative study of tranylcypromine and paragyline. *Psychopharmacologia.* 1964;6:295-298.

 Methoxyflurane (*Penthrane*)

Secobarbital

SUMMARY: Barbiturates like secobarbital may enhance the nephrotoxic effect of methoxyflurane.

RISK FACTORS: No specific risk factors are known.

RELATED DRUGS: Based upon the mechanism, one would expect all barbiturates to inter-act similarly with methoxyflurane.

MANAGEMENT OPTIONS:

➡ *Consider Alternative.* Consider anesthetics other than methoxyflurane in patients who are receiving enzyme inducers such as barbiturates. Remember that enzyme induction dissipates slowly following discontinuation of the inducing agent, so the enhanced metabolic activity usually returns to normal within 2 to 3 weeks.

➡ *Monitor.* Monitor for nephrotoxicity if the combination is given.

REFERENCES:

Churchill D, et al. Toxic nephropathy after low-dose methoxyflurane anesthesia: drug interaction with secobarbital? *Can Med Assoc J.* 1976;114:326-328,333.

Cousins MJ, et al. Methoxyflurane nephrotoxicity. A study of dose response in man. *JAMA.* 1973;225:1611-1616.

Methoxyflurane (*Penthrane*)
Tetracycline

SUMMARY: Patients receiving methoxyflurane anesthesia appear to be at increased risk of developing renal toxicity if they are treated with tetracycline.

RISK FACTORS: No specific risk factors are known.

RELATED DRUGS: Other antibiotics, including kanamycin (eg, *Kantrex*) and gentamicin (eg, *Garamycin*), have been implicated in similar nephrotoxic effects in patients who receive methoxyflurane.

MANAGEMENT OPTIONS:

➡ *Use Alternative.* The severe consequences of this possible interaction warrant great caution in administering tetracycline (and perhaps other nephrotoxic antibiotics) to patients who will soon undergo or have recently undergone methoxyflurane anesthesia. Avoid the use of tetracycline with methoxyflurane.

REFERENCES:

Kuzucu EY. Methoxyflurane, tetracycline, and renal failure. *JAMA*. 1970;211:1162.

Churchill D. Persisting renal insufficiency after methoxyflurane anesthesia. Report of two cases and review of literature. *Am J Med*. 1974;56:575.

Dryden GE. Incidence of tubular degeneration with microlithiasis following methoxyflurane compared with other anesthetic agents. *Anesth Analg*. 1974;53:383.

Stoelting RK, et al. Effect of tetracycline therapy on renal function after methoxyflurane anesthesia. *Anesth Analg*. 1973;52:431.

Albers DD, et al. Renal failure following prostatovesticulectomy related to methoxyflurane anesthesia and tetracycline complicated by candida infection. *J Urol*. 1971;106:348.

Proctor EA, et al. Polyuric acute renal failure after methoxyflurane and tetracycline. *BMJ*. 1971;4:661.

Mazze RI, et al. Renal dysfunction associated with methoxyflurane anesthesia. A randomized, prospective clinical evaluation. *JAMA*. 1971;216:278.

Cousins MJ. Tetracycline, methoxyflurane anesthesia, and renal dysfunction. *Lancet*. 1972;1:751.

Methyldopa (eg, *Aldomet*)
Norepinephrine (Levarterenol; *Levophed*)

SUMMARY: Methyldopa therapy may prolong the pressor response to norepinephrine.

RISK FACTORS: No specific risk factors are known.

RELATED DRUGS: No information is available.

MANAGEMENT OPTIONS:

➡ *Monitor.* Monitor for increased blood pressure response to norepinephrine in patients receiving methyldopa.

REFERENCES:

Dollery CT. Physiological and pharmacological interactions of antihypertensive drugs. *Proc R Soc Med*. 1965;58:983.

Dollery CT, et al. Haemodynamic studies with methyldopa: effect on cardiac output and response to pressor amines. *Br Heart J*. 1963;25:670.

Methylprednisolone (eg, *Medrol*)

Troleandomycin (*Tao*)

SUMMARY: Troleandomycin markedly enhances methylprednisolone effects and may enhance prednisolone effect in some patients.

RISK FACTORS: No specific risk factors are known.

RELATED DRUGS: Although prednisolone (eg, *Prelone*) disposition was not affected by troleandomycin in 3 steroid-dependent asthmatics, troleandomycin did reduce prednisolone elimination somewhat in the presence of phenobarbital (eg, *Solfoton*). Little is known regarding the effect of troleandomycin on other corticosteroids in humans. Erythromycin and clarithromycin (*Biaxin*) are likely to produce a similar effect on methylprednisolone. Azithromycin (*Zithromax*) and dirithromycin (*Dynabac*) would be unlikely to enhance the effects of methylprednisolone.

MANAGEMENT OPTIONS:

➡ ***Monitor.*** A considerable reduction in methylprednisolone dosage requirement is likely in the presence of troleandomycin. Monitor patients on other corticosteroids for the need to adjust corticosteroid doses when troleandomycin is started or stopped.

REFERENCES:

Szefler SJ, et al. The effect of troleandomycin on methylprednisolone elimination. *J Allergy Clin Immunol.* 1980;66:447.

Selenke W, et al. Nonantibiotic effects of macrolide antibiotics of the oleandomycin-erythromycin group with special reference to their "steroid-sparing" effects. *J Allergy Clin Immunol.* 1980;65:454.

Nelson HS, et al. A double-blind study of troleandomycin and methylprednisolone in asthmatic subjects who require daily corticosteroids. *Am Rev Respir Dis.* 1993;147:398.

Szefler SJ, et al. Steroid-specific and anticonvulsant interaction aspects of troleandomycin-steroid therapy. *J Allergy Clin Immunol.* 1982;69:455.

Metoprolol (eg, *Lopressor*)

Propafenone (*Rythmol*)

SUMMARY: Metoprolol or propranolol (eg, *Inderal*) concentrations may significantly increase after administration of propafenone.

RISK FACTORS: No specific risk factors are known.

RELATED DRUGS: Propafenone 225 mg every 8 hours for 7 days in healthy subjects resulted in an 83% and 213% increase in propranolol peak and steady-state serum concentrations, respectively. Beta blocking effects were minimally enhanced during combination therapy. Beta blockers that are renally eliminated such as atenolol (eg, *Tenormin*) or nadolol (eg, *Corgard*) would be unlikely to be affected by propafenone.

MANAGEMENT OPTIONS:

➠ *Monitor.* Monitor patients receiving metoprolol or propranolol for increased beta blockade (eg, bradycardia, hypotension, heart failure) when propafenone is added to their therapy and for a reduced effect when it is withdrawn.

REFERENCES:

Wegner F, et al. Drug interaction between propafenone and metoprolol. *Br J Clin Pharmacol.* 1987;24:213.
Kowey PR, et al. Interaction between propranolol and propafenone in healthy volunteers. *J Clin Pharmacol.* 1989;29:512.

Metoprolol (eg, *Lopressor*)

Propoxyphene (eg, *Darvon*)

SUMMARY: Propoxyphene may increase the plasma concentration of highly metabolized beta blockers such as metoprolol; increased beta blocker effects may occur.

RISK FACTORS: No specific risk factors are known.

RELATED DRUGS: Propranolol interacts similarly with propoxyphene. It is unlikely that beta blockers excreted primarily by the kidneys (eg, atenolol [eg, *Tenormin*], nadolol [eg, *Corgard*], and sotalol [eg, *Betapace*]) would be affected by propoxyphene.

MANAGEMENT OPTIONS:

➠ *Monitor.* Until more information is available, be aware of increased response to metoprolol and propranolol when propoxyphene is initiated and a decreased response when it is discontinued.

REFERENCES:

Lundborg P, et al. The effect of propoxyphene pretreatment on the disposition of metoprolol and propranolol. *Clin Pharmacol Ther.* 1981;29:263.

Metoprolol (eg, *Lopressor*)

Quinidine

SUMMARY: Quinidine may increase the plasma concentration of metoprolol, but the incidence of adverse effects due to the interactions is unknown.

RISK FACTORS:

➠ *Pharmacogenetics.* Patients who are rapid metabolizers of metoprolol are at increased risk for the interaction.

RELATED DRUGS: Quinidine also decreases the metabolism of propranolol (eg, *Inderal*), and timolol (eg, *Blocadren*). Preliminary evidence suggests that quinidine has no effect on labetalol (eg, *Normodyne*) pharmacokinetics or pharmacodynamics. Atenolol (eg, *Tenormin*) and other renally excreted beta blockers are less likely to interact.

MANAGEMENT OPTIONS:

➠ *Consider Alternative.* Renally excreted beta blockers (eg, atenolol [eg, *Tenormin*]) should be less likely to interact with quinidine, because their clearance is unlikely to be affected by quinidine. Nevertheless, additive cardiac depressant effects cannot be overlooked.

➡ **Monitor.** Concomitant use of quinidine and metoprolol should be undertaken with careful monitoring. Watch for bradycardia, heart failure, and arrhythmias.

REFERENCES:

Leeman NT, et al. Single dose quinidine treatment inhibits metoprolol oxidation in extensive metabolizers. *Eur J Clin Pharmacol.* 1986;29:739.

Schlanz KD, et al. Loss of stereoselective metoprolol metabolism following quinidine inhibition of P450IID6. *Pharmacotherapy.* 1991;11:271. Abstract.

Schlanz KD, et al. Metoprolol pharmacodynamics and quinidine-induced inhibition of polymorphic drug metabolism. *Pharmacotherapy.* 1990;10:232. Abstract.

Gearhart MO, et al. Lack of effects on labetalol pharmacodynamics with quinidine inhibition of P450IID6. *Pharmacotherapy.* 1991;11:P-36. Abstract.

Metoprolol (eg, *Lopressor*)

Rifampin (eg, *Rifadin*)

SUMMARY: Plasma concentrations of beta blockers that are metabolized in the liver, such as metoprolol, may decline with concomitant rifampin therapy.

RISK FACTORS: No specific risk factors are known.

RELATED DRUGS: Rifampin is likely to increase the clearance of all beta blockers that are oxidatively metabolized by the liver, such as propranolol and bisprolol. Atenolol (eg, *Tenormin*) and other renally excreted beta blockers are less likely to interact.

MANAGEMENT OPTIONS:

➡ **Consider Alternative.** Beta-adrenergic blockers that are primarily eliminated by the kidneys, such as atenolol, could be used.

➡ **Circumvent/Minimize.** Beta blocker dosages may need to be increased when rifampin therapy is initiated and decreased when rifampin is discontinued.

➡ **Monitor.** Watch for reduced beta-adrenergic effects if rifampin is administered with beta-adrenergic blockers that are eliminated by hepatic metabolism.

REFERENCES:

Shaheen O, et al. Effect of debrisoquine phenotype on the inducibility of propranolol metabolism. *Clin Pharmacol Ther.* 1989;45:439.

Bennett PN, et al. Effects of rifampin on metoprolol and antipyrine kinetics. *Br J Clin Pharmacol.* 1982;13:387.

Kirch W, et al. Interaction of bisoprolol with cimetidine and rifampicin. *Eur J Clin Pharmacol.* 1986;31:59.

Metoprolol (eg, *Lopressor*)

Terbutaline (eg, *Brethaire*)

SUMMARY: Beta blocker-induced bronchoconstriction may antagonize the bronchodilating effect of beta-agonists; metoprolol increases terbutaline serum concentrations. The use of β_1-selective beta blockers is preferable in asthmatics receiving beta-agonists.

RISK FACTORS:

➡ **Pharmacogenetics.** Patients who are slow metoprolol metabolizers are at increased risk for the interaction.

RELATED DRUGS: Nonspecific beta blockers, such as propranolol (eg, *Inderal*), would appear more likely to antagonize bronchodilators, such as terbutaline. Practolol does not appear to impair the bronchodilator activity of terbutaline.

MANAGEMENT OPTIONS:

➥ *Use Alternative.* If possible, beta blockers should be avoided in patients receiving beta-agonists or theophylline for bronchospastic pulmonary disease. If beta blockers are required, cardioselective agents are preferable. If a cardioselective beta blocker is administered to a patient with asthma taking a beta agonist, observe the patient for worsening asthma.

REFERENCES:

Formgren H, et al. Effects of practolol in combination with terbutaline in the treatment of hypertension and arrhythmics in asthmatic patients. *Scand J Respir Dis.* 1975;56:217.

Jonkers RE, et al. Debrisoquine phenotype and the pharmacokinetics and beta-2 receptor pharmacodynamics of metoprolol and its enantiomers. *J Pharmacol Exp Ther.* 1991;256:959.

Metronidazole (eg, *Flagyl*)

Phenytoin (*Dilantin*)

SUMMARY: Metronidazole may moderately increase phenytoin serum concentrations.

RISK FACTORS: No specific risk factors are known.

RELATED DRUGS: No information is available.

MANAGEMENT OPTIONS:

➥ *Monitor.* Patients who have serum phenytoin concentrations near the upper limit of the therapeutic range should be monitored more carefully for increased phenytoin effect when metronidazole is added to their therapy.

REFERENCES:

Blyden GT, et al. Metronidazole impairs clearance of phenytoin but not alprazolam or lorazepam. *J Clin Pharmacol.* 1988;28:240.

Metronidazole (eg, *Flagyl*)

Trimethoprim-Sulfamethoxazole (eg, *Bactrim*)

SUMMARY: Metronidazole may produce a disulfiram-like reaction when administered with IV trimethoprim-sulfamethoxazole (TMP-SMX).

RISK FACTORS:

➥ *Route of Administration.* Administration of IV TMP-SMX increases the risk for the interaction.

RELATED DRUGS: The coadministration of metronidazole and IV drugs containing ethanol (eg, phenytoin [*Dilantin*], phenobarbital [eg, *Solfoton*], diazepam [eg, *Valium*], and nitroglycerin [eg, *Tridil*]) may result in flushing and vomiting. Disulfiram (eg, *Antabuse*) may react with IV TMP-SMX.

MANAGEMENT OPTIONS:

➡ *Circumvent/Minimize.* The use of oral dosage forms of these agents will prevent this interaction.

➡ *Monitor.* Watch for signs of disulfiram-like reaction when metronidazole is administered with IV drugs containing ethanol.

REFERENCES:

Edwards DL, et al. Disulfiram-like reaction associated with intravenous trimethoprim-sulfamethoxazole and metronidazole. *Clin Pharm.* 1986;5:999.

Metronidazole (eg, *Flagyl*)

Warfarin (eg, *Coumadin*)

SUMMARY: Metronidazole increases the hypoprothrombinemic response to warfarin, and bleeding has occurred in some patients receiving both drugs. Adjustments in warfarin dosage may be needed during cotherapy.

RISK FACTORS: No specific risk factors are known.

RELATED DRUGS: No information is available.

MANAGEMENT OPTIONS:

➡ *Avoid Unless Benefit Outweighs Risk.* Concomitant use of metronidazole and oral anticoagulants should be avoided if possible.

➡ *Monitor.* Patients receiving oral anticoagulants should be monitored for an increased anticoagulant effect when metronidazole is started and the converse when it is stopped. If oral anticoagulant therapy is begun in a patient receiving metronidazole, use conservative doses until the maintenance dose is established.

REFERENCES:

O'Reilly RA. The stereoselective interaction of warfarin and metronidazole in man. *N Engl J Med.* 1976;295:354.

Kazmier FJ. A significant interaction between metronidazole and warfarin. *Mayo Clin Proc.* 1976;51:782.

Dean RP, et al. Bleeding associated with concurrent warfarin and metronidazole therapy. *Drug Intell Clin Pharm.* 1980;14:864.

Metyrapone (*Metopirone*)

Phenytoin (*Dilantin*)

SUMMARY: Phenytoin lowers blood metyrapone concentrations and invalidates the metyrapone test.

RISK FACTORS: No specific risk factors are known.

RELATED DRUGS: Other enzyme inducers also may interfere with metyrapone tests.

MANAGEMENT OPTIONS:

➡ *Circumvent/Minimize.* The standard oral metyrapone test will be invalid in patients receiving chronic phenytoin therapy. Doubling the oral metyrapone dose in such patients may produce valid results.

➦ *Monitor.* Be alert for evidence of invalid metyrapone tests if phenytoin or other enzyme inducers are used.

REFERENCES:
Meikle AW, et al. Effect of diphenylhydantoin on the metabolism of metyrapone and release of ACTH in man. *J Clin Endocrinol Metab.* 1969;29:1553.

Werk EE, Jr et al. Failure of metyrapone to inhibit 11-hydroxylation of 11-deoxycortisol during drug therapy. *J Clin Endocrinol Metab.* 1967;27:1358.

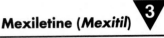

Mexiletine (*Mexitil*)
Phenytoin (*Dilantin*)

SUMMARY: A study in healthy subjects suggests that phenytoin substantially reduces mexiletine concentrations.

RISK FACTORS: No specific risk factors are known.

RELATED DRUGS: No information is available.

MANAGEMENT OPTIONS:

➦ *Circumvent/Minimize.* Mexiletine dosage requirements are likely to increase when phenytoin is administered and decrease when it is discontinued.

➦ *Monitor.* Measurement of mexiletine concentrations would be helpful to assure that dosage adjustments are adequate. Monitor patients for a decreased therapeutic response when phenytoin is used concurrently and an increased response if phenytoin is discontinued.

REFERENCES:
Begg EJ, et al. Enhanced metabolism of mexiletine after phenytoin administration. *Br J Clin Pharmacol.* 1982;14:219.

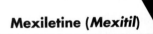

Mexiletine (*Mexitil*)
Quinidine

SUMMARY: Quinidine administration increases mexiletine concentrations and increases its antiarrhythmic effects.

RISK FACTORS:

➦ *Pharmacogenetics.* Patients who are extensive mexiletine metabolizers are at increased risk for the interaction.

RELATED DRUGS: No information is available.

MANAGEMENT OPTIONS:

➦ *Monitor.* Patients stabilized on mexiletine should be monitored for increased serum concentrations and electrophysiologic effects of mexiletine when quinidine is administered.

REFERENCES:
Turgeon J, et al. Influence of debrisoquine phenotype and of quinidine on mexiletine disposition in man. *J Pharmacol Exper Ther.* 1991;259:789.

Duff HJ, et al. Role of quinidine in the mexiletine-quinidine interaction: electrophysiologic correlates of enhanced antiarrhythmic efficacy. *J Cardiovasc Pharmacol.* 1990;16:685.

Duff HJ, et al. Electropharmacologic synergism with mexiletine and quinidine. *J Cardiovasc Pharmacol.* 1986;8:840.

Duff HJ, et al. Mexiletine/quinidine combination therapy: electrophysiology correlates of anti-arrhythmic efficacy. *Clin Invest Med.* 1991;14:476.

Mexiletine (*Mexitil*)

Sodium Bicarbonate

SUMMARY: An increase in urine pH could result in clinically significant increases in mexiletine concentrations.

RISK FACTORS: No specific risk factors are known.

RELATED DRUGS: Other agents that alkalinize the urine (eg, acetazolamide) would be expected to produce a similar interaction with mexiletine.

MANAGEMENT OPTIONS:

➡ *Monitor.* Patients receiving mexiletine who have large changes in their urine pH as a result of concurrent drug therapy should be monitored for changes in mexiletine plasma concentration.

REFERENCES:

Begg EJ, et al. Enhanced metabolism of mexiletine after phenytoin administration. *Br J Clin Pharmacol.* 1982;14:219.

Pentikainen PJ, et al. Effect of rifampicin treatment on the kinetics of mexiletine. *Eur J Clin Pharmacol.* 1982;23:261.

Kiddie MA, et al. The influence of urinary pH on the elimination of mexiletine. *Br J Clin Pharmacol.* 1974;1:229.

Mexiletine (*Mexitil*)

Theophylline (eg, *Theolair*)

SUMMARY: Patients maintained on theophylline may develop elevated theophylline serum concentrations and toxicity after initiating concomitant mexiletine therapy.

RISK FACTORS: No specific risk factors are known.

RELATED DRUGS: No information is available.

MANAGEMENT OPTIONS:

➡ *Use Alternative.* Patients taking mexiletine should avoid receiving theophylline. The use of a beta-agonist or steroid should be considered. An alternative to mexiletine should be considered in patients receiving theophylline. Patients stabilized on theophylline who receive mexiletine should be carefully monitored for increased theophylline concentrations and potentially toxic symptoms, including tachycardia, arrhythmias, GI upset, and seizures.

REFERENCES:

Katz A, et al. Oral mexiletine-theophylline interaction. *Int J Cardiol.* 1987;17:227.

Stanley R, et al. Mexiletine-theophylline interaction. *Am J Med.* 1989;86:733.

Kessler KM, et al. Proarrhythmia related to a kinetic and dynamic interaction of mexiletine and theophylline. *Am Heart J.* 1989;117:964.

Loi CM, et al. Effect of mexiletine on theophylline metabolism. *Clin Pharmacol Ther.* 1990;47:130. Abstract.

Kendall JD, et al. Theophylline-mexiletine interaction: a case report. *Pharmacotherapy.* 1992;12:416.

Hurwitz, A et al. Mexiletine effects on theophylline disposition. *Clin Pharmacol Ther.* 1991;50:299.

Stoysich AM, et al. Influence of mexiletine on the pharmacokinetics of theophylline in healthy volunteers. *J Clin Pharmacol.* 1991;31:354.

Mibefradil

Simvastatin (*Zocor*)

SUMMARY: Mibefradil coadministration with simvastatin or lovastatin (*Mevacor*) may increase the risk of rhabdomyolysis. Pending further data, the combination should be avoided.

RISK FACTORS: No specific risk factors are known.

RELATED DRUGS: Because lovastatin is metabolized similarly to simvastatin, mibefradil would be expected to reduce lovastatin's clearance and potentially induce muscle toxicity. While no data are currently available, atorvastatin and cerivastatin (*Baycol*) metabolism also may be reduced by mibefradil administration. Mibefradil is unlikely to reduce the clearance of fluvastatin (*Lescol*) or pravastatin (*Pravachol*). Verapamil (eg, *Isoptin*) and diltiazem (eg, *Cardizem*) are also likely to reduce lovastatin, simvastatin, atorvastatin, and cerivastatin clearance.

MANAGEMENT OPTIONS:

➡ ***Use Alternative.*** Patients taking mibefradil who require a HMG-CoA reductase inhibitor should receive fluvastatin or pravastatin.

REFERENCES:
Product information. Mibefradil (*Posicor*). Roche Laboratories, Inc. 1997.

Mibefradil

Terfenadine

SUMMARY: Terfenadine concentrations can increase during mibefradil coadministration; cardiac arrhythmias may result. Avoid concurrent use of terfenadine and mibefradil.

RISK FACTORS: No specific risk factors are known.

RELATED DRUGS: It is likely that mibefradil administration would cause an accumulation of astemizole and potentially produce cardiac toxicity. Other calcium channel blockers (eg, amlodipine [*Norvasc*], nifedipine [eg, *Procardia*], nicardipine [eg, *Cardene*]) would not be expected to change terfenadine plasma concentrations. The metabolism of fexofenadine (*Allegra*), cetirizine (*Zyrtec*), and loratadine (*Claritin*) would be unlikely to be affected by concomitant mibefradil administration.

MANAGEMENT OPTIONS:

➡ ***Use Alternative.*** Due to the risk of a possibly serious arrhythmia, the combination of mibefradil and terfenadine (or astemizole) should be avoided. Noninteracting antihistamines are available and should be used in patients receiving mibefradil.

REFERENCES:
Product information. Mibefradil (*Posicor*). Roche Laboratories, Inc. 1997.

Miconazole (eg, *Monistat*)

Tobramycin (eg, *Nebcin*)

SUMMARY: Miconazole reduces tobramycin peak serum concentrations; dosage adjustments may be required to maintain adequate serum concentrations.

RISK FACTORS: No specific risk factors are known.

RELATED DRUGS: Other aminoglycosides may be affected similarly by miconazole or related azole antifungals such as ketoconazole (eg, *Nizoral*) or itraconazole (*Sporanox*).

MANAGEMENT OPTIONS:

➡ ***Consider Alternative.*** Choose an alternative antifungal agent. Note that amphotericin can produce increased nephrotoxicity when administered with aminoglycosides. The effects of other antifungal agents on aminoglycoside pharmacokinetics are unknown.

➡ ***Monitor.*** Aminoglycoside concentrations should be monitored in patients receiving miconazole and aminoglycosides.

REFERENCES:

Hatfield SM, et al. Miconazole-induced alteration in tobramycin pharmacokinetics. *Clin Pharm.* 1986;5:415.

Miconazole (eg, *Monistat*)

Warfarin (eg, *Coumadin*)

SUMMARY: Miconazole given systemically and as an oral gel has been associated with enhanced hypoprothrombinemia and bleeding in some patients receiving oral anticoagulants.

RISK FACTORS: No specific risk factors are known.

RELATED DRUGS: The effect of miconazole on oral anticoagulants other than warfarin is not known, but be alert for a similar effect with all oral anticoagulants until information to the contrary is available.

MANAGEMENT OPTIONS:

➡ ***Monitor.*** Monitor for altered oral anticoagulant effect if miconazole is initiated, discontinued, or changed in dosage. Adjust the anticoagulant dose as needed.

REFERENCES:

Watson PG, et al. Drug interaction with coumarin derivative anticoagulants. *BMJ.* 1982;285:1045.

Goenen M, et al. A case of *Candida albicans* endocarditis 3 years after an aortic valve replacement: successful combined medical and surgical therapy. *J Cardiovasc Surg.* 1977;18:391.

Deresinski SC, et al. Miconazole treatment of human coccidioidomycosis: status report. In: Ajello L, ed. Coccidioidomycosis—Current Clinical and Diagnostic Status. Proceedings of the Third International Coccidioidomycosis Symposium. Tucson:1976 November. Miami Symposia Specialists. 1977;267-92.

Coloquhorn MC, et al. Interaction between warfarin and miconazole oral gel. *Lancet.* 1987;1:695.

Shenfield GM, et al. Potentiation of warfarin action by miconazole oral gel. *Aust N Z J Med.* 1991;21:928. Letter.

Midazolam (*Versed*)

Phenytoin (*Dilantin*)

SUMMARY: Phenytoin markedly reduces the effect of oral midazolam, but parenteral midazolam is likely to be less affected.

RISK FACTORS:

➡ *Route of Administration.* Because the majority of the interaction is likely caused by increased presystemic metabolism of oral midazolam by the gut wall and liver, parenteral midazolam is likely to be much less affected.

RELATED DRUGS: Carbamazepine (eg, *Tegretol*) interacts similarly with midazolam. Triazolam (eg, *Halcion*), alprazolam (eg, *Xanax*), and to some extent diazepam (eg, *Valium*) also are metabolized by CYP3A4 and would be expected to interact with enzyme inducers in a manner similar to midazolam.

MANAGEMENT OPTIONS:

➡ *Consider Alternative.* When midazolam is used orally as a sedative-hypnotic (as it is in several countries), patients receiving enzyme inducers such as phenytoin are unlikely to respond unless very large doses of midazolam are used. Thus, it may be preferable to use alternative sedative-hypnotics in such patients.

➡ *Monitor.* Although parenteral midazolam is likely to be much less affected, monitor for inadequate midazolam effect and increase its dose if needed.

REFERENCES:

Backman JT, et al. Concentrations and effects of oral midazolam are greatly reduced in patients treated with carbamazepine or phenytoin. *Epilepsia.* 1996;37:253.

Midazolam (*Versed*)

Rifampin (eg, *Rifadin*)

SUMMARY: Rifampin administration results in a marked reduction in midazolam plasma concentrations; loss of efficacy is likely to occur.

RISK FACTORS: No specific risk factors are known.

RELATED DRUGS: Rifampin will affect other benzodiazepines undergoing high first-pass metabolism via CYP3A4 such as triazolam (*Halcion*), and diazepam (*Valium*). Rifabutin (*Mycobutin*) is likely to interact in a similar manner with midazolam.

MANAGEMENT OPTIONS:

➡ *Consider Alternative.* Selection of a benzodiazepine that is not a CYP3A4 substrate such as temazepam (eg, *Restoril*) or oxazepam (eg, *Serax*) would avoid the interaction.

➡ **Monitor.** Monitor patients receiving rifampin for reduced midazolam efficacy. If rifampin is discontinued in a patient receiving both agents, the dose of midazolam will require reduction during the next week or 10 days to avoid excess sedation.

REFERENCES:

Backman JT, et al. Rifampin drastically reduces plasma concentrations and effects of oral midazolam. *Clin Pharmacol Ther.* 1996;59:7.

Gorski JC, et al. The effect of rifampin on intestinal and hepatic CYP3A activity. *Clin Pharmacol Ther.* 2000;67:133.

Midazolam (*Versed*)

Saquinavir (*Fortovase*)

SUMMARY: Saquinavir increases midazolam concentrations, particularly following oral midazolam. Increased midazolam-induced sedation is likely to result.

RISK FACTORS:

➡ **Route of Administration.** The effect of saquinavir on midazolam clearance is increased when midazolam is administered orally.

RELATED DRUGS: Benzodiazepines such as triazolam (eg, *Halcion*) or zolpidem (*Ambien*) that are metabolized by CYP3A4 would be expected to interact with saquinavir in a similar manner. Other protease inhibitors that have been reported to inhibit CYP3A4 (eg, ritonavir [*Norvir*], nelfinavir [*Viracept*], amprenavir [*Agenerase*], and indinavir [*Crixivan*]) would be expected to inhibit the metabolism of midazolam.

MANAGEMENT OPTIONS:

➡ **Consider Alternative.** An anxiolytic that is not metabolized by CYP3A4, such as oxazepam (eg, *Serax*) or lorazepam (eg, *Ativan*), could be considered as an alternative to midazolam for some indications.

➡ **Monitor.** Patients who are receiving saquinavir will probably require lower doses of oral or IV midazolam and may remain sedated for a longer period of time following a single dose of midazolam or the discontinuation of chronic midazolam therapy.

REFERENCES:

Palkama VJ, et al. Effect of saquinavir on the pharmacokinetics and pharmacodynamics of oral and intravenous midazolam. *Clin Pharmacol Ther.* 1999;66:33.

Merry C, et al. Saquinavir interaction with midazolam: pharmacokinetic considerations when prescribing protease inhibitors for patients with HIV disease. *AIDS.* 1997;11:268.

 ## Misoprostol (*Cytotec*)

Phenylbutazone

SUMMARY: The combined use of phenylbutazone and misoprostol has been associated with adverse effects (eg, tingling, headache, hot flushes, dizziness, nausea) in some patients, but a causal relationship is not established.

RISK FACTORS: No specific risk factors are known.

RELATED DRUGS: Naproxen and etodolac do not appear to affect misoprostol. The effect of other nonsteroidal anti-inflammatory drugs on misoprostol is not established.

MANAGEMENT OPTIONS:

➡ *Monitor.* Until more information is available, be alert for adverse effects such as tingling, headache, hot flushes, dizziness, and nausea when misoprostol is used in patients receiving phenylbutazone.

REFERENCES:

Chassagne P, et al. Neurosensory adverse effects after combined phenylbutazone and misoprostol. *Br J Rheumatol.* 1991;30:392. Letter.

Jacquemier JM, et al. Neurosensory adverse effects after phenylbutazone and misoprostol combined treatment. *Lancet.* 1989;2:1283. Letter.

Mitomycin (*Mutamycin*)
Vinblastine (eg, *Velban*)

SUMMARY: Administration of vinblastine following treatment with mitomycin has been associated with acute bronchospasm and dyspnea.

RISK FACTORS: No specific risk factors are known.

RELATED DRUGS: No information is available.

MANAGEMENT OPTIONS:

➡ *Avoid Unless Benefit Outweighs Risk.* Although most patients do not appear to develop pulmonary toxicity, the severity of the reaction dictates that the combination generally should be avoided.

➡ *Monitor.* In instances where the combination is felt to be necessary, advise patients to contact their physician or go to the emergency room immediately if they develop difficulty in breathing. Both drugs should be discontinued immediately at the first sign of respiratory compromise. Avoid further therapy with this combination in patients who experience dyspnea, as it appears to recur upon repeated administration.

REFERENCES:

Israel RH, et al. Pulmonary edema associated with intravenous vinblastine. *JAMA.* 1978;240:1585. Letter.

Konits PH, et al. Possible pulmonary toxicity secondary to vinblastine. *Cancer.* 1982;50:277.

Ozols RF, et al. MVP (mitomycin, vinblastine, and progesterone): a second-line regimen in ovarian cancer with a high incidence of pulmonary toxicity. *Cancer Treat Rep.* 1983;67:721.

Dyke RW. Acute bronchospasm after vinca alkaloid in patients previously treated with mitomycin. *N Engl J Med.* 1984;310:389.

Kris MG, et al. Dyspnea following vinblastine or vindesine administration in patients receiving mitomycin plus vinca alkaloid combination therapy. *Cancer Treat Rep.* 1984;68:1029.

Rao SX, et al. Fatal acute respiratory failure after vinblastine-mitomycin therapy in lung carcinoma. *Arch Intern Med.* 1985;145:1905.

Hoelzer KL. Vinblastine-associated pulmonary toxicity in patients receiving combination therapy with mitomycin and cisplatin. *Drug Intell Clin Pharm.* 1986;20:287.

Mitotane (*Lysodren*)

AVOID **Spironolactone (eg, *Aldactone*)**

SUMMARY: Spironolactone may antagonize the activity of mitotane.

RISK FACTORS: No specific risk factors are known.

RELATED DRUGS: No information is available.

MANAGEMENT OPTIONS:

➡ *AVOID COMBINATION.* Patients on mitotane should not receive concurrent spironolactone.

REFERENCES:
Wortsman J, et al. Mitotane. Spironolactone antagonism in Cushing's syndrome. *JAMA*. 1977;238:2527.

 Mitotane (*Lysodren*)

Warfarin (eg, *Coumadin*)

SUMMARY: Mitotane appears to inhibit the hypoprothrombinemic response to warfarin and probably other oral anticoagulants as well. Oral anticoagulant dose requirements may be increased in patients taking both drugs.

RISK FACTORS: No specific risk factors are known.

RELATED DRUGS: The effect of mitotane on oral anticoagulants other than warfarin is not
known, but be alert for a similar effect with all oral anticoagulants until information to the contrary is available.

MANAGEMENT OPTIONS:

➡ *Monitor.* Monitor for altered oral anticoagulant effect if mitotane is initiated, discontinued, or changed in dosage. Adjust the anticoagulant dose as needed.

REFERENCES:
Cuddy PG, et al. Influence of mitotane on the hypoprothrombinemic effect of warfarin. *South Med J.*
1986;79:387.

 Moclobemide[†]

Rizatriptan (*Maxalt*)

SUMMARY: Moclobemide substantially increases plasma concentrations of rizatriptan and its active metabolite; concurrent use is generally not recommended, although adverse clinical outcomes have not been reported.

RISK FACTORS: No specific risk factors are known.

RELATED DRUGS: Theoretically, any selective MAO-A inhibitor or nonselective MAO-A/
MAO-B inhibitor such as phenelzine (*Nardil*) or tranylcypromine (*Parnate*) would
also substantially increase rizatriptan plasma concentrations. Sumatriptan (*Imitrex*)
and zolmitriptan (*Zomig*), like rizatriptan, are metabolized by MAO-A. They
would be expected to interact similarly with MAO-A inhibitors such as
moclobemide or nonselective MAO-A/MAO-B inhibitors such as phenelzine or
tranylcypromine.

MANAGEMENT OPTIONS:

➡ *Use Alternative.* Use an alternative to moclobemide (ie, a non-MAO-A inhibitor) or rizatriptan (ie, a non-MAO-A substrate). Naratriptan (*Amerge*) is predominantly eliminated in the urine, and theoretically would be less likely than other "triptans" to interact with moclobemide or nonselective MAO inhibitors.

➡ *Monitor.* Theoretically, the combination of moclobemide and rizatriptan could result in excessive vasoconstriction. If the combination is used, monitor for increased blood pressure and other evidence of vasoconstriction.

REFERENCES:

van Haarst AD, et al. The effects of moclobemide on the pharmacokinetics of the 5-HT$_{1B/1D}$ agonist rizatriptan in healthy volunteers. *Br J Clin Pharmacol.* 1999;48:190-96

† Not available in the US.

Moclobemide†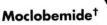

Selegiline (eg, *Eldepryl*)

SUMMARY: Combined use of selegiline and moclobemide substantially increases the pressor effect of tyramine over either drug used alone.

RISK FACTORS: No specific risk factors are known.

RELATED DRUGS: This interaction is likely to occur with any combination of an MAO-B and MAO-A inhibitor.

MANAGEMENT OPTIONS:

➡ *Consider Alternative.* Given the likely increase in risk of adverse drug or food interactions, consider using an antidepressant other than moclobemide in patients receiving MAO-B inhibitors such as selegiline.

➡ *Circumvent/Minimize.* Until more data are available, give patients receiving combined therapy with moclobemide and selegiline (or any other combination of an MAO-A and MAO-B inhibitor) the same dietary and drug interaction instructions as patients receiving nonselective MAOI such as phenelzine or tranylcypromine.

➡ *Monitor.* Monitor for evidence of tyramine-induced hypertension if the combination is used.

REFERENCES:

Dingemanse J. An update of recent moclobemide interaction data. *Int Clin Psychopharmacol.* 1993;7:167.

† Not available in the US.

Moclobemide†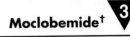

Tyramine

SUMMARY: Moclobemide may increase the pressor response to large amounts of tyramine; avoid high-tyramine foods (eg, aged cheese).

RISK FACTORS: No specific risk factors are known.

RELATED DRUGS: Other MAO-A inhibitors may interact similarly with tyramine.

MANAGEMENT OPTIONS:

➡ *Circumvent/Minimize.* Although moclobemide appears much less likely to interact with dietary tyramine than nonselective MAOIs, it would be prudent to avoid foods with high tyramine content. It also has been suggested that moclobemide be taken after meals to minimize the interaction, but more study is needed to assess the value of this precaution.

➡ *Monitor.* Monitor blood pressure if the interaction is suspected.

REFERENCES:

Dingemanse J. An update of recent moclobemide interaction data. *Int Clin Psychopharmacol.* 1993;7:167.

Simpson GM, et al. Comparison of the pressor effect of tyramine after treatment with phenelzine and moclobemide in healthy male volunteers. *Clin Pharmacol Ther.* 1992;52:286.

Freeman H. Moclobemide. *Lancet.* 1993;342:1528.

† Not available in the US.

Modafinil (*Provigil*)

Contraceptives, Oral (eg, *Ortho-Novum*)

SUMMARY: Modafinil appears to modestly reduce ethinyl estradiol plasma concentrations; reduced contraceptive efficacy may occur in some patients.

RISK FACTORS: No specific risk factors are known.

RELATED DRUGS: No information is available.

MANAGEMENT OPTIONS:

➡ *Consider Alternative.* In patients on modafinil, consider using contraceptive methods other than oral contraceptives.

➡ *Circumvent/Minimize.* If oral contraceptives are used in conjunction with modafinil therapy, it would be prudent to use additional methods of contraceptive during and for 1 month after stopping modafinil.

➡ *Monitor.* If oral contraceptives are used in conjunction with modafinil therapy, be alert for evidence of reduced contraceptive effect such as menstrual irregularities (eg, spotting, breakthrough bleeding).

REFERENCES:

Robertson P, et al. Effect of modafinil on the pharmacokinetics of ethinyl estradiol and triazolam in healthy volunteers. *Clin Pharmacol Ther.* 2002;71:46-56.

Modafinil (*Provigil*)

Triazolam (*Halcion*)

SUMMARY: Modafinil appears to substantially reduce triazolam plasma concentrations, and may reduce its hypnotic effect.

RISK FACTORS: No specific risk factors are known.

RELATED DRUGS: No information is available.

MANAGEMENT OPTIONS:

➡ *Monitor.* Be alert for evidence of reduced triazolam effect if modafinil is given concurrently. A larger dose of triazolam may be needed.

REFERENCES:

Robertson P, et al. Effect of modafinil on the pharmacokinetics of ethinyl estradiol and triazolam in healthy volunteers. *Clin Pharmacol Ther.* 2002;71:46-56.

Moricizine (*Ethmozine*)
Theophylline (eg, *Theolair*)

SUMMARY: Moricizine reduces theophylline serum concentrations; the clinical effects of this pharmacokinetic interaction have not been described.

RISK FACTORS: No specific risk factors are known.

RELATED DRUGS: No information is available.

MANAGEMENT OPTIONS:

➡ *Monitor.* Monitor patients taking theophylline for reduced theophylline concentrations and potential loss of effect when moricizine is added to their therapy.

REFERENCES:

Pieniaszek HJ, et al. Effect of moricizine on the pharmacokinetics of single-dose theophylline in healthy subjects. *Ther Drug Monit.* 1993;15:199.

Morphine (eg, *Roxanol*)
Rifampin (eg, *Rifadin*)

SUMMARY: Rifampin administration reduces the concentrations of morphine and 2 of its metabolites, as well as its analgesic efficacy.

RISK FACTORS: No specific risk factors are known.

RELATED DRUGS: Rifampin also reduces the plasma concentrations of methadone (eg, *Dolophine*). Rifabutin (*Mycobutin*) does not appear to affect methadone pharmacokinetics. Its effects on morphine are unknown.

MANAGEMENT OPTIONS:

➡ *Circumvent/Minimize.* Increased doses of morphine are likely to be required during coadministration of rifampin. Adjustments in morphine doses should be anticipated. Patients receiving morphine and rifampin should have their morphine doses adjusted based upon analgesic response when rifampin is added or removed from their drug regimen.

➡ *Monitor.* Until specific analgesics that are not affected by rifampin are identified, patients taking rifampin and narcotic analgesics should be monitored for adequate analgesic effect.

REFERENCES:

Fromm MF, et al. Loss of analgesic effect of morphine due to coadministration of rifampin. *Pain.* 1997;72:261.

Morphine (eg, *Roxanol*)

Somatostatin (*Zecnil*)

SUMMARY: Limited clinical evidence suggests that somatostatin inhibits the analgesic effect of morphine.

RISK FACTORS: No specific risk factors are known.

RELATED DRUGS: It is not known whether the somatostatin analog octreotide (*Sandostatin*) also inhibits morphine analgesia, but one should be alert to the possibility. Somatostatin has also been reported to inhibit methadone analgesia (see Methadone/Somatostatin), but its effect on other opioids is not established.

MANAGEMENT OPTIONS:

 Monitor. Watch for evidence of reduced analgesia if somatostatin is used with morphine or other opioid analgesics. If morphine analgesia appears diminished, it would be prudent to stop the somatostatin. If somatostatin cannot be stopped, current evidence suggests that it may be difficult to achieve adequate analgesia.

REFERENCES:
Ripamonti C, et al. Can somatostatin be administered in association with morphine in advanced cancer patients with pain? *Ann Oncol.* 1998;9:921. Letter.

Morphine (eg, *Roxanol*)

Trovafloxacin (*Trovan*)

SUMMARY: Intravenous morphine reduces the serum concentration of orally administered trovafloxacin. Reduced antibiotic efficacy may result.

RISK FACTORS:

➡ ***Route of Administration.*** This interaction has only been reported to occur with intravenous morphine and oral trovafloxacin.

RELATED DRUGS: No information is available regarding the interaction of other quinolones with morphine.

MANAGEMENT OPTIONS:

➡ ***Monitor.*** Patients receiving trovafloxacin and intravenous morphine should be monitored for possible reduced trovafloxacin efficacy.

REFERENCES:
Product information. Trovafloxacin (*Trovan*). Pfizer Inc. 1998.

❷ Moxalactam

Warfarin (eg, *Coumadin*)

SUMMARY: Moxalactam may produce hypoprothrombinemia and thus may enhance the anticoagulant effect of warfarin and other oral anticoagulants.

RISK FACTORS:

➡ ***Concurrent Diseases.*** Renal dysfunction, hepatic dysfunction, and reduced dietary vitamin K can place one at risk.

RELATED DRUGS: IV cefonicid (*Monocid*) 2 mg/day for 7 days did not affect the hypoprothrombinemic response.

MANAGEMENT OPTIONS:

➡ *Use Alternative.* Moxalactam, cefoperazone, cefamandole, cefotetan, and cefmetazole probably should be avoided in patients taking warfarin. Intravenous cefonicid may be an alternative.

REFERENCES:
Brown RB, et al. Enhanced bleeding with cefoxitin or moxalactam: statistical analysis within a defined population of 1493 patients. *Arch Intern Med.* 1986;146:2159.

Freedy HR Jr, et al. Cefoperazone-induced coagulopathy. *Drug Intell Clin Pharm.* 1986;20:281.

Rymer W, et al. Hypoprothrombinemia associated with cefamandole. *Drug Intell Clin Pharm.* 1980;14:780.

Conjura A, et al. Cefotetan and hypoprothrombinemia. *Ann Intern Med.* 1988;108:644.

Angaran DM, et al. The comparative influence of prophylactic antibiotics on the prothrombin response to warfarin in the postoperative prosthetic cardiac valve patient: cefamandole, cefazolin, vancomycin. *Ann Surg.* 1987;206:155.

Dupuis LL, et al. Cefazolin-induced coagulopathy. *Clin Pharmacol Ther.* 1984;35:237. Abstract.

Anagaran DM, et al. Effect of cefonicid (CN) on prothrombin time (PT) in outpatients (OP) receiving warfarin (W) therapy. *Pharmacotherapy.* 1988;8:120. Abstract.

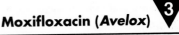

Moxifloxacin (*Avelox*)
Sucralfate (*Carafate*)

SUMMARY: Sucralfate reduces the plasma concentrations of moxifloxacin; a reduction in moxifloxacin efficacy is likely to occur in some patients.

RISK FACTORS: No specific risk factors are known.

RELATED DRUGS: Other quinolone antibiotics such as ciprofloxacin (*Cipro*) and ofloxacin (*Floxin*) are affected in a similar manner by sucralfate.

MANAGEMENT OPTIONS:

➡ *Consider Alternative.* Because it may be difficult to separate the doses of sucralfate and moxifloxacin sufficiently to prevent the interaction, consider using H_2-receptor antagonists or proton pump inhibitors in patients requiring gastric acid suppression.

➡ *Circumvent/Minimize.* Pending further information, avoid the coadministration of sucralfate and moxifloxacin. Administer moxifloxacin several hours before sucralfate; however, some degree of reduction in moxifloxacin plasma concentration may still occur.

➡ *Monitor.* Watch for reduced antibiotic efficacy if moxifloxacin and antacids are coadministered.

REFERENCES:
Stass H, et al. Effects of sucralfate on the oral bioavailability of moxifloxacin, a novel 8-methoxyfluoroquinolone, in healthy volunteers. *Clin Pharmacokinet.* 2001;40(suppl 1):49.

② Moxifloxacin (*Avelox*)

Ziprasidone (*Geodon*)

SUMMARY: Ziprasidone and moxifloxacin can prolong the corrected QT (QTc) interval on the electrocardiogram (ECG). Theoretically, this could increase the risk of ventricular arrhythmias such as torsades de pointes.

RISK FACTORS:

➡ **Hypokalemia.** The QTc on the ECG may be prolonged in patients with hypokalemia, increasing the risk of this interaction.

➡ **Miscellaneous.** Other factors that may prolong the QTc interval (eg, hypomagnesemia, bradycardia, impaired liver function, hypothyroidism) also may increase the risk of ventricular arrhythmias.

RELATED DRUGS: Available data suggest that ziprasidone produces less QTc prolongation than thioridazine (*Mellaril*) but about twice that of quetiapine (*Seroquel*), risperidone (*Risperdal*), haloperidol (*Haldol*), and olanzapine (*Zyprexa*). Sparfloxacin (*Zagam*), like moxifloxacin, can prolong the QTc interval substantially, but other fluoroquinolones such as levofloxacin (*Levaquin*), ofloxacin (*Floxin*), gatifloxacin (*Tequin*), and ciprofloxacin (*Cipro*) usually produce only minimal effects.

MANAGEMENT OPTIONS:

➡ **Use Alternative.** Given the theoretical risk and the fact that moxifloxacin is listed in the ziprasidone product information as "contraindicated," it would be prudent to use an alternative to one of the drugs (see Related Drugs).

➡ **Monitor.** If moxifloxacin and ziprasidone are used concurrently, monitor for evidence of arrhythmias (eg, syncope) and for prolonged QT intervals.

REFERENCES:

De Ponti F, et al. QT-interval prolongation by non-cardiac drugs: lessons to be learned from recent experience. *Eur J Clin Pharmacol.* 2000;56:1.

Product information. Ziprasidone (*Geodon*). Pfizer Pharmaceuticals. 2001.

Briefing Information, Psychopharmacological Drugs Advisory Committee, U.S. Food and Drug Administration, July 19, 2000.

Nabumetone (*Relafen*)

Warfarin (eg, *Coumadin*)

SUMMARY: Preliminary data suggest that nabumetone does not affect the hypoprothrombinemic response to warfarin, but cotherapy requires caution because of possible detrimental effects of nabumetone on the gastric mucosa and platelet function.

RISK FACTORS:

➡ **Concurrent Diseases.** Patients with peptic ulcer disease (PUD) or a history of GI bleeding are probably at greater risk.

RELATED DRUGS: All NSAIDs inhibit platelet function, cause gastric erosions, and probably increase the risk of GI bleeding.

MANAGEMENT OPTIONS:

➡ **Avoid Unless Benefit Outweighs Risk.** Because all NSAIDs probably increase the risk of GI bleeding in patients on oral anticoagulants, use the combination only after careful consideration of the benefit vs risk. If the NSAID is being used as an analgesic or antipyretic, acetaminophen probably is safer to use with oral anticoagulants. Nonacetylated salicylates (eg, choline salicylate, magnesium salicylate, salsalate, sodium salicylate) probably also are safer with oral anticoagulants than NSAIDs since they have minimal effects on platelet function and the gastric mucosa.

➡ **Monitor.** If any NSAID is used with an oral anticoagulant, one should monitor carefully the prothrombin time and watch for evidence of bleeding, especially from the GI tract.

REFERENCES:

Hilleman DE, et al. Hypoprothrombinemic effect of nabumetone in warfarin-treated patients. *Pharmacotherapy*. 1993;13:270. Abstract.

Shorr RI, et al. Concurrent use of nonsteroidal anti-inflammatory drugs and oral anticoagulants places elderly persons at high risk for hemorrhagic peptic ulcer disease. *Arch Intern Med*. 1993;153:1665.

Nafcillin (eg, *Unipen*)

Nifedipine (*Procardia*)

SUMMARY: Nafcillin administration results in a large reduction in the plasma concentration of nifedipine; loss of efficacy is likely to result.

RISK FACTORS:

➡ **Route of Administration.** The administration of nafcillin or the calcium channel blocker, nifedipine, orally would increase the magnitude of this interaction.

RELATED DRUGS: Nafcillin would be expected to reduce the plasma concentrations of other calcium channel blockers including felodipine (*Plendil*), nicardipine (eg, *Cardene*), verapamil (eg, *Calan*), and diltiazem (eg, *Cardizem*). There is no evidence that other penicillins affect nifedipine.

MANAGEMENT OPTIONS:

➡ **Avoid Unless Benefit Outweighs Risk.** The combination of nafcillin and nifedipine, or other calcium channel blockers, should be avoided. Selection of an alternative antibiotic should be considered.

➡ **Monitor.** Patients stabilized on nifedipine or other calcium channel blockers should be monitored for loss of efficacy during the administration of nafcillin.

REFERENCES:

Jamal SK, et al. Nafcillin is a potent inducer of cytochrome P4503A activity in humans. *Clin Pharmacol Ther*. 1998;63:151. Abstract.

Nafcillin (eg, *Unipen*)

Warfarin (eg, *Coumadin*)

SUMMARY: Several case reports suggest that nafcillin may inhibit the hypoprothrombinemic response to warfarin.

RISK FACTORS: No specific risk factors are known.

RELATED DRUGS: Dicloxacillin (eg, *Dynapen*) also may inhibit the hypoprothrombinemic response to warfarin, but data are limited.

MANAGEMENT OPTIONS:

➡ **Monitor.** In patients receiving warfarin or other oral anticoagulants, monitor for a decreased hypoprothrombinemic response whenever nafcillin or other penicillinase-resistant penicillins are given. Available evidence suggests that the onset of the interaction is delayed for several days after starting the penicillin, and the effect may persist for weeks after the penicillin is discontinued.

REFERENCES:

Qureshi GD, et al. Warfarin resistance with nafcillin therapy. *Ann Intern Med*. 1984;100:527.

Fraser GL, et al. Warfarin resistance associated with nafcillin therapy. *Am J Med*. 1989;87:237.

Davis RL, et al. Warfarin-nafcillin interaction. *J Pediatr*. 1991;118:300.

Shovick VA, et al. Decreased hypoprothrombinemic response to warfarin secondary to the warfarin-nafcillin interaction. *DICP*. 1991;25:598.

Nalidixic Acid (*NegGram*)

Warfarin (eg, *Coumadin*)

SUMMARY: Isolated case reports indicate that nalidixic acid enhances the hypoprothrombinemic response to warfarin and acenocoumarol,[†] but the incidence of this interaction in patients receiving the combination is unknown.

RISK FACTORS:

➡ **Concurrent Diseases.** Patients with fever or low albumin concentrations are at risk.

RELATED DRUGS: Acenocoumarol[†] interacts similarly with nalidixic acid. Little is known regarding the effect of nalidixic acid on other anticoagulants, but assume that an interaction may occur with all oral anticoagulants until evidence to the contrary is available.

MANAGEMENT OPTIONS:

➠ *Monitor.* Monitor patients for an altered hypoprothrombinemic response when nalidixic acid therapy is started or stopped in patients receiving oral anticoagulants.

REFERENCES:

Sellers EM, et al. Displacement of warfarin from human albumin by diazoxide and ethacrynic, mefenamic and nalidixic acids. *Clin Pharmacol Ther.* 1970;11:524.

Loeliger EA, et al. The biological disappearance rate of prothrombin and factors VII, IX and X from plasma in hypothyroidism, hyperthyroidism and during fever. *Thromb Diath Haemorrh.* 1964;10:267.

Hoffbrand BI. Interaction of nalidixic acid and warfarin. *BMJ.* 1974;2:666. Letter.

Potasman I, et al. Nicoumalone and nalidixic acid interaction. *Ann Intern Med.* 1980;92:572.

Leor J, et al. Interaction between nalidixic acid and warfarin. *Ann Intern Med.* 1987;107:601.

† Not available in the US.

Naproxen (eg, *Naprosyn*)

Warfarin (eg, *Coumadin*)

SUMMARY: Naproxen does not appear to affect the hypoprothrombinemic response to warfarin in most patients; however, naproxen should be used cautiously because of its possible detrimental effects on gastric mucosa and platelet function.

RISK FACTORS:

➠ *Concurrent Diseases.* Patients with peptic ulcer disease (PUD) or a history of GI bleeding are probably at greater risk.

RELATED DRUGS: All NSAIDs inhibit platelet function, cause gastric erosions, and probably increase the risk of GI bleeding.

MANAGEMENT OPTIONS:

➠ *Avoid Unless Benefit Outweighs Risk.* Because all NSAIDs probably increase the risk of GI bleeding in patients on oral anticoagulants, use the combination only after careful consideration of the benefit vs risk. If the NSAID is being used as an analgesic or antipyretic, acetaminophen probably is safer to use with oral anticoagulants. Nonacetylated salicylates (eg, choline salicylate, magnesium salicylate, salsalate, sodium salicylate) probably also are safer with oral anticoagulants than NSAIDs because they have minimal effects on platelet function and the gastric mucosa.

➠ *Monitor.* If any NSAID is used with an oral anticoagulant, one should monitor carefully the prothrombin time and watch for evidence of bleeding, especially from the GI tract.

REFERENCES:

Jain A, et al. Effect of naproxen on the steady-state serum concentration and anticoagulant activity of warfarin. *Clin Pharmacol Ther.* 1979;25:61.

Slattery JT, et al. Effect of naproxen on the kinetics of elimination and anticoagulant activity of single dose warfarin. *Clin Pharmacol Ther.* 1979;25:51.

Shorr RI, et al. Concurrent use of nonsteroidal anti-inflammatory drugs and oral anticoagulants places elderly persons at high risk for hemorrhagic peptic ulcer disease. *Arch Intern Med.* 1993;153:1665.

Nefazodone (*Serzone*)

Paroxetine (*Paxil*)

SUMMARY: A patient developed evidence of serotonin syndrome when paroxetine therapy was started soon after discontinuation of nefazodone.

RISK FACTORS: No specific risk factors are known.

RELATED DRUGS: Theoretically, combined therapy of nefazodone with other selective serotonin reuptake inhibitors (SSRIs) such as fluoxetine (*Prozac*), sertraline (*Zoloft*), fluvoxamine (*Luvox*), and citalopram (*Celexa*) also could result in serotonin syndrome, but reports of such interactions appear to be lacking.

MANAGEMENT OPTIONS:

➥ *Circumvent/Minimize.* When switching from nefazodone to a SSRI or visa versa, it may be prudent to begin the new agent with conservative doses to avoid excessive serotonergic effects.

➥ *Monitor.* In patients receiving nefazodone and paroxetine (or other SSRIs) be alert for evidence of serotonin syndrome. Serotonin syndrome can result in neurotoxicity (ie, myoclonus, tremors, rigidity, incoordination, hyperreflexia, seizures, coma), psychiatric symptoms (ie, agitation, confusion, hypomania, restlessness), and autonomic dysfunction (ie, fever, sweating, tachycardia, hypertension).

REFERENCES:

John L, et al. Serotonin syndrome associated with nefazodone and paroxetine. *Ann Emerg Med.* 1997;29:287–89.

Sternbach H. The serotonin syndrome. *Am J Psychiatry.* 1991;148:705-13.

Nefazodone (eg, *Serzone*)

Pimozide (*Orap*)

SUMMARY: Elevated pimozide concentrations and cardiac arrhythmias may occur if pimozide and nefazodone are coadministered.

RISK FACTORS: No specific risk factors are known.

RELATED DRUGS: In vitro studies indicate that paroxetine (eg, *Paxil*), sertraline (*Zoloft*), fluoxetine (eg, *Prozac*), and fluvoxamine (eg, *Luvox*) do not inhibit the metabolism of pimozide. However, fluvoxamine is known to produce some inhibition of CYP3A4 and CYP1A2, a lesser pathway of pimozide metabolism. Pending in vivo studies, avoid coadministration of pimozide and fluvoxamine.

MANAGEMENT OPTIONS:

➥ *Use Alternative.* Do not administer nefazodone to patients receiving pimozide. Consider other SSRI antidepressants that do not affect CYP3A4, but avoid fluvoxamine.

➥ *Monitor.* If nefazodone is coadministered with pimozide, monitor the ECG for evidence of QTc prolongation.

REFERENCES:

Product Information. Pimozide (*Orap*). Gate Pharmaceuticals. 1999.

Desta Z, et al. In vitro inhibition of pimozide N-dealkylation by selective serotonin reuptake inhibitors and azithromycin. *J Clin Psychopharmacol.* 2002;22:162-168.

Nefazodone (*Serzone*)

Simvastatin (*Zocor*)

SUMMARY: A patient on simvastatin developed muscle damage (myositis and rhabdomyolysis) after starting nefazodone therapy.

RISK FACTORS:

➡ ***Dosage Regimen.*** The ability of simvastatin to produce damage to skeletal muscle appears to be dose related. Thus, the risk of combined therapy with nefazodone is probably higher in patients on larger doses of simvastatin.

RELATED DRUGS: Lovastatin (*Mevacor*) is also known to result in muscle damage when given with CYP3A4 inhibitors; pravastatin (*Pravachol*), fluvastatin (*Lescol*), and atorvastatin (*Lipitor*) may be less likely to do so. Fluoxetine (eg, *Prozac*) may inhibit CYP3A4 to a lesser extent than nefazodone (see Management Options).

MANAGEMENT OPTIONS:

➡ ***Use Alternative.*** The use of an HMG-CoA reductase inhibitor other than simvastatin or lovastatin probably reduces the risk. Nefazodone is probably one of the most potent CYP3A4 inhibitors among antidepressants, so using an alternative antidepressant may reduce the interaction. Fluoxetine also may inhibit CYP3A4, but probably to a lesser extent than nefazodone. If the combination is used, be alert for evidence of muscle damage (eg, muscle pain, weakness, darkened urine, elevated muscle enzymes such as creatine kinase). It would be prudent to use conservative doses of simvastatin or lovastatin when they are used with a CYP3A4 inhibitor such as nefazodone.

REFERENCES:
Jacobson RH, et al. Myositis and rhabdomyolysis associated with concurrent use of simvastatin and nefazodone. *JAMA.* 1997;277:296. Letter.

Nefazodone (*Serzone*)

Tacrolimus (*Prograf*)

SUMMARY: A patient on tacrolimus developed evidence of nephrotoxicity and neurotoxicity 1 week after nefazodone was started.

RISK FACTORS: No specific risk factors are known.

RELATED DRUGS: Nefazodone probably also inhibits the metabolism of cyclosporine (eg, *Neoral*), because the latter drug is also metabolized by CYP3A4. Most selective serotonin reuptake inhibitors (eg, sertraline [*Zoloft*], paroxetine [*Paxil*], citalopram [*Celexa*]) have little or no effect on CYP3A4. Fluoxetine (eg, *Prozac*) is a weak inhibitor of CYP3A4, and would be expected to have only a small effect on tacrolimus, but fluvoxamine (eg, *Luvox*) appears to be a moderate inhibitor of CYP3A4 and might interact with tacrolimus to some degree.

MANAGEMENT OPTIONS:

➡ ***Consider Alternative.*** In patients receiving tacrolimus (or cyclosporine), it is preferable to use an antidepressant that has little or no effect on CYP3A4 (see Related Drugs).

➥ **Monitor.** Be alert for altered tacrolimus effect if nefazodone is initiated, discontinued, or changed in dosage. Possible evidence of tacrolimus toxicity includes decreased renal function, headache, confusion, and visual disturbances.

REFERENCES:

Olyaei AJ, et al. Interaction between tacrolimus and nefazodone in a stable renal transplant recipient. *Pharmacotherapy.* 1998;18:1356.

 Nelfinavir (*Viracept*)

Nevirapine (*Viramune*)

SUMMARY: Nevirapine administration reduces the concentration of nelfinavir; reduction in antiviral activity may result.

RISK FACTORS: No specific risk factors are known.

RELATED DRUGS: Nevirapine may produce similar effects on other protease inhibitors (eg, ritonavir [eg, *Norvir*], saquinavir [*Fortovase*], and indinavir [*Crixivan*]). Delavirdine (*Rescriptor*) is an inhibitor of CYP3A4 and, if it has any effect on nelfinavir, it would be expected to increase nelfinavir concentrations.

MANAGEMENT OPTIONS:

➥ **Monitor.** When nevirapine is started or discontinued in a patient taking nelfinavir, monitor serum concentrations of nelfinavir to assure they are maintained in the therapeutic range.

REFERENCES:

Merry C, et al. The pharmacokinetics of combination therapy with nelfinavir plus nevirapine. *AIDS.* 1998;12:1163.

 Nelfinavir (*Viracept*)

Rifampin (eg, *Rifadin*)

SUMMARY: Rifampin increases nelfinavir clearance; loss of efficacy is likely to result.

RISK FACTORS: No specific risk factors are known.

RELATED DRUGS: Rifampin increases the clearance of ritonavir (eg, *Norvir*), indinavir (*Crixivan*), and saquinavir (*Fortovase*). Rifabutin (*Mycobutin*) would be expected to have a similar affect on nelfinavir clearance.

MANAGEMENT OPTIONS:

➥ **Use Alternative.** Based on the magnitude of this interaction, it would be difficult to administer an effective dose of nelfinavir. Because other protease inhibitors are also likely to be affected, consider an alternative to rifampin.

REFERENCES:

Yuen GJ, et al. The pharmacokinetics of nelfinavir administration alone and with rifampin in healthy volunteers. *Clin Pharmacol Ther.* 1997;61:147. Abstract.

Nelfinavir (*Viracept*)

Saquinavir (eg, *Fortovase*)

SUMMARY: Nelfinavir appears to cause a large increase in saquinavir plasma concentrations; increased saquinavir toxicity may occur.

RISK FACTORS: No specific risk factors are known.

RELATED DRUGS: Nelfinavir may increase the concentrations of other protease inhibitors that undergo CYP3A4 mediated metabolism, such as indinavir or ritonavir.

MANAGEMENT OPTIONS:

➡ *Monitor.* Pending further information on this interaction, carefully monitor patients taking saquinavir whenever nelfinavir is initiated or discontinued from their antiretroviral drug regimen.

REFERENCES:
Product information. Nelfinavir (*Viracept*). Agouron Pharmaceuticals, Inc., 2001.

Nelfinavir (*Viracept*)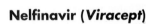

Sildenafil (*Viagra*)

SUMMARY: Nelfinavir may increase sildenafil plasma concentrations; increased sildenafil toxicity may occur. Sildenafil does not affect nelfinavir plasma concentrations.

RISK FACTORS: No specific risk factors are known.

RELATED DRUGS: Other protease inhibitors that inhibit CYP3A4 such as ritonavir may increase sildenafil concentrations.

MANAGEMENT OPTIONS:

➡ *Monitor.* Pending further information on this interaction, carefully monitor patients taking nelfinavir and sildenafil for increased sildenafil response.

REFERENCES:
Product information. Viracept (*Nelfinavir*). Agouron Pharmaceuticals, Inc, 2001.
Bratt G, et al. Sildenafil does not alter nelfinavir pharmacokinetics. *Ther Drug Monit.* 2003;25:240-242.

Nelfinavir (*Viracept*)

Simvastatin (*Zocor*)

SUMMARY: Nelfinavir administration markedly increases simvastatin concentrations; some patients may experience increased side effects.

RISK FACTORS: No specific risk factors are known.

RELATED DRUGS: Other protease inhibitors such as ritonavir (*Norvir*), amprenavir (*Agenerase*), indinavir (*Crixivan*), and saquinavir (eg, *Invirase*) would be expected to affect simvastatin in a similar manner. The clearance of other statins that are metabolized by CYP3A4 would likely be reduced by nelfinavir. Lovastatin (*Mevacor*) is likely to be affected to a similar degree as simvastatin by nelfinavir.

MANAGEMENT OPTIONS:

➡ *Use Alternative.* Because pravastatin (*Pravachol*) and fluvastatin (*Lescol*) are not metabolized by CYP3A4, consider using one of these agents in patients taking protease inhibitors. The affect of nelfinavir on atorvastatin (*Lipitor*) is less than that observed with simvastatin; low doses of atorvastatin with close monitoring could be considered in patients taking nelfinavir.

➡ *Monitor.* Monitor patients taking any statin that is metabolized by CYP3A4 and a protease inhibitor for side effects including myopathy and myoglobinuria.

REFERENCES:

Hsyu PH et al. Pharmacokinetic interactions between nelfinavir and 3-hydroxy-3-methylglutaryl coenzyme A reductase inhibitors atorvastatin and simvastatin. *Antimicrob Agents Chemother.* 2001;45:3445-3450.

Neomycin (eg, *Neo-fradin*)

Penicillin V (eg, *Veetids*)

SUMMARY: Neomycin reduces the serum concentration of penicillin V and may reduce its efficacy.

RISK FACTORS: No specific risk factors are known.

RELATED DRUGS: Penicillin G may be affected similarly by neomycin.

MANAGEMENT OPTIONS:

➡ *Circumvent/Minimize.* Administer the penicillin parenterally to avoid this interaction or select an alternative oral antibiotic.

➡ *Monitor.* Monitor patients taking oral neomycin and oral penicillin for reduced penicillin effect.

REFERENCES:

Cheng SH, et al. Effect of orally administered neomycin on the absorption of penicillin V. *N Engl J Med.* 1962;267:1296.

Neomycin (eg, *Neo-Tabs*)

Warfarin (eg, *Coumadin*)

SUMMARY: Oral administration of aminoglycosides like neomycin appears to enhance the hypoprothrombinemic response to oral anticoagulants like warfarin in certain predisposed patients.

RISK FACTORS:

➡ *Concurrent Diseases.* Deficiency of dietary vitamin K and impaired liver function place a patient at greater risk.

➡ *Dosage Regimen.* Large oral aminoglycoside doses produce a greater risk.

RELATED DRUGS: Other orally administered aminoglycosides may increase hypoprothrombinemic response to warfarin.

MANAGEMENT OPTIONS:

➡ *Monitor.* Careful monitoring of hypoprothrombinemia appears warranted when an oral aminoglycoside is coadministered for more than 1 to 2 days, particularly when a patient is predisposed to a dietary vitamin K deficiency.

REFERENCES:

Stenbjerg S, et al. A circulating factor V inhibitor: possible side effect of treatment with streptomycin. *Scand J Haematol.* 1975;14:280.

Remmel RP, et al. The effect of broad-spectrum antibiotics on warfarin excretion and metabolism in the rat. *Res Commun Chem Pathol Pharmacol.* 1981;34:503.

Rodriguez-Erdmann F, et al. Interaction of antibiotics with vitamin K. *JAMA.* 1981;246:937.

Schade RWB, et al. A comparative study of the effects of cholestyramine and neomycin in the treatment of type II hyperlipoproteinaemia. *Acta Med Scand.* 1976;199:175.

Kippel AP, et al. Hypoprothrombinemia secondary to antibiotic therapy and manifested by massive gastrointestinal hemorrhage. Report of three cases. *Arch Surg.* 1968;96:266.

Udall JA. Drug interference with warfarin therapy. *Clin Med.* 1970;77:20.

Finegold SM. Interaction of antimicrobial therapy and intestinal flora. *Am J Clin Nutr.* 1970;23:1466.

Messinger WJ, et al. The effect of a bowel sterilizing antibiotic on blood coagulation mechanisms. *Angiology.* 1965;16:29.

Neostigmine (eg, *Prostigmin*)

Procainamide (eg, *Procan*)

SUMMARY: In patients receiving cholinergic agents for myasthenia gravis, symptoms may be exacerbated by procainamide administration.

RISK FACTORS: No specific risk factors are known.

RELATED DRUGS: Although lidocaine (eg, *Xylocaine*) and propranolol (eg, *Inderal*) also might be expected to worsen myasthesia, limited use of lidocaine in 2 myasthenic patients did not result in aggravation of symptoms.

MANAGEMENT OPTIONS:

➡ *Monitor.* Watch for increased weakness in patients with myasthenia gravis if procainamide is coadministered.

REFERENCES:

Flacke W. Treatment of myasthenia gravis. *N Engl J Med.* 1973; 288:27.

Kornfeld P, et al. Myasthenia gravis unmasked by antiarrhythmic agents. *Mt Sinai J Med.* 1976;43:10.

Neostigmine (eg, *Prostigmin*)

Propranolol (eg, *Inderal*)

SUMMARY: Both neostigmine and beta-adrenergic blockers, such as propranolol, can slow the heart rate; additive bradycardia would be expected, but the risk of adverse consequences from the combination is not known.

RISK FACTORS: No specific risk factors are known.

RELATED DRUGS: Other beta blockers (eg, atenolol, nadolol) may produce similar effects. Physostigmine affects propranolol similarly.

MANAGEMENT OPTIONS:

➡ *Monitor.* Monitor for excessive bradycardia in patients receiving beta-adrenergic blockers concurrently with neostigmine or other cholinergic agents.

REFERENCES:

Sprague DH. Severe bradycardia after neostigmine in a patient taking propranolol to control paroxysmal atrial tachycardia. *Anesthesiology*. 1975;42:208.

Seidl DC, Martin DE. Prolonged bradycardia after neostigmine administration in a patient taking nadolol. *Anesth Analg*. 1984;63:365.

Baraka A, Dajani A. Severe bradycardia following physostigmine in the presence of beta-adrenergic blockade. *Middle East J Anesthesiol*. 1984;7:291.

Eldor J, et al. Prolonged bradycardia and hypotension after neostigmine administration in a patient receiving atenolol. *Anesthesia*. 1987;42:1294.

Nicardipine (eg, *Cardene*)

Propranolol (eg, *Inderal*)

SUMMARY: Nicardipine administration increases propranolol concentrations; an increase in beta blocker effect may occur in some patients.

RISK FACTORS: No specific risk factors are known.

RELATED DRUGS: A single dose of nicardipine 30 mg had no effect on the pharmacokinetics of atenolol (eg, *Tenormin*). Nicardipine increased metoprolol (eg, *Lopressor*) concentration by approximately 25%. Nimodipine (*Nimotop*) and propranolol had minimal effect on each other's plasma concentrations. Nisoldipine (*Sular*) and nifedipine (eg, *Procardia*) increased the AUC of propranolol., Conversely, nisoldipine AUC and peak serum concentrations were increased 30% and 57%, respectively, by propranolol. Others found no change in drug concentrations during chronic nisoldipine and propranolol dosing. Propranolol also blunted the increase in cardiac output observed following nisoldipine alone. Isradipine (*DynaCirc*) 10 mg increased the AUC of propranolol 28% and its peak concentration 60%.

MANAGEMENT OPTIONS:

➡ *Monitor.* Monitor patients receiving combined therapy with propranolol and nicardipine for enhanced effects resulting from pharmacokinetic or pharmacodynamic interactions.

REFERENCES:

Levine MA, et al. Pharmacokinetic and pharmacodynamic interactions between nisoldipine and propranolol. *Clin Pharmacol Ther*. 1988;43:39-48.

Rocha P, et al. Kinetics and hemodynamic effects of intravenous nicardipine modified by previous propranolol oral treatment. *Cardiovasc Drugs Ther*. 1990;4:1525-1532.

Funck-Brentano C, et al. Influence of CYP2D6-dependent metabolism on the steady-state pharmacokinetics and pharmacodynamics of metoprolol and nicardipine, alone and in combination. *Br J Clin Pharmacol*. 1993;36:531.

Packer M, et al. Hemodynamic consequences of combined beta-adrenergic and slow calcium channel blockade in man. *Circulation*. 1982;65:660-668.

Winniford MD, et al. Hemodynamic and electrophysiologic effects of verapamil and nifedipine in patients on propranolol. *Am J Cardiol*. 1982;50:704-710.

Vercruysse I, et al. Nicardipine does not influence the pharmacokinetics and pharmacodynamics of atenolol. *Br J Clin Pharmacol*. 1990;30:499-500.

Breuel HP, et al. Chronic administration of nimodipine and propranolol in elderly normotensive subjects—an interaction study. *Int J Clin Pharmacol Ther*. 1995;33:103-108.

Vinceneux PH, et al. Pharmacokinetic and pharmacodynamic interactions between nifedipine and propranolol or betaxolol. *Int J Clin Pharmacol Ther Toxicol.* 1986;24:153-158.

Shaw-Stiffel TA, et al. Pharmacokinetic and pharmacodynamic interactions during multiple-dose administration of nisoldipine and propranolol. *Clin Pharmacol Ther.* 1994;55:661-669.

Rosenkranz B, et al. Interaction between nifedipine and atenolol: pharmacokinetics and pharmacodynamics in normotensive volunteers. *J Cardiovasc Pharmacol.* 1986;8:943-949.

Nifedipine (eg, *Procardia*)
Phenobarbital (eg, *Solfoton*)

SUMMARY: Phenobarbital substantially reduces the plasma concentrations of nifedipine.

RISK FACTORS: No specific risk factors are known.

RELATED DRUGS: Phenobarbital also increases the metabolism of verapamil (eg, *Calan*). Other calcium channel blockers may be affected similarly by phenobarbital.

MANAGEMENT OPTIONS:

➡ *Circumvent/Minimize.* Patients receiving phenobarbital may require higher than usual doses of nifedipine.

➡ *Monitor.* Patients stabilized on nifedipine should be monitored for the possibility of decreased effectiveness when phenobarbital is administered concomitantly.

REFERENCES:

Schellens JHM, et al. Influence of enzyme induction and inhibition on the oxidation of nifedipine, sparteine, mephenytoin and antipyrine in humans as assessed by a cocktail study design. *J Pharmacol Exp Ther.* 1989;249:638.

Nifedipine (eg, *Procardia*)
Phenytoin (eg, *Dilantin*)

SUMMARY: Nifedipine was associated with increased plasma phenytoin concentration in 1 case; more study is needed.

RISK FACTORS: No specific risk factors are known.

RELATED DRUGS: The bioavailability of most calcium channel blockers appears to be reduced by enzyme inducers such as phenytoin.

MANAGEMENT OPTIONS:

➡ *Monitor.* Until more information regarding this potential interaction is available, patients receiving phenytoin should be monitored carefully when nifedipine or diltiazem is added to or removed from their regimen.

REFERENCES:

Ahmad S. Nifedipine-phenytoin interaction. *J Am Coll Cardiol.* 1984;3:1581.

Nifedipine (eg, *Procardia*)

Propranolol (eg, *Inderal*)

SUMMARY: The combination of nifedipine and propranolol may result in hypotension; nifedipine can increase propranolol concentrations.

RISK FACTORS: No specific risk factors are known.

RELATED DRUGS: Atenolol (eg, *Tenormin*) and metoprolol may interact similarly with nifedipine. Felodipine (*Plendil*) 10 mg twice daily increased the AUC of metoprolol 31%, but the AUC of felodipine was not altered by chronic metoprolol or atenolol therapy. Nisoldipine (*Sular*) 20 mg increased the propranolol AUC by approximately 50%. Conversely, nisoldipine AUC and peak serum concentrations were increased 30% and 57%, respectively, by propranolol. Propranolol also blunted the increase in cardiac output observed following nisoldipine alone. Isradipine (*DynaCirc*) 10 mg increased the AUC of propranolol 28% and its peak concentration 60%.

MANAGEMENT OPTIONS:

➡ ***Monitor.*** Patients receiving combined therapy with propranolol and nifedipine should be monitored for enhanced effects resulting from pharmacokinetic or pharmacodynamic interactions.

REFERENCES:

Levine MAH, et al. Pharmacokinetic and pharmacodynamic interactions between nisoldipine and propranolol. *Clin Pharmacol Ther.* 1988;43:39.

Dargie HJ, et al. Nifedipine and propranolol: a beneficial drug interaction. *Am J Med.* 1981;71:676.

Pfisterer M, et al. Combined acebutolol/nifedipine therapy in patients with chronic coronary artery disease: additional improvement of ischemia-induced left ventricular dysfunction. *Am J Cardiol.* 1982;49:1259.

Eggertsen R, et al. Effects of treatment with nifedipine and metoprolol in essential hypertension. *Eur J Clin Pharmacol.* 1982;21:389.

Robson RH, et al. Nifedipine and beta-blockade as a cause of cardiac failure. *BMJ.* 1982;284:104.

Anastassiades CJ. Nifedipine and beta blocker drugs. *BMJ.* 1980;281:1251.

Vinceneux PH, et al. Pharmacokinetic and pharmacodynamic interactions between nifedipine and propranolol or betaxolol. *Int J Clin Pharmacol Ther Toxicol.* 1986;24:153.

Gangji D, et al. Study of the influence of nifedipine on the pharmacokinetics and pharmacodynamics of propranolol, metoprolol and atenolol. *Br J Clin Pharmacol.* 1984;17:29S.

Rosenkranz B, et al. Interaction between nifedipine and atenolol: pharmacokinetics and pharmacodynamics in normotensive volunteers. *J Cardiovasc Pharmacol.* 1986;8:943.

Kleinbloesem CH, et al. Pharmacokinetic and haemodynamic interaction between nifedipine and propranolol. *Br J Clin Pharmacol.* 1985;19:537.

Smith SR, et al. Pharmacokinetic interactions between felodipine and metoprolol. *Eur J Clin Pharmacol.* 1987;31:575.

Shepherd AMM, et al. Pharmacokinetic interaction between isradipine and propranolol. *Clin Pharmacol Ther.* 1988;43:194. Abstract.

Bengtsson-Hasselgren B, et al. Haemodynamic effects and pharmacokinetics of felodipine at rest and during exercise in hypertensive patients treated with metoprolol. *Eur J Clin Pharmacol.* 1989;37:459.

Bauer LA, et al. Influence of nifedipine therapy on indocyanine green and oral propranolol pharmacokinetics. *Eur J Clin Pharmacol.* 1989;37:257.

Elliott HL, et al. The interactions between nisoldipine and two betaadrenoceptor antagonists-atenolol and propranolol. *Br J Clin Pharmacol.* 1991;32:379.

Nifedipine (eg, *Procardia*)
Quinidine (eg, *Quinora*)

SUMMARY: Nifedipine appears to reduce the serum concentrations of quinidine, and quinidine appears to increase the serum concentration of nifedipine.

RISK FACTORS: No specific risk factors are known.

RELATED DRUGS: Verapamil (eg, *Calan*) increases quinidine concentrations. Diltiazem (eg, *Cardizem*) 120 mg/day had no effect on quinidine concentrations.

MANAGEMENT OPTIONS:

➡ *Circumvent/Minimize.* Quinidine doses may require upward adjustment when nifedipine is added or downward adjustment if quinidine is discontinued.

➡ *Monitor.* Nifedipine and quinidine coadministration may reduce quinidine concentration and increase nifedipine concentration; monitor patients carefully.

REFERENCES:

Farringer JA, et al. Nifedipine-induced alterations in serum quinidine concentrations. *Am Heart J.* 1984;108:1570.

Van Lith RM, et al. Quinidine-nifedipine interaction. *Drug Intell Clin Pharm.* 1985;19:829.

Green JA, et al. Nifedipine-quinidine interaction. *Clin Pharm.* 1983;2:461.

Munger MA, et al. Elucidation of the nifedipine-quinidine interaction. *Clin Pharmacol Ther.* 1989;45:411.

Oates NS, et al. Influence of quinidine on nifedipine plasma pharmacokinetics. *Br J Clin Pharmacol.* 1988;25:675.

Schellens JHM, et al. Differential effects of quinidine on the disposition of nifedipine, sparteine, and mephenytoin in humans. *Clin Pharmacol Ther.* 1991;50:520.

Matera MG, et al. Quinidine-diltiazem: pharmacokinetic interaction in humans. *Curr Ther Res.* 1986;40:653.

Bowles SK, et al. Evaluation of the pharmacokinetic and pharmacodynamic interaction between quinidine and nifedipine. *J Clin Pharmacol.* 1993;33:727.

Bailey DG, et al. Quinidine interaction with nifedipine and felodipine: pharmacokinetic and pharmacodynamic evaluation. *Clin Pharmacol Ther.* 1993;53:354.

Nifedipine (eg, *Procardia*)
Quinupristin/Dalfopristin (*Synercid*)

SUMMARY: The plasma concentration of nifedipine is increased by the coadministration of quinupristin/dalfopristin; reduced doses of nifedipine may be necessary.

RISK FACTORS: No specific risk factors are known.

RELATED DRUGS: The metabolism of other calcium channel blockers, all of which are metabolized by CYP3A4, would likely be reduced by quinupristin/dalfopristin.

MANAGEMENT OPTIONS:

➡ *Consider Alternative.* If appropriate for the disease being treated, consider a noncalcium channel blocker for patients taking quinupristin/dalfopristin. In patients requiring calcium channel blockers, consider an alternative antibiotic that does not affect CYP3A4 activity.

➥ *Monitor.* Carefully monitor patients stabilized on nifedipine for increasing nifedipine response, such as hypotension, when quinupristin/dalfopristin is added.

REFERENCES:

Product information. Quinupristin/dalfopristin (*Synercid*). Rhone-Poulenc Rorer. 1999.

Nifedipine (eg, *Procardia*)
Rifampin (eg, *Rifadin*)

SUMMARY: Rifampin decreases nifedipine plasma concentrations; loss of therapeutic effect may result.

RISK FACTORS: No specific risk factors are known.

RELATED DRUGS: Rifampin probably affects other calcium channel blockers in a similar manner. Rifabutin (*Mycobutin*) would be expected to affect nifedipine in a similar manner.

MANAGEMENT OPTIONS:

➥ *Consider Alternative.* Because this interaction is likely to reduce the efficacy of nifedipine, consider an alternative agent for nifedipine. Other calcium channel blockers also may be affected; a therapeutic substitution to a different class of agent may be required.

➥ *Circumvent/Minimize.* Larger doses of calcium channel blockers (particularly those administered orally) may be required when rifampin is coadministered.

➥ *Monitor.* Monitor patients taking calcium channel blockers for a reduction in efficacy when rifampin is given.

REFERENCES:

Tsuchihashi K, et al. A case of variant angina exacerbated by administration of rifampicin. *Heart Vessels*. 1987;3:214-217.

Tada Y, et al. Case report: nifedipine-rifampicin interaction attenuates the effect on blood pressure in a patient with essential hypertension. *Am J Med Sci*. 1992;303:25-27.

† Not available in the US.

Nifedipine (eg, *Procardia*)
St. John's Wort

SUMMARY: St. John's wort reduces the plasma concentration of nifedipine; some loss of efficacy is likely to result.

RISK FACTORS: No specific risk factors are known.

RELATED DRUGS: St. John's wort would be likely to increase the metabolism of other calcium channel blockers because all are metabolized by CYP3A4.

MANAGEMENT OPTIONS:

➥ *Monitor.* Pending more complete data on this interaction, monitor patients for reduction in nifedipine effect if St. John's wort is coadministered.

REFERENCES:

Smith M, et al. An open trial of nifedipine-herb interactions: nifedipine with St. John's wort, ginseng or ginkgo biloba. *Clin Pharmacol Ther*. 2001;69:P86.

Nifedipine (*eg, Procardia*)

Tacrolimus (*Prograf*)

SUMMARY: Nifedipine administration reduced the dosage requirements of tacrolimus; tacrolimus dosage adjustments may be required.

RISK FACTORS: No specific risk factors are known.

RELATED DRUGS: Other calcium channel blocking drugs may affect tacrolimus in a similar manner. Nifedipine appears to have limited effect on cyclosporine (eg, *Neoral*) concentrations.

MANAGEMENT OPTIONS:

➡ *Monitor.* Pending further study of this interaction, observe patients receiving tacrolimus and nifedipine for reduced tacrolimus dose requirements.

REFERENCES:

Seifeldin RA, et al. Nifedipine interaction with tacrolimus in liver transplant recipients. *Ann Pharmacother.* 1997;31:571-575.

Nifedipine (*eg, Procardia*)

Vincristine (eg, *Oncovin*)

SUMMARY: Nifedipine appeared to increase markedly the half-life of vincristine; the clinical significance is unknown.

RISK FACTORS: No specific risk factors are known.

RELATED DRUGS: Little is known regarding the effect of other calcium channel blockers on vincristine, but consider the possibility that they also interact.

MANAGEMENT OPTIONS:

➡ *Monitor.* Until further information is available, monitor patients receiving vincristine and nifedipine concomitantly for enhanced pharmacodynamic effects of vincristine. It may be necessary to adjust vincristine dose.

REFERENCES:

Tsuruo T, et al. Potentiation of vincristine and adriamycin effects in human hemopoietic tumor cell lines by calcium antagonists and calmodulin inhibitors. *Cancer Res.* 1983;43:2267-2272.

Fedeli L, et al. Pharmacokinetics of vincristine in cancer patients treated with nifedipine. *Cancer.* 1989;64:1805-1811.

Nimodipine (*Nimotop*)

Valproic Acid (eg, *Depakene*)

SUMMARY: Valproic acid increases the area under the plasma concentration-time curve of nimodipine with no effect on the elimination half-life.

RISK FACTORS: No specific risk factors are known.

RELATED DRUGS: No information is available.

MANAGEMENT OPTIONS:

➡ *Monitor.* Monitor patients receiving nimodipine and valproic acid for altered nimodipine effect if valproic acid is initiated, discontinued, or changed in dosage.

REFERENCES:

Tartara A, et al. Differential effects of valproic acid and enzyme-inducing anticonvulsants on nimodipine pharmacokinetics in epileptic patients. *Br J Clin Pharmacol.* 1991;32:335-340.

Norepinephrine (*Levarterenol*)

Phenelzine (*Nardil*)

SUMMARY: Monoamine oxidase inhibitors (MAOIs) may slightly increase the pressor response to norepinephrine.

RISK FACTORS: No specific risk factors are known.

RELATED DRUGS: Theoretically other nonselective MAOIs, including isocarboxazid (*Marplan*), would interact with norepinephrine in a similar manner.

MANAGEMENT OPTIONS:

➡ *Monitor.* Monitor blood pressure carefully if patients on nonselective MAOIs receive norepinephrine. Remember that the effects of nonselective MAOIs should be assumed to persist for 2 weeks after they are discontinued.

REFERENCES:

Boakes AJ, et al. Interactions between sympathomimetic amines and antidepressant agents in man. *BMJ.* 1973;1:311.

Boakes AJ. Sympathomimetic amines and antidepressant agents. *BMJ.* 1973;2:114. Letter.

Goldberg LI. Monoamine oxidase inhibitors: adverse reactions and possible mechanisms. *JAMA.* 1964;190: 456.

Sjoqvist F. Psychotropic drugs (2). Interaction between monoamine oxidase (MAO) inhibitors and other substances. *Proc R Soc Med.* 1965;58:967.

Ellis J, et al. Modification by monoamine oxidase inhibitors of the effect of some sympathomimetics on blood pressure. *BMJ.* 1967;2:75.

Norfloxacin (*Noroxin*)

Sucralfate (eg, *Carafate*)

SUMMARY: The administration of sucralfate markedly reduces the serum and urine concentrations of norfloxacin and may reduce its clinical efficacy.

RISK FACTORS: No specific risk factors are known.

RELATED DRUGS: Aluminum-containing antacids also reduce the absorption of norfloxacin. Sucralfate inhibits the absorption of ciprofloxacin (*Cipro*), fleroxacin,[†] and ofloxacin (*Floxin*).

MANAGEMENT OPTIONS:

➡ *Consider Alternative.* If dosage separation is not possible, an alternative to sucralfate (eg, H$_2$-receptor antagonist, omeprazole [*Prilosec*], but not an antacid) should be considered.

➡ *Circumvent/Minimize.* Until further information is available, the coadministration of norfloxacin and sucralfate should be avoided. Norfloxacin should be administered several hours before sucralfate.

➡ *Monitor.* If sucralfate and a quinolone are coadministered, monitor the patient for reduced antibiotic efficacy.

REFERENCES:

Parpia SH, et al. Sucralfate reduces the gastrointestinal absorption of norfloxacin. *Antimicrob Agents Chemother.* 1989;33:99.

Lehto P, et al. Effect of sucralfate on absorption of norfloxacin and ofloxacin. *Antimicrob Agents Chemother.* 1994;38:248.

† Not available in the US.

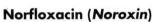

Norfloxacin (*Noroxin*)

Theophylline (eg, *Theolair*)

SUMMARY: Norfloxacin may increase the serum concentration of theophylline; however, the increase is unlikely to result in the development of theophylline toxicity in most patients.

RISK FACTORS: No specific risk factors are known.

RELATED DRUGS: Quinolones reported to inhibit the metabolism of drugs include ciprofloxacin (*Cipro*), enoxacin (*Penetrex*), pipemidic acid, and pefloxacin.†

MANAGEMENT OPTIONS:

➡ *Consider Alternative.* Quinolones reported to produce no or minor changes in theophylline pharmacokinetics include fleroxacin,† lomefloxacin (*Maxaquin*), ofloxacin (*Floxin*), rufloxacin,† and sparfloxacin, (*Zagam*).

➡ *Monitor.* Patients maintained on theophylline are at limited risk to develop theophylline toxicity (palpitations, tachycardia, nausea, tremor) during concomitant administrations of norfloxacin.

REFERENCES:

Bowles SK, et al. Effect of norfloxacin on theophylline pharmacokinetics at steady state. *Antimicrob Agents Chemother.* 1988;32:510.

Ho G, et al. Evaluation of the effect of norfloxacin on the pharmacokinetics of theophylline. *Clin Pharmacol Ther.* 1989;44:35.

Prince RA, et al. The effect of quinolone antibiotics on theophylline pharmacokinetics. *J Clin Pharmacol.* 1989;20:650.

Davis RL, et al. The effect of norfloxacin on theophylline metabolism. *Antimicrob Agents Chemother.* 1989;33:212.

Sano M, et al. Comparative pharmacokinetics of theophylline following two fluoroquinolones co-administration. *Eur J Clin Pharmacol.* 1987;32:431.

† Not available in the US.

Norfloxacin (*Noroxin*)

Warfarin (eg, *Coumadin*)

SUMMARY: A patient on chronic warfarin therapy developed excessive hypoprothrombinemia and fatal hemorrhage during therapy with norfloxacin, but a study in healthy subjects suggests that norfloxacin does not affect warfarin response.

RISK FACTORS:

➡ **Concurrent Diseases.** Fever may place a patient at increased risk.

RELATED DRUGS: Ciprofloxacin (*Cipro*) and ofloxacin (*Floxin*) have been noted to increase INRs in a few case reports.

MANAGEMENT OPTIONS:

➡ **Monitor.** Until additional information is available, monitor the prothrombin time carefully if norfloxacin therapy is initiated or discontinued in a patient receiving warfarin or other anticoagulants.

REFERENCES:

Linville T, et al. Norfloxacin and warfarin. *Ann Intern Med.* 1989;110:751. Letter.

Vlasses PH, et al. Warfarin in healthy men. *Pharmacotherapy.* 1988;8:120. Abstract.

Nortriptyline (eg, *Pamelor*)

Pentobarbital (eg, *Nembutal*)

SUMMARY: Pentobarbital may substantially reduce nortriptyline serum concentrations, and probably reduces its therapeutic response.

RISK FACTORS: No specific risk factors are known.

RELATED DRUGS: Other barbiturates probably have a similar effect on nortriptyline. Other tricyclic antidepressants have also been shown to interact with various barbiturates, and one should assume that all barbiturates reduce serum concentrations of all tricyclic antidepressants until proved otherwise.

MANAGEMENT OPTIONS:

➡ **Monitor.** Monitor for altered nortriptyline effect if pentobarbital is initiated, discontinued, or changed in dosage. The same precautions apply to any other combination of a tricyclic antidepressant and a barbiturate.

REFERENCES:

von Bahr C, et al. Time course of enzyme induction in humans: effect of pentobarbital on nortriptyline metabolism. *Clin Pharmacol Ther.* 1998;64:18.

Nortriptyline (eg, *Pamelor*)

Rifampin (eg, *Rifadin*)

SUMMARY: Rifampin and isoniazid (eg, *Rifater*) administration appeared to decrease nortriptyline concentrations in 1 patient; the significance of this interaction is not known.

RISK FACTORS: No specific risk factors are known.

RELATED DRUGS: If this interaction is confirmed, other cyclic antidepressants also may be affected by rifampin administration.

MANAGEMENT OPTIONS:

➡ *Circumvent/Minimize.* The dose of nortriptyline may have to be adjusted when rifampin is started or discontinued.

➡ *Monitor.* Until information is available, patients taking both nortriptyline and rifampin should be monitored for reduced nortriptyline concentration and effect. Discontinuation of rifampin may result in toxic antidepressant concentrations.

REFERENCES:

Bebchuk JM, et al. Drug interaction between rifampin and nortriptyline: a case report. *Int J Psychiatry Med.* 1991;21:183.

Ofloxacin (Floxin)

Procainamide (eg, Procanbid)

SUMMARY: Ofloxacin administration increases procainamide concentrations; it is possible that some patients may experience clinically significant increases in procainamide effects.

RISK FACTORS: No specific risk factors are known.

RELATED DRUGS: Lomefloxacin (*Maxaquin*) also is partially eliminated by the organic cationic transport system and may affect procainamide renal clearance to some degree. The effects of other quinolone antibiotics on procainamide renal clearance are unknown.

MANAGEMENT OPTIONS:

➡ *Monitor.* Patients stabilized on procainamide therapy should have procainamide plasma concentrations monitored during coadministration of ofloxacin. Electrocardiogram monitoring for widened QRS and QTc intervals would be warranted.

REFERENCES:

Martin DE, et al. Effects of ofloxacin on the pharmacokinetics and pharmacodynamics of procainamide. *J Clin Pharmacol.* 1996;36:85-91.

Hoffler D, et al. Pharmacokinetics of lomefloxacin in normal and impaired renal function. *Acta Ther.* 1989;15:321.

Ofloxacin (Floxin)

Sucralfate (Carafate)

SUMMARY: The cadministration of sucralfate with ofloxacin results in a marked reduction in ofloxacin serum concentrations and potentially reduced clinical efficacy.

RISK FACTORS: No specific risk factors are known.

RELATED DRUGS: Sucralfate also inhibits the absorption of ciprofloxacin (*Cipro*), fleroxacin,[†] and norfloxacin (*Noroxin*). Aluminum-containing antacids also reduce ofloxacin absorption.

MANAGEMENT OPTIONS:

➡ *Consider Alternative.* If dosage separation is not possible, consider an alternative to sucralfate (eg, H_2-receptor antagonist, omeprazole [*Prilosec*], but not an antacid).

➡ *Circumvent/Minimize.* Patients prescribed sucralfate and ofloxacin should avoid coadministration of the 2 agents. To avoid the interaction, the ofloxacin should be taken 2 hours before the sucralfate dose.

➡ *Monitor.* If sucralfate and a quinolone are coadministered, monitor the patient for reduced antibiotic efficacy.

REFERENCES:

Lehto P, et al. Effect of sucralfate on absorption of norfloxacin and ofloxacin. *Antimicrob Agents Chemother.* 1994;38:248-251.

Kawakami J, et al. The effect of food on the interaction of ofloxacin with sucralfate in healthy volunteers. *Eur J Clin Pharmacol.* 1994;47:67-69.

† Not available in the US.

Ofloxacin (*Floxin*)

Warfarin (eg, *Coumadin*)

SUMMARY: Ofloxacin therapy was associated with an increased hypoprothrombinemic response to warfarin in 2 patients, but a causal relationship was not established.

RISK FACTORS:

➡ *Concurrent Diseases.* Fever may place a patient at increased risk.

RELATED DRUGS: Ciprofloxacin (*Cipro*) and norfloxacin (*Noroxin*) have been noted to increase international normalized ratios in a few case reports.

MANAGEMENT OPTIONS:

➡ *Monitor.* Until more information is available, monitor patients for an altered hypoprothrombinemic response to warfarin if ofloxacin is initiated, discontinued, or changed in dosage.

REFERENCES:

Leor J, et al. Ofloxacin and warfarin. *Ann Intern Med.* 1988;109:761.

Baciewicz AM, et al. Interaction of ofloxacin and warfarin. *Ann Intern Med.* 1993;119:1223.

Olanzapine (eg, *Zyprexa*)

Ritonavir (*Norvir*)

SUMMARY: Ritonavir may reduce olanzapine serum concentrations, but it is not know how often this effect would reduce the therapeutic effect of olanzapine.

RISK FACTORS: No specific risk factors are known.

RELATED DRUGS: No information is available.

MANAGEMENT OPTIONS:

➡ *Monitor.* If ritonavir and olanzapine are used concurrently, monitor for reduced olanzapine effect and adjust olanzapine dose as needed.

REFERENCES:

Penzak SR, et al. Influence of ritonavir on olanzapine pharmacokinetics in healthy volunteers. *J Clin Psychopharmacol.* 2002;22:366-370.

Omeprazole (*Prilosec*)

Phenytoin (eg, *Dilantin*)

SUMMARY: Omeprazole increases plasma phenytoin concentrations modestly in healthy subjects given single oral or IV doses of phenytoin, but the importance of the interaction in patients on chronic phenytoin therapy is not established.

RISK FACTORS:

➡ *Dosage Regimen.* Omeprazole doses at least 40 mg/day may inhibit phenytoin metabolism.

RELATED DRUGS: The effect of lansoprazole (*Prevacid*) on phenytoin is not established, but lansoprazole generally is less likely to inhibit drug metabolism than omeprazole.

MANAGEMENT OPTIONS:

➥ **Monitor.** Until data from patients on chronic phenytoin therapy are available, monitor for an excessive phenytoin response when omeprazole is started and for a reduced phenytoin response when omeprazole is stopped. It may be necessary to adjust the phenytoin dose in some cases.

REFERENCES:

Andersson T, et al. Identification of human liver cytochrome P450 isoforms mediating secondary omeprazole metabolism. *Br J Clin Pharmacol.* 1994;37:597.

Andersson T. Omeprazole drug interaction studies. *Clin Pharmacokinet.* 1991;21:195.

Gugler R, et al. Omeprazole inhibits oxidative drug metabolism: studies with diazepam and phenytoin in vivo and 7-ethoxycoumarin in vitro. *Gastroenterology.* 1985;89:1235.

Prichard PJ, et al. Oral phenytoin pharmacokinetics during omeprazole therapy. *Br J Clin Pharmacol.* 1987;24:543.

Omeprazole (*Prilosec*)

Voriconazole (*Vfend*)

SUMMARY: Voriconazole increases omeprazole plasma concentrations; some increase in side effects may be expected.

RISK FACTORS:

➥ **Pharmacogenetics.** Patients who are poor metabolizers for CYP2C19 will have higher voriconazole and omeprazole concentrations, and thus are likely to have an interaction of larger magnitude.

RELATED DRUGS: Esomeprazole (*Nexium*), lansoprazole (eg, *Prevacid*), and pantoprazole (*Protonix*) are also metabolized by both CYP2C19 and CYP3A4 and probably are affected by voriconazole in a similar manner. Rabeprazole (*Aciphex*) has minimal dependence on CYP2C19 and CYP3A4 for its metabolism and would probably be less affected by voriconazole coadministration. Ketoconazole (eg, *Nizoral*), itraconazole (eg, *Sporanox*), and fluconazole (*Diflucan*) may increase omeprazole plasma concentrations.

MANAGEMENT OPTIONS:

➥ **Circumvent/Minimize.** Reduction of the dose of the PPIs may be necessary. The use of rabeprazole may lessen the likelihood of adverse effects occurring during voriconazole coadministration.

➥ **Monitor.** While the PPIs are generally well tolerated, be alert for increased side effects (eg, headache, diarrhea) if voriconazole is administered to patients taking PPIs metabolized by CYP2C19 or CYP3A4.

REFERENCES:

Product information. Voriconazole (*Vfend*). Pfizer, Inc. 2002.

Ondansetron (*Zofran*)

Rifampin (eg, *Rifadin*)

SUMMARY: Rifampin increases the metabolism of ondansetron; a loss of antiemetic activity may result.

RISK FACTORS: No specific risk factors are known.

RELATED DRUGS: Rifabutin (*Mycobutin*) would be likely to affect ondansetron in a similar manner.

MANAGEMENT OPTIONS:

➡ ***Monitor.*** Observe patients receiving ondansetron and rifampin or other potent inducers of CYP3A4 or CYP1A2 for reduced antiemetic effect. Increased ondansetron doses may be required for effective antiemetic control.

REFERENCES:
Villikka K, et al. The effect of rifampin on the pharmacokinetics of oral and intravenous ondansetron. *Clin Pharmacol Ther.* 1999;65:377-381.

Orange Juice

Fexofenadine (*Allegra*)

SUMMARY: Ingestion of large amounts of orange juice reduces the absorption of fexofenadine, and may reduce fexofenadine efficacy.

RISK FACTORS: No specific risk factors are known.

RELATED DRUGS: Apple juice and grapefruit juice also appear to reduce fexofenadine bioavailability.

MANAGEMENT OPTIONS:

➡ ***Circumvent/Minimize.*** Until more data are available, take fexofenadine with water rather than orange juice or other fruit juices.

REFERENCES:
Dresser GK, et al. Fruit juices inhibit organic anion transporting polypeptide-mediated drug uptake to decrease the oral availability of fexofenadine. *Clin Pharmacol Ther.* 2002;71:11-20.

Orlistat (*Xenical*)

Cyclosporine (eg, *Neoral*)

SUMMARY: Pharmacokinetic studies and case reports suggest that orlistat can reduce cyclosporine blood concentrations; avoid concurrent therapy.

RISK FACTORS: No specific risk factors are known.

RELATED DRUGS: The effect of orlistat on tacrolimus (*Prograf*) and sirolimus (*Rapamune*) is not established.

MANAGEMENT OPTIONS:

➡ ***Avoid Unless Benefit Outweighs Risk.*** Because alterations in cyclosporine blood concentrations can have serious consequences, it would be best to avoid this combination.

➥ **Monitor.** If the combination is used, monitor cyclosporine blood concentrations carefully and adjust cyclosporine dosage as needed.

REFERENCES:

Zhi J, et al. Pharmacokinetic evaluation of the possible interaction between selected concomitant medications and orlistat at steady state in healthy subjects. *J Clin Pharmacol.* 2002;42:1011-1019.

Colman E, et al. Reduction in blood cyclosporine concentrations by orlistat. *N Engl J Med.* 2000;342:1141-1142.

 Oxymetholone (Anadrol)

Warfarin (eg, Coumadin)

SUMMARY: Several anabolic steroids have been shown to enhance the hypoprothrombinemic response to oral anticoagulants; bleeding episodes have been reported in some cases.

RISK FACTORS: No specific risk factors are known.

RELATED DRUGS: Some evidence indicates that 17-alpha-alkylated anabolic steroids such as methandrostenolone (*Dianabol*), norethandrolone, methyltestosterone (*Metandren*), and stanozolol (*Winstrol*) are more likely to potentiate oral anticoagulants than anabolic steroids that are not so substituted. Testosterone also interacts with warfarin.

MANAGEMENT OPTIONS:

➥ **Avoid Unless Benefit Outweighs Risk.** Concomitant use of oral anticoagulants and anabolic steroids should be avoided if possible.

➥ **Monitor.** If the combination is necessary, monitor patients carefully for altered anticoagulant response when the anabolic steroid is initiated, discontinued, or changed in dosage.

REFERENCES:

Lorentz SM, et al. Potentiation of warfarin anticoagulation by topical testosterone ointment. *Clin Pharm.* 1985;4:333.

Murakami M, et al. Effects of anabolic steroids on anticoagulant requirements. *Jpn Circ J.* 1965;29:243.

Schrogie JJ, et al. The anticoagulant response to bishydroxycoumarin II: the effect of D-thyroxine, clofibrate, and norethandrolone. *Clin Pharmacol Ther.* 1967;8:70.

Dresdale FC, et al. Potential dangers in the combined use of methandrostenolone and sodium warfarin. *J Med Soc NJ.* 1967;64:609.

Robinson BHB, et al. Decreased anticoagulant tolerance with oxymetholone. *Lancet.* 1971;1:1356. Letter.

Longridge RGM, et al. Decreased anticoagulant tolerance with oxymetholone. *Lancet.* 1971;2:90. Letter.

Edwards MS, et al. Decreased anticoagulant tolerance with oxymetholone. *Lancet.* 1971;2:221. Letter.

De Oya JC, et al. Decreased anticoagulant tolerance with oxymetholone in paroxysmal nocturnal haemoglobinuria. *Lancet.* 1971;2:259. Letter.

Husted S, et al. Increased sensitivity to phenprocoumon during methyltestosterone therapy. *Eur J Clin Pharmacol.* 1976;10:209.

Acomb C, et al. A significant interaction between warfarin and stanozolol. *Pharmaceutical J.* 1985;234;73.

McLaughlin GE, et al. Hemarthrosis complicating anticoagulant therapy: report of three cases. *JAMA.* 1966;196:1020.

Shaw PW, et al. Possible interaction of warfarin and stanozolol. *Clin Pharm.* 1987;6:500.

Paclitaxel (eg, *Taxol*)

Saquinavir (eg, *Fortovase*)

SUMMARY: Two patients on combined therapy with saquinavir and delavirdine (*Rescriptor*) developed unexpectedly severe paclitaxel toxicity, but a causal relationship was not established.

RISK FACTORS: No specific risk factors are known.

RELATED DRUGS: Little is known about the effect of other antiretroviral agents on paclitaxel toxicity. Theoretically, any antiretroviral agents that inhibit CYP2A4 may be expected to increase paclitaxel serum concentrations, including ritonavir (*Norvir*), indinavir, nelfinavir (*Viracept*), and amprenavir (*Agenerase*).

MANAGEMENT OPTIONS:

➤ *Monitor.* Monitor patients on saquinavir or other antiretroviral agents that inhibit CYP3A4 and may be expected to increase paclitaxel toxicity, and reduce paclitaxel doses if necessary.

REFERENCES:

Schwartz JD, et al. Potential interaction of antiretroviral therapy with paclitaxel in patients with AIDS-related Kaposi's sarcoma. *AIDS.* 1999;13:283.

Pancuronium (*Pavulon*)

Polymyxin

SUMMARY: Polymyxin may prolong apnea following the use of muscle relaxants such as pancuronium.

RISK FACTORS: No specific risk factors are known.

RELATED DRUGS: Other neuromuscular blockers may interact with polymyxin.

MANAGEMENT OPTIONS:

➤ *Avoid Unless Benefit Outweighs Risk.* Only give polymyxin with caution during surgery or in the postoperative period.

➤ *Monitor.* If the polymyxin and neuromuscular blocking drugs are used together, monitor the patient carefully for enhanced neuromuscular blockade.

REFERENCES:

Pohlmann G. Respiratory arrest associated with intravenous administration of polymyxin B sulfate. *JAMA.* 1966;196:181.

Levi RA, et al. Polymyxin B-induced respiratory paralysis reversed by intravenous calcium chloride. *J Mt Sinai Hosp.* 1969;36:380.

Pittinger CB, et al. Antibiotic-induced paralysis. *Anesth Analg.* 1970;49:487.

Fogdall RP, et al. Prolongation of a pancuronium-induced neuronmuscular blockade by polymyxin B. *Anesthesiology.* 1974;40:84.

Para-Aminobenzoic Acid (eg, *Potaba*)

Sulfamethoxazole (*Gantanol*)

SUMMARY: Para-aminobenzoic acid (PABA) may interfere with the antibacterial activity of sulfonamides.

RISK FACTORS: No specific risk factors are known.

RELATED DRUGS: Do not administer PABA to patients receiving antibacterial sulfonamides.

MANAGEMENT OPTIONS:

➡ *Use Alternative.* Do not administer PABA to patients receiving antibacterial sulfonamides.

REFERENCES:

Mandell GL, et al. Antimicrobial agents. Sulfonamides, trimethoprim-sulfamethoxazole, quinolones, and agents for urinary tract infections. In: Gilmann AG, et al., eds. *The Pharmacological Basis of Therapeutics.* 8th ed. New York: Pergamon; 1990:1048.

 Paroxetine (*Paxil*)

Thioridazine (eg, *Mellaril*)

SUMMARY: Paroxetine may increase thioridazine serum concentrations, and thus may increase the risk of ventricular arrhythmias; avoid concurrent use.

RISK FACTORS:

➡ *Pharmacogenetics.* Only patients with the extensive metabolizer CYP2D6 phenotype (EMs) would be expected to experience this interaction. Poor metabolizers (PMs) do not have the gene for production of CYP2D6, and would likely already have high serum concentrations of thioridazine. Approximately 8% of whites are deficient in CYP2D6, but the deficiency is rare in Asians – usually no more than 1%.

➡ *Hypokalemia.* The corrected QT interval (QTc) may be prolonged in patients with hypokalemia, thus increasing the risk of this interaction. Any other factor that may prolong the QTc interval would also increase the risk of this interaction.

RELATED DRUGS: Fluoxetine (eg, *Prozac*), like paroxetine, is a potent inhibitor of CYP2D6, and also inhibits CYP2C19; it would also be expected to increase the risk of arrhythmias. Fluvoxamine (eg, *Luvox*), although not a significant CYP2D6 inhibitor, also increases thioridazine serum concentrations, possibly by inhibiting CYP2C19 and CYP1A2. Other SSRIs such as citalopram (eg, *Celexa*), and sertraline (eg, *Zoloft*) are less likely to significantly inhibit CYP2D6, CYP2C19, or CYP1A2. Theoretically, they would be less likely to interact with thioridazine, but little clinical information is available. Although a number of antipsychotic drugs, like thioridazine, have been shown to prolong the QT interval, clinical evidence suggests that thioridazine may produce the greatest risk.

MANAGEMENT OPTIONS:

➡ *Use Alternative.* Although the risk of this combination is not well established, it would be prudent to use alternatives for 1 of the drugs (see Related Drugs).

➡ *Monitor.* If the combination must be used, monitor the ECG for evidence of QT prolongation, and monitor for clinical evidence of arrhythmias (eg, syncope).

REFERENCES:

Hartigan-Go K, et al. Concentration-related pharmacodynamic effects of thioridazine and its metabolites in humans. *Clin Pharmacol Ther.* 1996;60:543-53.

'Dear Doctor or Pharmacist' Letter, Novartis Pharmaceuticals, July 7, 2000.

Paroxetine (*Paxil*)

Tramadol (*Ultram*)

SUMMARY: A patient on paroxetine and tramadol developed serotonin syndrome, but it is unknown how often this occurs in patients receiving the combination. Theoretically, paroxetine would partially inhibit the analgesic effect of tramadol.

RISK FACTORS: No specific risk factors are known.

RELATED DRUGS: The combination of sertraline (*Zoloft*) and tramadol also has been reported to produce serotonin syndrome. It is possible that other selective serotonin reuptake inhibitors such as fluoxetine, fluvoxamine (*Luvox*), and citalopram (*Celexa*) also may increase the risk of serotonin syndrome if combined with tramadol. However, inhibition of tramadol analgesia caused by inhibition of CYP2D6 would likely apply only to fluoxetine and paroxetine because the other selective serotonin reuptake inhibitors have only minimal effects of CYP2D6. Meperidine (eg, *Demerol*) may interact similarly with the SSRIs.

MANAGEMENT OPTIONS:

➡ *Consider Alternative.* In patients on paroxetine or other selective serotonin reuptake inhibitors, consider the use of an analgesic that is not serotonergic (eg, an agent other than tramadol or meperidine) to minimize the risk of serotonin syndrome. To avoid the possibility of reduced tramadol analgesia caused by inhibition of CYP2D6, consider the use of fluvoxamine or sertraline in place of paroxetine or fluoxetine.

➡ *Monitor.* In patients receiving tramadol and paroxetine (or other SSRIs) be alert for evidence of serotonin syndrome. Serotonin syndrome can result in neurotoxicity (myoclonus, tremors, rigidity, incoordination, hyperreflexia, seizures, coma), psychiatric symptoms (agitation, confusion, hypomania, restlessness), and autonomic dysfunction (fever, sweating, tachycardia, hypertension). If the SSRI used is paroxetine or fluoxetine, monitor for reduced tramadol analgesia.

REFERENCES:

Egberts AC, et al. Serotonin syndrome attributed to tramadol addition to paroxetine therapy. *Int Clin Psychopharmacol.* 1997;12:181-82.

Sternbach H. The serotonin syndrome. *Am J Psychiatry.* 1991;148:705-13.

Poulsen L, et al. The hypoalgesic effect of tramadol in relation to CYP2D6. *Clin Pharmacol Ther.* 1996;60:636-44.

Paroxetine (*Paxil*)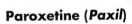

Warfarin (eg, *Coumadin*)

SUMMARY: Although paroxetine does not appear to affect the hypoprothrombinemic response to warfarin in most people, the combination may increase the risk of bleeding.

RISK FACTORS: No specific risk factors are known.

RELATED DRUGS: The effect of paroxetine on the response to other oral anticoagulants is not established, but the same precautions would apply until data are available. Data are insufficient to determine the relative risk of paroxetine versus other selective serotonin reuptake inhibitors (SSRIs) in anticoagulated patients.

MANAGEMENT OPTIONS:

➡ *Consider Alternative.* Although the ability of paroxetine to increase the risk of bleeding in patients on warfarin is not well established, it would be prudent to avoid the combination when possible. The use of an SSRI other than paroxetine may or may not reduce the risk.

➡ *Monitor.* If the combination is used, monitor for altered hypoprothrombinemic response to warfarin if paroxetine is initiated, discontinued, or changed in dosage. Note an increased bleeding risk may occur in the absence of excessive hypoprothrombinemia.

REFERENCES:

Bannister SJ, et al. Evaluation of the potential for interactions of paroxetine with diazepam, cimetidine, warfarin, and digoxin. *Acta Psychiatr Scand.* 1989;80(Suppl. 350):102.

Pefloxacin

Theophylline

SUMMARY: Pefloxacin increases the serum concentration of theophylline; this may result in the development of theophylline toxicity.

RISK FACTORS: No specific risk factors are known.

RELATED DRUGS: Quinolones reported to inhibit the metabolism of drugs include ciprofloxacin (*Cipro*), enoxacin (*Penetrex*), norfloxacin (*Noroxin*), pipemidic acid, and pefloxacin. Quinolones reported to produce no or minor changes in theophylline pharmacokinetics include fleroxacin, flosequinan, lomefloxacin (*Maxaquin*), ofloxacin (*Floxin*), rufloxacin, sparfloxacin, and temafloxacin.

MANAGEMENT OPTIONS:

➡ *Consider Alternative.* Consider using a quinolone which does not produce changes in theophylline metabolism (eg, fleroxacin, flosequinan, lomefloxacin, ofloxacin, rufloxacin, sparfloxacin, temafloxacin).

➡ *Monitor.* Monitor patients maintained on theophylline for elevated theophylline concentrations and signs of toxicity (eg, palpitations, tachycardia, nausea, tremor) during coadministration of pefloxacin.

REFERENCES:

Wijnands WJA, et al. The influence of quinolone derivatives of theophylline clearance. *Br J Clin Pharmacol.* 1986;22:677.

Wijnands WJA, et al. Steady-state kinetics of the quinolone derivatives ofloxacin, enoxacin, ciprofloxacin, and pefloxacin during maintenance treatment with theophylline. *Drugs.* 1987;34(Suppl. 1):159.

Penicillin G

Tetracycline

SUMMARY: Tetracycline administration may impair the efficacy of penicillin (eg, penicillin G) therapy.

RISK FACTORS: No specific risk factors are known.

RELATED DRUGS: Other penicillins may interact similarly.

MANAGEMENT OPTIONS:

➡ *Circumvent/Minimize.* When a penicillin is used with a tetracycline, be certain that adequate amounts of each agent are given because antagonism is most likely to occur when minimal doses of each agent are administered. If possible, begin penicillin administration a few hours before tetracycline administration.

➡ *Monitor.* If penicillin and tetracycline are coadministered, watch for reduced antibiotic efficacy.

REFERENCES:

Garrod LP. Causes of failure in antibiotic treatment. *BMJ.* 1972;4:441.

Kabins SA. Interactions among antibiotics and other drugs. *JAMA.* 1972;219:206.

Jawetz E. The use of combinations of antimicrobial drugs. *Ann Rev Pharmacol.* 1968;8:151.

Mills J, et al. Clinical use of antimicrobials. In: Katzung BG. Basic and Clinical Pharmacology. 4th ed. Los Altos: Lange Medical Publications; 1989:624.

Jawetz E. Synergism and antagonism among antimicrobial drugs, a personal perspective. *West J Med.* 1975;123:87.

Olsson RA, et al. Pneumococcal meningitis in the adult. *Ann Intern Med.* 1961;55:545.

Pentoxifylline (eg, *Trental*)

Theophylline

SUMMARY: Pentoxifylline increased plasma theophylline concentrations in healthy subjects; theophylline toxicity may be increased in patients receiving the combination, but more study is needed.

RISK FACTORS: No specific risk factors are known.

RELATED DRUGS: Whether other forms of theophylline would be affected similarly by pentoxifylline is unknown. If the mechanism of the interaction is inhibition of theophylline elimination, the interaction is likely to be similar with all forms of theophylline. If another mechanism is involved (eg, increased theophylline absorption), the interaction may or may not be similar for other theophylline dosage forms.

MANAGEMENT OPTIONS:

➡ *Monitor.* Monitor for evidence of altered theophylline effect if pentoxifylline therapy is initiated and for decreased theophylline effect if it is discontinued. Alteration of theophylline dose may be needed.

REFERENCES:

Ellison MJ, et al. Influence of pentoxifylline on steady-state theophylline serum concentrations from sustained-release formulation. *Pharmacotherapy.* 1990;10:383.

Cummings DM, et al. Interference potential of pentoxifylline and its major metabolite with theophylline assays. *Am J Hosp Pharm.* 1985;42:2717.

Cohen IA, et al. Effect of pentoxifylline and its metabolites on three theophylline assays. *Clin Pharm.* 1988;7:457.

1 Phenelzine (*Nardil*)

AVOID **Phenylephrine (*Neo-Synephrine*)**

SUMMARY: Monoamine oxidase (MAO) inhibitors such as phenelzine enhance the effects of phenylephrine, especially when it is administered orally. Concomitant use of these drugs may result in hypertensive reactions.

RISK FACTORS:

➡ ***Route of Administration.*** The interaction is likely to be much greater with oral than with parenteral phenylephrine.

RELATED DRUGS: All nonselective MAO inhibitors including isocarboxazid (*Marplan*) and tranylcypromine (*Parnate*) would be expected to interact with phenylephrine.

MANAGEMENT OPTIONS:

➡ ***AVOID COMBINATION.*** Avoid oral phenylephrine in patients taking an MAO inhibitor. Note that phenylephrine is found in many OTC cold remedies. Use parenteral phenylephrine with great care in patients on an MAO inhibitor. The effect of phenylephrine-containing nasal sprays in those taking an MAO inhibitor has not been studied, but avoid them until information on their safety is available. Remember that effects of nonselective MAO inhibitors should be assumed to persist for 2 weeks after they are discontinued.

REFERENCES:

Elis J, et al. Modification by monoamine oxidase inhibitors of the effect of some sympathomimetics on blood pressure. *BMJ.* 1967;2:75-78.

Boakes AJ, et al. Interactions between sympathomimetic amines and antidepressant agents in man. *BMJ.* 1973;1:311-315.

Davies B, et al. Pressor amines and monoamine-oxidase inhibitors for treatment of postural hypotension in autonomic failure. Limitations and hazards. *Lancet.* 1978;1:172-175.

Harrison WM, et al. MAOIs and hypertensive crises: the role of OTC drugs. *J Clin Psychiatry.* 1989;50:64-65.

1 Phenelzine (*Nardil*)

AVOID **Pseudoephedrine (eg, *Sudafed*)**

SUMMARY: Indirect-acting sympathomimetics, such as pseudoephedrine, may produce severe hypertension when administered to patients receiving a monoamine oxidase (MAO) inhibitor such as phenelzine.

RISK FACTORS: No specific risk factors are known.

RELATED DRUGS: All nonselective MAO inhibitors including isocarboxazid (*Marplan*) and tranylcypromine (*Parnate*) would be expected to interact with pseudoephedrine (as well as other indirect-acting sympathomimetics and phenylephrine [*Neo-Synephrine*]).

MANAGEMENT OPTIONS:

➡ ***AVOID COMBINATION.*** Do not give pseudoephedrine to patients receiving nonselective MAO inhibitors. Remember that the effects of nonselective MAO inhibitors should be assumed to persist for 2 weeks after they are discontinued.

REFERENCES:

Wright SP. Hazards with monoamine-oxidase inhibitors: a persistent problem. *Lancet.* 1978;1:284-285.

Harrison WM, et al. MAOIs and hypertensive crises: the role of OTC drugs. *J Clin Psychiatry.* 1989;50:64-65.

Phenelzine (*Nardil*) ▼ 3

Reserpine (*Serpalan*)

SUMMARY: Reserpine reportedly may cause a hypertensive reaction in patients receiving a monoamine oxidase inhibitor (MAOI) like phenelzine, but supporting clinical evidence is scanty.

RISK FACTORS:

➠ *Order of Drug Administration.* Theoretically, this interaction is most likely to occur in a patient who has been taking nonselective MAOIs who then is started on reserpine (rather than the reverse order of administration).

RELATED DRUGS: Theoretically, all nonselective MAOIs including isocarboxazid (*Marplan*) and tranylcypromine (*Parnate*) would be expected to interact with reserpine.

MANAGEMENT OPTIONS:

➠ *Consider Alternative.* Although more clinical information is needed to clarify this interaction, it would be prudent to consider antihypertensive therapy other than reserpine in patients on nonselective MAOIs. Remember that the effects of nonselective MAOIs should be assumed to persist for 2 weeks after they are discontinued.

➠ *Monitor.* Monitor for evidence of hypertensive reaction if the combination is given.

REFERENCES:

Goldberg LI. Monoamine oxidase inhibitors. Adverse reactions and possible mechanisms. *JAMA.* 1964;190:456.

Phenelzine (*Nardil*)

Sibutramine (*Meridia*) AVOID

SUMMARY: Given the theoretical risk of serotonin syndrome, sibutramine should not be given concurrently with monoamine oxidase inhibitors (MAOIs).

RISK FACTORS: No specific risk factors are known.

RELATED DRUGS: Avoid sibutramine with other MAOIs such as tranylcypromine (*Parnate*) and selegiline (*Eldepryl*)

MANAGEMENT OPTIONS:

➠ *AVOID COMBINATION.* Do not give sibutramine concurrently with MAOIs.

REFERENCES:

Knoll Pharmaceuticals. *Meridia* product information. Mount Olive, NJ. 1997.

Mills KC. Serotonin syndrome: a clinical update. *Crit Care Clin.* 1997;13:763.

Phenelzine (*Nardil*)

Succinylcholine (eg, *Anectine*)

SUMMARY: Phenelzine may prolong the muscle relaxation caused by succinylcholine administration.

RISK FACTORS: No specific risk factors are known.

RELATED DRUGS: Based upon information from this preliminary study, other monoamine oxidase inhibitors do not appear to affect pseudocholinesterase.

MANAGEMENT OPTIONS:

➡ *Monitor.* Monitor for prolonged succinylcholine effect in patients receiving phenelzine. Remember that the effects of phenelzine should be assumed to persist for 2 weeks after it is discontinued.

REFERENCES:

Bodley PO, et al. Low serum pseudocholinesterase levels complicating treatment with phenelzine. *BMJ.* 1969;3:510.

Phenelzine (*Nardil*)

AVOID Venlafaxine (*Effexor*)

SUMMARY: Severe serotonin syndrome can occur when venlafaxine is used with or within 2 weeks of discontinuation of phenelzine or other nonselective monoamine oxidase inhibitors (MAOIs). Strictly avoid the combination.

RISK FACTORS: No specific risk factors are known.

RELATED DRUGS: All nonselective MAOIs should be expected to result in serotonin syndrome if combined with venlafaxine. This would include tranylcypromine (*Parnate*) and isocarboxazid (*Marplan*); selegiline (*Eldepryl*) can act as a nonselective MAOI in some patients, especially if large doses are used.

MANAGEMENT OPTIONS:

➡ *AVOID COMBINATION.* Avoid combined use of venlafaxine with phenelzine (or any other nonselective MAOIs). This would include the use of venlafaxine within 2 weeks of discontinuation of a MAOI.

REFERENCES:

Weiner LA, et al. Serotonin syndrome secondary to phenelzine-venlafaxine interaction. *Pharmacotherapy.* 1998;18:399.

Diamond S, et al. Serotonin syndrome induced by transitioning from phenelzine to venlafaxine: four patient reports. *Neurology.* 1998;51:274.

Heisler MA, et al. Serotonin syndrome induced by administration of venlafaxine and phenelzine. *Ann Pharmacother.* 1996;30:84. Letter.

Phillips SD, Ringo P. Phenelzine and venlafaxine interaction. *Am J Psychiatry.* 1995;152:1400. Letter.

Phenobarbital ▼ 3

Phenytoin (eg, *Dilantin*)

SUMMARY: Phenobarbital tends to decrease serum phenytoin concentrations; it occasionally does not change and sometimes even increases the serum phenytoin concentration. Combined use of barbiturates and phenytoin can be beneficial in many patients; however, the phenytoin serum concentration can be affected when phenobarbital is started or stopped.

RISK FACTORS: No specific risk factors are known.

RELATED DRUGS: Little is known regarding the effect of barbiturates other than phenobarbital on phenytoin, but they probably will reduce phenytoin serum concentrations.

MANAGEMENT OPTIONS:

➡ *Circumvent/Minimize.* Avoid large doses of phenobarbital probably in patients with high blood levels of phenytoin because of the potential for competitive inhibition of phenytoin metabolism.

➡ *Monitor.* Observe patients maintained on phenytoin and a barbiturate for signs of phenytoin intoxication if the barbiturate therapy is stopped. Epileptic patients who manifest decreases in phenytoin blood concentrations caused by phenobarbital administration do not appear to be adversely affected clinically, and no action is required.

REFERENCES:

Gallagher BB, et al. Primidone, diphenylhydantoin and phenobarbital. Aspects of acute and chronic toxicity. *Neurology.* 1973;23:145.

Garrettson LK, et al. Disappearance of phenobarbital and diphenylhydantoin from serum of children. *Clin Pharmacol Ther.* 1970;11:674.

Buchanan RA, et al. Diphenylhydantoin and phenobarbital blood levels of epileptic children. *Neurology.* 1971;21:866.

Hahn TJ, et al. Effect of chronic anticonvulsant therapy on serum 25-hydroxy calciferol levels in adults. *N Engl J Med.* 1972;287:900.

Hansten PD. Interactions between anticonvulsant drugs: primidone, diphenylhydantoin and phenobarbital. *Northwest Med J.* 1974;1:17.

Cucinell SA, et al. Drug interactions in man. I. Lowering effect of phenobarbital on plasma levels of bishydroxycoumarin (*Dicumarol*) and diphenylhydantoin (*Dilantin*). *Clin Pharmacol Ther.* 1965;6:420.

Kutt H, et al. The effect of phenobarbital on plasma diphenylhydantoin level and metabolism in man and in rat liver microsomes. *Neurology.* 1969;19:611.

Buchanan RA, et al. The effect of phenobarbital on diphenylhydantoin metabolism in children. *Pediatrics.* 1969;43:114.

Kutt H, et al. The effect of phenobarbital upon diphenylhydantoin metabolism in man. *Neurology.* 1965;15:274. Abstract.

Kokenge R, et al. Neurological sequelae following *Dilantin* overdose in a patient and in experimental animals. *Neurology.* 1965;15:823.

Tudhope GR. Advances in medicine. *Practitioner.* 1969;203:405.

Diamond WD, et al. A clinical study of the effect of phenobarbital on diphenylhydantoin plasma levels. *J Clin Pharmacol.* 1970;10:306.

Sotaniemi E, et al. The clinical significance of microsomal enzyme induction in the therapy of epileptic patients. *Ann Clin Res.* 1970;2:223.

Booker HE, et al. Concurrent administration of phenobarbital and diphenylhydantoin: lack of an interference effect. *Neurology.* 1971;21:383.

Buchthal F, et al. Serum concentrations of diphenylhydantoin (phenytoin) and phenobarbital and their relation to therapeutic and toxic effects. *Psychiatr Neurol Neurochir.* 1971;74:117.

Morselli PL, et al. Interaction between phenobarbital and diphenylhydantoin in animals and in epileptic patients. *Ann NY Acad Sci.* 1971;179:88.

Rizzo M, et al. Further observations on the interactions between phenobarbital and diphenylhydantoin during chronic treatment in the rat. *Biochem Pharmacol.* 1972;21:449.

Callaghan N, et al. The effect of anticonvulsant drugs which induce liver enzymes on derived and ingested phenobarbitone levels. *Acta Neurol Scand.* 1977;56:1.

Lambie DG, et al. Therapeutic and pharmacokinetic effects of increasing phenytoin in chronic epileptics on multiple drug therapy. *Lancet.* 1976;2:386.

Cuzzolin L, et al. Phenytoin-phenobarbital interaction: importance of free plasma phenytoin monitoring. *Pharmacol Res Commun.* 1988;20:627.

Phenobarbital (eg, *Bellatal*)

Prednisone (eg, *Deltasone*)

SUMMARY: Barbiturates may reduce serum concentrations of prednisone and other corticosteroids sufficiently to impair their therapeutic effect.

RISK FACTORS: No specific risk factors are known.

RELATED DRUGS: Dexamethasone, prednisolone, and methylprednisolone interact similarly with phenobarbital. Assume that all combinations of barbiturates and corticosteroids interact until proven otherwise.

MANAGEMENT OPTIONS:

➡ *Consider Alternative.* If appropriate, consider possible alternatives to barbiturates (eg, benzodiazepines).

➡ *Monitor.* Monitor for altered corticosteroid effect if a barbiturate is initiated, discontinued, or changed in dosage; substantial adjustments in corticosteroid dosage may be needed.

REFERENCES:

Falliers CJ. Corticosteroids and phenobarbital in asthma. *N Engl J Med.* 1972;287:201.

Berman ML, et al. Acute stimulation of cortisol metabolism by pentobarbital in man. *Anesthesiology.* 1971;34:365.

Southren AL, et al. Effect of N-phenylbarbital (phetharbital) on the metabolism of testosterone and cortisol in man. *J Clin Endocrinol Metab.* 1969;29:251.

Brooks PM, et al. Effects of enzyme induction on metabolism of prednisolone. Clinical and laboratory study. *Ann Rheum Dis.* 1976;35:339.

Brooks SM, et al. Adverse effects of phenobarbital on corticosteroid metabolism in patients with bronchial asthma. *N Engl J Med.* 1972;286:1125.

Gambertoglio J, et al. Enhancement of prednisolone elimination by anticonvulsants in renal transplant recipients. *Clin Pharmacol Ther.* 1982;31:228.

Wassner SJ, et al. The adverse effect of anticonvulsant therapy on renal allograft survival. *J Pediatr.* 1976;88:134.

Stjernholm MR, et al. Effects of diphenylhydantoin, phenobarbital, and diazepam on the metabolism of methylprednisolone and its sodium succinate. *J Clin Endocrinol Metab.* 1975;41:887.

Phenobarbital (eg, *Bellatal*)

Primidone (*Mysoline*)

SUMMARY: The combination of primidone and phenobarbital may result in excessive serum phenobarbital concentrations.

RISK FACTORS: No specific risk factors are known.

RELATED DRUGS: No information is available.

MANAGEMENT OPTIONS:

➡ *Consider Alternative.* For most patients, do not use primidone and phenobarbital concomitantly.

➡ *Monitor.* If the combination is used, monitor the patient for excessive phenobarbital serum concentrations.

REFERENCES:

Griffin GD, et al. Primidone-phenobarbital intoxication. *Drug Ther.* 1976;60:76.

Fincham RW, et al. The influence of diphenylhydantoin on primidone metabolism. *Arch Neurol.* 1974;30:259.

Wilson JT, et al. Chronic and severe phenobarbital intoxication in a child treated with primidone and diphenylhydantoin. *J Pediatr.* 1973;83:484.

Gallagher BB, et al. Primidone, diphenylhydantoin and phenobarbital. Aspects of acute and chronic toxicity. *Neurology.* 1973;23:145.

Phenobarbital (eg, *Bellatal*)

Propafenone (*Rythmol*)

SUMMARY: Phenobarbital increases the metabolism of propafenone and reduces its plasma concentrations in healthy subjects; the clinical importance of this interaction is not established.

RISK FACTORS: No specific risk factors are known.

RELATED DRUGS: No information is available.

MANAGEMENT OPTIONS:

➡ *Monitor.* Until this interaction is studied in patients receiving chronic propafenone and phenobarbital, monitor patients for diminished propafenone efficacy and toxicity when phenobarbital is added to or removed from the drug regimen.

REFERENCES:

Chan GL-Y, et al. The effect of phenobarbital on the pharmacokinetics of propafenone in man. *Pharm Res.* 1988;5:S-153.

Phenobarbital

Protriptyline (eg, *Vivactil*)

SUMMARY: Phenobarbital and other barbiturates may reduce serum concentrations of protriptyline and other tricyclic antidepressants (TCAs); the therapeutic response to the antidepressants probably is reduced in some patients.

RISK FACTORS:

➡ *Dosage Regimen.* Barbiturate-induced enzyme induction is known to be dose related; small or occasional doses are unlikely to significantly affect drug metabolism. Depending upon the barbiturate, it may take 1 to 2 weeks or more for the maximal reduction in serum concentrations of the affected drug.

RELATED DRUGS: Other barbiturates may reduce serum concentrations of protriptyline and other TCAs. Unlike barbiturates, benzodiazepines do not appear likely to affect TCA serum concentrations.

MANAGEMENT OPTIONS:

➡ *Consider Alternative.* Patients on TCAs probably respond better without barbiturates, and it has been recommended that barbiturates be avoided in such patients.

➡ *Monitor.* Monitor for altered TCA effect if barbiturate therapy is initiated, discontinued, or changed in dosage; adjust tricyclic antidepressant dose as needed.

REFERENCES:

Moody JP, et al. Pharmacokinetic aspects of protriptyline plasma levels. *Eur J Clin Pharmacol.* 1977;11:51.

Burrows GD, et al. Antidepressants and barbiturates. *BMJ.* 1971;4:113. Letter.

Silverman G, et al. Interaction of benzodiazepines with tricyclic antidepressants. *BMJ.* 1972;4:111. Letter.

Borden EC, et al. Recovery from massive amitriptyline overdosage. *Lancet.* 1968;1:1256. Letter.

Alexanderson B, et al. Steady state plasma levels of nortriptyline in twins: influence of genetic factors and drug therapy. *BMJ.* 1969;4:764.

Crocker, et al. Tricyclic (antidepressant) drug toxicity. *Clin Toxicol.* 1969;2:397.

Noble, et al. Acute poisoning by tricyclic antidepressants: clinical features and management of 100 patients. *Clin Toxicol.* 1969;2:403.

Sjoqvist F, et al. Plasma level of monomethylated tricyclic antidepressants and side-effects in man. In: Toxicity and Side-Effects of Psychotropic Drugs. Amsterdam: Excerpta Medica Foundation; 1968:246–57.

Hammer W, et al. A comparative study of the metabolism of desmethylimipramine, nortriptyline, and oxyphenbutazone in man. *Clin Pharmacol Ther.* 1969;10:44.

Metabolism of drugs. *BMJ.* 1970;1:767.

Royds R, et al. Tricyclic antidepressant poisoning. *Practitioner.* 1970;204:282.

Phenobarbital

Quinidine

SUMMARY: Barbiturates can reduce quinidine plasma concentrations; loss of efficacy could result.

RISK FACTORS: No specific risk factors are known.

RELATED DRUGS: Other barbiturates would be expected to produce a similar response.

MANAGEMENT OPTIONS:

➡ *Circumvent/Minimize.* Initiation or discontinuation of phenobarbital therapy in patients taking quinidine may necessitate a change in quinidine dosage.

➡ *Monitor.* Quinidine response and plasma concentrations may be reduced when barbiturates are added or increased when phenobarbital is discontinued.

REFERENCES:

Data JL, et al. Interaction of quinidine with anticonvulsant drugs. *N Engl J Med.* 1976;294:699.

Chapron DJ, et al. Apparent quinidine-induced digoxin toxicity after withdrawal of pentobarbital. A case of sequential drug interactions. *Arch Intern Med.* 1979;139:363.

Kroboth FJ, et al. Phenytoin-theophylline-quinidine interaction. *N Engl J Med.* 1983;308:725. Letter.

Phenobarbital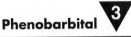

Theophylline

SUMMARY: Barbiturates like phenobarbital may reduce serum theophylline concentrations; in some patients, the effect may be large enough to reduce the therapeutic response to theophylline.

RISK FACTORS: No specific risk factors are known.

RELATED DRUGS: Pentobarbital and secobarbital interact similarly with theophylline. All barbiturates probably have a similar effect on theophylline.

MANAGEMENT OPTIONS:

➡ *Monitor.* Monitor patients receiving chronic theophylline therapy for altered theophylline effect when barbiturate therapy is started or stopped.

REFERENCES:

Gibson GA, et al. Influence of high-dose pentobarbital theophylline pharmacokinetics: a case study. *Ther Drug Monit.* 1985;7:181.

Paladino JA, et al. Effect of secobarbital on theophylline clearance. *Ther Drug Monit.* 1983;5:135.

Piafsky KM, et al. Effect of phenobarbital on the disposition of intravenous theophylline. *Clin Pharmacol Ther.* 1977;22:336.

Landay RA, et al. Effect of phenobarbital on theophylline disposition. *J Allergy Clin Immunol.* 1978;62:27.

Phenobarbital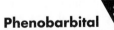

Valproic Acid (eg, *Depakene*)

SUMMARY: Valproic acid increases serum phenobarbital concentrations; phenobarbital intoxication may occur in some patients.

RISK FACTORS: No specific risk factors are known.

RELATED DRUGS: No information is available.

MANAGEMENT OPTIONS:

➡ *Monitor.* Monitor for excessive phenobarbital effect when valproic acid is given concurrently; reductions in the phenobarbital dose may be necessary for many patients.

REFERENCES:

Wilder BJ, et al. Valproic acid: interaction with other anticonvulsant drugs. *Neurology.* 1978;28:892.

Patel IH, et al. Phenobarbital-valproic acid interaction. *Clin Pharmacol Ther.* 1980;27:515.

Bruni J, et al. Valproic acid and plasma levels of phenobarbital. *Neurology.* 1980;30:94.

Phenobarbital

Verapamil (eg, *Calan*)

SUMMARY: Phenobarbital substantially reduces the plasma concentrations of verapamil, especially when verapamil is given orally.

RISK FACTORS:

➠ *Route of Administration.* Oral verapamil dosing can increase the risk of interaction.

RELATED DRUGS: Phenobarbital also increases the metabolism of nifedipine (eg, *Procardia*). Other calcium channel blockers may be similarly affected by phenobarbital and other barbiturates.

MANAGEMENT OPTIONS:

➠ *Circumvent/Minimize.* Patients receiving phenobarbital may require higher than usual doses of verapamil, especially if the verapamil is administered orally.

➠ *Monitor.* Monitor patients stabilized on verapamil (especially if taken orally) for the possibility of decreased effectiveness when phenobarbital is administered concomitantly.

REFERENCES:

Rutledge DR, et al. Effects of chronic phenobarbital on verapamil disposition in humans. *J Pharmacol Exp Ther.* 1988;246:7.

Phenobarbital

Warfarin (eg, *Coumadin*)

SUMMARY: Barbiturates inhibit the hypoprothrombinemic response to oral anticoagulants like warfarin. Fatal bleeding episodes have occurred when barbiturates were discontinued in patients stabilized on an anticoagulant.

RISK FACTORS:

➠ *Dosage Regimen.* The effect of barbiturates on anticoagulants may be dose related. For example, plasma warfarin did not change in 1 patient when 100 mg/day of secobarbital was given, but it decreased considerably when the dosage was increased to 200 mg/day. However, in 6 healthy subjects, 100 mg/day of secobarbital was sufficient to enhance warfarin metabolism. A decrease in the anticoagulant response usually develops gradually after a barbiturate is initiated, with maximal effects occurring at about 2 weeks. The time course following discontinuation of the barbiturate is similar; the results of enzyme induction usually begin to diminish within a week, with little induction remaining by 2 to 3 weeks. Note that the onset and offset of enzyme induction by barbiturates will vary depending upon the half-life of the specific barbiturate.

RELATED DRUGS: Phenobarbital (eg, *Solfoton*), butabarbital (eg, *Butisol*), heptabarbital, pentobarbital (eg, *Nembutal*), secobarbital (*Seconal*), and amobarbital (*Amytal*) have all been shown to decrease the response to coumarin anticoagulants. Most barbiturates (including primidone [eg, *Mysoline*], which is metabolized to phenobarbital) probably have this ability. Most of the interaction studies have involved warfarin or dicumarol, but barbiturates also appear to increase the metabolism of other anticoagulants such as phenprocoumon, acenocoumarol, and ethyl biscoumacetate.

MANAGEMENT OPTIONS:

➡ *Avoid Unless Benefit Outweighs Risk.* If the barbiturate is being used as a sedative/ hypnotic, its use with an oral anticoagulant generally should be avoided. Alternative sedative/hypnotic drugs unlikely to interact with oral anticoagulants include flurazepam (*Dalmane*), chlordiazepoxide (*Librium*), diazepam (eg, *Valium*), or diphenhydramine (eg, *Benadryl*). Nonetheless, the consistent use of stable doses of barbiturates, as in epileptic patients, does not appear to interfere significantly with anticoagulant control.

➡ *Monitor.* If a barbiturate is used in a patient receiving an oral anticoagulant, monitor for altered hypoprothrombinemic response if the barbiturate is initiated, discontinued, or changed in dosage. Moreover, advise patients stabilized on a barbiturate and an oral anticoagulant not to stop taking the barbiturate or change its dosage without consulting with their physician for careful monitoring of their anticoagulant response.

REFERENCES:

Aggeler PM, et al. Effect of heptabarbital on the response to bishydroxycoumarin in man. *J Lab Clin Med.* 1969;74:229.

Lewis RJ. Effect of barbiturates on anticoagulant therapy. *N Engl J Med.* 1966;274:110. Letter.

Whitfield JB, et al. Changes in plasma gamma-glutamyl transpeptidase activity associated with alterations in drug metabolism in man. *BMJ.* 1973;1:316.

O'Reilly RA, et al. Interaction of secobarbital with warfarin pseudoracemates. *Clin Pharmacol Ther.* 1980;28:187.

Williams JRB, et al. Effect of concomitantly administered drugs on the control of long term anticoagulant therapy. *Q J Med.* 1976;45:63.

Starr KJ, et al. Drug interactions in patients on long term oral anticoagulant and antihypertensive adrenergic neuron-blocking drugs. *BMJ.* 1972;4:133.

Zaroslinski J, et al. Effect of subacute administration of methaqualone, phenobarbital and glutethimide on plasma levels of bishydroxycoumarin. *Arch Int Pharmacodyn Ther.* 1972;195:185.

Therapeutic conferences. Drug interaction. *BMJ.* 1971;1:389.

Breckenridge A, et al. Dose-dependent enzyme induction. *Clin Pharmacol Ther.* 1973;14:514.

Cucinell SA, et al. Drug interactions in man. I. Lowering effect of phenobarbital on plasma levels of bishydroxycoumarin (*Dicumarol*) and diphenylhydantoin (*Dilantin*). *Clin Pharmacol Ther.* 1965;6:420.

Corn M. Effect of phenobarbital and glutethimide on biological halflife of warfarin. *Thromb Diath Haemorrh.* 1966;16:606.

Robinson DS, et al. The effect of phenobarbital administration on the control of coagulation achieved during warfarin therapy in man. *J Pharmacol Exp Ther.* 1966;153:250.

Robinson DS, et al. Interaction of commonly prescribed drugs and warfarin. *Ann Intern Med.* 1970;72:853.

Hunninghake DB, et al. Drug interactions with warfarin. *Arch Intern Med.* 1968;121:349.

Antlitz AM, et al. Effect of butabarbital on orally administered anticoagulants. *Curr Ther Res.* 1968;10:70.

MacDonald MG, et al. Clinical observations of possible barbiturate interference with anticoagulation. *JAMA.* 1968;204:97.

MacDonald MG, et al. The effects of phenobarbital, chloral betaine, and glutethimide administration on warfarin plasma levels and hypoprothrombinemic responses in man. *Clin Pharmacol Ther.* 1969;10:80.

Goss JE, et al. Increased bishydroxycoumarin requirements in patients receiving phenobarbital. *N Engl J Med.* 1965;273:1094.

Levy G, et al. Pharmacokinetic analysis of the effect of barbiturate on the anticoagulant action of warfarin in man. *Clin Pharmacol Ther.* 1970;11:372.

Udall JA. Clinical implications of warfarin interactions with five sedatives. *Am J Cardiol.* 1975;35:67.

Dayton PG, et al. The influence of barbiturates on coumarin plasma levels and prothrombin response. *J Clin Invest.* 1961;40:1797.

Kroon C, et al. Interaction between single dose acenocoumarol and cimetidine or pentobarbitone: validation of a single dose model to predict interactions in steady state. *Br J Clin Pharmacol.* 1990;29:643P.

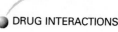
 Phenylbutazone (*Butazolidin*)

Phenytoin (eg, *Dilantin*)

SUMMARY: Phenylbutazone appears to increase serum phenytoin concentrations, but the incidence of phenytoin intoxication in patients on this combination is unknown.

RISK FACTORS: No specific risk factors are known.

RELATED DRUGS: Although oxyphenbutazone probably interacts with phenytoin in a similar manner, the effect of other nonsteroidal anti-inflammatory drugs is not established.

MANAGEMENT OPTIONS:

➡ *Consider Alternative.* *Butazolidin* is no longer available for human use in the US, so alternative NSAIDs would be used in any case.

➡ *Monitor.* Closely watch patients receiving both phenylbutazone and phenytoin for signs of phenytoin intoxication (eg, ataxia, nystagmus, mental impairment, involuntary muscular movements, seizures). Serum phenytoin determinations may be useful for monitoring this interaction, but any given total phenytoin concentration may correspond to a higher-than-normal free serum phenytoin level when phenylbutazone is given concurrently (caused by possible displacement of phenytoin from plasma protein binding).

REFERENCES:

Andreasen PB, et al. Diphenylhydantoin half life in man and its inhibition by phenylbutazone: the role of genetic factors. *Acta Med Scand.* 1973;193:561.

Hansen JM, et al. Dicumarol-induced diphenylhydantoin intoxication. *Lancet.* 1966;2:265.

Lucas BG. "*Dilantin*" overdosage. *Med J Aust.* 1968;2:639. Letter.

Lunde PKM, et al. Plasma protein binding of diphenylhydantoin in man. Interaction with other drugs and the effect of temperature and plasma dilution. *Clin Pharmacol Ther.* 1970;11:846.

Lunde PKM. Plasma protein binding of diphenylhydantoin in man. *Acta Pharmacol Toxicol.* 1971;29:152.

Neuvonen PJ, et al. Antipyretic analgesics in patients on antiepileptic drug therapy. *Eur J Clin Pharmacol.* 1979;15:263.

 Phenylbutazone (*Butazolidin*)

Tolbutamide (*Orinase*)

SUMMARY: Phenylbutazone increases the serum concentrations of tolbutamide and several other oral hypoglycemic drugs and may increase their hypoglycemic action.

RISK FACTORS: No specific risk factors are known.

RELATED DRUGS: It is not known whether other oral hypoglycemics are affected by phenylbutazone. Other nonsteroidal anti-inflammatory drugs appear to be safer than phenylbutazone to use with hypoglycemic drugs.

MANAGEMENT OPTIONS:

➡ *Use Alternative.* Do not administer phenylbutazone to patients taking oral hypoglycemic agents. Other nonsteroidal anti-inflammatory drugs appear to be acceptable alternatives.

REFERENCES:

Field JB, et al. Potentiation of acetohexamide hypoglycemia by phenylbutazone. *N Engl J Med.* 1967;277:889.

Slade IH, et al. Fatal hypoglycemic coma from the use of tolbutamide in elderly patients: report of two cases. *J Am Geriatr Soc.* 1967;15:948.

Harris EL. Adverse reactions to oral antidiabetic agents. *BMJ.* 1971;3:29.

Metz R. Bulletin of the Mason Clinic (Case Notes). 1976;30:38.

Pond SM, et al. Mechanisms of inhibition of tolbutamide metabolism: phenylbutazone, oxyphenbutazone, sulfaphenazole. *Clin Pharmacol Ther.* 1977;22:573.

Morrison PJ, et al. Effect of pirprofen on glibenclamide kinetics and response. *Br J Clin Pharmacol.* 1982;14:123.

Stoeckel K, et al. Lack of effect of tenoxicam on glibornuride kinetics and response. *Br J Clin Pharmacol.* 1985;19:249.

Verbeeck RK, et al. Clinical pharmacokinetics of nonsteroidal anti-inflammatory drugs. *Clin Pharmackin.* 1983;8:297.

Day RO, et al. The effect of tenoxicam on tolbutamide pharmacokinetics and glucose concentrations in healthy volunteers. *Int J Clin Pharmacol Ther.* 1995;33:308

Diwan PV, et al. Potentiation of hypoglycemic response of glibenclamide by piroxicam in rats and humans. *Indian J Exp Biol.* 1992;30:317.

Phenylbutazone (*Butazolidin*)

Warfarin (eg, *Coumadin*) AVOID

SUMMARY: Phenylbutazone dramatically enhances the hypoprothrombinemic response to warfarin, leading to severe bleeding in some patients. Avoid this combination.

RISK FACTORS:

➡ *Concurrent Diseases.* Patients with peptic ulcer disease (PUD) or a history of GI bleeding are probably at greater risk.

RELATED DRUGS: All NSAIDs inhibit platelet function, cause gastric erosions, and probably increase the risk of GI bleeding. However, some NSAIDs such as ibuprofen (eg, *Motrin*), naproxen (eg, *Naprosyn*), or diclofenac (*Voltaren*) may be less likely to increase oral anticoagulant-induced hypoprothrombinemia than other NSAIDs.

MANAGEMENT OPTIONS:

➡ *AVOID COMBINATION.* Avoid phenylbutazone in patients receiving oral anticoagulants. Probably no condition exists in which the benefit of phenylbutazone therapy outweighs the serious risk of concomitant therapy with oral anticoagulants. It would be prudent to use NSAIDs that are unlikely to affect the hypoprothrombinemic response to oral anticoagulants. If the NSAID is being used as an analgesic or antipyretic, acetaminophen is probably safer to use with oral anticoagulants. Nonacetylated salicylates (eg, choline salicylate, magnesium salicylate, salsalate, sodium salicylate) probably also are safer with oral anticoagulants than NSAIDs because such salicylates have minimal effects on platelet function and the gastric mucosa. If any NSAID is used with an oral anticoagulant, carefully monitor the prothrombin time and watch for evidence of bleeding, especially from the GI tract.

REFERENCES:

Udall JA. Drug interference with warfarin therapy. *Clin Med.* 1970;77:20.

Brozovic M, et al. Prothrombin during warfarin treatment. *Br J Haematol.* 1973;24:579.

Packham MA, et al. Alteration of the response of platelets to surface stimuli by pyrazole compounds. *J Exp Med.* 1967;126:171.

Wosilait WD, et al. The effect of oxyphenbutazone on the excretion of 14 C-warfarin in the bile of rat. *Res Commun Chem Pathol Pharmacol.* 1972;4:413.

Weiner M, et al. Drug interactions: the effect of combined administration of the half-life of coumarin and pyrazolone drugs in man. *Fed Proc.* 165;24:153. Abstract.

O'Reilly RA. The binding of sodium warfarin to plasma albumin and its displacement by phenylbutazone. *Ann NY Acad Sci.* 1973;226:293.

Aggeler PM, et al. Potentiation of anticoagulant effect of warfarin by phenylbutazone. *N Engl J Med.* 1967;276:496.

Hoffbrand BI, et al. Potentiation of anticoagulants. *BMJ.* 1967;2:838. Letter.

Kleinman PD, et al. Studies of the epidemiology of anticoagulant-drug interactions. *Arch Intern Med.* 1970;126:522.

Zucker MB, et al. Effect of acetylsalicylic acid, other nonsteroidal antiinflammatory agents, and dipyridamole on human blood platelets. *J Lab Clin Med.* 1970;76:66.

Lewis RJ, et al. Warfarin. Stereochemical aspects of its metabolism and the interaction with phenylbutazone. *J Clin Invest.* 1974;53:1607.

Bull J, et al. Phenylbutazone and anticoagulant control. *Practitioner.* 1975;215:767.

Chierichetti S, et al. Comparison of feprazone and phenylbutazone interaction with warfarin in man. *Curr Ther Res.* 1975;18:568.

O'Reilly RA. Phenylbutazone and sulfinpyrazone interaction with oral anticoagulant phenprocoumon. *Arch Int Med.* 1982;142:1634.

O'Reilly RA, et al. Comparative interaction of sulfinpyrazone and phenylbutazone with racemic warfarin: alteration in vivo of free fraction of plasma warfarin. *J Pharmacol Exp Ther.* 1981;219:691.

O'Reilly RA, et al. Stereoselective interaction of phenylbutazone with 12 C/ 13C warfarin pseudoracemates in man. *J Clin Invest.* 1980;68:746.

Shorr RI, et al. Concurrent use of nonsteroidal anti-inflammatory drugs and oral anticoagulants places elderly persons at high risk for hemorrhagic peptic ulcer disease. *Arch Intern Med.* 1993;153:1665.

 Phenylephrine (*Neo-Synephrine*)

Propranolol (eg, *Inderal*)

SUMMARY: Very limited evidence suggests that propranolol may predispose patients to acute hypertensive episodes when phenylephrine is administered.

RISK FACTORS:

➡ ***Dosage Regimen.*** IV or intraocularly administered phenylephrine increases the risk of interaction.

RELATED DRUGS: If the interaction between beta blockers and phenylephrine occurs, it is likely to be most important with nonselective beta blockers, such as propranolol, nadolol (eg, *Corgard*), timolol (eg, *Blocadren*), or pindolol (eg, *Visken*). Metoprolol does not interact.

MANAGEMENT OPTIONS:

➡ ***Consider Alternative.*** The use of cardioselective beta blockers (eg, metoprolol) may minimize the risk of this interaction.

➡ *Monitor.* Until this potential interaction is substantiated or disproved, carefully monitor the blood pressure when phenylephrine is given to patients receiving beta blockers, particularly when the phenylephrine is administered IV or intraocularly.

REFERENCES:

Cass E, et al. Hazards of phenylephrine topical medication in persons taking propranolol. *Can Med Assoc J.* 1979;120:1261-1262.

Brown MM, et al. Lack of side effects from topically administered 10% phenylephrine eyedrops. A controlled study. *Arch Ophthalmol.* 1980;98:487-489.

Adler AG, et al. Systemic effects of eye drops. *Arch Intern Med.* 1982;142:2293-2294.

Shephard AM, et al. Dependence of phenylephrine dose/blood responses on autonomic activity in humans. *Clin Pharmacol Ther.* 1989;45:168.

Myers MG, et al. Intranasally administered phenylephrine and blood pressure. *Can Med Assoc J.* 1982;127:365-368.

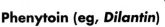

Phenytoin (eg, *Dilantin*)

Primidone (eg, *Mysoline*)

SUMMARY: Phenytoin appears to enhance the conversion of primidone to phenobarbital. Excessive phenobarbital serum concentrations may occur in some patients.

RISK FACTORS:

➡ *Other Drugs.* Concurrent therapy with phenobarbital or carbamazepine can increase the magnitude of this interaction.

RELATED DRUGS: No information is available.

MANAGEMENT OPTIONS:

➡ *Monitor.* No special precautions are necessary with the concomitant use of phenytoin and primidone, although relatively high concentrations of phenobarbital can be generated. The finding of supratherapeutic concentrations of phenobarbital in patients receiving phenytoin, primidone, and phenobarbital sheds doubt on the advantage of adding phenobarbital to a regimen of phenytoin and primidone.

REFERENCES:

Windorfer A. Drug interaction during anticonvulsive therapy. *Int J Clin Pharmacol.* 1976;14:236.

Fincham RW, et al. The influence of diphenylhydantoin on primidone metabolism. *Arch Neurol.* 1974;30:259-262.

Callaghan N, et al. The effect of anticonvulsant drugs which induce liver enzymes on derived and ingested phenobarbitone levels. *Acta Neurol Scand.* 1977;56:1-6.

Gallagher BB, et al. Primidone, diphenylhydantoin and phenobarbital. Aspects of acute and chronic toxicity. *Neurology.* 1973;23:145-149.

Wilson JT, et al. Chronic and severe phenobarbital intoxication in a child treated with primidone and diphenylhydantoin. *J Pediatr.* 1973;83:484-489.

Phenytoin (eg, *Dilantin*)

Pyridoxine (Vitamin B₆)

SUMMARY: There is limited evidence that large doses of pyridoxine may reduce phenytoin serum concentrations.

RISK FACTORS:

➡ ***Dosage Regimen.*** The potential effect was seen with very large doses of pyridoxine; smaller doses, such as in multivitamins, probably have a minimal effect.

RELATED DRUGS: No information is available.

MANAGEMENT OPTIONS:

➡ ***Monitor.*** No special precautions appear necessary when small doses of pyridoxine (as in multivitamins) are given to patients receiving phenytoin. Monitoring for reduced serum phenytoin concentrations is probably warranted if large doses of pyridoxine are used.

REFERENCES:

Hansson O, et al. Pyridoxine and serum concentrations of phenytoin and phenobarbitone. *Lancet.* 1976;1:256.

Phenytoin (eg, *Dilantin*)

Quetiapine (*Seroquel*)

SUMMARY: Preliminary results suggest that phenytoin substantially increases the elimination of quetiapine; reduced quetiapine effect would be expected, but more study is needed.

RISK FACTORS: No specific risk factors are known.

RELATED DRUGS: No information is available.

MANAGEMENT OPTIONS:

➡ ***Monitor.*** Observe patient for altered quetiapine response if phenytoin is initiated, discontinued, or changed in dosage.

REFERENCES:

Product information. Quetiapine (*Seroquel*). Zeneca Pharmaceuticals. 1997.

Phenytoin (eg, *Dilantin*)

Quinidine

SUMMARY: Phenytoin may substantially decrease quinidine serum concentrations.

RISK FACTORS: No specific risk factors are known.

RELATED DRUGS: No information is available.

MANAGEMENT OPTIONS:

➡ ***Monitor.*** Starting or stopping phenytoin therapy in patients receiving quinidine may necessitate a change in quinidine dosage.

REFERENCES:

Data JL, et al. Interaction of quinidine with anticonvulsant drugs. *N Engl J Med.* 1976;294:699-702.

Urbano AM. Phenytoin-quinidine interaction in a patient with recurrent ventricular tachyarrhythmias. *N Engl J Med*. 1982;308:225.

Kroboth FJ, et al. Phenytoin-theophylline-quinidine interaction. *N Engl J Med*. 1983;308:725.

Phenytoin (eg, *Dilantin*)

Rifampin (eg, *Rifadin*)

SUMMARY: Pharmacokinetic data and a case report indicate that rifampin decreases serum phenytoin concentrations; adjustments in the phenytoin dose may be needed.

RISK FACTORS: No specific risk factors are known.

RELATED DRUGS: No information is available.

MANAGEMENT OPTIONS:

➡ *Circumvent/Minimize.* The phenytoin dose may require adjustment if rifampin is added or removed from a patient's regimen.

➡ *Monitor.* Carefully monitor patients on phenytoin therapy who receive rifampin for reduced serum phenytoin concentrations.

REFERENCES:

Kay L, et al. Influence of rifampicin and isoniazid on the kinetics of phenytoin. *Br J Clin Pharmacol*. 1985;20:323-326.

Wagner JC. Rifampin-phenytoin drug interaction. *Drug Intell Clin Pharm*. 1984;18:497.

Phenytoin (eg, *Dilantin*)

Simvastatin (*Zocor*)

SUMMARY: A woman on simvastatin developed increased total cholesterol after phenytoin was added to her therapy. Although the effect is consistent with the known interactive properties of the drugs, additional information is needed to determine the clinical importance of this interaction.

RISK FACTORS: No specific risk factors are known.

RELATED DRUGS: Like simvastatin, lovastatin (*Mevacor*) is extensively metabolized by CYP3A4, and would be expected to interact with phenytoin in a similar manner. Atorvastatin does not undergo as much first pass metabolism by CYP3A4 as simvastatin or lovastatin, and would not be expected to interact to the same degree. Fluvastatin is metabolized primarily by CYP2A9, an isozyme which, like CYP3A4, is susceptible to enzyme induction. Pravastatin (*Pravachol*) is not metabolized to a clinically important extent by cytochrome P450 isozymes, and would not be expected to interact with phenytoin or other enzyme inducers.

MANAGEMENT OPTIONS:

➡ *Consider Alternative.* If phenytoin or another enzyme inducer appears to be inhibiting the effect of simvastatin or lovastatin, consider using pravastatin as an alternative. Theoretically, enzyme inducers would not affect pravastatin. The effect of atorvastatin may be reduced by enzyme inducers, but probably to a lesser extent than simvastatin and lovastatin.

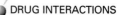

➡ **Monitor.** Monitor patients receiving simvastatin or lovastatin with phenytoin or other enzyme inducers for reduced cholesterol-lowering effect.

REFERENCES:

Murphy MJ, et al. Efficacy of statin therapy: possible effect of phenytoin. *Postgrad Med J.* 1999;75;359-360.

Phenytoin (eg, *Dilantin*)
Sucralfate (*Carafate*)

SUMMARY: Sucralfate modestly reduces the GI absorption of phenytoin, but the clinical importance of this effect is not established.

RISK FACTORS: No specific risk factors are known.

RELATED DRUGS: No information is available.

MANAGEMENT OPTIONS:

➡ **Circumvent/Minimize.** Although any reduction in phenytoin absorption is likely to be modest, it would be prudent to give phenytoin 2 hours before or 6 hours after sucralfate and keep the interval between the drugs as constant as possible.

➡ **Monitor.** Monitor for altered phenytoin response if sucralfate is initiated, discontinued, or if the interval between the drugs is changed.

REFERENCES:

Smart HL, et al. The effects of sucralfate upon phenytoin absorption in man. *Br J Clin Pharmacol.* 1985;20:238-240.

Hall TG, et al. Effect of sucralfate on phenytoin bioavailability. *Drug Intell Clin Pharm.* 1986;20:607–611.

Phenytoin (eg, *Dilantin*)
Sulfaphenazole

SUMMARY: Some sulfonamides, including sulfaphenazole, appears to increase serum phenytoin concentrations; adjustment of the phenytoin dose may be required.

RISK FACTORS: No specific risk factors are known.

RELATED DRUGS: Sulfamethoxazole (*Gantanol*) appears to increase phenytoin half-life only modestly. Phenytoin half-life increased from an average of 11.3 hours before, to 20.5 hours after, sulfamethizole administration (4 g/day for 7 days). Sulfamethizole also inhibits phenytoin metabolism. Sulfisoxazole, sulfadimethoxine, and sulfamethoxypyridazine do not appear to inhibit phenytoin metabolism.

MANAGEMENT OPTIONS:

➡ **Consider Alternative.** Consider using a sulfonamide that does not inhibit phenytoin metabolism.

➡ **Monitor.** Monitor patients for increased phenytoin serum concentrations and signs of phenytoin toxicity (eg, ataxia, nystagmus, mental impairment) when sulfamethizole or sulfaphenazole is started. Stopping these sulfonamides may cause a fall in serum phenytoin concentrations.

REFERENCES:

Siersbaek-Nielsen K, et al. Sulfamethizole-induced inhibition of diphenylhydantoin and tolbutamide metabolism in man. *Clin Pharmacol Ther*. 1973;14:148. Abstract.

Hansen JM, et al. Dicumarol-induced diphenylhydantoin intoxication. *Lancet*. 1966;2:265.

Christensen LK, et al. Inhibition of drug metabolism by chloramphenicol. *Lancet*. 1969;2:1397.

Lunde PKM, et al. Plasma protein binding of diphenylhydantoin in man. Interaction with other drugs and the effect of temperature and plasma dilution. *Clin Pharmacol Ther*. 1970;11:846.

Lumholtz B, et al. Sulfamethizole-induced inhibition of diphenylhydantoin, tolbutamide, and warfarin metabolism. *Clin Pharmacol Ther*. 1975;17:731.

Hansen JM, et al. The effect of different sulfonamides on phenytoin metabolism in man. *Acta Med Scand*. 1979;624(Suppl.):106.

Phenytoin (eg, *Dilantin*)
Sulthiame (*Ospolot*)

SUMMARY: Sulthiame may increase serum phenytoin concentrations; phenytoin intoxication has occurred in some patients receiving both drugs.

RISK FACTORS: No specific risk factors are known.

RELATED DRUGS: No information is available.

MANAGEMENT OPTIONS:

➡ *Monitor.* Monitor patients receiving both sulthiame and phenytoin for signs of phenytoin intoxication (eg, ataxia, nystagmus, mental impairment, involuntary muscular movements, seizures); reduce the phenytoin dose if necessary.

REFERENCES:

Richens A, et al. Phenytoin intoxication caused by sulthiame. *Lancet*. 1973;2:1442. Letter.

Morselli PL, et al. Effect of sulthiame on blood and brain levels of diphenylhydantoin in the rat. *Biochem Pharmacol*. 1970;19:1846.

Hansen JM, et al. Sulthiame (*Ospolot*) as inhibitor of diphenylhydantoin metabolism. *Epilepsia*. 1968;9:17.

Kariks J, et al. Serum folic acid and phenytoin levels in permanently hospitalized epileptic patients receiving anticonvulsant drug therapy. *Med J Aust*. 1971;2:368.

Houghton GW, et al. Phenytoin intoxication induced by sulthiame in epileptic patients. *J Neurol Neurosurg Psychiatry*. 1974;37:275.

Phenytoin (eg, *Dilantin*)
Tacrolimus (*Prograf*)

SUMMARY: Phenytoin probably reduces tacrolimus blood concentrations; increased tacrolimus dosage may be needed.

RISK FACTORS: No specific risk factors are known.

RELATED DRUGS: Other enzyme inducers such as aminoglutethimide (*Cytadren*), barbiturates, carbamazepine (eg, *Tegretol*), glutethimide (*Doriden*), primidone (eg, *Mysoline*), rifabutin (*Mycobutin*), and rifampin (eg, *Rifadin*) also may reduce tacrolimus blood concentrations.

MANAGEMENT OPTIONS:

➡ *Monitor.* Monitor for subtherapeutic tacrolimus blood concentrations if phenytoin or other enzyme inducers are used concurrently.

REFERENCES:

Thompson PA, et al. Tacrolimus-phenytoin interaction. *Ann Pharmacother*. 1996;30:544. Letter.

 Phenytoin (eg, *Dilantin*)

Teniposide (*Vumon*)

SUMMARY: Phenytoin substantially increased the systemic clearance of teniposide and may reduce teniposide's efficacy.

RISK FACTORS: No specific risk factors are known.

RELATED DRUGS: No information is available.

MANAGEMENT OPTIONS:

➡ *Monitor.* Monitor for altered teniposide effect if phenytoin is initiated, discontinued, or changed in dosage; adjust teniposide dose as needed.

REFERENCES:

Baker, et al. Increased teniposide clearance with concomitant anticonvulsant therapy. *J Clin Oncol*. 1992;10:311.

 Phenytoin (eg, *Dilantin*)

Theophylline (eg, *Theo-Dur*)

SUMMARY: Phenytoin reduces serum theophylline concentrations and may increase theophylline dosage requirements. Also, theophylline may decrease serum phenytoin concentrations, but the clinical importance of this latter effect is not established.

RISK FACTORS: No specific risk factors are known.

RELATED DRUGS: Other enzyme inducers also are likely to enhance theophylline metabolism.

MANAGEMENT OPTIONS:

➡ *Monitor.* Be alert for the need to increase the theophylline dose when phenytoin is started and decrease the dose when phenytoin is stopped. Patients on chronic phenytoin therapy may require larger-than-expected theophylline doses. Also monitor for a reduced phenytoin response in patients receiving theophylline.

REFERENCES:

Miller M, et al. Influence of phenytoin on theophylline clearance. *Clin Pharmacol Ther*. 1984;35:666.

Marquis JF, et al. Phenytoin-theophylline interaction. *N Engl J Med*. 1982;307:1189.

Taylor JW, et al. The interaction of phenytoin and theophylline. *Drug Intell Clin Pharm*. 1980;14:638.

Reed RC, et al. Phenytoin-theophylline-quinidine interaction. *N Engl J Med*. 1983;308:724.

Sklar SJ, et al. Enhanced theophylline clearance secondary to phenytoin therapy. *Drug Intell Clin Pharm*. 1985;19:34.

Phenytoin (eg, *Dilantin*)

Thyroid

SUMMARY: Limited evidence indicates phenytoin may increase thyroid replacement dose requirements in some patients.

RISK FACTORS: No specific risk factors are known.

RELATED DRUGS: No information is available.

MANAGEMENT OPTIONS:

➡ *Monitor.* In patients on thyroid replacement, starting or stopping phenytoin therapy may increase or decrease thyroid dose requirements, respectively. Also, give patients requiring thyroid replacement therapy IV phenytoin with caution, especially if they also have a cardiac disease.

REFERENCES:

Fulop M, et al. Possible diphenylhydantoin-induced arrhythmia in hypothyroidism. *JAMA.* 1966;196:454.

Blackshear JL, et al. Thyroxine replacement requirements in hypothyroid patients receiving phenytoin. *Ann Intern Med.* 1983;99:341.

Phenytoin (eg, *Dilantin*)

Ticlopidine (*Ticlid*)

SUMMARY: Patients have developed phenytoin toxicity after ticlopidine was added to their therapy; it may be necessary to reduce phenytoin dose in the presence of ticlopidine.

RISK FACTORS: No specific risk factors are known.

RELATED DRUGS: No information is available.

MANAGEMENT OPTIONS:

➡ *Monitor.* Monitor for altered phenytoin effect if ticlopidine is initiated, discontinued, or changed in dosage; adjust phenytoin dose as needed. If phenytoin is initiated in the presence of ticlopidine therapy, it would be prudent to begin with conservative doses of phenytoin.

REFERENCES:

Rindone JP, et al. Phenytoin toxicity associated with ticlopidine administration. *Arch Intern Med.* 1996;156:1113. Letter.

Privitera M, et al. Axute phenytoin toxicity followed by seizure break-though from a ticlopidine-phenytoin interaction. *Arch Neurol.* 1996;53:1191.

Riva R, et al. Ticlopidine impairs phenytoin clearance: a case report. *Neurology.* 1996;46:1172.

Phenytoin (eg, *Dilantin*)

Tolbutamide (eg, *Orinase*)

SUMMARY: Although excessive phenytoin doses may result in hyperglycemia, alteration in glucose tolerance appears unlikely in patients with free serum phenytoin concentrations within the usual therapeutic range. Tolbutamide may transiently increase free serum phenytoin concentrations, but the incidence of toxicity from this effect is unknown.

RISK FACTORS: No specific risk factors are known.

RELATED DRUGS: The effect of other sulfonylureas on phenytoin is not well established, although one possible case of tolazamide (eg, *Tolinase*)-induced phenytoin toxicity has been reported.

MANAGEMENT OPTIONS:

➡ ***Monitor.*** Monitor for alterations in antidiabetic drug requirements if phenytoin therapy is started, stopped, or changed in dosage. Warn patients stabilized on phenytoin of the possibility of transient phenytoin toxicity (eg, ataxia, dizziness, nausea, headache) when tolbutamide therapy is begun.

REFERENCES:

Klein JP. Diphenylhydantoin intoxication associated with hyperglycemia. *J Pediatr.* 1966;69:463.

Dahl JR. Diphenylhydantoin toxic psychosis with associated hyperglycemia. *Calif Med.* 1967;107:345.

Peters BH, et al. Hyperglycemia with relative hypoinsulinemia in diphenylhydantoin toxicity. *N Engl J Med.* 1969;281:91.

Sanbar SS, et al. Diabetogenic effect of *Dilantin* (diphenylhydantoin). *Diabetes.* 1967;16:533.

Fariss BL, et al. Diphenylhydantoin-induced hyperglycemia and impaired insulin release. *Diabetes.* 1971;20:177.

Malherbe C, et al. Effect of diphenylhydantoin on insulin secretion in man. *N Engl J Med.* 1972;286:339.

Saudek CD, et al. Phenytoin in the treatment of diabetic symmetrical polyneuropathy. *Clin Pharmacol Ther.* 1977;22:196.

Millichap JG. Hyperglycemic effect of diphenylhydantoin. *N Engl J Med.* 1969;281:447.

Wesseling H, et al. Diphenylhydantoin (DPH) and tolbutamide in man. *Eur J Clin Pharmacol.* 1975;8:75.

Beech E, et al. Phenytoin toxicity produced by tolbutamide. *BMJ.* 1988;297:1613.

Phenytoin (eg, *Dilantin*)

Trimethoprim (eg, *Proloprim*)

SUMMARY: Trimethoprim may increase serum phenytoin concentrations; phenytoin toxicity may occur in some patients.

RISK FACTORS: No specific risk factors are known.

RELATED DRUGS: Phenytoin half-life was similarly prolonged by trimethoprim-sulfamethoxazole (eg, *Bactrim*), but sulfamethoxazole (*Gantanol*) alone produced only a small increase in phenytoin half-life.

MANAGEMENT OPTIONS:

➡ **Monitor.** Monitor for signs of phenytoin toxicity (eg, nystagmus, ataxia, mental impairment) when trimethoprim is given concurrently with phenytoin. Serum phenytoin determinations would be useful if the interaction is suspected.

REFERENCES:

Hansen JM, et al. The effect of different sulfonamides on phenytoin metabolism in man. *Acta Med Scand.* 1979;624(Suppl.):106.

Phenytoin (eg, *Dilantin*)

Valproic Acid (eg, *Depakene*)

SUMMARY: Valproic acid can increase, decrease, or have no effect on total phenytoin plasma concentrations. Phenytoin may decrease serum valproic acid concentrations.

RISK FACTORS: No specific risk factors are known.

RELATED DRUGS: No information is available.

MANAGEMENT OPTIONS:

➡ **Monitor.** Patients receiving phenytoin may not require an alteration in the dose of phenytoin when valproic acid therapy is initiated because the free serum concentration of phenytoin may not change. Nevertheless, watch for signs of phenytoin toxicity (eg, ataxia, nystagmus, mental impairment, involuntary muscular movements, seizures) when valproic acid is used concurrently. The decreased total serum phenytoin concentrations seen during the first few weeks of valproic acid therapy should not prompt an increase in phenytoin dose unless poor seizure control occurs concurrently. Free phenytoin in plasma concentrations should be followed whenever possible because total phenytoin concentrations may be altered without a change in the free phenytoin plasma concentration.

REFERENCES:

Bardy A, et al. Valproate may lower serum-phenytoin. *Lancet.* 1976;2:1297. Letter.

Patsalos PN, et al. Valproate may lower serum-phenytoin. *Lancet.* 1977;1:50. Letter.

Patsalos PN, et al. Effect of sodium valproate on plasma protein binding of diphenylhydantoin. *J Neurol Neurosurg Psychiatr.* 1977;40:570.

Windorfer A, et al. Elevation of diphenylhydantoin and primidone serum concentration by addition of dipropylacetate, a new anticonvulsant drug. *Acta Paediatr Scand.* 1975;64:771.

Reunanen MI, et al. Low serum valproic acid concentrations in epileptic patients on combination therapy. *Curr Ther Res.* 1980;28:456.

Dahlqvist R, et al. Decreased plasma protein binding of phenytoin in patients on valproic acid. *Br J Clin Pharmacol.* 1979;8:547.

Sansom LN, et al. Interaction between phenytoin and valproate. *Med J Aust.* 1980;2:212.

Monks A, et al. Effect of single doses of sodium valproate on serum phenytoin levels and protein binding in epileptic patients. *Clin Pharmacol Ther.* 1980;27:89.

Bruni J, et al. Interactions of valproic acid with phenytoin. *Neurology.* 1980;30:1233.

Miles MV, et al. Predictability of unbound antiepileptic drug concentrations in children treated with valproic acid and phenytoin. *Clin Pharm.* 1988;7:688.

Phenytoin (eg, *Dilantin*)

Vigabatrin (*Sabril*)

SUMMARY: Vigabatrin has been found to decrease the serum concentrations of phenytoin 20% to 30%.

RISK FACTORS: No specific risk factors are known.

RELATED DRUGS: No information is available.

MANAGEMENT OPTIONS:

➡ ***Monitor.*** Monitor phenytoin plasma concentrations for 1 month after initiation or removal of vigabatrin therapy. Patients receiving phenytoin may require an increase in the dose of phenytoin when vigabatrin therapy is initiated.

REFERENCES:

Rimmer EM, et al. Double blind study of gamma-vinyl-GABA in patients with refractory epilepsy. *Lancet.* 1984;i:189.

Tartara A, et al. Vigabatrin in the treatment of epilepsy: a long-term follow-up study. *J Neurol Neurosurg Psych.* 1989;52:467.

Rimmer EM, et al. Interaction between vigabatrin and phenytoin. *Br J Clin Pharmacol.* 1989;27(Suppl. 1):S27.

Gatti G, et al. Vigabatrin induced decrease in serum phenytoin concentration does not involve a change in phenytoin bioavailability. *Br J Clin Pharmacol.* 1993;35:603.

 Phenytoin (eg, *Dilantin*)

Warfarin (eg, *Coumadin*)

SUMMARY: Initiation of phenytoin therapy may transiently increase the hypoprothrombinemic response to warfarin (and probably other oral anticoagulants). This is followed within 1 to 2 weeks by an inhibition of the hypoprothrombinemic response. Patients on chronic phenytoin therapy may require larger-than-expected doses of oral anticoagulants. Dicumarol and phenprocoumon may increase serum phenytoin concentrations, whereas warfarin does not appear to do so.

RISK FACTORS: No specific risk factors are known.

RELATED DRUGS: Interactions of phenytoin with oral anticoagulants other than warfarin, dicumarol, and phenprocoumon are not established.

MANAGEMENT OPTIONS:

➡ ***Consider Alternative.*** Warfarin is preferable to dicumarol in patients receiving phenytoin because warfarin does not appear to affect phenytoin serum concentrations.

➡ ***Monitor.*** Monitor for altered oral anticoagulant effect if phenytoin is initiated, discontinued, or changed in dosage. Adjust the anticoagulant dose as needed. If an oral anticoagulant is started in the presence of phenytoin therapy, remember that the anticoagulant dosage requirements may be greater than usual.

REFERENCES:

Andreasen PB, et al. Abnormalities in liver function tests during long-term diphenylhydantoin therapy in epileptic outpatients. *Acta Med Scand.* 1973;194:261-264.

Solomon GE, et al. Coagulation defects caused by diphenylhydantoin. *Neurology.* 1972;22:1165-1171.

Nappi JM. Warfarin and phenytoin interaction. *Ann Intern Med.* 1979;90:852.

Taylor JW, et al. Oral anticoagulant-phenytoin interactions. *Drug Intell Clin Pharm.* 1980;14:669.

Hansen JM, et al. Dicumarol-induced diphenylhydantoin intoxication. *Lancet*. 1966;2:265-266.

Hansen JM, et al. Effect of diphenylhydantoin on the metabolism of dicumarol in man. *Acta Med Scand*. 1971;189:15-19.

Rothermich NO. Diphenylhydantoin intoxication. *Lancet*. 1966;2:640.

Skovsted L, et al. The effect of different oral anticoagulants on diphenylhydantoin (DPH) and tolbutamide metabolism. *Acta Med Scand*. 1976;199:513-515.

Pimozide (*Orap*)

Ritonavir (*Norvir*)

SUMMARY: Elevated pimozide concentrations and cardiac arrhythmias may occur if pimozide and ritonavir are coadministered.

RISK FACTORS: No specific risk factors are known.

RELATED DRUGS: Other antiviral agents that inhibit CYP3A4 (eg, amprenavir [*Agenerase*], delavirdine [*Rescriptor*], indinavir [*Crixivan*], nelfinavir [*Viracept*], saquinavir [eg, *Fortovase*]) should be avoided in patients taking pimozide.

MANAGEMENT OPTIONS:

➡ *Use Alternative.* Do not administer ritonavir or other antiviral agents that inhibit CYP3A4 to patients receiving pimozide.

➡ *Monitor.* If ritonavir is coadministered with pimozide, monitor the ECG for evidence of QTc prolongation.

REFERENCES:
Product Information. Pimozide (*Orap*). Gate Pharmaceuticals. 1999.

Pimozide (*Orap*)

Thioridazine (eg, *Mellaril*) AVOID

SUMMARY: Pimozide may produce additive prolongation of the QT interval with thioridazine and thus may increase the risk of ventricular arrhythmias; avoid concurrent use.

RISK FACTORS:

➡ *Hypokalemia.* The corrected QT interval (QTc) may be prolonged in patients with hypokalemia, increasing the risk of this interaction. Any other factor that may prolong the QTc interval would also increase the risk of this interaction.

RELATED DRUGS: Several phenothiazines have been associated with prolongation of the QT interval, but clinical evidence suggests that the risk of excessive prolongation is greater with thioridazine than other phenothiazines.

MANAGEMENT OPTIONS:

➡ *AVOID COMBINATION.* Although the risk of this combination is not well established, it would be prudent to avoid concurrent use.

REFERENCES:
Hartigan-Go K, et al. Concentration-related pharmacodynamic effects of thioridazine and its metabolites in humans. *Clin Pharmacol Ther*. 1996;60:543-553.

"Dear Doctor or Pharmacist" Letter, Novartis Pharmaceuticals, July 7, 2000.

Pimozide (*Orap*)

Verapamil (eg, *Calan*)

SUMMARY: Elevated pimozide concentrations and cardiac arrhythmias may occur if pimozide and verapamil are coadministered.

RISK FACTORS: No specific risk factors are known.

RELATED DRUGS: Diltiazem (eg, *Cardizem*) also inhibits CYP3A4 and should be avoided in patients taking pimozide. The dihydropyridine calcium channel blockers do not appear to inhibit CYP3A4.

MANAGEMENT OPTIONS:

➡ **Use Alternative.** Treat patients receiving pimozide who require treatment with a calcium channel blocker with a dihydropyridine calcium channel blocker such as amlodipine (*Norvasc*) or felodipine (*Plendil*).

➡ **Monitor.** If verapamil or diltiazem is coadministered with pimozide, monitor the ECG for evidence of QTc prolongation.

REFERENCES:

Product Information. Pimozide (*Orap*). Gate Pharmaceuticals. 1999.

Pimozide (*Orap*)

Ziprasidone (*Geodon*)

SUMMARY: Ziprasidone and pimozide can prolong the corrected QT interval (QTc) interval on the electrocardiogram (ECG). Theoretically, this could increase the risk of ventricular arrhythmias such as torsades de pointes.

RISK FACTORS:

➡ **Hypokalemia.** The QTc on the ECG may be prolonged in patients with hypokalemia, increasing the risk of this interaction.

➡ **Miscellaneous.** Other factors that may prolong the QTc interval (eg, hypomagnesemia, bradycardia, impaired liver function, hypothyroidism) also may increase the risk of ventricular arrhythmias.

RELATED DRUGS: Available data suggest that ziprasidone produces less QTc prolongation than thioridazine (*Mellaril*), but about twice that of quetiapine (*Seroquel*), risperidone (*Risperdal*), haloperidol (*Haldol*), and olanzapine (*Zyprexa*).

MANAGEMENT OPTIONS:

➡ **Use Alternative.** Given the theoretical risk and the fact that pimozide is listed in the ziprasidone product information as "contraindicated," it would be prudent to use an alternative to one of the drugs (see Related Drugs).

➡ **Monitor.** If pimozide and ziprasidone are used concurrently, monitor for evidence of arrhythmias (eg, syncope) and for prolonged QT intervals.

REFERENCES:

De Ponti F, et al. QT-interval prolongation by non-cardiac drugs: lessons to be learned from recent experience. *Eur J Clin Pharmacol.* 2000;56:1-18.

Product information. Ziprasidone (*Geodon*). Pfizer Pharmaceuticals. 2001.

Briefing Information, Psychopharmacological Drugs Advisory Committee, U.S. Food and Drug Administration, July 19, 2000.

Pirmenol ▼ ③

Rifampin (eg, *Rifadin*)

SUMMARY: Pirmenol serum concentrations are markedly reduced by rifampin administration; the changes are likely to be clinically significant.

RISK FACTORS: No specific risk factors are known.

RELATED DRUGS: No information is available.

MANAGEMENT OPTIONS:

➡ *Monitor.* Carefully monitor patients stabilized on pirmenol for loss of antiarrhythmic efficacy during rifampin administration. Increased pirmenol doses may be required.

REFERENCES:

Stringer KA, et al. Enhanced pirmenol elimination by rifampin. *J Clin Pharmacol.* 1988;28:1094-1097.

Piroxicam (*Feldene*)

Warfarin (eg, *Coumadin*)

SUMMARY: Preliminary clinical evidence indicates that piroxicam may increase the hypoprothrombinemic response to warfarin, acenocoumarol, and possibly other oral anticoagulants.

RISK FACTORS:

➡ *Concurrent Diseases.* Patients with peptic ulcer disease (PUD) or a history of GI bleeding are probably at greater risk.

RELATED DRUGS: All NSAIDs inhibit platelet function, cause gastric erosions, and probably increase the risk of GI bleeding. However, some NSAIDs such as ibuprofen (eg, *Advil*), naproxen (eg, *Naprosyn*), or diclofenac (*Voltaren*) may be less likely to increase oral anticoagulant-induced hypoprothrombinemia than other NSAIDs.

MANAGEMENT OPTIONS:

➡ *Avoid Unless Benefit Outweighs Risk.* Since all NSAIDs probably increase the risk of GI bleeding in patients on oral anticoagulants, use the combination only after careful consideration of the benefit vs risk. If an NSAID must be used with an oral anticoagulant, it would be prudent to use NSAIDs that are unlikely to affect the hypoprothrombinemic response to oral anticoagulants. (See Related Drugs). If the NSAID is being used as an analgesic or antipyretic, acetaminophen is probably safer to use with oral anticoagulants. Nonacetylated salicylates (eg, choline salicylate, magnesium salicylate, salsalate, sodium salicylate) are probably also safer with oral anticoagulants than NSAIDs because such salicylates have minimal effects on platelet function and the gastric mucosa.

➡ *Monitor.* If any NSAID is used with an oral anticoagulant, monitor carefully the prothrombin time and watch for evidence of bleeding, especially from the GI tract.

REFERENCES:

Dahl SL. Pharmacology, clinical efficacy, and adverse effects of piroxicam, a new nonsteroidal antiinflammatory agent. *Pharmacotherapy.* 1982;2:80.

Rhodes RS, et al. A warfarin-piroxicam drug interaction. *Drug Intell Clin Pharm.* 1985;19:556.

Emery P. Gastrointestinal blood loss and piroxicam. *Lancet.* 1982;1:1302.

Shorr R,I et al. Concurrent use of nonsteroidal anti-inflammatory drugs and oral anticoagulants places elderly persons at high risk for hemorrhagic peptic ulcer disease. *Arch Intern Med.* 1993;153:1665.

2 Potassium

Spironolactone (eg, *Aldactone*)

SUMMARY: Coadministration of potassium supplements and spironolactone may result in severe hyperkalemia.

RISK FACTORS:

➡ *Other Drugs.* Coadministration of ACE inhibitors may enhance the risk.

➡ *Concurrent Diseases.* Patients with impaired renal function or severe diabetes may be at greater risk. Patients with diet-controlled diabetes do not appear to be predisposed particularly to potassium-sparing diuretic-induced hyperkalemia if no other predisposing factors are present.

➡ *Effects of Age.* The elderly may be at a greater risk.

➡ *Diet/Food.* A high potassium diet (including salt substitutes) may enhance the risk of hyperkalemia.

RELATED DRUGS: Amiloride (*Midamor*) and triamterene (*Dyrenium*) also can result in hyperkalemia when combined with potassium supplements.

MANAGEMENT OPTIONS:

➡ *Avoid Unless Benefit Outweighs Risk.* Use the combination of potassium-sparing diuretics and potassium supplementation only for severe or refractory hypokalemia. Particular caution is needed in predisposed patients (eg, an elderly diabetic with impaired renal function).

➡ *Monitor.* If the combination is used, monitor serum potassium concentrations carefully.

REFERENCES:

Mashford ML, et al. Spironolactone and ammonium and potassium chloride. *BMJ.* 1972;4:299. Letter.

Kalbian VV. Iatrogenic hyperkalemic paralysis with electrocardiographic changes. *South Med J.* 1974;67:342.

Shapiro S, et al. Fatal reactions among medical inpatients. *JAMA.* 1972;216:467.

Greenblatt DJ. Adverse reactions to spironolactone: a report from the Boston Collaborative Drug Surveillance Program. *Clin Pharmacol Ther.* 1973;14:136. Abstract.

Simborg DN. Medication prescribing on a university medical service—the incidence of drug combinations with potential adverse interactions. *Johns Hopkins Med J.* 1976;139:23.

Lowenthal DT, et al. Effects of amiloride on oral glucose loading, serum potassium, renin, and aldosterone in diet-controlled diabetes. *Clin Pharmacol Ther.* 1980;27:671.

Potassium

Triamterene (*Dyrenium*)

SUMMARY: Potassium supplementation in patients taking triamterene may result in severe hyperkalemia.

RISK FACTORS:

➡ *Other Drugs.* Coadministration of angiotensin-converting enzyme inhibitors may increase the risk.

➡ *Concurrent Diseases.* Patients with impaired renal function or severe diabetes may be at a greater risk. Patients with diet-controlled diabetes do not appear to be particularly predisposed to potassium-sparing, diuretic-induced hyperkalemia if no other predisposing factors are present.

➡ *Effects of Age.* Elderly patients may be at a greater risk.

➡ *Diet/Food.* A high-potassium diet (including salt substitutes) may place a patient at greater risk.

RELATED DRUGS: Amiloride (*Midamor*) and spironolactone (eg, *Aldactone*) also can result in hyperkalemia when combined with potassium supplements.

MANAGEMENT OPTIONS:

➡ *Avoid Unless Benefit Outweighs Risk.* Use the combination of potassium-sparing diuretics and potassium supplementation only for severe or refractory hypokalemia. Particular caution is needed in predisposed patients (eg, an elderly diabetic patient with impaired renal function).

➡ *Monitor.* If the combination is used, monitor serum potassium concentrations carefully.

REFERENCES:

Lowenthal DT, et al. Effects of amiloride on oral glucose loading, serum potassium, renin, and aldosterone in diet-controlled diabetes. *Clin Pharmacol Ther.* 1980;27:671–676.

O'Reilly MV, et al. Transvenous pacemaker failure induced by hyperkalemia. *JAMA.* 1974;228:336–337.

Prazosin (eg, *Minipress*)

Propranolol (eg, *Inderal*)

SUMMARY: The first-dose syncopal response to prazosin may be enhanced by beta blockade.

RISK FACTORS: No specific risk factors are known.

RELATED DRUGS: A similar increase in the incidence of first-dose hypotensive reaction was observed with combined use of prazosin and alprenolol in hypertensive patients. The combination of other beta blockers and alpha blockers (eg, terazosin [*Hytrin*]) may produce acute postural hypotension.

MANAGEMENT OPTIONS:

➡ *Circumvent/Minimize.* The addition of propranolol to patients stabilized on prazosin will lessen the likelihood of a syncopal episode. However, monitor for orthostatic blood pressure changes.

➥ *Monitor.* In patients receiving beta blockers, initiate prazosin therapy with caution and with conservative (eg, 50% of normal) doses. Taking the initial prazosin dose at bedtime would be prudent.

REFERENCES:

Seideman P, et al. Prazosin first dose phenomenon during combined treatment with a beta-adrenoceptor in hypertensive patients. *Br J Clin Pharmacol.* 1982;13:865–870.

Rubin P, et al. Studies on the clinical pharmacology of prazosin. II: The influence of indomethacin and of propranolol on the action and disposition of prazosin. *Br J Clin Pharmacol.* 1980;10:33–39.

Graham RM, et al. Prazosin: the first-dose phenomenon. *BMJ.* 1976;4:1293–1294.

Elliott HL, et al. Immediate cardiovascular responses to oral prazosin—effects of concurrent beta-blockers. *Clin Pharmacol Ther.* 1981;29:303–309.

Prazosin (eg, *Minipress*)

Verapamil (eg, *Calan*)

SUMMARY: The combination of verapamil with prazosin can enhance hypotensive effects.

RISK FACTORS: No specific risk factors are known.

RELATED DRUGS: The combination of verapamil and terazosin (*Hytrin*) also has been noted to produce increased pharmacodynamic effect. Verapamil apparently reduces the first-pass metabolism of terazosin. Other calcium channel blockers may have additive hypotensive effects when administered with prazosin, terazosin, or doxazosin (*Cardura*).

MANAGEMENT OPTIONS:

➥ *Circumvent/Minimize.* Smaller doses of prazosin may be indicated when verapamil is coadministered.

➥ *Monitor.* The combination of verapamil and prazosin appears to produce a potent antihypertensive effect. Carefully monitor patients stabilized on one of these drugs for hypotension during the institution of the second drug.

REFERENCES:

Pasanisi F, et al. Combined alpha-adrenoceptor antagonism and calcium channel blockade in normal subjects. *Clin Pharmacol Ther.* 1984;36:716.

Elliott HL, et al. Verapamil and prazosin in essential hypertension: evidence of synergistic combination? *J Cardiovasc Pharmacol.* 1987;10(Suppl. 10):108.

Lenz M, et al. Combined terazosin and verapamil therapy in essential hypertension; haemodynamic interactions. *Clin Pharmacol Ther.* 1991;49:146. Abstract.

Varghese A, et al. Combined terazosin and verapamil therapy in essential hypertension; pharmacokinetic interactions. *Clin Pharmacol Ther.* 1991;49:130. Abstract.

Meredith PA, et al. An additive or synergistic drug interaction: application of concentration-effect modeling. *Clin Pharmacol Ther.* 1992;51:708.

Prednisolone

Rifampin (eg, *Rifadin*)

SUMMARY: Rifampin appears to reduce the effect of corticosteroids like prednisolone significantly in some patients.

RISK FACTORS: No specific risk factors are known.

RELATED DRUGS: It is likely that most corticosteroids would be affected similarly by rifampin.

MANAGEMENT OPTIONS:

➡ *Circumvent/Minimize.* The dose of corticosteroid may require an increase.

➡ *Monitor.* It does not seem necessary to avoid concomitant use of corticosteroids and rifampin, but be alert for evidence of reduced corticosteroid effect.

REFERENCES:

Maisey DN, et al. Rifampicin and cortisone replacement therapy. *Lancet.* 1974;2:896.

Yamada S, et al. Induction of hepatic cortisol-6-hydroxylase by rifampicin. *Lancet.* 1976;2:366.

Edwards OM, et al. Changes in cortisol metabolism following rifampicin therapy. *Lancet.* 1974;2:549.

Buffington GA, et al. Interaction of rifampin and glucocorticoids. *JAMA.* 1976;236:1958.

van Marle W, et al. Concurrent steroid and rifampicin therapy. *BMJ.* 1979;1:1029.

Carrie F, et al. Rifampin-induced nonresponsiveness of giant cell arteritis to prednisone treatment. *Arch Intern Med.* 1994;154:1521.

Primidone (*Mysoline*)

Valproic Acid (*Depakene*)

SUMMARY: Valproic acid may increase serum concentrations of the phenobarbital that is produced from primidone; excessive phenobarbital response may occur.

RISK FACTORS: No specific risk factors are known.

RELATED DRUGS: No information is available.

MANAGEMENT OPTIONS:

➡ *Monitor.* Monitor patients receiving primidone for signs of phenobarbital toxicity when valproate is given concomitantly.

REFERENCES:

Windorfer A, et al. Elevation of diphenylhydantoin and primidone serum concentration by addition of dipropylacetate, a new anticonvulsant drug. *Acta Paediatr Scand.* 1975;64:771.

Probenecid (*Benemid*)

Thiopental (eg, *Pentothal*)

SUMMARY: Probenecid may prolong thiopental anesthesia.

RISK FACTORS: No specific risk factors are known.

RELATED DRUGS: No information is available.

MANAGEMENT OPTIONS:

➡ *Monitor.* Monitor for prolonged anesthesia in patients receiving probenecid.

REFERENCES:

Kaukinen S, et al. Prolongation of thiopentone anaesthesia by probenecid. *Br J Anæsth.* 1980;52:603.

Probenecid (eg, *Benemid*)

Zidovudine (*Retrovir*)

SUMMARY: Probenecid increases the plasma concentration of zidovudine and may allow zidovudine to be administered less frequently and in lower doses.

RISK FACTORS: No specific risk factors are known.

RELATED DRUGS: No information is available.

MANAGEMENT OPTIONS:

➡ ***Circumvent/Minimize.*** Reduce the dose of zidovudine when probenecid is administered concomitantly. The coadministration of probenecid with zidovudine may enable every 8 hours dosing of zidovudine that would be more convenient than taking zidovudine every 4 hours. The decreased total daily dose of zidovudine also would decrease the financial expenditure for this costly medication.

➡ ***Monitor.*** Observe patients for rash and other side effects when both agents are administered.

REFERENCES:

Hedaya MA, et al. Probenecid inhibits the metabolic and renal clearances of zidovudine (AZT) in human volunteers. *Pharm Res.* 1990;7:411.

Kornhauser DM, et al. Probenecid and zidovudine metabolism. *Lancet.* 1989;2:473.

de Mirande P, et al. Alterations of zidovudine pharmacokinetics by probenecid in patients with AIDS or AIDS-related complex. *Clin Pharmacol Ther.* 1989;46:494.

Campion JJ, et al. Effect of probenecid on the pharmacokinetics of zidovudine and zidovudine glucuronide. *Pharmacotherapy.* 1990;10:235. Abstract.

Petty BG, et al. Zidovudine with probenecid: a warning. *Lancet.* 1990;335:1044.

Duckworth AS, et al. Zidovudine with probenecid. *Lancet.* 1990;336:441. Letter.

 Procainamide (eg, *Procan SR*)

Quinidine

SUMMARY: Quinidine markedly increased procainamide serum concentrations in 1 patient; more study is needed.

RISK FACTORS: No specific risk factors are known.

RELATED DRUGS: No information is available.

MANAGEMENT OPTIONS:

➡ ***Circumvent/Minimize.*** Until further data are available, avoid the concomitant use of procainamide and quinidine.

➡ ***Monitor.*** Monitor patients receiving procainamide for antiarrhythmic therapy for an increased response, increased serum concentrations, and toxicity (wide QRS, QT interval) when quinidine is added to their drug regimens. Discontinuing quinidine may reduce the serum concentration and efficacy of coadministered procainamide.

REFERENCES:

Hughes B, et al. Increased procainamide plasma concentrations caused by quinidine: a new drug interaction. *Am Heart J.* 1987;114:908.

Procainamide (eg, *Pronestyl*)

Thioridazine (eg, *Mellaril*)

SUMMARY: Procainamide may produce additive prolongation of the QT interval with thioridazine, and thus may increase the risk of ventricular arrhythmias; avoid concurrent use.

RISK FACTORS:

➡ *Hypokalemia.* The corrected QT interval (QTc) may be prolonged in patients with hypokalemia, thus increasing the risk of this interaction. Any other factor that may prolong the QTc interval would also increase the risk of this interaction.

RELATED DRUGS: Other antiarrhythmics such as amiodarone (eg, *Cordarone*), disopyramide (eg, *Norpace*), and quinidine can also increase the QT interval, and may increase the risk of arrhythmias. Also, amiodarone, propafenone (*Rythmol*), and quinidine are known inhibitors of CYP2D6, and may increase thioridazine serum concentrations. Although a number of antipsychotic drugs have, like thioridazine, have shown to prolong the QT interval, clinical evidence suggests that thioridazine may produce the greatest risk.

MANAGEMENT OPTIONS:

➡ *Use Alternative.* Although the risk of this combination is not well established, it would be prudent to use alternatives for 1 of the drugs (see Related Drugs).

➡ *Monitor.* If the combination must be used, monitor the ECG for evidence of QT prolongation, and monitor for clinical evidence of arrhythmias (eg, syncope).

REFERENCES:

Hartigan-Go K, et al. Concentration-related pharmacodynamic effects of thioridazine and its metabolites in humans. *Clin Pharmacol Ther.* 1996;60:543-53.

"Dear Doctor or Pharmacist" Letter, Novartis Pharmaceuticals, July 7, 2000.

Procainamide (eg, *Pronestyl*)

Trimethoprim (eg, *Proloprim*)

SUMMARY: Trimethoprim significantly increases serum concentrations of procainamide and N-acetylprocainamide (NAPA); cardiac toxicity may result.

RISK FACTORS: No specific risk factors are known.

RELATED DRUGS: No information is available.

MANAGEMENT OPTIONS:

➡ *Monitor.* Monitor serum procainamide and NAPA concentrations. Observe patients for procainamide toxicity (wide QRS, QT interval) when trimethoprim is coadministered.

REFERENCES:

Kosoglou T, et al. Trimethoprim alters the disposition of procainamide and N-acetylprocainamide. *Clin Pharmacol Ther.* 1988;44:467.

Vlasses PH, et al. Trimethoprim inhibition of the renal clearance of procainamide and N-acetylprocainamide. *Arch Intern Med.* 1989;149:1350.

Procarbazine (*Matulane*)

Prochlorperazine (eg, *Compazine*)

SUMMARY: Use of phenothiazines in patients receiving procarbazine has been associated with increased sedation and possibly with increased severity of extrapyramidal symptoms.

RISK FACTORS: No specific risk factors are known.

RELATED DRUGS: Procarbazine purportedly can increase sedation from opiates and barbiturates, but cases in humans are lacking.

MANAGEMENT OPTIONS:

➡ *Monitor.* Instruct patients and families to watch for increased sedation and changes in extrapyramidal symptoms if phenothiazines are used with procarbazine.

REFERENCES:

Brunner KW, et al. A methylhydrazine derivative in Hodgkin's disease and other malignant neoplasms. Therapeutic and toxic effects studied in 51 patients. *Ann Int Med.* 1965;63:69.

Sicher K, et al. Experiences with methylhydrazine. *BMJ.* 1965;1:858.

Sicher K, et al. Methyl-hydrazine in malignant disease. *Lancet.* 1963;2:1278.

Todd ID. Natulan in management of late Hodgkin's disease, other lymphoreticular neoplasms, and malignant melanoma. *BMJ.* 1965;1:628.

Poster DS. Procarbazine-prochlorperazine interaction: an underreported phenomenon. *J Med.* 1978;9:519.

Weiss HD, et al. Neurotoxicity of commonly used antineoplastic agents. *N Engl J Med.* 1974;291:127.

Propafenone (eg, *Rythmol*)

Quinidine

SUMMARY: Quinidine increases propafenone serum concentrations and reduces the serum concentrations of its active metabolite. The result may be no net change in response.

RISK FACTORS:

➡ *Pharmacogenetics.* Rapid propafenone metabolizers may be at increased risk for the interaction.

RELATED DRUGS: No information is available.

MANAGEMENT OPTIONS:

➡ *Circumvent/Minimize.* Take note that in this group of patients, doses of propafenone were reduced an average of 45% before quinidine was initiated. In all likelihood, this attenuated the increase in propafenone concentration and the potential for toxicity to occur. Prophylactic reduction of the propafenone dose may be the most judicious approach.

➡ *Monitor.* Until more data are available, carefully monitor patients stabilized on propafenone for toxicity when quinidine is added.

REFERENCES:

Funck-Brentano C, et al. Genetically-determined interaction between propafenone and low dose quinidine: role of active metabolites in modulating net drug effect. *Br J Clin Pharmacol.* 1989;27:435.

Siddoway LA, et al. Polymorphism of propafenone metabolism and disposition in man: clinical and pharmacokinetic consequences. *Circulation.* 1987;75:785.

Morike KE, et al. Quinidine-enhanced beta-blockade during treatment with propafenone in extensive metabolizer human subjects. *Clin Pharmacol Ther.* 1994;55:28.

Propafenone (eg, *Rythmol*)

Rifampin (eg, *Rifadin*)

SUMMARY: Rifampin significantly reduces propafenone plasma concentrations; loss of antiarrhythmic activity may occur.

RISK FACTORS: No specific risk factors are known.

RELATED DRUGS: Rifabutin (*Mycobutin*) may not be as potent an inducer as rifampin and would be less likely to produce a large reduction in propafenone concentrations.

MANAGEMENT OPTIONS:

➥ *Monitor.* Monitor propafenone plasma concentrations in patients when rifampin is initiated or discontinued. Up to 2 weeks may be required to observe the maximum change in propafenone concentration after rifampin is initiated or discontinued.

REFERENCES:

Dilger K, et al. Consequences of rifampicin on propafenone disposition in extensive and poor metabolizers of CYP2D6. *Pharmacogenetics.* 1999;9:551.

Castel JM, et al. Rifampicin lowers plasma concentrations of propafenone and its antiarrhythmic effect. *Br J Clin Pharmacol.* 1990;30:155.

Propafenone (*Rythmol*)

Theophylline (eg, *Theo-Dur*)

SUMMARY: Case reports suggest that propafenone elevates theophylline plasma concentrations and may produce symptoms of theophylline toxicity.

RISK FACTORS: No specific risk factors are known.

RELATED DRUGS: No information is available.

MANAGEMENT OPTIONS:

➥ *Circumvent/Minimize.* Theophylline doses may require reduction following the addition of propafenone.

➥ *Monitor.* Monitor patients stabilized on theophylline for elevated theophylline concentrations and signs of theophylline toxicity (eg, nausea, anorexia, tremor, tachycardia) if propafenone therapy is added. Discontinuing propafenone may result in subtherapeutic theophylline concentrations.

REFERENCES:

Lee BL, et al. Theophylline toxicity after propafenone treatment: evidence for drug interaction. *Clin Pharmacol Ther.* 1992;51:353-55.

Spinler SA, et al. Propafenone-theophylline interaction. *Pharmacotherapy.* 1993;13:68-71.

2 **Propafenone (*Rythmol*)**

Thioridazine (eg, *Mellaril*)

SUMMARY: Propafenone may increase thioridazine serum concentrations, and thus may increase the risk of ventricular arrhythmias; avoid concurrent use.

RISK FACTORS:

➥ *Pharmacogenetics.* Only patients with the extensive metabolizer CYP2D6 phenotype (EMs) would be expected to experience this interaction. Poor metabolizers (PMs) do not have the gene for production of CYP2D6, and would likely already have high serum concentrations of thioridazine. Approximately 8% of whites are deficient in CYP2D6, but the deficiency is rare in Asians – usually no more than 1%.

➥ *Hypokalemia.* The corrected QT interval (QTc) may be prolonged in patients with hypokalemia, thus increasing the risk of this interaction. Any other factor that may prolong the QTc interval would also increase the risk of this interaction.

RELATED DRUGS: Antiarrhythmics such as amiodarone (eg, *Cordarone*), disopyramide (eg, *Norpace*), procainamide (eg, *Procan SR*), and quinidine can increase the QT interval, and may also increase the risk of arrhythmias. Amiodarone and quinidine, known inhibitors of CYP2D6, may increase thioridazine serum concentrations. Although a number of antipsychotic drugs have, like thioridazine, been shown to prolong the QT interval, clinical evidence suggests that thioridazine may produce the greatest risk.

MANAGEMENT OPTIONS:

➥ *Use Alternative.* Although the risk of this combination is not well established, it would be prudent to use alternatives for 1 of the drugs (see Related Drugs).

➥ *Monitor.* If the combination must be used, monitor the ECG for evidence of QT prolongation, and monitor for clinical evidence of arrhythmias (eg, syncope).

REFERENCES:

Hartigan-Go K, et al. Concentration-related pharmacodynamic effects of thioridazine and its metabolites in humans. *Clin Pharmacol Ther.* 1996;60:543-53.

'Dear Doctor or Pharmacist' Letter, Novartis Pharmaceuticals, July 7, 2000.

3 **Propafenone (*Rythmol*)**

Warfarin (eg, *Coumadin*)

SUMMARY: Propafenone increases warfarin serum concentrations and prolongs the prothrombin time in subjects taking low doses of both drugs.

RISK FACTORS: No specific risk factors are known.

RELATED DRUGS: In a case report, a similar enhancement of anticoagulant effect was noted in a patient taking phenprocoumon and propafenone.

MANAGEMENT OPTIONS:

➥ *Monitor.* Although data from therapeutically anticoagulated patients are limited, the administration of propafenone in antiarrhythmic doses could enhance the anticoagulation effect of warfarin significantly. Monitor patients stabilized on warfarin if propafenone is added or withdrawn from therapy.

REFERENCES:

Kates RE, et al. Interaction between warfarin and propafenone in healthy volunteer subjects. *Clin Pharmacol Ther.* 1987;42:305-11.

Korst HA, et al. Warning: propafenone potentiates the effect of oral anticoagulants. *Med Klin.* 1981;72:349. German

Propoxyphene (eg, *Darvocet-N*)

Warfarin (eg, *Coumadin*)

SUMMARY: Several cases of enhanced hypoprothrombinemic response to warfarin have been reported during the use of a propoxyphene-acetaminophen preparation, but an effect of propoxyphene alone on oral anticoagulant response has not been documented.

RISK FACTORS: No specific risk factors are known.

RELATED DRUGS: No information is available.

MANAGEMENT OPTIONS:

➡ *Monitor.* Although this interaction is not well established, monitor for altered oral anticoagulant effect if propoxyphene is initiated, discontinued, or changed in dosage. Adjust the anticoagulant dose as needed.

REFERENCES:

Orme M, et al. Warfarin and distalgesic interaction. *BMJ.* 1976;1:200.

Jones RV. Warfarin and distalgesic interaction. *BMJ.* 1976;1:460. Letter.

Smith R, et al. Propoxyphene and warfarin interaction. *Drug Intell Clin Pharm.* 1984;18:822.

Justice JL, et al. Analgesic and warfarin. A case that brings up questions and cautions. *Postgrad Med.* 1988;83:217-18.

Propranolol (eg, *Inderal*)

Quinidine

SUMMARY: Quinidine may increase the plasma concentration of propranolol, but the incidence of adverse effects caused by these interactions is unknown. Propranolol does not affect quinidine kinetics.

RISK FACTORS:

➡ *Pharmacogenetics.* Rapid metabolizers of propranolol may be at increased risk to develop the interaction.

RELATED DRUGS: Quinidine decreases the metabolism of metoprolol (*Lopressor*), and timolol (eg, *Blocadren*).

MANAGEMENT OPTIONS:

➡ *Consider Alternative.* Preliminary evidence suggests no effect of quinidine on labetalol pharmacokinetics or pharmacodynamics. Renally excreted beta blockers (eg, atenolol [*Tenormin*]) should be less likely to interact with quinidine because their metabolism is unlikely to be affected by quinidine. Nevertheless, additive cardiac depressant effects cannot be overlooked.

➡ **Monitor.** Carefully monitor concomitant use of quinidine and propranolol. Watch for bradycardia, heart failure, and arrhythmias.

REFERENCES:

Dreifus LS, et al. Propranolol and quinidine in the management of ventricular tachycardia. *JAMA.* 1986;204:736.

Hillestad L, et al. Conversion of chronic atrial fibrillation to sinus rhythm with combined propranolol and quinidine treatment. *Am Heart J.* 1969;77:137.

Kates RE, et al. Disposition kinetics of oral quinidine when administered concurrently with propranolol. *J Clin Pharmacol.* 1979;19:378.

Fors WJ, et al. Evaluation of propranolol and quinidine in the treatment of quinidine-resistant arrhythmias. *Am J Cardiol.* 1971;27:190.

Kessler KM, et al. Quinidine pharmacokinetics in patients with cirrhosis or receiving propranolol. *Am Heart J.* 1978;96:627.

Fenster P, et al. Kinetic evaluation of the propranolol-quinidine combination. *Clin Pharmacol Ther.* 1980;27:450.

Loon NR, et al. Orthostatic hypotension due to quinidine and propranolol. *Am J Med.* 1986;81:1101.

Yasuhara M, et al. Alteration of propranolol pharmacokinetics and pharmacodynamics by quinidine in man. *J Pharmacobiodyn.* 1990;13:681.

Zhou H-H, et al. Quinidine reduces clearance of ± propranolol more than ± propranolol through marked reduction in 4-hydroxylation. *Clin Pharmacol Ther.* 1990;47:686.

Gearhart MO, et al. Lack of effects on labetalol pharmacodynamics with quinidine inhibition of P450IID6. *Pharmacotherapy.* 1991;11:P36. Abstract.

Propranolol (*Inderal*)

Rizatriptan (*Maxalt*)

SUMMARY: Propranolol increases the plasma concentration of rizatriptan.

RISK FACTORS: No specific risk factors are known.

RELATED DRUGS: Metoprolol (*Lopressor*) 100 mg every 12 hours and nadolol (*Corgard*) 80 mg every 12 hours did not interact with rizatriptan. In vitro studies suggest that timolol (*Blocadren*) and atenolol (*Tenormin*) will not interact with rizatriptan. Propranolol has been reported to have no interaction with sumatriptan (*Imitrex*). The effects of other 5-HT agonists and propranolol are not known.

MANAGEMENT OPTIONS:

➡ **Consider Alternative.** The use of metoprolol or nadolol could be considered for patients taking rizatriptan.

➡ **Circumvent/Minimize.** Reduce the dose of rizatriptan to 5 mg for patients receiving propranolol.

➡ **Monitor.** Be alert for increased myocardial ischemia, vasospasms, elevated blood pressure, or dizziness when propranolol and rizatriptan are coadministered.

REFERENCES:

Product information. Rixaptriptan (*Maxalt*). Merck & Co., Inc. 1998.

Scott AK, et al. Lack of an interaction between propranolol and sumatriptan. *Br J Clin Pharmacol.* 1991;32:581.

Propranolol (eg, *Inderal*)

Tacrine (*Cognex*)

SUMMARY: Both tacrine and propranolol can slow the heart rate. Additive bradycardia would be expected, but the risk of adverse consequences from the combination is not known.

RISK FACTORS: No specific risk factors are known.

RELATED DRUGS: Other beta blockers (eg, atenolol, nadolol) may produce similar additive bradycardia.

MANAGEMENT OPTIONS:

➡ *Monitor.* Monitor for excessive bradycardia in patients receiving beta-adrenergic blockers concurrently with tacrine or other cholinergic agents.

REFERENCES:

Sprague DH. Severe bradycardia after neostigmine in a patient taking propranolol to control paroxysmal atrial tachycardia. *Anesthesiology.* 1975;42:208-210.

Seidl DC, et al. Prolonged bradycardia after neostigmine administration in a patient taking nadolol. *Anesth Analg.* 1984;63:365-367.

Baraka A, et al. Severe bradycardia following physostigmine in the presence of beta-adrenergic blockade — a case report. *Middle East J Anesthesiol.* 1984;7:291-293.

Eldor J, et al. Prolonged bradycardia and hypotension after neostigmine administration in a patient receiving atenolol. *Anaesthesia.* 1987;42:1294-1297.

Taylor P. Agents acting at the neuromuscular junction and autonomic ganglia. In: Gilman AG, Rall TW, Nies AS, Taylor P, eds. The Pharmacological Basis of Therapeutics. 8th ed. New York: Pergamon Press; 1990:166–186.

Hartvig P, et al. Pharmacokinetics and effects of 9-amino-1,2,3,4-tetrahydroacridine in the immediate postoperative period in neurosurgical patients. *J Clin Anesth.* 1991;3:137-142.

Propranolol (eg, *Inderal*)

Tetracaine (*Pontocaine*)

SUMMARY: The use of propranolol with tetracaine or other local anesthetics, particularly those containing epinephrine, may enhance sympathomimetic side effects resulting in hypertensive reactions. Acute discontinuation of beta blockers before local anesthesia may increase the risk of side effects caused by the anesthetic.

RISK FACTORS:

➡ *Anesthetic Combinations.* Local anesthetics containing epinephrine may be at risk for hypertensive reactions.

RELATED DRUGS: Bupivacaine and lidocaine appear to interact similarly with propranolol. Cardioselective beta blocker (eg, metoprolol [*Lopressor*], acebutolol [*Sectral*], atenolol [*Tenormin*]) are probably less likely to predispose patients to epinephrine-induced hypertension.

MANAGEMENT OPTIONS:

➡ *Consider Alternative.* If possible, avoid local anesthetics containing epinephrine in patients receiving propranolol or other nonselective beta blockers, such as nadolol, pindolol, or timolol.

➡ **Circumvent/Minimize.** These studies indicate that chronic beta blocker therapy should not be discontinued before the use of local anesthetics such as tetracaine or bupivacaine, although be alert for evidence of cardiodepression.

➡ **Monitor.** If local anesthetics and beta blockers are coadministered, monitor for hypertensive or cardiotoxic reactions.

REFERENCES:

Ponten J, et al. Beta-receptor blockade and spinal anesthesia. Withdrawal versus continuation of long-term therapy. *Acta Anesthesiol Scand.* 1982;76:62-69.

Ponten J, et al. Bupivacaine for intercostal nerve blockade in patients on long-term beta-receptor blocking therapy. *Acta Anesthesiol Scand. Suppl.* 1982;76:70-77.

Roitman K, et al. Enhancement of bupivacaine cardiotoxicity with cardiac glycosides and beta-adrenergic blockers: a case report. *Anesth Analg.* 1993;76:658-661.

Foster CA, et al. Propranolol-epinephrine interaction: a potential disaster. *Plast Reconstr Surg.* 1983;72:74-78.

Dzubow LM. The interaction between propranolol and epinephrine as observed in patients undergoing Mohs'surgery. *J Am Acad Dermatol.* 1986;15:71-75.

Propranolol (eg, *Inderal*)

Theophylline

SUMMARY: Propranolol increases theophylline serum concentrations in a dose-dependent manner. Theophylline and beta blockers have antagonistic pharmacodynamic effects.

RISK FACTORS:

➡ **Dosage Regimen.** Higher doses of propranolol may reduce theophylline clearance.

RELATED DRUGS: Metoprolol appears to interact similarly with theophylline. Atenolol (*Tenormin*) and nadolol (*Corgard*) do not appear to alter the theophylline pharmacokinetics but may interact pharmacodynamically. Other beta blockers may produce similar antagonistic effects with theophylline.

MANAGEMENT OPTIONS:

➡ **Use Alternative.** If possible, avoid beta blockers in patients receiving theophylline for bronchospastic pulmonary disease. If beta blockers are required, cardioselective agents are preferable.

➡ **Monitor.** If cardioselective beta blockers are administered to asthmatics, monitor carefully for reduced bronchodilator response.

REFERENCES:

Miners JO, et al. Selectivity and dose-dependency of the inhibitory effect of propranolol on theophylline. *Br J Clin Pharmacol.* 1985;20:219.

Lombardi TP, et al. The effects of a beta₂ agonist and a nonselective beta antagonist on theophylline clearance. *Drug Intell Clin Pharm.* 1986;20:455.

Deacon CS, et al. Inhibition of oxidative drug metabolism by betaadrenoreceptor antagonists is related to their lipid solubility. *Br J Clin Pharmacol.* 1981;12:429.

Greenblatt DJ, et al. Impairment of antipyrine clearance in humans by propranolol. *Circulation.* 1978;57:1161.

Conrad KA, et al. Effects of metoprolol and propranolol on theophylline elimination. *Clin Pharmacol Ther.* 1980;28:463.

Conrad KA, et al. Cardiovascular effects of theophylline. Partial attenuation by beta-blockade. *Eur J Clin Pharmacol.* 1981;21:109.

Bax NDS, et al. Inhibition of antipyrine metabolism by beta-adrenoceptor antagonists. *Br J Clin Pharmacol.* 1981;12:779.

Daneshmend TK, et al. The short term effects of propranolol, atenolol, and labetalol on antipyrine kinetics in normal subjects. *Br J Clin Pharmacol.* 1982;13:817.

Cerasa LA, et al. Lack of effect of atenolol on the pharmacokinetics of theophylline. *Br J Clin Pharmacol.* 1988;26:800.

Corsi CM, et al. Lack of effect of atenolol and nadolol on the metabolism of theophylline. *Br J Clin Pharmacol.* 1990;29:265.

Propranolol (eg, *Inderal*)

Verapamil (eg, *Calan*)

SUMMARY: Propranolol serum concentrations may be increased by verapamil; beta blocker and verapamil combinations may result in a greater risk of bradycardia or hypotension than when either is used alone.

RISK FACTORS: No specific risk factors are known.

RELATED DRUGS: Atenolol, metoprolol, and timolol appear to interact similarly with verapamil. Diltiazem (eg, *Cardizem*) reduces the metabolism of several beta blockers.

MANAGEMENT OPTIONS:

➡ *Circumvent/Minimize.* The use of beta blockers that are not metabolized (eg, atenolol) should minimize pharmacokinetic (but not pharmacodynamic) interactions with verapamil.

➡ *Monitor.* Monitor patients receiving therapy with beta blockers and verapamil for enhanced effects, particularly atrioventricular conduction slowing, resulting from pharmacokinetic or pharmacodynamic interactions.

REFERENCES:

McLean AJ, et al. Clearance-based oral drug interaction between verapamil and metoprolol and comparison with atenolol. *Am J Cardiol.* 1985;55:1628.

Keech AC, et al. Pharmacokinetic interaction between oral metoprolol and verapamil for angina pectoris. *Am J Cardiol.* 1986;58:551.

Carruthers SG, et al. Synergistic adverse hemodynamic interaction between oral verapamil and propranolol. *Clin Pharmacol Ther.* 1989;46:469.

Warrington SJ, et al. Pharmacokinetics and pharmacodynamics of verapamil in combination with atenolol, metoprolol and propranolol. *Br J Clin Pharmacol.* 1984;17:37S.

Pringle SD, et al. Severe bradycardia due to interaction of timolol eye drops and verapamil. *BMJ.* 1987;294:155.

Packer M, et al. Hemodynamic and clinical effects of combined verapamil and propranolol therapy in angina pectoris. *Am J Cardiol.* 1982;50:903.

Winniford MD, et al. Randomized, double-blind comparison of propranolol alone and a propranolol-verapamil combination in patients with severe angina of effort. *J Am Coll Cardiol.* 1983;1:492.

Winniford MD, et al. Hemodynamic and electrophysiologic effects of verapamil and nifedipine in patients on propranolol. *Am J Cardiol.* 1982;50:704.

Keech AC, et al. Extent and pharmacokinetic mechanisms of oral atenolol-verapamil interaction in man. *Eur J Clin Pharmacol.* 1988;35:363.

McCourty JC, et al. The effect of combined therapy on the pharmacokinetics and pharmacodynamics of verapamil and propranolol in patients with angina pectoris. *Br J Clin Pharmacol.* 1988;25:349.

Pieper JA, et al. Pharmacokinetic interaction between verapamil and propranolol. *Drug Intell Clin Pharm.* 1987;21:16A. Abstract.

Murdoch DL, et al. Evaluation of potential pharmacodynamic and pharmacokinetic interactions between verapamil and propranolol in normal subjects. *Br J Clin Pharmacol.* 1991;31:323.

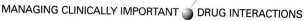

Hunt BA, et al. Effects of calcium channel blockers on the pharmacokinetics of propranolol stereoisomers. *Clin Pharmacol Ther.* 1990;47:584.

Bailey DG, et al. Interaction between oral verapamil and beta-blockers during submaximal exercise: relevance of ancillary properties. *Clin Pharmacol Ther.* 1991:49:370.

Propylthiouracil

Warfarin (eg, *Coumadin*)

SUMMARY: A reduction in thyrometabolic status caused by antithyroid drugs, such as propylthiouracil (PTU) and methimazole or any other factor tends to reduce the hypoprothrombinemic response to oral anticoagulants.

RISK FACTORS: No specific risk factors are known.

RELATED DRUGS: In 1 patient receiving warfarin, the discontinuation of methimazole (*Tapazole*) resulted in a return of thyrotoxicosis and a marked increase in prothrombin time on 2 occasions. Any agent that reduces the thyrometabolic status of the patient would be expected to reduce the hypoprothrombinemic response to any oral anticoagulant.

MANAGEMENT OPTIONS:

➡ *Monitor.* Be alert for evidence of an altered hypoprothrombinemic response to oral anticoagulants when antithyroid drugs are initiated, discontinued, or changed in dosage. Monitor prothrombin time carefully and adjust the oral anticoagulant dose as needed.

REFERENCES:

Loeliger EA, et al. The biological disappearance rate of prothrombin and factors VII, IX and X from plasma in hypothyroidism, hyperthyroidism and during fever. *Thromb Diath Haemorrh.* 1964;10:267.

Vagenakis AG, et al. Enhancement of warfarin-induced hypoprothrombinemia by thyrotoxicosis. *Johns Hopkins Med J.* 1972;131:69.

McIntosh TJ, et al. Increased sensitivity to warfarin in thyrotoxicosis. *J Clin Invest.* 1970;49:63a. Abstract.

Self T, et al. Warfarin-induced hypoprothrombinemia: potentiation by hyperthyroidism. *JAMA.* 1975;231:1165.

Hansten PD. Oral anticoagulants and drugs which alter thyroid function. *Drug Intell Clin Pharm.* 1980;14:331.

Walters MB. The relationship between thyroid function and anticoagulant therapy. *Am J Cardiol.* 1963;11:112.

Rice AJ, et al. Decreased sensitivity to warfarin in patients with myxedema. *Am J Med Sci.* 1971;262:211.

Naeye RL, et al. Hemorrhagic state after therapy with propylthiouracil. *Am J Clin Path.* 1960;34:254.

Gotta AW, et al. Prolonged intraoperative bleeding caused by propylthiouracil-induced hypoprothrombinemia. *Anesthesiology.* 1972;37:562.

D'Angelo G, et al. Severe hypoprothrombinaemia after propylthiouracil therapy. *Can Med Assoc J.* 1959;81:479.

Greenstein RH. Hypoprothrombinemia due to propylthiouracil therapy. *JAMA.* 1960;173:1014.

Quinidine (eg, *Quinora*)

Rifampin (eg, *Rifadin*)

SUMMARY: Rifampin markedly reduces quinidine plasma concentrations.

RISK FACTORS: No specific risk factors are known.

RELATED DRUGS: Theoretically rifabutin (*Mycobutin*) would affect quinidine in a similar manner.

MANAGEMENT OPTIONS:

➡ *Circumvent/Minimize.* In patients receiving rifampin, the quinidine dose may have to be increased substantially to maintain therapeutic efficacy. Discontinuation of rifampin will result in increased quinidine concentrations.

➡ *Monitor.* Plasma quinidine determinations can be used to achieve the optimal dose of quinidine in the presence of rifampin. Carefully observe patients for changes in quinidine response for several days to 2 weeks following the addition or removal of rifampin therapy.

REFERENCES:

Ahmad D, et al. Rifampicin-quinidine interaction. *Br J Dis Chest.* 1979;73:409.

Schwartz A, et al. Quinidine-rifampin interaction. *Am Heart J.* 1984;107:789.

Bussey HI, et al. Influence of rifampin on quinidine and digoxin. *Arch Intern Med.* 1984;144:1021.

Twum-Barima Y, et al. Quinidine-rifampin interaction. *N Engl J Med.* 1981;304:1466.

Quinidine (eg, *Quinora*)

Sodium Bicarbonate

SUMMARY: Sodium bicarbonate can increase quinidine concentrations; toxicity could result.

RISK FACTORS: No specific risk factors are known.

RELATED DRUGS: Other agents that alkalinize the urine (eg, antacids, acetazolamide [eg, *Diamox*]) would be expected to produce similar results.

MANAGEMENT OPTIONS:

➡ *Monitor.* When a urinary alkalizer such as sodium bicarbonate is initiated, the quinidine dose may have to be reduced to avoid toxicity.

REFERENCES:

Knouss RF, et al. Variation in quinidine excretion with changing urine pH. *Ann Intern Med.* 1968;68:1157.

Milne MD. Influence of acid-base balance on the efficacy and toxicity of drugs. *Proc R Soc Med.* 1965;58:961.

Quinidine

AVOID **Thioridazine (eg, *Mellaril*)**

SUMMARY: Quinidine may increase thioridazine serum concentrations and also may produce additive prolongation of the QT interval, thus increasing the risk of ventricular arrhythmias; avoid concurrent use.

RISK FACTORS:

➡ ***Pharmacogenetics.*** Only patients with the extensive metabolizer CYP2D6 phenotype (EMs) would be expected to experience increased thioridazine serum concentrations. Poor metabolizers (PMs) do not have the gene for production of CYP2D6, and would likely already have high serum concentrations of thioridazine. Approximately 8% of whites are deficient in CYP2D6, but the deficiency is rare in Asians – usually no more than 1%.

➡ ***Hypokalemia:.*** The corrected QT interval (QTc) may be prolonged in patients with hypokalemia, thus increasing the risk of this interaction. Any other factor that may prolong the QTc interval would also increase the risk of this interaction.

RELATED DRUGS: Other antiarrhythmics such as amiodarone (eg, *Cordarone*), disopyramide (eg, *Norpace*), and procainamide (eg, *Procan SR*) can also increase the QT interval, and may increase the risk of arrhythmias. Also, amiodarone and propafenone (*Rythmol*) are known inhibitors of CYP2D6, and may increase thioridazine serum concentrations. Although a number of antipsychotic drugs have, like thioridazine, been shown to prolong the QT interval, clinical evidence suggests that thioridazine may produce the greatest risk.

MANAGEMENT OPTIONS:

➡ ***AVOID COMBINATION.*** Although the risk of this combination is not well established, it would be prudent to avoid concurrent use.

REFERENCES:

Hartigan-Go K, et al. Concentration-related pharmacodynamic effects of thioridazine and its metabolites in humans. *Clin Pharmacol Ther.* 1996;60:543-53.

'Dear Doctor or Pharmacist' Letter, Novartis Pharmaceuticals, July 7, 2000.

 Quinidine (eg, *Quinora*)

Timolol (eg, *Blocadren*)

SUMMARY: Quinidine may increase the plasma concentration of timolol, but the incidence of adverse effects due to these interactions is unknown.

RISK FACTORS:

➡ ***Pharmacogenetics.*** Patients who are rapid metabolizers of timolol are at increased risk for the interaction.

RELATED DRUGS: Quinidine also decreases the metabolism of metoprolol (eg, *Lopressor*) and propranolol (eg, *Inderal*). It would not likely affect renally eliminated beta blockers such as atenolol (eg, *Tenormin*). Preliminary evidence suggests no effect of quinidine on labetalol (eg, *Normodyne*) pharmacokinetics or pharmacodynamics.

MANAGEMENT OPTIONS:

➥ **Consider Alternative.** Renally excreted beta blockers (eg, atenolol) should be less likely to interact with quinidine, since their metabolism is unlikely to be affected by quinidine. Nevertheless, additive cardiac depressant effects cannot be overlooked.

➥ **Monitor.** Concomitant use of quinidine and timolol should be undertaken with careful monitoring. Watch for bradycardia, heart failure, and arrhythmias.

REFERENCES:

Dinai Y, et al. Bradycardia induced by interaction between quinidine and ophthalmic timolol. *Ann Intern Med*. 1985;103:890.

Kaila T, et al. Beta blocking effects of timolol at low plasma concentrations. *Clin Pharmacol Ther*. 1991;49:53.

Gearhart MO, et al. Lack of effects on labetalol pharmacodynamics with quinidine inhibition of P450IID6. *Pharmacotherapy*. 1991;11:P36. Abstract.

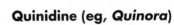

Quinidine (eg, *Quinora*)

Tubocurarine

SUMMARY: Quinidine administration may enhance the effects of tubocurarine and other neuromuscular blockers.

RISK FACTORS: No specific risk factors are known.

RELATED DRUGS: A similar effect might be seen with other neuromuscular blockers (eg, succinylcholine).

MANAGEMENT OPTIONS:

➥ **Monitor.** If possible, quinidine should be avoided in the immediate postoperative period when the effects of muscle relaxants still may be present. If quinidine must be used, the need for respiratory support should be anticipated.

REFERENCES:

Way WL, et al. Recurarization with quinidine. *JAMA*. 1967;200:153.

Schmidt JL, et al. The effect of quinidine on the action of muscle relaxants. *JAMA*. 1963;183:669.

Cuthbert MF. The effect of quinidine and procainamide on the neuromuscular blocking action of suxamethonium. *Br J Anaesth*. 1966;38:775.

Kambam JR, et al. Effect of quinidine on plasma cholinesterase activity and succinylcholine neuromuscular blockade. *Anesthesiology*. 1987;67:858.

Quinidine (eg, *Quinora*)

Verapamil (eg, *Calan*)

SUMMARY: Verapamil administration with quinidine increases quinidine concentrations and may result in quinidine toxicity.

RISK FACTORS: No specific risk factors are known.

RELATED DRUGS: Nifedipine (eg, *Procardia*) reduces quinidine concentrations. Diltiazem (eg, *Cardizem*) 120 mg/day had no effect on quinidine concentrations.

MANAGEMENT OPTIONS:

➥ **Circumvent/Minimize.** The addition of verapamil to quinidine therapy may necessitate a reduction in the dose of quinidine.

➡ *Monitor.* If quinidine and verapamil are coadministered, monitor for quinidine toxicity including hypotension, arrhythmia, and heart block.

REFERENCES:

Trohman RG, et al. Increased quinidine plasma concentrations during administration of verapamil: a new quinidine-verapamil interaction. *Am J Cardiol.* 1986;57:706.

Edwards DJ, et al. The effect of co-administration of verapamil on the pharmacokinetics and metabolism of quinidine. *Clin Pharmacol Ther.* 1987;41:68.

Matera MG, et al. Quinidine-diltiazem: pharmacokinetic interaction in humans. *Curr Ther Res.* 1986;40:653.

Quinidine (eg, *Quinora*)

Warfarin (eg, *Coumadin*)

SUMMARY: A few patients experienced enhanced anticoagulation after quinidine was added to warfarin therapy. Prospective studies do not indicate that the interaction is widespread or of substantial magnitude.

RISK FACTORS: No specific risk factors are known.

RELATED DRUGS: Theoretically, the same effect could be seen with other oral anticoagulants.

MANAGEMENT OPTIONS:

➡ *Monitor.* Closely observe patients on oral anticoagulants who subsequently receive quinidine for prolonged prothrombin times and signs of bleeding.

REFERENCES:

Koch-Weser J. Quinidine-induced hypoprothrombinemic hemorrhage in patients on chronic warfarin therapy. *Ann Intern Med.* 1968;68:511-517.

Gazzaniga AB, et al. Possible quinidine-induced hemorrhage in a patient on warfarin sodium. *N Engl J Med.* 1969;280:711-712.

Sopher IM, et al. Fatal corpus luteum hemorrhage during anticoagulant therapy. *Obstet Gynecol.* 1971;37:695-697.

Udall JA. Drug interference with warfarin therapy. *Clin Med.* 1970;77:20.

Quinidine (eg, *Quinora*)

Ziprasidone (*Geodon*)

SUMMARY: Both ziprasidone and quinidine can prolong the QTc interval on the electrocardiogram (ECG). Theoretically, this could increase the risk of ventricular arrhythmias such as torsades de pointes.

RISK FACTORS:

➡ *Hypokalemia.* The corrected QT interval (QTc) on the ECG may be prolonged in patients with hypokalemia, increasing the risk of this interaction.

➡ *Miscellaneous.* Other factors that may prolong the QTc interval (eg, hypomagnesemia, bradycardia, impaired liver function, hypothyroidism) also may increase the risk of ventricular arrhythmias.

RELATED DRUGS: Available data suggest that ziprasidone produces less QTc prolongation than thioridazine (*Mellaril*), but about twice that of quetiapine (*Seroquel*), risperidone (*Risperdal*), haloperidol (*Haldol*), and olanzapine (*Zyprexa*).

MANAGEMENT OPTIONS:

➡ *Use Alternative.* Given the theoretical risk and the fact that quinidine is listed in the ziprasidone product information as "contraindicated," it would be prudent to use an alternative to one of the drugs (see Related Drugs).

➡ *Monitor.* If quinidine and ziprasidone are used concurrently, monitor for evidence of arrhythmias (eg, syncope) and for prolonged QT intervals.

REFERENCES:

De Ponti F, et al. QT-interval prolongation by non-cardiac drugs: lessons to be learned from recent experience. *Eur J Clin Pharmacol.* 2000;56:1-18.

Product information. Ziprasidone (*Geodon*). Pfizer Pharmaceuticals. 2001.

Briefing Information, Psychopharmacological Drugs Advisory Committee, U.S. Food and Drug Administration, July 19, 2000.

Radioactive Iodine (I^{131})

Theophylline (eg, *Theolair*)

SUMMARY: A patient developed theophylline toxicity following I^{131} therapy for thyrotoxicosis; this response is consistent with the known effect of thyroid function on theophylline elimination.

RISK FACTORS:

➠ **Concurrent Diseases.** Patients who develop hypothyroidism following I^{131} are at increased risk for the interaction.

RELATED DRUGS: Theoretically, antithyroid drugs such as methimazole (eg, *Tapazole*) and propylthiouracil would produce an effect similar to that of I^{131} (an increase in serum theophylline concentrations).

MANAGEMENT OPTIONS:

➠ **Monitor.** Monitor for theophylline toxicity in patients who receive I^{131} therapy for hyperthyroidism. Although hypothyroidism following I^{131} therapy is not unusual, it may take months or years to occur; thus, the time course of any increase in serum theophylline concentrations would be highly variable.

REFERENCES:

Johnson CE, et al. Theophylline toxicity after iodine 131 treatment for hyperthyroidism. *Clin Pharm.* 1988;7:620-622.

Raloxifene (*Evista*)

Levothyroxine (eg, *Synthroid*)

SUMMARY: A patient on levothyroxine developed increased thyroid requirements after starting raloxifene. The interaction was well documented in this patient, but the incidence and magnitude of the interaction is not established.

RISK FACTORS: No specific risk factors are known.

RELATED DRUGS: Until additional information is available, assume that all thyroid replacement would interact in a similar manner.

MANAGEMENT OPTIONS:

➠ **Circumvent/Minimize.** Pending additional information, separate doses of levothyroxine (or other thyroid replacement) from raloxifene by as much as possible. It would also be prudent to keep the interval between doses of levothyroxine and raloxifene as consistent as possible to minimize fluctuation in levothyroxine response.

➠ **Monitor.** Monitor thyroid function and adjust levothyroxine dose as needed in patients taking raloxifene and levothyroxine (or other thyroid replacement). Monitoring is especially important when raloxifene is started, stopped, changed in dosage, or if the interval between administration of levothyroxine and raloxifene is changed. Note that changes in levothyroxine effect are likely to be gradual and may take place over many weeks.

REFERENCES:

Siraj ES, et al. Raloxifene causing malabsorption of levothyroxine. *Arch Intern Med.* 2003;163:1367-1370.

Repaglinide (*Prandin*)

Rifampin (eg, *Rimactane*)

SUMMARY: Rifampin reduces repaglinide plasma concentrations and its glucose lowering effect.

RISK FACTORS: No specific risk factors are known.

RELATED DRUGS: Rifabutin (*Mycobutin*) is likely to reduce the concentrations of repaglinide. Other oral hypoglycemic drugs that are metabolized by CYP3A4 or CYP2C9 (eg, glimepiride [*Amaryl*], glipizide [*Glucotrol*], nateglinide [*Starlix*], tolbutamide [*Orinase*]) may have their efficacy reduced by coadministration of rifampin.

MANAGEMENT OPTIONS:

➡ *Circumvent/Minimize.* Patients stabilized on repaglinide who initiate rifampin may require increased repaglinide doses. Adjust repaglinide doses based on blood glucose response.

➡ *Monitor.* Monitor blood glucose concentrations in patients maintained on repaglinide for several weeks after starting or stopping rifampin, or other inducers of CYP3A4, to determine if a repaglinide dose adjustment will be necessary.

REFERENCES:

Niemi M, et al. Rifampin decreases the plasma concentrations and effects of repaglinide. *Clin Pharmacol Ther.* 2000;68:495-500.

Product information. Repaglinide (*Prandin*). Novo Nordisk. 2002.

Ribavirin (eg, *Rebetol*)

Warfarin (eg, *Coumadin*)

SUMMARY: A patient on warfarin developed reduced anticoagulant effect when ribavirin was added. Although a causal relationship was well established in this case, it is not known how often other patients would be similarly affected.

RISK FACTORS: No specific risk factors are known.

RELATED DRUGS: No information is available.

MANAGEMENT OPTIONS:

➡ *Monitor.* Monitor for altered anticoagulant effect of warfarin if ribavirin is initiated, discontinued, or changed in dosage. Adjust warfarin dose as needed.

REFERENCES:

Schulman S. Inhibition of warfarin activity by ribavirin. *Ann Pharmacother.* 2002;36:72-74.

Rifabutin (*Mycobutin*)

Ritonavir (*Norvir*)

SUMMARY: Ritonavir administration produces marked increases in rifabutin concentrations; rifabutin toxicity may result.

RISK FACTORS: No specific risk factors are known.

RELATED DRUGS: Indinavir (*Crixivan*) also inhibits the metabolism of rifabutin. Rifabutin decreases the area under the concentration-time curve of saquinavir (*Fortovase*). The effects of saquinavir and nelfinavir (*Viracept*) on rifabutin are unknown.

MANAGEMENT OPTIONS:

➥ *Consider Alternative.* If monotherapy for *Mycobacterium avium* complex (MAC) is required, consider azithromycin or clarithromycin. Note that ritonavir inhibits the metabolism of clarithromycin, and lower doses of clarithromycin may be required.

➥ *Circumvent/Minimize.* Pending further information on this interaction, avoid the use of ritonavir and rifabutin if possible. Rifabutin dose and frequency may require reduction during coadministration with ritonavir.

➥ *Monitor.* If ritonavir and rifabutin are coadministered, watch for signs of rifabutin toxicity including arthralgia, dyspepsia, anemia, or skin discoloration. Be alert for subtherapeutic rifabutin concentrations when ritonavir is discontinued.

REFERENCES:
Product information. Ritonavir (*Norvir*). Abbott Laboratories. 1996.

Rifabutin (*Mycobutin*)

Saquinavir (eg, *Invirase*)

SUMMARY: Rifabutin markedly reduces the serum concentration of saquinavir; loss of efficacy or development of resistant organisms may result.

RISK FACTORS: No specific risk factors are known.

RELATED DRUGS: Rifabutin reduces the concentrations of other protease inhibitors including ritonavir (*Norvir*), indinavir (*Crixivan*), and probably nelfinavir (*Viracept*). Rifampin (eg, *Rifadin*) also reduces saquinavir serum concentrations.

MANAGEMENT OPTIONS:

➥ *Circumvent/Minimize.* The dose of saquinavir may require a substantial increase to produce therapeutic serum concentrations. If possible, monitor saquinavir serum concentrations if dosage adjustments are attempted.

➥ *Monitor.* Watch for loss of saquinavir efficacy during rifabutin coadministration.

REFERENCES:
Product information. Saquinavir (*Invirase*). Hoffman-La Roche, Inc. 1995.

Rifabutin (*Mycobutin*)

Voriconazole (*Vfend*)

SUMMARY: Rifabutin reduces the plasma concentration of voriconazole; a loss of antifungal activity may result. Voriconazole increases the concentration of rifabutin; watch for evidence of rifabutin toxicity.

RISK FACTORS:

➥ *Pharmacogenetics.* Patients who are poor metabolizers for CYP2C19 will have higher voriconazole concentrations, and thus are likely to have an interaction of larger magnitude.

RELATED DRUGS: Rifampin (eg, *Rifadin*) is known to be an inducer of cytochrome P450 enzymes and also reduces the plasma concentration of voriconazole. Rifabutin may also reduce the concentrations of ketoconazole (eg, *Nizoral*), fluconazole (*Diflucan*), and itraconazole (eg, *Sporanox*) in a similar manner.

MANAGEMENT OPTIONS:

➡ *Circumvent/Minimize.* The dose of voriconazole may need to be increased substantially when rifabutin is coadministered. Rifabutin doses may need to be reduced during voriconazole coadministration.

➡ *Monitor.* It will be difficult to predict the outcome of this drug combination. Careful monitoring for decreased voriconazole efficacy and rifabutin toxicity (eg, uveitis, bone marrow depression) is necessary if voriconazole and rifabutin are coadministered.

REFERENCES:
Product information. Voriconazole (*Vfend*). Pfizer, Inc. 2002.

Rifampin (eg, *Rifadin*)
Ritonavir (*Norvir*)

SUMMARY: Rifampin appears to reduce ritonavir plasma concentrations; loss of antiviral efficacy may result.

RISK FACTORS: No specific risk factors are known.

RELATED DRUGS: Rifabutin (*Mycobutin*) also may reduce the concentrations of ritonavir. Other protease inhibitors such as indinavir (*Crixivan*), saquinavir (eg, *Invirase*), and nelfinavir (*Viracept*) may be affected by rifampin in a similar manner.

MANAGEMENT OPTIONS:

➡ *Circumvent/Minimize.* Pending further clinical data, consider increasing the dosage of ritonavir during coadministration of rifampin.

➡ *Monitor.* Monitor for reduced ritonavir efficacy.

REFERENCES:
Product information. Ritonavir (*Norvir*). Abbott Laboratories. 1996.

Rifampin (eg, *Rifadin*)
Ropivacaine (*Naropin*)

SUMMARY: Rifampin increased the metabolism of ropivacaine; a reduction in anesthetic effect may occur in some patients.

RISK FACTORS: No specific risk factors are known.

RELATED DRUGS: While no data are available, rifabutin (*Mycobutin*) also may increase the metabolism of ropivacaine.

MANAGEMENT OPTIONS:

➡ **Monitor.** Monitor patients taking rifampin for a potential reduction in anesthetic effect if ropivacaine is used for local anesthesia.

REFERENCES:

Jokinen MJ, et al. Effect of rifampin and tobacco smoking on the pharmacokinetics of ropivacaine. *Clin Pharmacol Ther.* 2001;70:344-350.

② Rifampin (eg, *Rifadin*)

Saquinavir (eg, *Invirase*)

SUMMARY: Rifampin markedly reduces the serum concentration of saquinavir; loss of efficacy or development of resistant organisms may result.

RISK FACTORS: No specific risk factors are known.

RELATED DRUGS: Rifampin reduces the concentrations of other protease inhibitors including ritonavir (*Norvir*), indinavir (*Crixivan*), and nelfinavir (*Viracept*). Rifabutin (*Mycobutin*) also reduces saquinavir serum concentrations.

MANAGEMENT OPTIONS:

➡ **Use Alternative.** Based on the magnitude of this interaction, it would be difficult to administer an effective dose of saquinavir. Because other protease inhibitors also are likely to be affected, consider an alternative to rifampin.

REFERENCES:

Product information. Saquinavir (*Invirase*). Hoffman-La Roche, Inc. 1995.

② Rifampin (eg, *Rifadin*)

Simvastatin (*Zocor*)

SUMMARY: Rifampin produces a profound reduction in simvastatin and simvastatin acid plasma concentrations; therapeutic failure is likely to occur.

RISK FACTORS: No specific risk factors are known.

RELATED DRUGS: Lovastatin (eg, *Mevacor*), because of its similar metabolism to simvastatin, would be expected to display a similar interaction with rifampin. Other statins that are metabolized by CYP3A4 or CYP2C9 (eg, atorvastatin [*Lipitor*], fluvastatin [eg, *Lescol*]) probably would be affected by rifampin but perhaps to a lesser extent. Because pravastatin (*Pravachol*) is not a CYP3A4 substrate, rifampin may have limited effect on its pharmacokinetics. Rifabutin (*Mycobutin*) also is known to induce CYP3A4 and would be expected to reduce simvastatin concentrations, although perhaps to a lesser extent.

MANAGEMENT OPTIONS:

➡ **Use Alternative.** For patients taking rifampin, select cholesterol-lowering drugs that are not dependent on CYP3A4 or CYP2C9 for their metabolism.

➡ *Monitor.* Monitor serum cholesterol in patients taking statins when rifampin is administered for more than a few weeks.

REFERENCES:
Kyrklund C, et al. Rifampin greatly reduces plasma simvastatin and simvastatin acid concentrations. *Clin Pharmacol Ther.* 2000;68:592–597.

Rifampin (eg, *Rifadin*)

Tacrolimus (*Prograf*)

SUMMARY: Rifampin sufficiently decreased tacrolimus plasma concentrations to reduce its immunosuppressive efficacy.

RISK FACTORS: No specific risk factors are known.

RELATED DRUGS: Rifampin is known to increase the metabolism of cyclosporine (eg, *Neoral*). Sirolimus (*Rapamune*) may be affected in a similar manner. Rifabutin (*Mycobutin*) would probably reduce the concentration of tacrolimus.

MANAGEMENT OPTIONS:

➡ *Monitor.* If rifampin is started or stopped, monitor patients taking tacrolimus for altered tacrolimus concentrations.

REFERENCES:
Hebert MF, et al. Effects of rifampin on tacrolimus pharmacokinetics in healthy volunteers. *J Clin Pharmacol.* 1999;39(1):91-96.

Furlan V, et al. Interactions between FK506 and rifampicin or erythromycin in pediatric liver recipients. *Transplantation.* 1995;59(8):1217-18.

Rifampin (eg, *Rifadin*)

Tamoxifen (eg, *Nolvadex*)

SUMMARY: Rifampin administration markedly reduces tamoxifen concentration; loss of tamoxifen's antiestrogenic effect is likely.

RISK FACTORS: No specific risk factors are known.

RELATED DRUGS: Rifabutin (*Mycobutin*) would be likely to affect tamoxifen and toremifene metabolism similarly.

MANAGEMENT OPTIONS:

➡ *Monitor.* Monitor patients taking tamoxifen for loss of efficacy if rifampin is coadministered. The dosage of tamoxifen may need to be increased.

REFERENCES:
Kivisto KT, et al. Tamoxifen and toremifene concentrations in plasma are greatly decreased by rifampin. *Clin Pharmacol Ther.* 1998;64:648-54.

Rifampin (eg, *Rifadin*)

Theophylline

SUMMARY: Rifampin lowers the plasma concentration of theophylline; a reduction of theophylline efficacy may result.

RISK FACTORS: No specific risk factors are known.

RELATED DRUGS: No information is available.

MANAGEMENT OPTIONS:

➡ ***Monitor.*** Be alert for the need to adjust the theophylline dose when rifampin therapy is started or stopped. Theophylline dose requirement may be higher in patients receiving rifampin.

REFERENCES:

Robson RA, et al. Theophylline-rifampin interaction: non-selective induction of theophylline metabolic pathways. *Br J Clin Pharmacol.* 1984;18:455.

Hauser AR, et al. The effect of rifampin on theophylline disposition. *Clin Pharmacol Ther.* 1983;33:254.

Straughn AB, et al. Effect of rifampin on theophylline disposition. *Ther Drug Monit.* 1984;6:153.

Boyce EG, et al. The effect of rifampin on theophylline kinetics. *Clin Pharmacol Ther.* 1985;37:183.

Brocks DR, et al. Theophylline-rifampin interaction in a pediatric patient. *Clin Pharm.* 1986;5:602.

Rifampin (eg, *Rifadin*)

Tocainide (*Tonocard*)

SUMMARY: Rifampin administration to healthy subjects reduces tocainide serum concentrations considerably. There appears to be a potential for a loss of efficacy resulting from diminished tocainide concentrations.

RISK FACTORS: No specific risk factors are known.

RELATED DRUGS: No information is available.

MANAGEMENT OPTIONS:

➡ ***Monitor.*** Monitor patients stabilized on tocainide for a decreased response and serum concentrations if rifampin is instituted. Discontinuing concomitant rifampin therapy could result in an increased tocainide concentration and effect.

REFERENCES:

Rice TL, et al. Influence of rifampin on tocainide pharmacokinetics in humans. *Clin Pharm.* 1989;8:200.

Edgar B, et al. The pharmacokinetics of r-and s-tocainide in healthy subjects. *Br J Clin Pharmacol.* 1984;17:216P.

Hoffmann KJ, et al. Stereoselective disposition of RS-tocainide in man. *Eur J Drug Metab Pharmacokinet.* 1984;9:215.

Rifampin (eg, *Rifadin*)

Tolbutamide (eg, *Orinase*)

SUMMARY: Rifampin reduces tolbutamide and glyburide serum concentrations and may reduce hypoglycemic activity.

RISK FACTORS: No specific risk factors are known.

RELATED DRUGS: A 67-year-old patient taking rifampin 600 mg/day and glyburide (eg, *DiaBeta*) 15 mg/day had glyburide concentrations between 30 and 40 ng/mL. After cessation of the rifampin therapy, the glyburide concentrations increased more than 160 ng/mL. Blood glucose concentrations did not appear to be altered by the change in glyburide concentrations. Little is known concerning the effect of rifampin on other oral antidiabetic drugs, but their metabolism also might be enhanced by rifampin. Rifabutin (*Mycobutin*) might affect tolbutamide in a similar manner.

MANAGEMENT OPTIONS:

➡ *Monitor.* When rifampin is coadministered with tolbutamide or glyburide and possibly other sulfonylureas, be alert for the potential for diminished hypoglycemic activity. Discontinuation of rifampin could result in hypoglycemia.

REFERENCES:

Zilly W, et al. Induction of drug metabolism in man after rifampicin treatment measured by increased hexobarbital and tolbutamide clearance. *Eur J Clin Pharmacol.* 1975;9:219.

Syvalahti E, et al. Effect of tuberculostatic agents on the response of serum growth hormone and immunoreactive insulin to intravenous tolbutamide, and on the half-life of tolbutamide. *Int J Clin Pharmacol Biopharm.* 1976;13:83.

Zilly W, et al. Stimulation of drug metabolism by rifampicin in patients with cirrhosis or cholestasis measured by increased hexobarbital and tolbutamide clearance. *Eur J Clin Pharmacol.* 1977;11:287.

Self TH, et al. Interaction of rifampin and glyburide. *Chest.* 1989;96:1443.

Rifampin (eg, *Rifadin*)

Triazolam (*Halcion*)

SUMMARY: Rifampin markedly reduces the plasma concentrations of triazolam; loss of triazolam effect is likely to occur during coadministration.

RISK FACTORS: No specific risk factors are known.

RELATED DRUGS: Rifabutin (*Mycobutin*) is likely to produce a similar effect on triazolam pharmacokinetics. Rifampin is known to increase the elimination of other benzodiazepines including midazolam (*Versed*) and diazepam (eg, *Valium*). Benzodiazepines that do not interact with rifampin include temazepam (eg, *Restoril*) and oxazepam (eg, *Serax*).

MANAGEMENT OPTIONS:

➡ *Consider Alternative.* Selection of a benzodiazepine that does not interact with rifampin would avoid the interaction (see Related Drugs).

➡ *Monitor.* Monitor patients receiving rifampin for reduced triazolam efficacy. If rifampin is discontinued in a patient receiving both agents, the dose of triazolam may require reduction during the next week or 2 to avoid excess sedation.

REFERENCES:

Villikka K, et al. Triazolam is ineffective in patients taking rifampin. *Clin Pharmacol Ther.* 1997;61:8.

Rifampin (eg, *Rifadin*)

Verapamil (eg, *Calan*)

SUMMARY: Rifampin decreases verapamil plasma concentrations; loss of therapeutic effect may result.

RISK FACTORS:

➡ *Route of Administration.* Administration of verapamil orally increases the magnitude of this interaction.

RELATED DRUGS: Rifampin is likely to affect other calcium channel blockers in a similar manner. Rifabutin (*Mycobutin*) might affect verapamil similarly.

MANAGEMENT OPTIONS:

➡ *Consider Alternative.* Because this interaction is likely to reduce the efficacy of verapamil, consider an alternative agent for verapamil. Other calcium channel blockers also may be affected; a therapeutic substitution to a different class of agent may be required.

➡ *Circumvent/Minimize.* Larger doses of calcium channel blockers (particularly those administered orally) may be required when rifampin is coadministered.

➡ *Monitor.* Monitor patients taking calcium channel blockers for a reduction in efficacy when rifampin is given.

REFERENCES:

Rahn KH, et al. Reduction of bioavailability of verapamil by rifampin. *N Engl J Med.* 1985;312:920-921.

Barbarash RA. Verapamil-rifampin interaction. *Drug Intell Clin Pharm.* 1985;19:559-560.

Barbarash RA, et al. Near-total reduction in verapamil bioavailability by rifampin. *Chest.* 1988;94:954-959.

Mooy J, et al. The influence of antituberculosis drugs on the plasma level of verapamil. *Eur J Clin Pharmacol.* 1987;32:107-109.

Pieper JA, et al. Rifampin alters serum albumin concentrations and verapamil protein binding. *Clin Pharmacol Ther.* 1988;43:146.

Rifampin (eg, *Rifadin*)

Voriconazole (*Vfend*)

SUMMARY: Do not administer rifampin with voriconazole; a loss of antifungal efficacy is likely to result.

RISK FACTORS: No specific risk factors are known.

RELATED DRUGS: Rifabutin (*Mycobutin*) is known to be an inducer of cytochrome P450 enzymes and also reduces the plasma concentration of voriconazole. Although data are limited, rifampin reduces the concentrations of ketoconazole (eg, *Nizoral*), fluconazole (*Diflucan*), and itraconazole (eg, *Sporanox*) in a similar manner.

MANAGEMENT OPTIONS:

➡ *Use Alternative.* If possible, avoid coadministration of voriconazole and rifampin. It is likely to be very difficult to obtain adequate antifungal concentrations of voriconazole in patients taking rifampin.

➡ *Monitor.* If rifampin and voriconazole are coadministered, voriconazole doses may have to be increased several fold. Monitor for lack of antifungal effect.

REFERENCES:
Product information. Voriconazole (*Vfend*). Pfizer, Inc. 2002.

Rifampin (eg, *Rifadin*)

Warfarin (eg, *Coumadin*)

SUMMARY: Rifampin reduces the hypoprothrombinemic effect of warfarin and other oral anticoagulants in most patients to a clinically significant extent; anticoagulant dosage adjustments are likely to be necessary during cotherapy with these drugs.

RISK FACTORS: No specific risk factors are known.

RELATED DRUGS: Phenprocoumon and acenocoumarol interact similarly with rifampin.

MANAGEMENT OPTIONS:

➡ *Avoid Unless Benefit Outweighs Risk.* Do not coadminister rifampin and oral anticoagulants unless no alternative is available.

➡ *Monitor.* If rifampin is administered to patients requiring warfarin, evaluate the patient's anticoagulant response carefully and readjust the anticoagulant dose as needed when rifampin is started, stopped, or changed in dosage.

REFERENCES:
Heimark LD, et al. The mechanism of the warfarin-rifampin drug interaction in humans. *Clin Pharmacol Ther.* 1987;42:388-394.
O'Reilly RA. Interaction of sodium warfarin and rifampin. Studies in man. *Ann Intern Med.* 1974;81:337-340.
O'Reilly RA. Interaction of chronic daily warfarin therapy and rifampin. *Ann Intern Med.* 1975;83:506-508.
Self TH, et al. Interaction of rifampin and warfarin. *Chest.* 1975;67:490-491.
Romankiewicz JA, et al. Rifampin and warfarin: a drug interaction. *Ann Intern Med.* 1975;82:224-225.
Boekhout-Mussert RJ, et al. Inhibition by rifampicin of the anticoagulant effect of phenprocoumon. *JAMA.* 1974;229:1903-1904.

Rifampin (eg, *Rifadin*)

Zaleplon (*Sonata*)

SUMMARY: Rifampin reduced the concentration of zaleplon to the point that loss of efficacy can result.

RISK FACTORS: No specific risk factors are known.

RELATED DRUGS: Rifabutin (*Mycobutin*) may have a similar effect on zaleplon.

MANAGEMENT OPTIONS:

➡ *Monitor.* Expect patients taking zaleplon and rifampin to demonstrate a reduced response to zaleplon. When rifampin is discontinued in patients receiving zaleplon, monitor for increased zaleplon effects, including sedation.

REFERENCES:
Product information. Zaleplon (*Sonata*). Wyeth-Ayerst Laboratories. 1999.

Rifampin (eg, *Rifadin*)

Zidovudine (*Retrovir*)

SUMMARY: Zidovudine plasma concentrations are reduced by the coadministration of rifampin; loss of efficacy could result.

RISK FACTORS: No specific risk factors are known.

RELATED DRUGS: No information is available.

MANAGEMENT OPTIONS:

➡ *Monitor.* Monitor zidovudine plasma concentrations of patients taking zidovudine and watch for a change in zidovudine response if rifampin therapy is added or discontinued. Zidovudine dose adjustments are likely to be necessary.

REFERENCES:

Burger DM, et al. Pharmacokinetic interation between rifampin and zidovudine. *Antimicrob Agents Chemother.* 1993;37:1426-1431.

Rifampin (eg, *Rifadin*)

Zolpidem (*Ambien*)

SUMMARY: Rifampin reduces the plasma concentration and effect of zolpidem; a reduction in efficacy may result.

RISK FACTORS: No specific risk factors are known.

RELATED DRUGS: Rifabutin (*Mycobutin*) would also be expected to induce the metabolism of zolpidem.

MANAGEMENT OPTIONS:

➡ *Monitor.* Patients taking rifampin may require an increase in their zolpidem dosage to produce adequate hypnotic effect.

REFERENCES:

Villikka K, et al. Tifampin reduces plasma concentrations and effects of zolpidem. *Clin Pharmacol Ther.* 1997;62:629.

Ritonavir (*Norvir*)

Saquinavir (eg, *Invirase*)

SUMMARY: Ritonavir increases saquinavir plasma concentrations; saquinavir toxicity may result.

RISK FACTORS: No specific risk factors are known.

RELATED DRUGS: Other protease inhibitors such as indinavir (*Crixivan*) and nelfinavir (*Viracept*) may affect saquinavir metabolism in a similar manner although the magnitude of the inhibition may be less than that observed with ritonavir. Ritonavir may inhibit the metabolism of other protease inhibitors such as indinavir and nelfinavir.

MANAGEMENT OPTIONS:

➡ *Consider Alternative.* Using another protease inhibitor instead of ritonavir may reduce but not eliminate the interaction. Be alert for evidence of increased saquinavir plasma concentrations.

➡ *Circumvent/Minimize.* Reduction of the saquinavir dose may be necessary to avoid toxicity such as GI upset and increased LFTs.

➡ *Monitor.* Monitor for GI upset and elevated liver function tests when saquinavir is administered with ritonavir.

REFERENCES:
Product information. Ritonavir (*Norvir*). Abbott Laboratories. 1996.
Product information. Saquinavir (*Invirase*). Hoffman-La Roche Inc. 1996.

Ritonavir (*Norvir*)

Sildenafil (*Viagra*)

SUMMARY: Ritonavir administration increases sildenafil plasma concentrations; observe patients for side effects.

RISK FACTORS: No specific risk factors are known.

RELATED DRUGS: Other protease inhibitors such as indinavir (*Crixivan*), saquinavir (eg, *Fortovase*), amprenavir (*Agenerase*), and nelfinavir (*Viracept*) are known to inhibit CYP3A4 and would be expected to interact with sildenafil.

MANAGEMENT OPTIONS:

➡ *Circumvent/Minimize.* Because of the potential for serious side effects, counsel patients taking protease inhibitors that are CYP3A4 inhibitors to avoid concurrent sildenafil administration. If sildenafil were coadministered to patients taking ritonavir, a starting dose of 25 mg would be prudent.

➡ *Monitor.* Carefully monitor patients treated with sildenafil for side effects (eg, headache, flushing, hypotension, abnormal vision) if ritonavir is prescribed.

REFERENCES:
Muirhead GJ, et al. Pharmacokinetic interactions between sildenafil and saquinavir/ritonavir. *Br J Clin Pharmacol.* 2000;50:99.

Ritonavir (*Norvir*)

Theophylline (eg, *Theolair*)

SUMMARY: Ritonavir reduces theophylline plasma concentrations; a reduction in theophylline efficacy may result.

RISK FACTORS: No specific risk factors are known.

RELATED DRUGS: The effect of other protease inhibitors such as indinavir (*Crixivan*), saquinavir (eg, *Fortovase*), and nelfinavir (*Viracept*) on theophylline metabolism is unknown.

MANAGEMENT OPTIONS:

➡ *Consider Alternative.* While specific information is not available, other protease inhibitors may avoid the interaction with theophylline.

➥ *Circumvent/Minimize.* The coadministration of theophylline and ritonavir may require increasing the dose of theophylline to maintain therapeutic concentrations.

➥ *Monitor.* Monitor theophylline concentrations to ensure adequate plasma levels are maintained during ritonavir administration. Watch for inadequate theophylline response such as bronchospasm or wheezing.

REFERENCES:

Product information. Ritonavir (*Norvir*). Abbott Laboratories. 1996.

Saquinavir (eg, *Fortovase*)

Sildenafil (*Viagra*)

SUMMARY: Saquinavir administration increases sildenafil plasma concentrations; observe patients for side effects.

RISK FACTORS: No specific risk factors are known.

RELATED DRUGS: Other protease inhibitors such as indinavir (*Crixivan*), ritonavir (*Norvir*), amprenavir (*Agenerase*), and nelfinavir (*Viracept*) are known to inhibit CYP3A4 and would be expected to interact with sildenafil.

MANAGEMENT OPTIONS:

➡ *Circumvent/Minimize.* Because of the potential for serious side effects, counsel patients taking protease inhibitors that are CYP3A4 inhibitors to avoid sildenafil coadministration. If sildenafil were coadministered to patients taking saquinavir, a starting dose of 25 mg would be prudent.

➡ *Monitor.* Carefully monitor patients treated with sildenafil for side effects (eg, headache, flushing, hypotension, abnormal vision) if saquinavir is prescribed.

REFERENCES:

Muirhead GJ, et al. Pharmacokinetic interactions between sildenafil and saquinavir/ritonavir. *Br J Clin Pharmacol.* 2000;50:99.

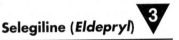

Selegiline (*Eldepryl*)

Tyramine

SUMMARY: Selegiline may increase the pressor response to food or drink containing tyramine, but the effect usually is not large.

RISK FACTORS:

➡ *Dosage Regimen.* Selegiline doses of up to 10 mg/day usually have only a small inhibitory effect on monoamine oxidase (MAO)-A, but larger doses can have a clinically important effect.

RELATED DRUGS: Mofegiline, another MAO-B inhibitor, does not appear to lose its MAO-B selectivity when large doses are used.

MANAGEMENT OPTIONS:

➡ *Circumvent/Minimize.* Although strict avoidance of tyramine-containing foods is not necessary, it would be prudent to avoid high-tyramine foods, especially if the patient is taking more than 10 mg/day of selegiline.

➡ *Monitor.* Monitor for evidence of tyramine-induced hypertension.

REFERENCES:

Elsworth JD, et al. Deprenyl administration in man: a selective monoamine oxidase B inhibitor without the "cheese effect." *Psychopharmacology.* 1978;57:33.

Schulz R, et al. Tyramine kinetics and pressor sensitivity during monoamine oxidase inhibition by selegiline. *Clin Pharmacol Ther.* 1989;46:528.

Sertraline (*Zoloft*)

Tramadol (*Ultram*)

SUMMARY: A patient on sertraline and tramadol developed serotonin syndrome, but it is unknown how often this occurs in patients receiving the combination.

RISK FACTORS: No specific risk factors are known.

RELATED DRUGS: The combination of paroxetine (*Paxil*) and tramadol also has been reported to produce serotonin syndrome. It is possible that other selective serotonin reuptake inhibitors (SSRIs) such as fluoxetine (eg, *Prozac*), fluvoxamine (*Luvox*), and citalopram also may increase the risk of serotonin syndrome if combined with tramadol. Meperidine (*Demerol*) may interact similarly with SSRIs.

MANAGEMENT OPTIONS:

➡ *Consider Alternative.* In patients on sertraline or other SSRIs, consider the use of an analgesic that is not serotonergic (eg, an agent other than tramadol or meperidine) to minimize the risk of serotonin syndrome.

➡ *Monitor.* In patients receiving tramadol and sertraline (or other SSRIs) be alert for evidence of serotonin syndrome. Serotonin syndrome can result in neurotoxicity (eg, myoclonus, tremors, rigidity, incoordination, hyperreflexia, seizures, coma), psychiatric symptoms (eg, agitation, confusion, hypomania, restlessness), and autonomic dysfunction (eg, fever, sweating, tachycardia, hypertension).

REFERENCES:

Mason BJ, et al. Possible serotonin syndrome associated with tramadol and sertraline coadministration. *Ann Pharmacother.* 1997;31:175-177.

Sternbach H. The serotonin syndrome. *Am J Psychiatry.* 1991;148:705-13.

Sertraline (*Zoloft*)

Warfarin (eg, *Coumadin*)

SUMMARY: A preliminary report suggests that sertraline may slightly increase the hypoprothrombinemic response to warfarin.

RISK FACTORS: No specific risk factors are known.

RELATED DRUGS: Some selective serotonin reuptake inhibitors (eg, fluoxetine [eg, *Prozac*], paroxetine [*Paxil*]) have been reported to have an intrinsic inhibitory effect on hemostasis, but it is not known if sertraline has a similar effect. The effect of sertraline on oral anticoagulants other than warfarin is not established.

MANAGEMENT OPTIONS:

➡ *Monitor.* Although data are scanty, be alert for evidence of an altered hypoprothrombinemic response to warfarin (or other anticoagulants) if sertraline is initiated, discontinued, or changed in dosage. Although not reported for sertraline, some SSRIs may impair hemostasis; thus, be alert for evidence of bleeding even if the hypoprothrombinemic response is in the desired range.

REFERENCES:

Wilner KD, et al. The effects of sertraline on the pharmacodynamics of warfarin in healthy volunteers. *Biol Psychiatry.* 1991;29:333S.

Sibutramine (*Meridia*)
Sumatriptan (*Imitrex*)

SUMMARY: The risk of serotonin syndrome would theoretically increase when sibutramine is combined with other serotonergic drugs such as sumatriptan.

RISK FACTORS: No specific risk factors are known.

RELATED DRUGS: Little is known regarding concurrent use of zolmitriptan (*Zomig*) and sibutramine, but it is possible that there may be an increase in the risk of serotonin syndrome.

MANAGEMENT OPTIONS:

➡ **Avoid Unless Benefit Outweighs Risk.** The manufacturer states that sibutramine should not be used with sumatriptan. This is a prudent recommendation until more information is available.

➡ **Monitor.** Serotonin syndrome can result in neurotoxicity (eg, myoclonus, tremors, rigidity, incoordination, restlessness, hyperreflexia, seizures, coma), psychiatric symptoms (eg, agitation, confusion, hypomania), and temperature regulation abnormalities (eg, fever, sweating). Note that mild forms of serotonin syndrome also have been reported, so consider any combination of the above symptoms possibly related to excessive serotonin activity.

REFERENCES:

Product information. Sibutramine (*Meridia*). Knoll Pharmaceuticals. 1997.

Mills KC. Serotonin syndrome: a clinical update. *Crit Care Clin.* 1997;13:763.

Sibutramine (*Meridia*)
Tryptophan (*Tryptacin*)

SUMMARY: The risk of serotonin syndrome would theoretically increase when sibutramine is combined with other serotonergic drugs such as tryptophan.

RISK FACTORS: No specific risk factors are known.

RELATED DRUGS: No information is available.

MANAGEMENT OPTIONS:

➡ **Avoid Unless Benefit Outweighs Risk.** The manufacturer states that sibutramine should not be used with tryptophan. This is a prudent recommendation until more information is available.

➡ **Monitor.** Serotonin syndrome can result in neurotoxicity (eg, myoclonus, tremors, rigidity, incoordination, restlessness, hyperreflexia, seizures, coma), psychiatric symptoms (eg, agitation, confusion, hypomania), and temperature regulation abnormalities (eg, fever, sweating). Note that mild forms of serotonin syndrome have also been reported, so any combination of the above symptoms should be considered possibly related to excessive serotonin activity.

REFERENCES:

Product information. Sibutramine (*Meridia*). Knoll Pharmaceuticals. 1997.

Mills KC. Serotonin syndrome: a clinical update. *Crit Care Clin.* 1997;13:763.

Simvastatin (*Zocor*)

Ritonavir (*Norvir*)

SUMMARY: Ritonavir administration appears to increase the risk of serious toxicity in patients taking simvastatin.

RISK FACTORS: No specific risk factors are known.

RELATED DRUGS: The clearance of other statins that are metabolized by CYP3A4 (eg, lovastatin [eg, *Mevacor*], atorvastatin [*Lipitor*]) would likely be reduced by ritonavir. Other protease inhibitors such as amprenavir (*Agenerase*), indinavir, nelfinavir (*Viracept*), and saquinavir (*Invirase*) would be expected to decrease simvastatin clearance.

MANAGEMENT OPTIONS:

➡ ***Use Alternative.*** Because pravastatin (*Pravachol*) and fluvastatin (*Lescol*) are not metabolized by CYP3A4, consider using one of these agents in patients taking protease inhibitors.

➡ ***Monitor.*** Monitor patients taking statins that are metabolized by CYP3A4 and a protease inhibitor for side effects including myopathy and myoglobinemia.

REFERENCES:

Cheng CH, et al. Rhabdomyolysis due to probable interaction between simvastatin and ritonavir. *Am J Health Syst Pharm.* 2002;59:728-730.

Burger DM, et al. Pharmacokinetic interaction between the proton pump inhibitor omeprazole and the HIV protease inhibitor indinavir. *AIDS.* 1998;12:2080-2082.

Simvastatin (*Zocor*)

St. John's Wort

SUMMARY: St. John's wort appears to substantially lower simvastatin plasma concentrations; consider using pravastatin as an alternative.

RISK FACTORS: No specific risk factors are known.

RELATED DRUGS: Theoretically, lovastatin (*Mevacor*) would interact with St. John's wort in a manner similar to simvastatin. Atorvastatin (*Lipitor*) also may interact, but probably to a lesser degree. Pravastatin (*Pravachol*) pharmacokinetics were not affected by St. John's wort.

MANAGEMENT OPTIONS:

➡ ***Consider Alternative.*** Pravastatin does not appear to interact with St. John's wort and would be preferable to simvastatin or lovastatin. An alternative antidepressant to St. John's wort also could be considered, but nefazodone (*Serzone*) would not be a good choice with any HMG-CoA reductase inhibitor that is metabolized by CYP3A4 (eg, simvastatin, lovastatin, atorvastatin).

➡ ***Monitor.*** If St. John's wort is used with simvastatin, lovastatin, or atorvastatin, monitor serum lipid concentrations for evidence of reduced effect.

REFERENCES:

Sugimoto K, et al. Different effects of St. John's wort on the pharmacokinetics of simvastatin and pravastatin. *Clin Pharmacol Ther.* 2001;70:518-524.

Simvastatin (*Zocor*)
Tacrolimus (*Prograf*)

SUMMARY: A patient on tacrolimus developed rhabdomyolysis after simvastatin was added, but a causal relationship was not established.

RISK FACTORS: No specific risk factors are known.

RELATED DRUGS: Theoretically, other statins metabolized by CYP3A4 such as atorvastatin (*Lipitor*) and lovastatin (*Mevacor*) would also interact with tacrolimus. Numerous cases of myopathy and rhabdomyolysis have been reported with concurrent use of simvastatin or lovastatin with cyclosporine (eg, *Neoral*), and isolated cases have been reported with atorvastatin and cyclosporine. On the other hand, pravastatin (*Pravachol*) and fluvastatin (*Lescol*) do not appear to interact with CYP3A4 inhibitors such as cyclosporine, and probably would not interact with tacrolimus.

MANAGEMENT OPTIONS:

➡ *Consider Alternative.* Although this interaction is not well documented, until more data are available it would be prudent to avoid simvastatin, lovastatin, or atorvastatin in patients receiving tacrolimus. Pravastatin and fluvastatin are unlikely to interact with tacrolimus, and would be preferred.

➡ *Monitor.* If simvastatin, lovastatin, or atorvastatin is used with tacrolimus, advise the patient to monitor for evidence of myopathy (eg, muscle pain or weakness, dark urine). Elevated creatine kinase (CK) levels are another indication of possible myopathy.

REFERENCES:
Kotanko P, et al. Rhabdomyolysis and acute renal graft impairment in a patient treated with simvastatin, tacrolimus, and fusidic acid. *Nephron.* 2002;90:234-235.

Simvastatin (*Zocor*) **②**
Verapamil (eg, *Calan*)

SUMMARY: Verapamil administration may increase simvastatin concentrations markedly; avoid using the drugs together for the risk of increased side effects.

RISK FACTORS: No specific risk factors are known.

RELATED DRUGS: Diltiazem (eg, *Cardizem*) may affect simvastatin metabolism in a similar manner. The effect of other calcium channel blockers on simvastatin metabolism is unknown but would not be expected to be significant. Verapamil will likely produce a similar increase in lovastatin (*Mevacor*) plasma concentrations. While no data are available, verapamil also may increase the plasma concentration of atorvastatin (*Lipitor*). The metabolism of pravastatin (*Pravachol*) and fluvastatin (*Lescol*) would not be expected to be affected by verapamil.

MANAGEMENT OPTIONS:

➡ *Use Alternative.* Consider the use of an HMG-CoA reductase inhibitor other than simvastatin or lovastatin for patients receiving verapamil. Atorvastatin and cerivastatin plasma concentrations are likely to be increased by a smaller amount during verapamil coadministration. Do not alter pravastatin and fluvastatin metabolism by verapamil.

REFERENCES:

Kantola T, et al. Erythromycin and verapamil considerably increase serum simvastatin and simvastatin acid concentrations. *Clin Pharmacol Ther.* 1998;64:177-182.

 Sirolimus (*Rapamune*)

Voriconazole (*Vfend*)

SUMMARY: Voriconazole administration with sirolimus causes a marked increase in sirolimus plasma concentrations, which are likely to result in toxicity such as bone marrow suppression.

RISK FACTORS:

➡ **Pharmacogenetics.** Patients who are poor metabolizers for CYP2C19 will have higher voriconazole concentrations, and thus are likely to have an interaction of larger magnitude.

RELATED DRUGS: Tacrolimus (eg, *Prograf*) and cyclosporine (eg, *Neoral*) metabolism is reduced by voriconazole administration. The metabolism of other immunosuppressants such as everolimus (*Certican*) (not available in the US) is likely to be decreased by voriconazole. Other azole antifungal agents including ketoconazole (eg, *Nizoral*) and itraconazole (eg, *Sporanox*) are known to reduce the metabolism of sirolimus. Fluconazole (*Diflucan*) also may reduce the metabolism of sirolimus.

MANAGEMENT OPTIONS:

➡ **Use Alternative.** If possible, avoid the coadministration of voriconazole and sirolimus.

REFERENCES:

Product information. Voriconazole (*Vfend*). Pfizer, Inc. 2002.

 Sotalol (eg, *Betapace*)

Ziprasidone (*Geodon*)

SUMMARY: Ziprasidone and sotalol can prolong the QTc interval on the electrocardiogram (ECG). Theoretically, this could increase the risk of ventricular arrhythmias such as torsades de pointes.

RISK FACTORS:

➡ **Hypokalemia.** The corrected QT interval (QTc) on the ECG may be prolonged in patients with hypokalemia, increasing the risk of this interaction.

➡ **Miscellaneous.** Other factors that may prolong the QTc interval (eg, hypomagnesemia, bradycardia, impaired liver function, hypothyroidism) also may increase the risk of ventricular arrhythmias.

RELATED DRUGS: Available data suggest that ziprasidone produces less QTc prolongation than thioridazine (*Mellaril*), but about twice that of quetiapine (*Seroquel*), risperidone (*Risperdal*), haloperidol (*Haldol*), and olanzapine (*Zyprexa*).

MANAGEMENT OPTIONS:

➡ *Use Alternative.* Given the theoretical risk and the fact that sotalol is listed in the ziprasidone product information as "contraindicated," it would be prudent to use an alternative to one of the drugs (see Related Drugs).

➡ *Monitor.* If sotalol and ziprasidone are used concurrently, monitor for evidence of arrhythmias (eg, syncope) and for prolonged QT intervals.

REFERENCES:

De Ponti F, et al. QT-interval prolongation by non-cardiac drugs: lessons to be learned from recent experience. *Eur J Clin Pharmacol.* 2000;56:1-18.

Product information. Ziprasidone (*Geodon*). Pfizer Pharmaceuticals. 2001.

Briefing Information, Psychopharmacological Drugs Advisory Committee, U.S. Food and Drug Administration, July 19, 2000.

Sparfloxacin (*Zagam*)
Sucralfate (eg, *Carafate*)

SUMMARY: Sucralfate reduces the plasma concentration of sparfloxacin; loss of efficacy may occur.

RISK FACTORS: No specific risk factors are known.

RELATED DRUGS: Aluminum-containing antacids (eg, *Maalox*) may produce a similar change in the absorption of sparfloxacin. Sucralfate is known to reduce the absorption of other quinolone antibiotics, such as ciprofloxacin (*Cipro*) and ofloxacin (*Floxin*).

MANAGEMENT OPTIONS:

➡ *Circumvent/Minimize.* While there are no direct data to support separating the doses of sparfloxacin and sucralfate, administration of sparfloxacin 2 to 3 hours prior to sucralfate dosing may minimize the interaction.

➡ *Monitor.* Monitor patients receiving sparfloxacin for reduction in antibiotic efficacy if sucralfate is coadministered.

REFERENCES:

Zix JA. Pharmacokinetics of sparfloxacin and interaction with cisapride and sucralfate. *Antimicrob Agents Chemother.* 1997;41:1668–1672.

Sparfloxacin (*Zagam*)
Ziprasidone (*Geodon*)

SUMMARY: Ziprasidone and sparfloxacin can prolong the corrected QT interval (QTc) interval on the electrocardiogram (ECG). Theoretically, this can increase the risk of ventricular arrhythmias such as torsades de pointes.

RISK FACTORS:

➡ *Hypokalemia.* The QTc on the ECG may be prolonged in patients with hypokalemia, increasing the risk of this interaction.

➡ *Miscellaneous.* Other factors that may prolong the QTc interval (eg, hypomagnesemia, bradycardia, impaired liver function, hypothyroidism) may also increase the risk of ventricular arrhythmias.

RELATED DRUGS: Available data suggest that ziprasidone produces less QTc prolongation than thioridazine (eg, *Mellaril*), but about twice that of quetiapine (*Seroquel*), risperidone (eg, *Risperdal*), haloperidol (eg, *Haldol*), and olanzapine (eg, *Zyprexa*). Moxifloxacin (eg, *Avelox*), like sparfloxacin, can prolong the QTc interval substantially, but other fluoroquinolones such as levofloxacin (*Levaquin*), ofloxacin (eg, *Floxin*), gatifloxacin (*Tequin*), and ciprofloxacin (eg, *Cipro*) usually produce only minimal effects.

MANAGEMENT OPTIONS:

➥ *Use Alternative.* Given the theoretical risk and the fact that sparfloxacin is listed in the ziprasidone product information as contraindicated, it would be prudent to use an alternative to one of the drugs (see Related Drugs).

➥ *Monitor.* If sparfloxacin and ziprasidone are used concurrently, monitor for evidence of arrhythmias (eg, syncope) and for prolonged QT intervals.

REFERENCES:

De Ponti F, et al. QT-interval prolongation by non-cardiac drugs: lessons to be learned from recent experience. *Eur J Clin Pharmacol.* 2000;56:1-18.

Product information. Ziprasidone (*Geodon*). Pfizer Pharmaceuticals. 2001.

Briefing Information, Psychopharmacological Drugs Advisory Committee, U.S. Food and Drug Administration, July 19, 2000.

Spironolactone (eg, *Aldactone*)

Candesartan (*Atacand*)

SUMMARY: Combining spironolactone with candesartan or other angiotensin II receptor blockers (ARBs) increases the risk of hyperkalemia, especially in patients with 1 or more risk factors.

RISK FACTORS:

➥ *Other Drugs.* In patients taking spironolactone and ARBs, the addition of other hyperkalemic drugs can increase the risk. Such drugs include potassium supplements, nonselective beta-adrenergic blockers, cyclosporine, tacrolimus, NSAIDs, COX-2 inhibitors, trimethoprim, and pentamidine.

➥ *Concurrent Diseases.* Diseases that increase the risk of hyperkalemia for this interaction include diabetes and significant renal impairment.

➥ *Dosage Regimen.* Patients receiving spironolactone in doses of 50 mg/day or more are at greater risk of hyperkalemia from this interaction.

➥ *Effects of Age.* Most of the patients who have developed hyperkalemia from this interaction have been elderly.

➥ *Diet/Food.* A diet high in potassium may increase the risk of hyperkalemia from this interaction. Some salt substitutes contain potassium.

RELATED DRUGS: Spironolactone would be expected to interact with other ARBs, including eprosartan (*Teveten*), irbesartan (*Avapro*), losartan (*Cozaar*), telmisartan (*Micardis*), and valsartan (*Diovan*).

MANAGEMENT OPTIONS:

➥ *Circumvent/Minimize.* Use the minimum effective dose of spironolactone; 25 mg/day may be enough for many patients.

➡️ *Monitor.* In patients receiving spironolactone and an ARB, monitor serum potassium and renal function, particularly if the patient has 1 or more of the risk factors listed above.

REFERENCES:

Wrenger E, et al. Interaction of spironolactone with ACE inhibitors or antiogensin receptor blockers: analysis of 44 cases. *BMJ*. 2003;327:147-149.

Schepkens H, et al. Life-threatening hyperkalemia during combined therapy with angiotensin-converting enzyme inhibitors and spironolactone: an analysis of 25 cases. *Am J Med*. 2001;110:438-441.

Berry C, et al. Life-threatening hyperkalemia during combined therapy with angiotensin-converting enzyme inhibitors and spironolactone. *Am J Med*. 2001;111:587.

Blaustein DA, et al. Estimation of glomerular filtration rate to prevent life-threatening hyperkalemia due to combined therapy with spironolactone and angiotensin-converting enzyme inhibition or angiotensin receptor blockade. *Am J Cardiol*. 2002;90:662-663.

Weber EW, et al. Incidence of hyperkalemia in chronic heart failure patients taking spironolactone in a VA medical center. *Pharmacotherapy*. 2003;23:391.

Spironolactone (eg, *Aldactone*)

Enalapril (eg, *Vasotec*)

SUMMARY: Combining spironolactone with enalapril or other ACE inhibitors increases the risk of hyperkalemia, especially in patients with 1 or more risk factors.

RISK FACTORS:

➡️ *Other Drugs.* In patients taking spironolactone and ACE inhibitors, the addition of other hyperkalemic drugs can increase the risk. Such drugs include potassium supplements, nonselective beta-adrenergic blockers, cyclosporine, tacrolimus, NSAIDs, COX-2 inhibitors, trimethoprim, and pentamidine.

➡️ *Concurrent Diseases.* Diseases that increase the risk of hyperkalemia for this interaction include diabetes and significant renal impairment.

➡️ *Dosage Regimen.* Patients receiving spironolactone in doses of 50 mg/day or more are at greater risk of hyperkalemia from this interaction.

➡️ *Effects of Age.* Most of the patients who have developed hyperkalemia from this interaction have been elderly.

➡️ *Diet/Food.* A diet high in potassium may increase the risk of hyperkalemia from this interaction. Some salt substitutes contain potassium.

RELATED DRUGS: Spironolactone would be expected to interact with other ACE inhibitors, including benazepril (*Lotensin*), captopril (eg, *Capoten*), fosinopril (*Monopril*), lisinopril (eg, *Prinivil*), moexipril (eg, *Univasc*), quinapril (*Accupril*), ramipril (*Altace*), and trandolapril (*Mavik*).

MANAGEMENT OPTIONS:

➡️ *Circumvent/Minimize.* Use the minimum effective dose of spironolactone; 25 mg/day may be enough for many patients.

➡ *Monitor.* In patients receiving spironolactone and an ACE inhibitor, monitor serum potassium and renal function, particularly if the patient has 1 or more of the risk factors listed above.

REFERENCES:

Pitt B, et al. The effect of spironolactone on morbidity and mortality in patients with severe heart failure. Randomized *Aldactone* Evaluation Study Investigators. *New Engl J Med.* 1999;341:709-717.

Schepkens H, et al. Life-threatening hyperkalemia during combined therapy with angiotensin-converting enzyme inhibitors and spironolactone. *Am J Med.* 2001;110:438-441.

Berry C, et al. Life-threatening hyperkalemia during combined therapy with angiotensin-converting enzyme inhibitors and spironolactone. *Am J Med.* 2001;111:587.

Blaustein DA, et al. Estimation of glomerular filtration rate to prevent life-threatening hyperkalemia due to combined therapy with spironolactone and angiotensin-converting enzyme inhibition or angiotensin receptor blockade. *Am J Cardiol.* 2002;90:662-663.

Wrenger E, et al. Interaction of spironolactone with ACE inhibitors or angiotensin receptor blockers: analysis of 44 cases. *BMJ.* 2003;327:147-149.

Weber EW, et al. Incidence of hyperkalemia in chronic heart failure patients taking spironolactone in a VA medical center. *Pharmacotherapy.* 2003;23:391.

St. John's Wort

Tacrolimus (*Prograf*)

SUMMARY: Preliminary clinical evidence suggests that St. John's wort substantially reduces tacrolimus plasma concentrations; avoid the combination.

RISK FACTORS: No specific risk factors are known.

RELATED DRUGS: It is well documented that St. John's wort reduces serum concentrations of cyclosporine and can lead to organ transplant rejection. Theoretically, St. John's wort would also reduce plasma concentrations of sirolimus (*Rapamune*).

MANAGEMENT OPTIONS:

➡ *Use Alternative.* In patients receiving tacrolimus, cyclosporine, and probably sirolimus, it would be preferable to use antidepressants other than St. John's wort. Selective serotonin reuptake inhibitors (SSRIs) and related antidepressants (eg, paroxetine [eg, *Paxil*], sertraline [*Zoloft*], citalopram [*Celexa*], venlafaxine [eg, *Effexor*]) are not known to induce or inhibit CYP3A4 to a clinically important extent. Fluoxetine (eg, *Prozac*) appears to be a weak inhibitor of CYP3A4. Fluvoxamine (eg, *Luvox*) is a moderate CYP3A4 inhibitor and nefazodone (eg, *Serzone*) is a potent inhibitor of CYP3A4.

➡ *Monitor.* If St. John's wort is used with tacrolimus, cyclosporine, or sirolimus, monitor the patient for reduced immunosuppressant effect.

REFERENCES:

Bauer S, et al. The influence of St. John's wort extract on blood concentrations of cyclosporine A, tacrolimus and mycophenolic acid in renal transplant patients. *Ther Drug Monit.* 2003;25:511.

St. John's Wort ▼
Warfarin (eg, *Coumadin*)

SUMMARY: Several cases of reduced warfarin response have been reported with the use of St. John's wort. Although a causal relationship has not been conclusively established, it would be prudent to carefully monitor a patient's warfarin response carefully if St. John's wort is used concurrently.

RISK FACTORS: No specific risk factors are known.

RELATED DRUGS: Theoretically, acenocoumarol (not available in the US) would interact similarly with St. John's wort, but data are lacking. Phenprocoumon (not available in the US) is metabolized primarily by glucuronide conjugation, a process that may be enhanced by enzyme induction.

MANAGEMENT OPTIONS:

➥ ***Consider Alternative.*** In patients receiving oral anticoagulants, consider using alternative antidepressants. Selective serotonin reuptake inhibitors (SSRIs) (eg, fluoxetine [eg, *Prozac*], paroxetine [*Paxil*], sertraline [*Zoloft*], citalopram [*Celexa*]) are not known to inhibit CYP2C9, the isozyme primarily responsible for the metabolism of S-warfarin. However, some SSRIs have been reported to increase the risk of bleeding in anticoagulated patients in the absence of an increase in the INR.

➥ ***Monitor.*** Monitor patients taking warfarin or other oral anticoagulants for altered hypoprothrombinemic response if St. John's wort is started, stopped, or changed in dosage.

REFERENCES:

Ruschitzka F, et al. Acute heart transplant rejection due to Saint John's wort. *Lancet.* 2000;355:548.

Piscitelli SC, et al. Indinavir concentrations and St. John's wort. *Lancet.* 2000;355:547.

Yue QY, et al. Safety of St. John's wort (*Hypericum perforatum*). *Lancet.* 2000;355(9203):576-77.

De Smet PA, et al. Safety of St. John's wort (*Hypericum perforatum*). *Lancet.* 2000;355:575.

Succinylcholine (eg, *Anectine*) ▼
Tacrine (*Cognex*)

SUMMARY: Tacrine may prolong the effect of depolarizing neuromuscular blockers such as succinylcholine and theoretically would antagonize the effect of nondepolarizing agents such as curare.

RISK FACTORS: No specific risk factors are known.

RELATED DRUGS: Theoretically, tacrine should antagonize the neuromuscular blockade of nondepolarizing neuromuscular blockers such as tubocurarine, although clinical evidence of the interaction appears to be lacking.

MANAGEMENT OPTIONS:

➥ ***Circumvent/Minimize.*** Because of the short half-life of tacrine, it should not be difficult to avoid tacrine interactions with neuromuscular blockers. Theoretically, the effect of tacrine should be minimal 10 to 12 hours after the last dose.

➠ *Monitor.* Be alert for altered neuromuscular blockade if tacrine has been given within the previous 24 hours.

REFERENCES:

Moriearty PL, et al. Estimation of plasma tacrine concentrations using an *in vitro* cholinesterase inhibition assay. *Alzheimer Dis Assoc Discord.* 1989;3:143.

Eldon MA, et al. Investigation of the central and peripheral cholinomimetic effects and plasma cholinesterase inhibition of tacrine. *Clin Pharmacol Ther.* 1992;51:175.

Ford JM, et al. Serum concentrations of tacrine hydrochloride predict its adverse effects in Alzheimer's disease. *Clin Pharmacol Ther.* 1993;53:691.

Oberoi GS et al. The use of tacrine (THA) and succinylcholine compared with alcuronium during laparoscopy. *P N G Med J.* 1990;33:25.

Taylor P. Agents acting at the neuromuscular junction and autonomic ganglia. In: Gilman AG, et al., eds. *The Pharmacological Basis of Therapeutics.* 8th ed. New York, NY: Pergamon Press; 1990:166.

Sucralfate (eg, *Carafate*)

Trovafloxacin (*Trovan*)

SUMMARY: Sucralfate reduces the bioavailability of trovafloxacin; a loss of therapeutic efficacy may occur in some patients.

RISK FACTORS: No specific risk factors are known.

RELATED DRUGS: Sucralfate similarly affects other quinolones such as ciprofloxacin (*Cipro*) and ofloxacin (*Floxin*).

MANAGEMENT OPTIONS:

➠ *Consider Alternative.* The use of H_2-receptor antagonists in place of sucralfate should be considered when trovafloxacin is being administered.

➠ *Circumvent/Minimize.* Administer the antibiotic at least 2 hours before the sucralfate.

➠ *Monitor.* Observe patients receiving trovafloxacin who are administered sucralfate for reduced antibiotic effect.

REFERENCES:

Product information. Trovafloxacin (*Trovan*). Pfizer Pharmaceuticals. 1998.

Sucralfate (eg, *Carafate*)

Warfarin (eg, *Coumadin*)

SUMMARY: In isolated cases, sucralfate appeared to inhibit the effect of warfarin, but subsequent studies have failed to demonstrate an interaction.

RISK FACTORS: No specific risk factors are known.

RELATED DRUGS: The effect of sucralfate on oral anticoagulants other than warfarin is not established. Ranitidine (eg, *Zantac*) and famotidine (eg, *Pepcid*) do not interact.

MANAGEMENT OPTIONS:

➠ *Consider Alternative.* Consider using a noninteracting H_2-receptor antagonist, such as ranitidine (*Zantac*) or famotidine (*Pepcid*).

➡ *Circumvent/Minimize.* Take oral anticoagulants at least 2 hours before or 6 hours after sucralfate and try to maintain a relatively constant interval and sequence of administration of the 2 drugs.

➡ *Monitor.* Although this interaction is not well established, monitor for altered oral anticoagulant effect if sucralfate is initiated, discontinued, or changed in dosage. Adjust the anticoagulant dose as needed.

REFERENCES:

Mungall D, et al. Sucralfate and warfarin. *Ann Intern Med.* 1983;98:557.

Talbert RL, et al. Effect of sucralfate on plasma warfarin concentration in patients requiring chronic warfarin therapy. *Drug Intell Clin Pharm.* 1985;19:456.

Neuvonen PJ, et al. Clinically significant sucralfate-warfarin interaction is not likely. *Br J Clin Pharmacol.* 1985;20:178.

Rey AM, et al. Altered absorption of digoxin, sustained-release quinidine, and warfarin with sucralfate administration. *DICP.* 1991;25:745.

Braverman SE, et al. Sucralfate-warfarin interaction. *Drug Intell Clin Pharm.* 1988;22:913. Letter.

Parrish RH, et al. Sucralfate-warfarin interaction. *Ann Pharmacother.* 1992;26:1015. Letter.

Sulfasalazine (eg, *Azulfidine*)

Talinolol

SUMMARY: Serum concentrations of the selective beta blocker, talinolol, are markedly reduced by the coadministration of sulfasalazine; reduced clinical efficacy is likely to result.

RISK FACTORS: No specific risk factors are known.

RELATED DRUGS: Other beta blockers may be similarly affected by sulfasalazine administration.

MANAGEMENT OPTIONS:

➡ *Circumvent/Minimize.* If binding in the GI tract is the mechanism for this interaction, giving the talinolol several hours before the sulfasalazine would minimize the interaction. Talinolol and, pending further studies, other beta blockers should be administered 2 to 3 hours before doses of sulfasalazine.

➡ *Monitor.* If talinolol and sulfasalazine are coadministered, be alert for a reduction in beta blocker activity.

REFERENCES:

Terhaag B, et al. Interaction of talinolol and sulfasalazine in the human GI tract. *Eur J Clin Pharmacol.* 1992;42:461.

Sulfinpyrazone (eg, *Anturane*)

Tolbutamide (eg, *Orinase*)

SUMMARY: Sulfinpyrazone may increase the hypoglycemic effects of tolbutamide.

RISK FACTORS: No specific risk factors are known.

RELATED DRUGS: Sulfinpyrazone could potentially affect other sulfonylureas.

MANAGEMENT OPTIONS:

➡ *Monitor.* Diabetic patients receiving tolbutamide may require dosage adjustments when therapy with sulfinpyrazone is initiated or withdrawn. Monitor blood glucose and watch for symptoms of hypoglycemia if sulfinpyrazone is initiated or hyperglycemia if it is withdrawn.

REFERENCES:

Miners JO. The effect of sulfinpyrazone on oxidative drug metabolism in man: inhibition of tolbutamide elimination. *Eur J Clin Pharmacol.* 1982;22:321.

 ## Sulfinpyrazone (eg, *Anturane*)

Warfarin (eg, *Coumadin*)

SUMMARY: Sulfinpyrazone markedly increases the hypoprothrombinemic response to warfarin, acenocoumarol, and possibly other oral anticoagulants. If the combination must be used, monitor carefully for excessive hypoprothrombinemia and clinical evidence of bleeding.

RISK FACTORS: No specific risk factors are known.

RELATED DRUGS: Acenocoumarol is affected similarly by sulfinpyrazone. Phenprocoumon does not appear to interact with sulfinpyrazone. The effect of sulfinpyrazone on other oral anticoagulants is unknown, but assume that they interact until proven otherwise.

MANAGEMENT OPTIONS:

➡ *Avoid Unless Benefit Outweighs Risk.* Do not use sulfinpyrazone in anticoagulated patients unless the potential benefit clearly outweighs the substantial risk.

➡ *Monitor.* If sulfinpyrazone is used, closely monitor the hypoprothrombinemic response. When warfarin therapy is initiated in patients receiving sulfinpyrazone, increased sensitivity to warfarin's hypoprothrombinemic effect may occur.

REFERENCES:

Weiss M. Potentiation of coumarin effect by sulfinpyrazone. *Lancet.* 1979;1:609.

Jamil A, et al. Interaction between sulfinpyrazone and warfarin. *Chest.* 1981;79:373.

Bailey RR, et al. Potentiation of warfarin action by sulfinpyrazone. *Lancet.* 1980;1:254.

Davis JW, et al. Possible interaction of sulfinpyrazone with coumarins. *N Engl J Med.* 1978;299:955.

Gallus A, et al. Sulfinpyrazone and warfarin: a probable drug interaction. *Lancet.* 1980;1:535.

Thompson PL, et al. Potentially serious interaction of warfarin with sulfinpyrazone. *Med J Aust.* 1981;1:41.

Nenci GG, et al. Biphasic sulfinpyrazone-warfarin interaction. *BMJ.* 1981;282:1361.

O'Reilly RA. Stereoselective interaction of sulfinpyrazone with racemic warfarin and its separated enantiomorphs in man. *Circulation.* 1982;65:202.

Girolami A, et al. Potentiation of anticoagulated response to warfarin by sulfinpyrazone: a double-blind study in patients with prosthetic heart values. *Clin Lab Haematol.* 1982;4:23.

Michot F, et al. Uber die Beeiflussung der Gerinnungshemmenden Wirkung von Acenocoumarol durch Sulfinpyrazon. *Schweiz Med Wochenschr.* 1981;111:255.

O'Reilly RA. Phenylbutazone and sulfinpyrazone interaction with oral anticoagulant phenprocoumon. *Arch Intern Med.* 1982;142:1634.

Sulindac (eg, *Clinoril*)

Warfarin (eg, *Coumadin*)

SUMMARY: Although sulindac did not affect the response to warfarin in healthy subjects, several patients receiving warfarin have developed excessive hypoprothrombinemia following sulindac therapy.

RISK FACTORS:

➡ ***Concurrent Diseases.*** Patients with peptic ulcer disease (PUD) or a history of GI bleeding probably are at a greater risk.

RELATED DRUGS: All NSAIDs inhibit platelet function, cause gastric erosions, and probably increase the risk of GI bleeding. However, some NSAIDs such as ibuprofen (eg, *Advil*), naproxen (eg, *Naprosyn*), or diclofenac (eg, *Voltaren*) may be less likely to increase oral anticoagulant-induced hypoprothrombinemia than other NSAIDs.

MANAGEMENT OPTIONS:

➡ ***Avoid Unless Benefit Outweighs Risk.*** Because all NSAIDs probably increase the risk of GI bleeding in patients on oral anticoagulants, use the combination only after careful consideration of the benefit vs risk. If an NSAID must be used with an oral anticoagulant, it would be prudent to use NSAIDs that are unlikely to affect the hypoprothrombinemic response to oral anticoagulants. If the NSAID is being used as an analgesic or antipyretic, acetaminophen (eg, *Tylenol*) is probably safer to use with oral anticoagulants. Nonacetylated salicylates (eg, choline salicylate, magnesium salicylate, salsalate, sodium salicylate) probably also are safer with oral anticoagulants than NSAIDs, since such salicylates have minimal effects on platelet function and the gastric mucosa.

➡ ***Monitor.*** If any NSAID is used with an oral anticoagulant, carefully monitor the prothrombin time and watch for evidence of bleeding, especially from the GI tract.

REFERENCES:

Loftin JP. Interaction between sulindac and warfarin: different results in normal subjects and in an unusual patient with a potassium-losing renal tubular defect. *J Clin Pharmacol.* 1979;19:733

Ross JRY, et al. Sulindac, prothrombin time, and anticoagulants. *Lancet.* 1979;2:1075.

Carter SA. Potential effect of sulindac on response of prothrombin time to oral anticoagulants. *Lancet.* 1979;2:698.

Shorr RI, et al. Concurrent use of nonsteroidal anti-inflammatory drugs and oral anticoagulants places elderly persons at high risk for hemorrhagic peptic ulcer disease. *Arch Intern Med.* 1993;153:1665.

Tacrine (*Cognex*)

Theophylline

SUMMARY: Tacrine can substantially increase theophylline plasma concentrations; reductions in theophylline dosage are likely to be necessary.

RISK FACTORS: No specific risk factors are known.

RELATED DRUGS: No information is available.

MANAGEMENT OPTIONS:

➡ *Consider Alternative.* In patients already receiving tacrine who are being started on theophylline, consider using alternatives to theophylline. If theophylline is used, it would be prudent to begin with smaller than usual doses until the response is determined.

➡ *Circumvent/Minimize.* Given the potential magnitude of the interaction, it may be prudent to adjust theophylline dosage prophylactically in patients at higher risk (eg, those with high pre-existing theophylline plasma concentrations).

➡ *Monitor.* In patients receiving theophylline, monitor clinical status and theophylline plasma concentrations if tacrine is initiated, discontinued, or changed in dosage.

REFERENCES:

Madden S, et al. An investigation into the formation of stable, proteinreactive and cytotoxic metabolites from tacrine *in vitro*: studies with human and rat liver microsomes. *Biochem Pharmacol*. 1993;46:13.

de Vries TM, et al. Effect of multiple-dose tacrine administration on single-dose pharmacokinetics of digoxin, diazepam, and theophylline. *Pharm Res*. 1993;10:S333. Abstract.

Product information. Tacrine (*Cognex*). Parke-Davis. 1993.

Tacrine (*Cognex*)

Trihexyphenidyl (*Artane*)

SUMMARY: Tacrine may inhibit the therapeutic effect of anticholinergic agents such as trihexyphenidyl, and centrally acting anticholinergics may inhibit the therapeutic effect of tacrine.

RISK FACTORS: No specific risk factors are known.

RELATED DRUGS: Although more study is needed, one would expect all centrally acting anticholinergic agents to inhibit tacrine response. Tacrine may inhibit the therapeutic effect of anticholinergics.

MANAGEMENT OPTIONS:

➡ *Consider Alternative.* It would be prudent to avoid centrally acting anticholinergic agents in patients receiving tacrine, because they would be expected to antagonize the favorable effects of tacrine in Alzheimer disease.

➡ *Monitor.* If the combination is used, monitor for reduced tacrine response.

REFERENCES:

Ott BR, et al. Exacerbation of Parkinsonism by tacrine. *Clin Neuropharmacol*. 1992;15:322.

Summers WK, et al. Use of THA in treatment of Alzheimer-like dementia: pilot study in twelve patients. *Biol Psychiatry*. 1981;16:145.

Tacrolimus (eg, *Prograf*)

Voriconazole (*Vfend*)

SUMMARY: Voriconazole administration increases tacrolimus concentrations; increased side effects may occur in some patients.

RISK FACTORS:

➡ ***Pharmacogenetics.*** Patients who are poor metabolizers for CYP2C19 will have higher voriconazole concentrations, and thus are likely to have an interaction of larger magnitude.

RELATED DRUGS: Sirolimus (*Rapamune*) and cyclosporine (eg, *Neoral*) metabolism is reduced by voriconazole administration. The metabolism of other immunosuppressants such as everolimus (*Certican*) (not available in the US) is likely to be decreased by voriconazole. Other azole antifungal agents including ketoconazole (eg, *Nizoral*), fluconazole (*Diflucan*), and itraconazole (eg, *Sporanox*) are known to reduce the metabolism of tacrolimus.

MANAGEMENT OPTIONS:

➡ ***Circumvent/Minimize.*** A reduction in the dose of tacrolimus may be required during coadministration of voriconazole.

➡ ***Monitor.*** Monitor tacrolimus plasma concentrations if voriconazole is prescribed concomitantly. When voriconazole is discontinued, monitor for decreasing tacrolimus concentrations.

REFERENCES:
Product information. Voriconazole (*Vfend*). Pfizer, Inc. 2002.

Terfenadine

Troleandomycin (*Tao*)

SUMMARY: The administration of troleandomycin with terfenadine may lead to arrhythmias.

RISK FACTORS: No specific risk factors are known.

RELATED DRUGS: Erythromycin and clarithromycin (eg, *Biaxin*) inhibit terfenadine metabolism. Astemizole (*Hismanal*) metabolism would be inhibited by troleandomycin. Azithromycin (*Zithromax*) and dirithromycin (*Dynabac*) do not alter terfenadine concentrations.

MANAGEMENT OPTIONS:

➡ ***Use Alternative.*** Avoid taking terfenadine and troleandomycin because of the risk of arrhythmias. Astemizole may not be a safe alternative to terfenadine since it has been associated with arrhythmias when administered with drugs that inhibit its metabolism. The use of sedating antihistamines, cetirizine (*Zyrtec*), or loratadine (eg, *Claritin*) may be preferable in patients who require antihistamine therapy during troleandomycin treatment.

REFERENCES:
Fournier P, et al. A new cause of torsades de pointes: combination of terfenadine and troleandomycin [in French]. *Ann Cardiol Angeiol* (Paris). 1993;42:249-252.

Terfenadine (*Seldane*)

Zafirlukast (*Accolate*)

SUMMARY: Studies in healthy subjects suggest that terfenadine substantially reduces the plasma concentrations of zafirlukast, but the degree to which this would reduce the therapeutic response of zafirlukast in asthmatic patients is not established.

RISK FACTORS: No specific risk factors are known.

RELATED DRUGS: The effect of other antihistamines on zafirlukast pharmacokinetics is not established. Because astemizole (*Hismanal*) has interactive properties similar to terfenadine, it might be expected to interact with zafirlukast in a similar manner. However, no information is available.

MANAGEMENT OPTIONS:

➡ *Consider Alternative.* In patients on zafirlukast, consider using antihistamines with fewer interactive properties than terfenadine or astemizole.

➡ *Monitor.* If the combination is used, monitor for reduced zafirlukast response (ie, uncontrolled asthma).

REFERENCES:

Product information. Zafirlukast (*Accolate*). Zeneca Pharmaceuticals. 1996.

Tetracycline

Zinc

SUMMARY: Zinc may reduce the serum concentration of tetracycline enough to reduce its antibacterial efficacy.

RISK FACTORS: No specific risk factors are known.

RELATED DRUGS: Doxycycline (eg, *Vibramycin*) absorption was not significantly affected by zinc coadministration.

MANAGEMENT OPTIONS:

➡ *Consider Alternative.* Doxycycline might be considered as an alternative.

➡ *Circumvent/Minimize.* When patients are receiving both tetracycline and zinc sulfate, the drugs should be taken as far apart as possible to minimize mixing in the GI tract. Take the tetracycline 2 to 3 hours before the zinc.

➡ *Monitor.* If tetracycline and foods or dairy products containing large amounts of cations are coadministered, be alert for reduced antibiotic effects.

REFERENCES:

Penttila O, et al. Effect of zinc sulphate on the absorption of tetracycline and doxycycline in man. *Eur J Clin Pharmacol.* 1975;9:131.

Mapp RK, et al. The effect of zinc sulphate and of bicitropeptide on tetracycline absorption. *S Afr Med J.* 1976;50:1829.

Andersson KE, et al. Inhibition of tetracycline absorption by zinc. *Eur J Clin Pharmacol.* 1976;10:59.

Theophylline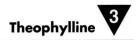

Thiabendazole (*Mintezol*)

SUMMARY: Case reports suggest that thiabendazole can substantially increase serum theophylline concentrations; theophylline toxicity may result.

RISK FACTORS: No specific risk factors are known.

RELATED DRUGS: Mebendazole does not interact.

MANAGEMENT OPTIONS:

➡ *Circumvent/Minimize.* Reduce theophylline dosages in patients who must take thiabendazole with theophylline. Consider alternative drugs for theophylline (eg, beta-agonists, steroids) during thiabendazole treatment.

➡ *Monitor.* Carefully monitor patients taking theophylline for increased theophylline concentrations and manifestations of theophylline toxicity (eg, tachycardia, nervousness, nausea) if they require a course of thiabendazole therapy.

REFERENCES:

Sugar AM, et al. Possible thiabendazole-induced theophylline toxicity. *Am Rev Respir Dis.* 1980;122:501.

Lew G, et al. Theophylline-thiabendazole drug interaction. *Clin Pharm.* 1989;8:225.

Schneider D, et al. Theophylline and antiparasitic drug interactions. A case report and study of the influence of thiabendazole and mebendazole on theophylline pharmacokinetics in adults. *Chest.* 1990;97:84.

Theophylline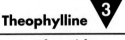

Thyroid

SUMMARY: Initiation of thyroid replacement therapy in patients receiving theophylline may reduce serum theophylline concentrations.

RISK FACTORS:

➡ *Order of Drug Administration.* Patients on theophylline therapy who are started on thyroid replacement are at increased risk for the interaction. (Patients stabilized on thyroid replacement before theophylline therapy is started probably are at minimal risk for the interaction.)

RELATED DRUGS: No information is available.

MANAGEMENT OPTIONS:

➡ *Monitor.* Monitor patients for a reduced theophylline response when thyroid replacement therapy is initiated for hypothyroidism.

REFERENCES:

Johnson CE, et al. Theophylline toxicity after iodine 131 treatment for hyperthyroidism. *Clin Pharm.* 1988;7:620.

Theophylline

Ticlopidine (eg, *Ticlid*)

SUMMARY: Ticlopidine substantially increased plasma theophylline concentrations in healthy subjects and may increase the risk of theophylline toxicity in patients.

RISK FACTORS: No specific risk factors are known.

RELATED DRUGS: No information is available.

MANAGEMENT OPTIONS:

➥ **Monitor.** Monitor for altered theophylline effect if ticlopidine therapy is initiated, discontinued, or changed in dosage; adjustments in theophylline dosage may be needed.

REFERENCES:

Colli A, et al. Ticlopidine-theophylline interaction. *Clin Pharmacol Ther.* 1987;41:358.

Theophylline

Troleandomycin (*Tao*)

SUMMARY: Troleandomycin may increase theophylline serum concentrations and the potential for theophylline toxicity.

RISK FACTORS:

➥ **Dosage Regimen.** Troleandomycin doses greater than 250 mg/day increases the risk for the interaction.

RELATED DRUGS: Erythromycin and clarithromycin (*Biaxin*) will inhibit theophylline metabolism. Azithromycin (*Zithromax*) has been shown to have no effect on theophylline metabolism.

MANAGEMENT OPTIONS:

➥ **Use Alternative.** Patients should avoid theophylline and troleandomycin administration. Azithromycin may be an alternative.

REFERENCES:

Weinberger M, et al. Inhibition of theophylline clearance by troleandomycin. *J Allergy Clin Immunol.* 1977;59:228.

Kamada AK, et al. Effect of low-dose troleandomycin on theophylline clearance: implications for therapeutic drug monitoring. *Pharmacotherapy.* 1992;12:98.

Theophylline

Verapamil (eg, *Calan*)

SUMMARY: Verapamil appears to increase plasma concentrations of theophylline. In some patients, the increases may be large enough to result in theophylline toxicity.

RISK FACTORS:

➥ **Pharmacogenetics.** Children and cigarette smokers are at increased risk for the interaction.

RELATED DRUGS: The clearance of theophylline was decreased approximately 20%, or not affected by diltiazem (eg, *Cardizem*). Diltiazem attenuated rifampin (*Rifadin*)-induced theophylline clearance but not smoking-induced clearance. Theophylline absorption was noted to be moderately reduced following felodipine (*Plendil*) administration. Additional study is needed to substantiate these findings and establish clinical significance. Isradipine (*DynaCirc*) and nifedipine (eg, *Procardia*) appear to have no or minimal effect on theophylline pharmacokinetics.

MANAGEMENT OPTIONS:

➡ *Consider Alternative.* Isradipine and nifedipine may be alternatives to verapamil.

➡ *Monitor.* Carefully monitor patients receiving verapamil and perhaps diltiazem for evidence of theophylline toxicity (eg, tachycardia, tremor, GI upset). Theophylline plasma concentration determinations may be helpful.

REFERENCES:

Burnakis TG, et al. Increased serum theophylline concentrations secondary to oral verapamil. *Clin Pharmacol.* 1983;2:458.

Parrillo SJ, et al. Elevated theophylline blood levels from institution of nifedipine therapy. *Ann Emerg Med.* 1984;13:216.

Harrod CS. Theophylline toxicity and nifedipine. *Ann Intern Med.* 1987;106:480.

Sirmans S, et al. Effect of calcium channel blockers on theophylline disposition. *Clin Pharmacol Ther.* 1988;44:29.

Nafziger AN, et al. Inhibition of theophylline elimination by diltiazem therapy. *J Clin Pharmacol.* 1987;27:862.

Jackson SHD, et al. The interaction between IV theophylline and chronic oral dosing with slow-release nifedipine in volunteers. *Br J Clin Pharmacol.* 1986;21:389.

Christopher MA, et al. Clinical relevance of the interaction of theophylline with diltiazem or nifedipine. *Chest.* 1989;95:309.

Garty M, et al. Effect of nifedipine and theophylline in asthma. *Clin Pharmacol Ther.* 1986;40:195.

Robson RA, et al. Selective inhibitory effects of nifedipine and verapamil on oxidative metabolism: effects of theophylline. *Br J Clin Pharmacol.* 1988;25:397.

Nielsen-Kudsk JE, et al. Verapamil-induced inhibition of theophylline elimination in healthy humans. *Pharmacol Toxicol.* 1990;66:101.

Gin AS, et al. The effect of verapamil on the pharmacokinetic disposition of theophylline in cigarette smokers. *J Clin Pharmacol.* 1989;29:728.

Adebayo GI, et al. Attenuation of rifampicin-induced theophylline metabolism by dilitiazem/rifampicin coadministration in healthy volunteers. *Eur J Clin Pharmacol.* 1989;37:127.

Bratel T, et al. Felodipine reduces the absorption of theophylline in man. *Eur J Clin Pharmacol.* 1989;36:481.

Abernethy DR, et al. Substrate-selective inhibition by verapamil and diltiazem: differential disposition of antipyrine and theophylline in humans. *J Pharmacol Exp Ther.* 1989;244:994.

Stringer KA, et al. The effect of three different oral doses of verapamil on the disposition of theophylline. *Eur J Clin Pharmacol.* 1992;43:35.

Yilmaz E, et al. Nifedipine alters serum theophylline levels in asthmatic patients with hypertension. *Fundam Clin Pharmacol.* 1991;5:341.

Perreault M, et al. The effect of isradipine on theophylline pharmacokinetics in healthy volunteers. *Pharmacotherapy.* 1993;13:149.

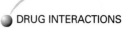

 Theophylline

Zafirlukast (*Accolate*)

SUMMARY: The manufacturer reports that theophylline can decrease plasma concentrations of zafirlukast; adjustments in zafirlukast dose may be needed.

RISK FACTORS: No specific risk factors are known.

RELATED DRUGS: No information is available.

MANAGEMENT OPTIONS:

➡ *Monitor.* Monitor for altered zafirlukast effect if theophylline is initiated, discontinued, or changed in dosage.

REFERENCES:

Product information. Zafirlukast (*Accolate*). Zeneca Pharmaceuticals. 1997.

 Thioridazine (*Mellaril*)

Ziprasidone (*Geodon*)

SUMMARY: Ziprasidone and thioridazine can prolong the QTc interval on the electrocardiogram (ECG). Theoretically, this could increase the risk of ventricular arrhythmias such as torsades de pointes.

RISK FACTORS:

➡ *Hypokalemia.* The corrected QT interval (QTc) on the ECG may be prolonged in patients with hypokalemia, increasing the risk of this interaction.

➡ *Miscellaneous.* Other factors that may prolong the QTc interval (eg, hypomagnesemia, bradycardia, impaired liver function, hypothyroidism) also may increase the risk of ventricular arrhythmias.

RELATED DRUGS: Available data suggest that the QTc prolongation following ziprasidone is about twice that of quetiapine (*Seroquel*), risperidone (*Risperdal*), haloperidol (*Haldol*), and olanzapine (*Zyprexa*).

MANAGEMENT OPTIONS:

➡ *Use Alternative.* Given the theoretical risk and the fact that thioridazine is listed in the ziprasidone product information as "contraindicated," it would be prudent to use an alternative to one of the drugs (see Related Drugs).

➡ *Monitor.* If thioridazine and ziprasidone are used concurrently, monitor for evidence of arrhythmias (eg, syncope) and for prolonged QT intervals.

REFERENCES:

De Ponti F, et al. QT-interval prolongation by non-cardiac drugs: lessons to be learned from recent experience. *Eur J Clin Pharmacol.* 2000;56:1-18.

Product information. Ziprasidone (*Geodon*). Pfizer Pharmaceuticals. 2001.

Briefing Information, Psychopharmacological Drugs Advisory Committee, U.S. Food and Drug Administration, July 19, 2000.

Thyroid

Warfarin (eg, *Coumadin*)

SUMMARY: The hypoprothrombinemic response to oral anticoagulants is altered by changes in clinical thyroid status; adjustments in anticoagulant dosage are likely to be required if the thyrometabolic status changes.

RISK FACTORS:

➡ *Order of Drug Administration.* The primary risk is in starting thyroid replacement therapy in the presence of chronic oral anticoagulants, while the risk appears small if the oral anticoagulant is started in the presence of chronic thyroid therapy.

RELATED DRUGS: Given the mechanism, it is likely that all oral anticoagulants are affected by all types of thyroid replacement.

MANAGEMENT OPTIONS:

➡ *Monitor.* Monitor for altered oral anticoagulant effect if thyroid replacement therapy is initiated, discontinued, or changed in dosage. Adjust the anticoagulant dose as needed. No special precautions appear necessary when oral anticoagulant therapy is begun in a patient already stabilized on maintenance thyroid replacement therapy.

REFERENCES:

Hansten PD. Oral anticoagulants and drugs which alter thyroid function. *Drug Intell Clin Pharm.* 1980;14:331.

Loeliger EA, et al. The biological disappearance rate of prothrombin and factors VII, IX and X from plasma in hypothyroidism, hyperthyroidism and during fever. *Thromb Diath Haemorrh.* 1964;10:267.

Walters MB. The relationship between thyroid function and anticoagulant therapy. *Am J Cardiol.* 1963;11:112.

Vagenakis AG, et al. Enhancement of warfarin-induced hypoprothrombinemia by thyrotoxicosis. *Johns Hopkins Med J.* 1972;131:69.

McIntosh TJ, et al. Increased sensitivity to warfarin in thyrotoxicosis. *J Clin Invest.* 1970;49:63a. Abstract.

Rice AJ, et al. Decreased sensitivity to warfarin in patients with myxedema. *Am J Med Sci.* 1971;262:211.

Self T, et al. Warfarin-induced hypoprothrombinemia: potentiation by hyperthyroidism. *JAMA.* 1975;231:1165.

Edson JR, et al. Low platelet adhesiveness and other hemostatic abnormalities in hypothyroidism. *Ann Intern Med.* 1975;82:342.

Self TH, et al. Effect of hyperthyroidism on hypoprothrombinemic response to warfarin. *Am J Hosp Pharm.* 1976;33:387.

Van Dosterom AT, et al. The influence of the thyroid function on the metabolic rate of prothrombin, factor VII, and factor X in the rat. *Thromb Haemost.* 1976;3:607.

Costigan DC, et al. Potentiation of oral anticoagulant effect by 1-thyroxine. *Clin Pediatr.* 1984;23:172.

Tolbutamide (eg, *Orinase*)

Trimethoprim-Sulfamethoxazole (eg, *Bactrim*)

SUMMARY: Several sulfonamides like trimethoprim-sulfamethoxazole (TMP-SMZ) can increase plasma concentration of oral antidiabetic agents like tolbutamide and enhance their hypoglycemic effects.

RISK FACTORS: No specific risk factors are known.

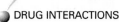

RELATED DRUGS: Glipizide, glyburide, and chlorpropamide are affected similarly by sulfonamides such as TMP-SMZ, sulfamethizole, sulfaphenazole, and sulfisoxazole. Sulfonamides have not been reported to affect the response to insulin.

MANAGEMENT OPTIONS:

➡ *Monitor.* TMP-SMZ and tolbutamide coadministration should be undertaken with the realization that enhanced hypoglycemic effects may occur. Sulfadiazine and sulfadimethoxine do not appear to have this effect.

REFERENCES:

Wing LMH, et al. Cotrimoxazole as an inhibitor of oxidative drug metabolism: effects of trimethoprim and sulphamethoxazole separately and combined on tolbutamide disposition. *Br J Clin Pharmacol.* 1985;20:482.

Christensen LK, et al. Sulfaphenazole-induced hypoglycemic attacks in tolbutamide-treated diabetics. *Lancet.* 1963;2:1298.

Soeldner JS, et al. Hypoglycemia in tolbutamide-treated diabetes. *JAMA.* 1965;193:398.

Dall JLC, et al. Hypoglycaemia due to chlorpropamide. *Scott Med J.* 1967;12:403.

Mihic M, et al. Effect of trimethoprim-sulfamethoxazole on blood insulin and glucose concentrations of diabetics. *Can Med Assoc J.* 1975;112:805.

Johnson JF, et al. Symptomatic hypoglycemia secondary to a glipizidetrimethoprim/sulfamethoxazole drug interaction. *DICP.* 1990;24:250.

Asplund K, et al. Glibenclamide-associated hypoglycemia: a report on 57 cases. *Diabetologia.* 1983;24:412.

Baciewicz AM, et al. Hypoglycemia induced by the interaction of chlorpropamide and co-trimoxazole. *Drug Intell Clin Pharm.* 1984;18:309.

 Tolmetin (eg, *Tolectin*)

Warfarin (eg, *Coumadin*)

SUMMARY: Tolmetin does not appear to affect the hypoprothrombinemic response to warfarin, but caution during cotherapy is indicated because of possible detrimental effects of tolmetin on the gastric mucosa and platelet function.

RISK FACTORS:

➡ *Concurrent Diseases.* Patients with peptic ulcer disease (PUD) or a history of GI bleeding probably are at greater risk for the interaction.

RELATED DRUGS: All NSAIDs inhibit platelet function, cause gastric erosions, and probably increase the risk of GI bleeding.

MANAGEMENT OPTIONS:

➡ *Avoid Unless Benefit Outweighs Risk.* Because all NSAIDs probably increase the risk of GI bleeding in patients on oral anticoagulants, use the combination only after careful consideration of the benefit vs risk. If the NSAID is being used as an analgesic or antipyretic, acetaminophen (eg, *Tylenol*) probably is safer to use with oral anticoagulants. Nonacetylated salicylates (eg, choline salicylate, magnesium salicylate, salsalate, sodium salicylate) probably also are safer with oral anticoagulants than NSAIDs since they have minimal effects on platelet function and the gastric mucosa.

➡ *Monitor.* If any NSAID is used with an oral anticoagulant, carefully monitor the prothrombin time and watch for evidence of bleeding, especially from the GI tract.

REFERENCES:

Pullar T. Interaction between oral anti-coagulant drugs and nonsteroidal anti-inflammatory agents: a review. *Scott Med J.* 1983;28:42.

Shorr RI, et al. Concurrent use of nonsteroidal anti-inflammatory drugs and oral anticoagulants places elderly persons at high risk for hemorrhagic peptic ulcer disease. *Arch Intern Med.* 1993;153:1665.

Toloxatone

Tyramine

SUMMARY: Large doses of toloxatone (a selective monoamine oxidase [MAO]-A inhibitor) may increase the pressor response to large amounts of tyramine; avoid high tyramine foods (eg, aged cheese).

RISK FACTORS: No specific risk factors are known.

RELATED DRUGS: Other MAO-A inhibitors, such as moclobemide, may interact similarly with tyramine.

MANAGEMENT OPTIONS:

➥ **Circumvent/Minimize.** Although toloxatone appears less likely to interact with dietary tyramine than nonselective MAOIs, it would be prudent to avoid foods with a high tyramine content.

➥ **Monitor.** Monitor blood pressure if the interaction is suspected.

REFERENCES:

Provost JC, et al. Pharmacokinetic and pharmacodynamic interaction between toloxatone, a new reversible monoamine oxidase-A inhibitor, and oral tyramine in healthy subjects. *Clin Pharmacol Ther.* 1992;52:384.

Freeman H. Moclobemide. *Lancet.* 1993;342:1528.

Simpson GM, et al. Comparison of the pressor effect of tyramine aftertreatment with phenelzine and moclobemide in healthy male volunteers. *Clin Pharmacol Ther.* 1992;52:286.

Tramadol (*Ultram*) ❷

Tranylcypromine (*Parnate*)

SUMMARY: Tramadol theoretically increases the risk of seizures and serotonin syndrome in patients taking monoamine oxidase inhibitors (MAOIs).

RISK FACTORS: No specific risk factors are known.

RELATED DRUGS: Until clinical data are available, all MAOIs, including phenelzine (*Nardil*) and isocarboxazid (*Marplan*), should be considered equally likely to interact with tramadol.

MANAGEMENT OPTIONS:

➥ **Avoid Unless Benefit Outweighs Risk.** Although published clinical information appears lacking, theoretical and medicolegal considerations suggest that the combination should generally be avoided.

➥ **Monitor.** If the combination is used, monitor for seizures and for early evidence of serotonin syndrome. Serotonin syndrome can result in neurotoxicity (eg, myoclonus, tremors, rigidity, incoordination, restlessness, hyperreflexia, seizures, coma), psychiatric symptoms (eg, agitation, confusion, hypomania), and temperature regulation abnormalities (eg, fever, sweating).

REFERENCES:

Product information. Tramadol (*Ultram*). McNeil Pharmaceutical. 1997.

Tranylcypromine (*Parnate*)

AVOID **Tyramine**

SUMMARY: The consumption of foods containing large amounts of tyramine can result in hypertensive reactions in patients taking monoamine oxidase inhibitors (MAOIs).

RISK FACTORS: No specific risk factors are known.

RELATED DRUGS: One patient receiving phenelzine (*Nardil*) developed a hypertensive reaction and headache following ingestion of a cup of miso soup. All nonselective MAOIs including isocarboxazid (*Marplan*) interact with tyramine-containing foods.

MANAGEMENT OPTIONS:

➡ *AVOID COMBINATION.* Instruct patients taking MAOIs to avoid foods that may have a high tyramine content. Remember that the effects of nonselective MAOIs should be assumed to persist for 2 weeks after they are discontinued. Estimates of the tyramine content of various foods and beverages have been published. Foods to be avoided include cheeses (especially aged), red wines, caviar, herring (dried or pickled), canned figs, fermented or spoiled meat (including salami, pepperoni, summer sausage), fava beans, yeast extracts, miso soup, and avocados (especially if overripe).

REFERENCES:

Blackwell B. Hypertensive crises due to monoamine-oxidase inhibitors. *Lancet.* 1963;2:849.

Hedberg DL, et al. Six cases of hypertensive crises in patients on tranylcypromine after eating chicken livers. *Am J Psychiatry.* 1966;122:933.

Nuessle WF, et al. Pickled herring and tranylcypromine reaction. *JAMA.* 1965;192:726. Letter.

Blackwell B, et al. Effects of yeast extract after monoamine oxidase inhibition. *Lancet.* 1965;1:940.

Shullman KI, et al. Dietary restriction, tyramine, and the use of monoamine oxidase inhibitors. *J Clin Psychopharmacol.* 1989;9:397.

Tedeschi DH, et al. Monoamine oxidase inhibitors: augmentation of pressor effects of peroral tyramine. *Science.* 1964;144:1225.

Cuthill JM, et al. Death associated with tranylcypromine and cheese. *Lancet.* 1964;1:1076.

Sen NP. Analysis and significance of tyramine in foods. *J Food Sci.* 1969;34:22.

Marley E, et al. Interactions of monoamine-oxidase inhibitors, amines, foodstuffs. *Adv Pharmacol Chemother.* 1970;8:185.

Anon. Monoamine oxidase inhibitors for depression. *Med Lett.* 1980;22:58.

Peet M, et al. The interaction of tyramine with a single dose of tranylcypromine in healthy volunteers. *Br J Clin Pharmacol.* 1981;11:212.

Brown C, et al. The monoamine oxidase inhibitor-tyramine interaction. *J Clin Pharmacol.* 1989;29:529.

Mesmer RE, et al. Don't mix miso with MAOIs. *JAMA.* 1987;258:3515.

 Tranylcypromine (*Parnate*)

AVOID **Venlafaxine (*Effexor*)**

SUMMARY: Severe serotonin syndrome can occur when venlafaxine is used with or within 2 weeks of discontinuation of tranylcypromine or other nonselective monoamine oxidase inhibitors (MAOIs). Avoid the combination.

RISK FACTORS: No specific risk factors are known.

RELATED DRUGS: Expect all nonselective MAOIs to result in serotonin syndrome if combined with venlafaxine. This would include phenelzine (*Nardil*) and isocarboxazid (*Marplan*); selegiline (*Eldepryl*) can act as a nonselective MAOI in some patients, especially if large doses are used.

MANAGEMENT OPTIONS:

➡ *AVOID COMBINATION.* Avoid combined use of venlafaxine with tranylcypromine (or any other nonselective MAOI). This would include the use of venlafaxine within 2 weeks of discontinuation of an MAOI.

REFERENCES:
Brubacher JR, et al. Serotonin syndrome from venlafaxine-tranylcypromine interaction. *Vet Hum Toxicol.* 1996;38:358–361.

Hodgman MJ, et al. Serotonin syndrome due to venlafaxine and maintenance tranylcypromine therapy. *Hum Exp Toxicol.* 1997;16:14–17.

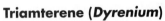

Triamterene (*Dyrenium*)

Candesartan (*Atacand*)

SUMMARY: Combining triamterene with candesartan or other angiotensin II receptor blockers (ARBs) may increase the risk of hyperkalemia, especially in patients with 1 or more risk factors.

RISK FACTORS:

➡ *Other Drugs.* The addition of other hyperkalemic drugs may increase the risk of hyperkalemia in patients taking triamterene and ARBs. Hyperkalemic drugs include ACE inhibitors, potassium supplements, cyclosporine, tacrolimus, NSAIDs, COX-2 inhibitors, nonselective beta-adrenergic blockers, trimethoprim, and pentamidine.

➡ *Concurrent Diseases.* Diseases that increase the risk of hyperkalemia for this interaction include diabetes and significant renal impairment.

➡ *Diet/Food.* A diet high in potassium may increase the risk of hyperkalemia from this interaction. Salt substitutes may contain potassium.

RELATED DRUGS: Triamterene would be expected to increase the risk of hyperkalemia when combined with other ARBs, including eprosartan (*Teveten*), irbesartan (*Avapro*), losartan (*Cozaar*), telmisartan (*Micardis*), and valsartan (*Diovan*).

MANAGEMENT OPTIONS:

➡ *Monitor.* In patients receiving triamterene and an ARB, monitor serum potassium and renal function, particularly if the patient has 1 or more of the risk factors listed before.

REFERENCES:
Wrenger E, et al. Interaction of spironolactone with ACE inhibitors or antiogensin receptor blockers: analysis of 44 cases. *BMJ.* 2003;327:147-149.

Triamterene *(Dyrenium)*

Enalapril (eg, *Vasotec*)

SUMMARY: Combining triamterene with enalapril or other ACE inhibitors increases the risk of hyperkalemia, especially in patients with 1 or more risk factors.

RISK FACTORS:

➡ ***Other Drugs.*** In patients taking triamterene and ACE inhibitors, the addition of other hyperkalemic drugs can increase the risk. Such drugs include potassium supplements, nonselective beta-adrenergic blockers, cyclosporine, tacrolimus, NSAIDs, COX-2 inhibitors, trimethoprim, and pentamidine.

➡ ***Concurrent Diseases.*** Diseases that increase the risk of hyperkalemia for this interaction include diabetes and significant renal impairment.

➡ ***Diet/Food.*** A diet high in potassium may increase the risk of hyperkalemia from this interaction. Some salt substitutes contain potassium.

RELATED DRUGS: Triamterene would also be expected to interact with other ACE inhibitors, including benazepril (*Lotensin*), captopril (eg, *Capoten*), fosinopril (*Monopril*), lisinopril (eg, *Prinivil*), moexipril (eg, *Univasc*), quinapril (*Accupril*), ramipril (*Altace*), and trandolapril (*Mavik*).

MANAGEMENT OPTIONS:

➡ ***Monitor.*** In patients receiving triamterene and an ACE inhibitor, monitor serum potassium and renal function, particularly if the patient has 1 or more of the risk factors listed above.

REFERENCES:

Pitt B, et al. The effect of spironolactone on morbidity and mortality in patients with severe heart failure. Randomized *Aldactone* Evaluation Study Investigators. *New Engl J Med.* 1999;341:709-717.

Schepkens H, et al. Life-threatening hyperkalemia during combined therapy with angiotensin-converting enzyme inhibitors and spironolactone: an analysis of 25 cases. *Am J Med.* 2001;110:438-441.

Berry C, et al. Life-threatening hyperkalemia during combined therapy with angiotensin-converting enzyme inhibitors and spironolactone. *Am J Med.* 2001;111:587.

Blaustein DA, et al. Estimation of glomerular filtration rate to prevent life-threatening hyperkalemia due to combined therapy with spironolactone and angiotensin-converting enzyme inhibition or angiotensin receptor blockade. *Am J Cardiol.* 2002;90:662-663.

Wrenger E, et al. Interaction of spironolactone with ACE inhibitors or angiotensin receptor blockers: analysis of 44 cases. *BMJ.* 2003;327:147-149.

Weber EW, et al. Incidence of hyperkalemia in chronic heart failure patients taking spironolactone in a VA medical center. *Pharmacotherapy.* 2003;23:391.

Triazolam (eg, *Halcion*)

Troleandomycin *(Tao)*

SUMMARY: Troleandomycin causes considerable increase in triazolam serum concentrations and increased sedation may result.

RISK FACTORS: No specific risk factors are known.

RELATED DRUGS: Erythromycin and clarithromycin (eg, *Biaxin*) may inhibit the metabolism of triazolam. Azithromycin (*Zithromax*) would not be expected to affect triazolam. Other benzodiazepines metabolized by CYP3A4 (eg, alprazolam [eg, *Xanax*], midazolam [eg, *Versed*], diazepam [eg, *Valium*]) may be inhibited similarly by troleandomycin.

MANAGEMENT OPTIONS:

➡ *Monitor.* Carefully observe patients receiving triazolam who are prescribed troleandomycin for enhanced triazolam effects. Several days may be required for the maximum effect of troleandomycin to become evident, and triazolam dosages may require adjustment after addition of the antibiotic and again when it is discontinued.

REFERENCES:

Warot D, et al. Troleandomycin-induced interaction in healthy volunteers: pharmacokinetic and psychometric evaluation. *Eur J Clin Pharmacol.* 1987;32:389-393.

Triclofos

Warfarin (eg, *Coumadin*)

SUMMARY: Because triclofos transiently increases the hypoprothrombinemic response to warfarin, alternative hypnotics are preferable in patients on oral anticoagulants.

RISK FACTORS: No specific risk factors are known.

RELATED DRUGS: Alternative sedative/hypnotic drugs unlikely to interact with oral anticoagulants include flurazepam (eg, *Dalmane*), chlordiazepoxide (eg, *Librium*), diazepam (eg, *Valium*), or diphenhydramine (eg, *Benadryl*).

MANAGEMENT OPTIONS:

➡ *Consider Alternative.* Consider an alternative sedative/hypnotic which is unlikely to interact, such as flurazepam, chlordiazepoxide, diazepam, or diphenhydramine.

➡ *Monitor.* If triclofos is used, monitor for altered oral anticoagulant effect when triclofos is initiated, discontinued, or changed in dosage. Adjust the anticoagulant dose as needed.

REFERENCES:

Beliles RP, et al. Interaction of bishydroxycoumarin with chloral hydrate and trichloroethyl phosphate. *Toxicol Appl Pharmacol.* 1974;27:225.

Sellers EM, et al. Enhancement of warfarin-induced hypoprothrombinemia by triclofos. *Clin Pharmacol Ther.* 1972;13:911.

Trimethoprim-Sulfamethoxazole (eg, *Bactrim*)

Warfarin (eg, *Coumadin*)

SUMMARY: Trimethoprim-sulfamethoxazole (TMP-SMZ) increases the hypoprothrombinemic response to warfarin; adjustments in warfarin dose may be required during cotherapy. Oral anticoagulants and other sulfonamides may also interact, but supporting evidence is limited.

RISK FACTORS:

➡ *Concurrent Diseases.* Fever may enhance the catabolism of clotting factors, thus increasing the interaction.

RELATED DRUGS: Preliminary clinical evidence indicates that sulfamethizole (*Thiosulfil*) inhibits warfarin metabolism and that sulfaphenazole (*Thiosulf*) enhances the hypoprothrombinemic response to phenindione. The effect on phenindione appeared to be more pronounced in patients with hypoalbuminemia.

MANAGEMENT OPTIONS:

➡ *Consider Alternative.* If possible, do not use TMP-SMZ in patients anticoagulated with oral agents. Consider a noninteracting antibiotic or heparin anticoagulation.

➡ *Monitor.* If the combination is used, monitor the patient carefully for an increased hypoprothrombinemic response and risk of bleeding during initiation and decreased effects upon discontinuation of TMP-SMZ.

REFERENCES:

Loeliger EA, et al. The biological disappearance rate of prothrombin and factors VII, IX and X from plasma in hypothyroidism, hyperthyroidism and during fever [in German]. *Thromb Diath Haemorrh Suppl.* 1964;10:267.

Tilstone WJ, et al. Interaction between warfarin and sulfamethoxazole. *Postgrad Med J.* 1977;53:388.

Kaufman JM, et al. Potentiation of warfarin by trimethoprim-sulfamethoxazole. *Urology.* 1980;16:601.

Errick JK, et al. Co-trimoxazole and warfarin: case report of an interaction. *Am J Hosp Pharm.* 1978;35:1399.

Greenlaw CW. Drug interaction between co-trimoxazole and warfarin. *Am J Hosp Pharm.* 1979;36:1155.

O'Reilly RA, et al. Racemic warfarin trimethoprim-sulfamethoxazole interaction in humans. *Ann Intern Med.* 1979;91:34.

O'Reilly RA. Stereoselective interaction of trimethoprim-sulfamethoxazole with the separated enantiomorphs of racemic warfarin in man. *N Engl J Med.* 1980;302:33.

Lumholtz B, et al. Sulfamethizole-induced inhibition of diphenylhydantoin, tolbutamite, and warfarin metabolsim. *Clin Pharmacol Ther.* 1975;17:731.

Varma DL, et al. Prothrombin response to phenindione during hypoalbuminaemia. *Br J Clin Pharmacol.* 1975;2:467.

Troleandomycin (*TAO*)

Clopidogrel (*Plavix*)

SUMMARY: Troleandomycin appears to inhibit the antiplatelet effects of clopidogrel, but the extent to which the therapeutic effects of clopidogrel are reduced is not known.

RISK FACTORS: No specific risk factors are known.

RELATED DRUGS: Erythromycin (*TAO*) also appears to inhibit the antiplatelet effects of clopidogrel. Clarithromycin (*Biaxin*) is also an inhibitor of CYP3A4 and would theoretically interact with clopidogrel in a similar manner.

MANAGEMENT OPTIONS:

➡ *Consider Alternative.* Theoretically, azithromycin (*Zithromax*) and dirithromycin (*Dynabac*) would be unlikely to interact with clopidogrel since they do not inhibit CYP3A4.

➡ *Monitor.* Consider monitoring platelet function if troleandomycin is initiated or discontinued. Adjustments in clopidogrel dose may be needed.

REFERENCES:

Clarke TA, et al. The metabolism of clopidogrel is catalyzed by human cytochrome P450 3A and is inhibited by atorvastatin. *Drug Metab Dispos.* 2003;31:53-59.

Lau WC, et al. Atorvastatin reduces the ability of clopidogrel to inhibit platelet aggregation: a new drug-drug interaction. *Circulation.* 2003;107:32-37.

Vecuronium (*Norcuron*) ▼3

Verapamil (eg, *Calan*)

SUMMARY: Verapamil (and perhaps other calcium channel blocking drugs) appears to prolong the neuromuscular blockade of nondepolarizing neuromuscular blockers such as vecuronium and pancuronium (*Pavulon*).

RISK FACTORS: No specific risk factors are known.

RELATED DRUGS: Other calcium channel blockers (eg, nicardipine, diltiazem) may produce similar interactions with vercuronium and other neuromuscular blockers (eg, pancuronium).

MANAGEMENT OPTIONS:

➡ *Circumvent/Minimize.* Reduction in the dose of muscle relaxant may be needed. Edrophonium may be required to reverse the muscle blockade.

➡ *Monitor.* Until additional information is available, patients receiving verapamil or other calcium channel blockers should be observed carefully for prolongation of neuromuscular blockade.

REFERENCES:

Van Poorten JF, et al. Verapamil and reversal of vecuronium neuromuscular blockade. *Anesth Analg.* 1984;63:155.

Jones RM, et al. Verapamil potentiation of neuromuscular blockade: failure of reversal with neostigmine but prompt reversal with edrophonium. *Anesth Analg.* 1985;64:1021.

Kazunaga K, et al. Decrease in vecuronium infusion dose requirements by nicardipine in humans. *Anesth Analg.* 1994;79:1159.

Sumikawa K, et al. Reduction in vecuronium infusion dose requirements by diltiazem in humans. *Anesthesiology.* 1992;77:A939. Abstract.

Vitamin C ▼3

Warfarin (eg, *Coumadin*)

SUMMARY: Isolated cases of impaired warfarin response associated with large doses of vitamin C have been reported, but this effect has not been confirmed.

RISK FACTORS: No specific risk factors are known.

RELATED DRUGS: The effect of vitamin C on oral anticoagulants other than warfarin is not established.

MANAGEMENT OPTIONS: No specific action is required, but be alert for evidence of the interaction.

REFERENCES:

Feetam CL, et al. Lack of a clinically important interaction between warfarin and ascorbic acid. *Toxicol Appl Pharmacol.* 1975;31:544.

Rosenthal G. Interaction of ascorbic acid and warfarin. *JAMA.* 1971;215:1671.

Smith EC, et al. Interaction of ascorbic acid and warfarin. *JAMA.* 1972;221:1166.

Hume R, et al. Interaction of ascorbic acid and warfarin. *JAMA.* 1972;219:1479.

Weintraub M, et al. Warfarin and ascorbic acid: lack of evidence for a drug interaction. *Toxicol Appl Parmacol.* 1974;28:53.

▼ Vitamin E

Warfarin (eg, *Coumadin*)

SUMMARY: Vitamin E may increase the hypoprothrombinemic response to warfarin and other oral anticoagulants. Although the incidence of this interaction in patients receiving the combination is not known, avoid vitamin E in anticoagulated patients.

RISK FACTORS:

➡ *Dosage Regimen.* The risk is probably greater with large doses of vitamin E than the small amounts normally present in multivitamin preparations.

RELATED DRUGS: Three healthy subjects showed a mild increase in hypoprothrombinemic response to dicumarol 150 mg when they were given vitamin E 42 IU/day for 30 days.

MANAGEMENT OPTIONS:

➡ *Monitor.* Monitor for altered oral anticoagulant effect if vitamin E is initiated, discontinued, or changed in dosage. Adjust the anticoagulant dose as needed.

REFERENCES:

Corrigan JJ, et al. Coagulopathy associated with vitamin E ingestion. *JAMA.* 1974;230:1300.

Vitamin K, vitamin E and the coumarin drugs. *Nutr Rev.* 1982;40:180.

Schrogie JJ, et al. Coagulopathy and fat-soluble vitamins. *JAMA.* 1975;232:19.

▼ Vitamin K

Warfarin (eg, *Coumadin*)

SUMMARY: Ingestion of large amounts of foods high in vitamin K may antagonize the hypoprothrombinemic effect of oral anticoagulants.

RISK FACTORS: No specific risk factors are known.

RELATED DRUGS: All oral anticoagulants would be similarly affected by vitamin K.

MANAGEMENT OPTIONS:

➡ *Circumvent/Minimize.* Patients on oral anticoagulants should avoid sudden increases in their intake of leafy vegetables or other foods high in vitamin K content. However, warfarin requirements should not change if patients are consistent in their intake of these foods.

➡ *Monitor.* Monitor for altered hypoprothrombinemic response if vitamin K intake changes substantially.

REFERENCES:

Quick A. Leafy vegetables in diet alter prothrombin time in patients taking anticoagulant drugs. *JAMA.* 1987;187:27.

Fletcher DC. Do clotting factors in vitamin K-rich vegetables hinder anticoagulant therapy? *JAMA.* 1977;237:1871.

Karlson B, et al. On the influence of vitamin K-rich vegetables and wine on the effectiveness of warfarin treatment. *Acta Med Scand.* 1986;220:347.

Kempin SJ. Warfarin resistance caused by broccoli. *N Engl J Med.* 1983;308:1229.

Chow WH, et al. Anticoagulation instability with life-threatening complication after dietary modification. *Postgrad Med J.* 1990;66:855.

Voriconazole (*Vfend*)

Warfarin (eg, *Coumadin*)

SUMMARY: Warfarin activity will be increased when voriconazole is added to a patient's drug regimen; excessive anticoagulation, and increased risk of bleeding may occur.

RISK FACTORS:

➡ ***Pharmacogenetics.*** Patients who are poor metabolizers for CYP2C19 will have higher voriconazole concentrations, and thus are likely to have an interaction of larger magnitude.

RELATED DRUGS: All other antifungal agents except (terbinafine [eg, *Lamisil*]) have been reported to increase the effect of warfarin.

MANAGEMENT OPTIONS:

➡ ***Monitor.*** Carefully monitor patients stabilized on warfarin for increased anticoagulant effect when voriconazole is initiated. Depending on the dosage regimen, 7 to 14 days may be required to observe the maximum change in the INR. Discontinuation of voriconazole is likely to result in decreased anticoagulant effect and warfarin doses may need to be increased.

REFERENCES:

Product information. Voriconazole (*Vfend*). Pfizer, Inc. 2002.

▼ Warfarin (eg, *Coumadin*)

Zafirlukast (*Accolate*)

SUMMARY: Zafirlukast appears to increase the hypoprothrombinemic response to warfarin; adjustments in warfarin dosage may be necessary.

RISK FACTORS: No specific risk factors are known.

RELATED DRUGS: The effect of zafirlukast on oral anticoagulants other than warfarin is not established. If the mechanism of the interaction is inhibition of CYP2C9, phenprocoumon (which is metabolized primarily by glucuronide conjugation) theoretically would be less likely to interact with zafirlukast than warfarin.

MANAGEMENT OPTIONS:

➡ ***Consider Alternative.*** Given the substantial effect of zafirlukast on warfarin response, consider using alternative antiasthmatic medications. In countries where phenprocoumon is available, consider it as an alternative to warfarin, which (theoretically) would be less likely to interact.

➡ ***Monitor.*** Monitor for altered hypoprothrombinemic response to warfarin if zafirlukast is initiated, discontinued, or changed in dosage; adjust warfarin dose as needed.

REFERENCES:

Product information. Zafirlukast (*Accolate*). Zeneca Pharmaceuticals. 1996.

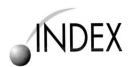

INDEX

GENERAL INDEX

The key to the effective use of *Hansten and Horn's Managing Clinically Important Drug Interactions* is in the index. The drug interaction monographs are listed in alphabetical order beginning on page 1.

All drug interaction monographs are listed by generic name except for combination products (eg, antacids, oral contraceptives) and drugs that interact equally within the class (eg, hormones, thiazide diuretics). The term "homogeneous interactions" is used within the text to refer to drug interactions that apply to all drugs equally within a pharmacological class. Descriptions of intervention categories are found in the Introduction and are provided below.

1 = Avoid Combination   **2** = Usually Avoid Combination   **3** = Minimize Risk

❶ = Avoid Combination   ❷ = Usually Avoid Combination   ▼❸ = Minimize Risk

Atorvastatin *(cont.)*
   3 erythromycin, 80
   3 gemfibrozil, 81
   3 itraconazole, 81
   3 nelfinavir, 82
Atracurium
   2 gentamicin, 83
Atromid-S
   see Clofibrate
Attapulgite
   3 promazine, 83
Avelox
   see Moxifloxacin
Axert
   see Almotriptan
Azapropazone
   2 methotrexate, 84
   2 warfarin, 85
Azathioprine
   2 allopurinol, 13
   3 captopril, 85
   3 phenprocoumon, 86
   3 warfarin, 86
Azulfidine
   see Sulfasalazine
Bactrim
   see Trimethoprim-
     Sulfamethoxazole
Baycol
   see Cerivastatin
Bayer
   see Aspirin
Baypress
   see Nitrendipine
Bellatal
   see Phenobarbital
Benadryl
   see Diphenhydramine
Benemid
   see Probenecid
Benylin DM
   see Dextromethorphan
Benztropine
   3 haloperidol, 87
Bepridil
   3 digoxin, 88
Betapace
   see Sotalol
Betaseron
   see Interferon
Bethanechol
   3 tacrine, 88
Bethanidine
   2 amitriptyline, 36

Bezafibrate
   3 dicumarol, 89
   3 warfarin, 89
Biaxin
   see Clarithromycin
BiCNU
   see Carmustine
Biltricide
   see Praziquantel
Bismuth
   2 doxycycline, 90
   2 tetracycline, 90
Blocadren
   see Timolol
Bosentan,
   3 warfarin, 90
Brethaire
   see Terbutaline
Bromfenac
   3 lithium, 91
   3 phenytoin, 91
   2 warfarin, 92
Bromocriptine
   3 erythromycin, 92
   1 isometheptene, 93
   3 thioridazine, 93
Bumetanide
   3 indomethacin, 94
Bumex
   see Bumetanide
Bunazosin
   3 enalapril, 94
Bupropion
   3 amantadine, 22
Buspar
   see Buspirone
Buspirone
   3 citalopram, 95
   3 diltiazem, 95
   3 erythromycin, 96
   3 fluoxetine, 96
   3 grapefruit juice, 97
   3 itraconazole, 97
   3 rifampin, 98
   3 ritonavir, 98
   3 trazodone, 99
   3 verapamil, 99
Butazolidin
   see Phenylbutazone
Caffeine
   3 ciprofloxacin, 100
   3 enoxacin, 100
   3 fluconazole, 101
   3 methotrexate, 101
   3 norfloxacin, 102
   3 pipemidic acid, 102

Calan
   see Verapamil
Calcium
   3 digoxin, 103
   3 thiazides, 103
   3 verapamil, 104
Candesartan
   3 amiloride, 23
   3 eplerenone, 341
   3 lithium, 104
   3 triamterene, 659
   3 spironolactone, 640
Capoten
   see Captopril
Captopril
   2 allopurinol, 14
   3 aspirin, 66
   3 azathioprine, 85
   3 insulin, 105
Carafate
   see Sucralfate
Carbamazepine
   3 cimetidine, 106
   3 citalopram, 106
   3 clarithromycin, 107
   3 clozapine, 107
   3 contraceptives, oral,
     108
   3 cyclosporine, 109
   2 danazol, 109
   2 diltiazem, 110
   3 doxycycline, 110
   3 erythromycin, 111
   3 felbamate, 112
   2 felodipine, 112
   3 fluconazole, 113
   3 fluoxetine, 113
   3 fluvoxamine, 114
   3 grapefruit juice, 114
   3 haloperidol, 115
   3 imipramine, 115
   3 isoniazid, 116
   3 isotretinoin, 116
   3 ketoconazole, 117
   3 lamotrigine, 117
   3 lithium, 118
   3 mebendazole, 118
   3 methadone, 119
   3 methylphenidate, 119
   3 metronidazole, 120
   3 midazolam, 120
   3 omeprazole, 121
   3 phenytoin, 121
   2 propoxyphene, 122
   3 risperidone, 122
   3 ritonavir, 123
   3 theophylline, 123
   3 thyroid, 123

❶ = Avoid Combination   ❷ = Usually Avoid Combination   ▼3 = Minimize Risk

❶= Avoid Combination　　❷= Usually Avoid Combination　　▼❸= Minimize Risk

Ciprofloxacin *(cont.)*
  3 foscarnet, 185
  3 iron, 185
  3 metoprolol, 186
  3 pentoxifylline, 187
  3 phenytoin, 187
  3 ropinirole, 188
  3 sucralfate, 188
  3 theophylline, 189
  3 warfarin, 189
  3 zinc, 190

Cisapride
  3 cimetidine, 160
  2 clarithromycin, 191
  2 erythromycin, 191
  2 grapefruit juice, 192
  2 indinavir, 192
  2 itraconazole, 193
  2 ketoconazole, 193
  2 mibefradil, 194
  2 miconazole, 194
  2 nefazodone, 195
  2 ritonavir, 195
  2 simvastatin, 196
  2 troleandomycin, 196

Cisplatin
  3 diazoxide, 197
  2 ethacrynic acid, 197
  3 gentamicin, 198
  3 phenytoin, 198

Citalopram
  3 buspirone, 95
  3 carbamazepine, 106
  3 cimetidine, 161
  2 moclobemide, 199

Clarithromycin
  3 atorvastatin, 79
  3 carbamazepine, 107
  2 cisapride, 191
  3 colchicine, 200
  3 cyclosporine, 200
  3 digoxin, 201
  3 disopyramide, 316
  2 ergotamine, 201
  3 indinavir, 202
  3 itraconazole, 202
  2 midazolam, 203
  3 pimozide, 203
  3 prednisone, 204
  1 rifabutin, 204
  3 rifampin, 205
  2 simvastatin, 206
  3 tacrolimus, 206
  2 terfenadine, 207
  3 triazolam, 207
  3 warfarin, 208

Claritin
  see Loratadine

Clinafloxacin
  3 theophylline, 208

Clinoril
  see Sulindac

Clobazam
  3 phenytoin, 209

Clofibrate
  3 chlorpropamide, 149
  3 furosemide, 209
  3 rifampin, 210
  2 warfarin, 210

Clomipramine
  3 fluvoxamine, 211
  3 grapefruit juice, 211
  3 ibuprofen, 212
  2 moclobemide, 213
  1 phenelzine, 213

Clonazepam
  3 valproic acid, 214

Clonidine
  3 chlorpromazine, 143
  3 cyclosporine, 214
  2 desipramine, 215
  3 insulin, 216
  2 mirtazapine, 216
  3 nitroprusside, 217
  3 propranolol, 217

Clopidogrel,
  3 atorvastatin, 80
  3 erythromycin, 343
  3 rifampin, 218
  3 troleandomycin, 662

Clotrimazole
  3 tacrolimus, 218

Clozapine
  3 carbamazepine, 107
  3 cimetidine, 161
  3 ciprofloxacin, 183
  3 diazepam, 219
  2 erythromycin, 219
  2 fluvoxamine, 220
  3 lorazepam, 220
  3 valproic acid, 221

Clozaril
  see Clozapine

Cocaine
  3 disulfiram, 221
  3 propranolol, 222

Codeine
  2 quinidine, 222

Cogentin
  see Benztropine

Cognex
  see Tacrine

Colchicine
  3 clarithromycin, 200
  3 cyclosporine, 223

Colchicine *(cont.)*
  3 erythromycin, 224

Colestid
  see Colestipol

Colestipol
  3 diclofenac, 224
  3 furosemide, 224
  3 gemfibrozil, 225
  3 tetracycline, 225
  3 thiazides, 226

Compazine
  see Prochlorperazine

Contraceptives, Oral
  3 ampicillin, 45
  3 carbamazepine, 108
  1 cigarette smoking, 158
  3 cyclosporine, 237
  3 felbamate, 226
  3 griseofulvin, 426
  3 modafinil, 540
  3 oxcarbazepine, 227
  3 phenobarbital, 227
  3 phenytoin, 228
  3 prednisolone, 229
  3 rifabutin, 230
  3 rifampin, 230
  3 ritonavir, 231
  3 selegiline, 231
  3 St. John's wort, 232
  3 tetracycline, 232
  3 topiramate, 233
  2 warfarin, 233

Contrast Media
  3 propranolol, 234

Cordarone
  see Amiodarone

Cortef
  see Hydrocortisone

Coumadin
  see Warfarin

Cozaar
  see Losartan

Crixivan
  see Indinavir

Cuprimine
  see Penicillamine

Cyclobenzaprine
  3 droperidol, 235
  3 fluoxetine, 235

Cyclophosphamide
  3 allopurinol, 15
  3 digoxin, 235
  3 succinylcholine, 236
  3 warfarin, 236

Cycloserine
  3 isoniazid, 237

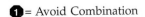 = Avoid Combination   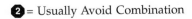 = Usually Avoid Combination   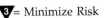 = Minimize Risk

① = Avoid Combination   **②** = Usually Avoid Combination   **▽③** = Minimize Risk

❶ = Avoid Combination   **❷** = Usually Avoid Combination   **▼❸** = Minimize Risk

➊= Avoid Combination ➋= Usually Avoid Combination ▼= Minimize Risk

1= Avoid Combination   **2**= Usually Avoid Combination   **3**= Minimize Risk

❶ = Avoid Combination   ❷ = Usually Avoid Combination   ▼❸ = Minimize Risk

1 = Avoid Combination   **2** = Usually Avoid Combination   **▼3** = Minimize Risk

❶ = Avoid Combination   **❷** = Usually Avoid Combination   **▼❸** = Minimize Risk

1 = Avoid Combination   **2** = Usually Avoid Combination   **3** = Minimize Risk

❶ = Avoid Combination   ❷ = Usually Avoid Combination   ▼❸ = Minimize Risk

Nembutal
  see Pentobarbital
Neo-Fradin
  see Neomycin
Neo-Synephrine
  see Phenylephrine
Neo-Tabs
  see Neomycin
Neomycin
  3 digoxin, 300
  1 methotrexate, 519
  3 penicillin V, 552
  3 warfarin, 552
Neoral
  see Cyclosporine
Neostigmine
  3 procainamide, 553
  3 propranolol, 553
Nevirapine
  3 methadone, 513
  3 nelfinavir, 550
Niacin
  see Nicotinic Acid
Nicardipine
  3 cyclosporine, 253
  3 propranolol, 554
Nicorette
  see Nicotine
Nicotine
  3 adenosine, 10
  3 cimetidine, 171
Nicotinic Acid
  3 lovastatin, 503
Nifedipine
  3 cimetidine, 171
  3 diltiazem, 310
  3 doxazosin, 325
  3 food, 404
  3 grapefruit juice, 422
  3 itraconazole, 465
  3 magnesium, 506
  2 nafcillin, 545
  3 phenobarbital, 555
  3 phenytoin, 555
  3 propranolol, 556
  3 quinidine, 557
  3 quinupristin/
      dalfopristin, 557
  3 rifampin, 558
  3 St. John's wort, 558
  3 tacrolimus, 559
  3 vincristine, 559
Nimodipine
  3 cimetidine, 172
  3 grapefruit juice, 423
  3 valproic acid, 559

Nimotop
  see Nimodipine
Nipride
  see Nitroprusside
Nisoldipine,
  3 cimetidine, 172
  3 grapefruit juice, 423
  3 ketoconazole, 474
Nitrendipine
  3 cimetidine, 173
Nitroglycerin
  2 ergotamine, 343
  3 ethanol, 359
Nitroprusside
  3 clonidine, 217
  3 diltiazem, 311
Nizoral
  see Ketoconazole
Nolvadex
  see Tamoxifen
Norepinephrine
  3 guanethidine, 428
  2 imipramine, 437
  3 methyldopa, 525
  3 phenelzine, 560
Norethindrone
  1 acitretin, 8
Norflex
  see Orphenadrine
Norfloxacin
  3 antacids, 56
  3 caffeine, 102
  3 iron, 456
  3 sucralfate, 560
  3 theophylline, 561
  3 warfarin, 562
Noroxin
  see Norfloxacin
Norpace
  see Disopyramide
Norpramin
  see Desipramine
Nortriptyline
  3 cimetidine, 173
  3 pentobarbital, 562
  3 rifampin, 562
Norvir
  see Ritonavir
Nydrazid
  see Isoniazid
Ofloxacin
  3 antacids, 57
  3 procainamide, 564
  3 sucralfate, 564
  3 warfarin, 565

Olanzapine
  3 fluvoxamine, 395
  3 ritonavir, 565
Omeprazole
  3 carbamazepine, 121
  3 delavirdine, 267
  3 diazepam, 284
  3 digoxin, 300
  3 indinavir, 441
  3 itraconazole, 466
  3 ketoconazole, 475
  3 methotrexate, 519
  3 phenytoin, 565
  3 voriconazole, 566
Omnipen-N
  see Ampicillin
Oncovin
  see Vincristine
Ondansetron
  3 rifampin, 567
Orange Juice,
  3 fexofenadine, 567
Orap
  see Pimozide
Orinase
  see Tolbutamide
Orlistat
  2 cyclosporine, 567
Orphenadrine
  3 chlorpromazine, 147
Ortho-Novum
  see Contraceptives, Oral
Ortho-Novum 1/35
  see Ethinyl Estradiol
Orudis
  see Ketoprofen
Ospolot
  see Sulthiame
Oxacillin,
  3 methotrexate, 519
Oxcarbazepine
  3 contraceptives, oral,
      227
Oxycodone
  3 carisoprodol, 130
Oxycontin
  see Oxycodone
Oxymetholone
  2 warfarin, 568
PABA
  see Para-Aminobenzoic
      Acid
Paclitaxel
  3 delavirdine, 267
  3 saquinavir, 569

❶ = Avoid Combination   ❷ = Usually Avoid Combination   ❸ = Minimize Risk

1 = Avoid Combination   **2** = Usually Avoid Combination   **3** = Minimize Risk

❶ = Avoid Combination   ❷ = Usually Avoid Combination   ▼❸= Minimize Risk

❶ = Avoid Combination ❷ = Usually Avoid Combination ▼3 = Minimize Risk

Rifampin *(cont.)*
3 amiodarone, 34
3 buspirone, 98
3 chloramphenicol, 139
3 clarithromycin, 205
3 clofibrate, 210
3 clopidogrel, 218
3 contraceptives, oral, 230
2 cyclosporine, 256
3 dapsone, 265
3 delavirdine, 268
3 diazepam, 284
3 digitoxin, 294
3 diltiazem, 313
3 disopyramide, 320
3 fluconazole, 379
3 fluvastatin, 394
3 glyburide, 418
3 hexobarbital, 433
3 isoniazid, 460
3 itraconazole, 468
3 ketoconazole, 477
3 lamotrigine, 487
3 lorcainide, 502
3 losartan, 503
3 methadone, 514
3 metoprolol, 528
3 midazolam, 535
3 morphine, 541
2 nelfinavir, 550
3 nifedipine, 558
3 nortriptyline, 562
3 ondansetron, 567
3 phenytoin, 589
3 pirmenol, 599
3 prednisolone, 602
3 propafenone, 607
3 quinidine, 615
3 repaglinide, 621
3 ritonavir, 623
3 ropivacaine, 623
2 saquinavir, 624
2 simvastatin, 624
3 tacrolimus, 625
3 tamoxifen, 625
3 theophylline, 626
3 tocainide, 626
3 tolbutamide, 626
3 triazolam, 627
3 verapamil, 628
2 voriconazole, 628
2 warfarin, 629
3 zaleplon, 629
3 zidovudine, 630
3 zolpidem, 630

Rimactane
see Rifampin

Risperdal
see Risperidone

Risperidone
3 carbamazepine, 122

Ritalin
see Methylphenidate

Ritonavir
3 buspirone, 98
3 carbamazepine, 123
2 cisapride, 195
3 contraceptives, oral, 231
3 desipramine, 271
3 digoxin, 304
3 efavirenz, 331
2 ergotamine, 343
3 erythromycin, 348
3 fentanyl, 372
3 indinavir, 442
3 ketoconazole, 478
3 methadone, 515
3 olanzapine, 565
2 pimozide, 597
3 rifabutin, 621
3 rifampin, 623
3 saquinavir, 630
3 sildenafil, 631
2 simvastatin, 636
3 theophylline, 631

Rizatriptan
2 moclobemide, 538
3 propranolol, 610

Robaxin
see Methocarbamol

Robinul
see Glycopyrrolate

Robitussin-DM
see Dextromethorphan

Rocephin
see Ceftriaxone

Rofecoxib
3 enalapril, 334
3 lisinopril, 493

Roferon-A
see Interferon Alfa-2a

Rondomycin
see Methacycline

Ropinirole
3 ciprofloxacin, 188

Ropivacaine,
3 rifampin, 623

Roxanol
see Morphine

Roxithromycin
3 cyclosporine, 257

Rythmol
see Propafenone

Sabril
see Vigabatrin

Sandimmune
see Cyclosporine

Sanorex
see Mazindol

Saquinavir
3 garlic, 409
3 ketoconazole, 478
3 midazolam, 536
3 nelfinavir, 551
3 paclitaxel, 569
3 rifabutin, 622
2 rifampin, 624
3 ritonavir, 630
3 sildenafil, 633

Secobarbital
3 methoxyflurane, 524

Seldane
see Terfenadine

Selegiline
3 contraceptives, oral, 231
2 dextromethorphan, 277
2 fluoxetine, 388
2 meperidine, 511
3 moclobemide, 539
3 tyramine, 633

Serax
see Oxazepam

Serlect
see Sertindole

Seromycin
see Cycloserine

Seroquel
see Quetiapine

Serpalan
see Reserpine

Sertraline
3 erythromycin, 348
3 tramadol, 634
3 warfarin, 634

Serzone
see Nefazodone

Sibutramine
2 dextromethorphan, 278
2 dihydroergotamine, 308
2 fluoxetine, 388
2 lithium, 498
2 meperidine, 511
1 phenelzine, 575
2 sumatriptan, 635
2 tryptophan, 635

Sildenafil
3 diltiazem, 313
3 erythromycin, 349
3 grapefruit juice, 424

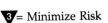

❶ = Avoid Combination   ❷ = Usually Avoid Combination   ▼❸ = Minimize Risk

❶ = Avoid Combination   ❷ = Usually Avoid Combination   ▼3 = Minimize Risk

Synthroid
see Levothyroxine

Tacrine
3 bethanechol, 88
3 cigarette smoking, 159
3 cimetidine, 179
3 enoxacin, 336
2 fluvoxamine, 397
3 levodopa, 491
3 propranolol, 611
3 succinylcholine, 643
3 theophylline, 648
3 trihexyphenidyl, 648

Tacrolimus
3 clarithromycin, 206
3 clotrimazole, 218
3 diltiazem, 314
3 erythromycin, 350
3 fluconazole, 379
3 itraconazole, 469
3 ketoconazole, 480
3 nefazodone, 549
3 nifedipine, 559
3 phenytoin, 591
3 rifampin, 625
3 simvastatin, 637
2 St. John's wort, 642
3 voriconazole, 649

Tagamet
see Cimetidine

Talinolol
3 sulfasalazine, 645

Talwin
see Pentazocine

Tambocor
see Flecainide

Tamoxifen
2 aminoglutethimide, 26
3 rifampin, 625

TAO
see Troleandomycin

Tapazole
see Methimazole

Taractan
see Chlorprothixene

Taxol
see Paclitaxel

Tegison
see Etretinate

Tegretol
see Carbamazepine

Telmisartan
3 digoxin, 306

Tenex
see Guanfacine

Teniposide
3 phenytoin, 592

Tenormin
see Atenolol

Tensilon
see Edrophonium

Tenuate
see Diethylpropion

Tequin
see Gatifloxacin

Terbinafine
3 dextromethorphan, 278

Terbutaline
3 furosemide, 407
2 metoprolol, 528

Terfenadine
2 clarithromycin, 207
1 erythromycin, 350
3 fluconazole, 380
2 fluoxetine, 389
1 fluvoxamine, 397
3 grapefruit juice, 425
1 itraconazole, 469
1 ketoconazole, 481
2 mibefradil, 533
2 troleandomycin, 649
3 zafirlukast, 650

Terramycin
see Oxytetracycline

Tetracaine
3 propranolol, 611

Tetracyclines
3 antacids, 61
2 bismuth, 90
3 colestipol, 225
3 contraceptives, oral, 232
3 digoxin, 306
3 food, 405
3 iron, 457
2 methoxyflurane, 525
3 penicillin G, 572
3 zinc, 650

Teveten
see Eprosartan

Thalomid
see Thalidomide

Theo-Dur
see Theophylline

Theolair
see Theophylline

Theophylline
3 adenosine, 10
3 allopurinol, 16
3 aminoglutethimide, 27
3 amiodarone, 35
3 carbamazepine, 123
3 cigarette smoking, 159
3 cimetidine, 179

Theophylline *(cont.)*
3 ciprofloxacin, 189
3 clinafloxacin, 208
3 disulfiram, 322
2 enoxacin, 337
3 erythromycin, 351
2 fluvoxamine, 398
3 imipenem, 437
3 interferon, 452
3 isoniazid, 460
3 lithium, 500
2 mexiletine, 532
3 moricizine, 541
3 norfloxacin, 561
3 pefloxacin, 572
3 pentoxifylline, 573
3 phenobarbital, 581
3 phenytoin, 592
3 propafenone, 607
2 propranolol, 612
3 radioactive iodine, 620
3 rifampin, 626
3 ritonavir, 631
3 tacrine, 648
3 thiabendazole, 651
3 thyroid, 651
3 ticlopidine, 652
2 troleandomycin, 652
3 verapamil, 652
3 zafirlukast, 654

Thiabendazole
3 theophylline, 651

Thiazides
3 calcium, 103
3 colestipol, 226
3 diazoxide, 286
3 insulin, 451
3 methotrexate, 522

Thiopental
3 probenecid, 603

Thioridazine
1 amiodarone, 35
3 bromocriptine, 93
3 cigarette smoking, 160
2 diphenhydramine, 316
2 disopyramide, 320
2 fluoxetine, 389
2 fluvoxamine, 399
2 paroxetine, 570
1 pimozide, 597
2 procainamide, 605
2 propafenone, 608
1 quinidine, 616
3 zafirlukast, 654
2 ziprasidone, 654

Thiothixene
3 guanethidine, 430

Thorazine
see Chlorpromazine

---

❶ = Avoid Combination   **❷** = Usually Avoid Combination   **❸** = Minimize Risk

❶ = Avoid Combination   ❷ = Usually Avoid Combination   ▼3 = Minimize Risk

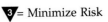

1 = Avoid Combination   **2** = Usually Avoid Combination   **3** = Minimize Risk

❶= Avoid Combination   ❷= Usually Avoid Combination   ▼= Minimize Risk